Advances in Experimental Medicine and Biology

Volume 1367

Advances in Experimental Medicine and Biology provides a platform for scientific contributions in the main disciplines of the biomedicine and the life sciences. This series publishes thematic volumes on contemporary research in the areas of microbiology, immunology, neurosciences, biochemistry, biomedical engineering, genetics, physiology, and cancer research. Covering emerging topics and techniques in basic and clinical science, it brings together clinicians and researchers from various fields.

Advances in Experimental Medicine and Biology has been publishing exceptional works in the field for over 40 years, and is indexed in SCOPUS, Medline (PubMed), Journal Citation Reports/Science Edition, Science Citation Index Expanded (SciSearch, Web of Science), EMBASE, BIOSIS, Reaxys, EMBiology, the Chemical Abstracts Service (CAS), and Pathway Studio.

2020 Impact Factor: 2.622

More information about this series at https://link.springer.com/bookseries/5584

Nima Rezaei • Fateme Rajabi
Editors

The Immunogenetics of Dermatologic Diseases

Springer

Editors
Nima Rezaei
Research Center for Immunodeficiencies
Children's Medical Center
Tehran University
of Medical Sciences
Tehran, Iran

Department of Immunology
School of Medicine
Tehran University of Medical Sciences
Tehran, Iran

Network of Immunity in Infection
Malignancy and Autoimmunity (NIIMA)
Universal Scientific Education and
Research Network (USERN)
Tehran, Iran

Fateme Rajabi
Center for Research and Training
in Skin Diseases and Leprosy
Tehran University
of Medical Sciences
Tehran, Iran

Network of Dermatology
Research (NDR)
Universal Scientific Education and
Research Network (USERN)
Tehran, Iran

ISSN 0065-2598 ISSN 2214-8019 (electronic)
Advances in Experimental Medicine and Biology
ISBN 978-3-030-92615-1 ISBN 978-3-030-92616-8 (eBook)
https://doi.org/10.1007/978-3-030-92616-8

This Springer imprint is published by the registered company Springer Nature Switzerland AG
The registered company address is: Gewerbestrasse 11, 6330 Cham, Switzerland

I wish to dedicate this book to my lovely family with the hope that progress in diagnosis and treatment of diseases may result in improved medical care for the next generations. Whatever I have learnt, comes from my mentors. This book is therefore dedicated also to all of them, but most importantly to the patients and their families whose continuous support has guided me during the years.

Nima Rezaei

I wish to dedicate this book to my father who has always been my role model and inspiration, my mother who encourages me to be a better person and has been a source of motivation and strength throughout my life, and to my husband for his unconditional love and support.

Fateme Rajabi

Preface

The concept of immunogenetics deals with the genetic regulation of immunological responses. Many dermatological conditions are influenced by the functions of the immune system. The dysregulation of the immune system is directly responsible for diseases such as pemphigus and partially accountable for conditions such as atopic dermatitis and psoriasis. Thus immunogenetic investigations can greatly benefit our understanding of dermatological diseases.

One of the main goals of immunogenetic studies is finding susceptibility genes for complex diseases. This can provide an insight into the pathogenesis of the condition in a way that is not easily achievable through other kinds of studies. Candidate gene and genome-wide association studies, though expansive, are pretty much easy to conduct. Their design is not as complicated as other types of investigation such as animal studies and the interpretation of the data they provide is straightforward. Thus they are a rational initial step for generating hypotheses about disease pathogenesis. This may especially benefit dermatology, a field notorious for having too many diseases with unknown etiologies.

Immunogenetic investigations have made targeted treatment strategies possible for diseases such as psoriasis and pemphigus. Even though these strategies have revolutionized the management of these chronic conditions, still there are a lot of unanswered questions. For instance, patients respond very differently to these modalities. This diversity could be partially explained by the differences in the sets of genes responsible for disease induction in each individual. Thus whole genome sequencing strategies, if feasible at individual levels, might help in tailoring these targeted treatments based on specific genetic backgrounds.

Our intention in preparing this book was to explore the broad spectrum of the genetic aspects of immunological processes involved in cutaneous diseases. We have tried to cover most areas of dermatology where enough studies were available to gather a chapter. Still, there is a substantial lack of knowledge on the immunogenetics of many dermatological conditions. We hope that this book would encourage the investigators to fill these gaps of knowledge.

This book is the result of the efforts of 35 authors from around the world and is organized into 18 chapters. The first chapter provides a general insight into genetic polymorphisms and the types of strategies employed to investigate them. The remaining chapters discuss the immunogenetics of specific dermatological conditions.

Finally, we hope that this book would be welcomed by scientists and clinicians who wish to extend their knowledge of the fast-growing intersection of dermatology, immunology, and genetics.

Tehran, Iran

Nima Rezaei
Fateme Rajabi

Contents

Contributors

Fahimeh Abdollahimajd Skin Research Center, Shahid Beheshti University or Medical Sciences, Tehran, Iran

Dalia G. Aly Dermatology and Venereology, National Research Centre, Cairo, Egypt

Kyle T. Amber Division of Dermatology, Rush University Medical Center, Chicago, USA;
Department of Internal Medicine, Rush University Medical Center, Chicago, USA

Rasheedunnisa Begum Department of Biochemistry, The Maharaja Sayajirao University of Baroda, Vadodara, Gujarat, India

Pooya Khan Mohammad Beigi Mismedicine Organization and Research Institute, Beverly Hills, CA, USA

Reza Chalangari Kasir Dermatology, Dallas, TX, USA

Tzu-Ying Chen Department of Dermatology, National Cheng Kung University Hospital, College of Medicine, Tainan, Taiwan

Elisa Cinotti Department of Medical, Surgical and Neurological Science, Dermatology Section, University of Siena, S. Maria Alle Scotte Hospital, Siena, Italy

Farzaneh Darbeheshti Departments of Medical Genetics, School of Medicine, Tehran University of Medical Sciences, Tehran, Iran;
Cancer Immunology Project (CIP), Universal Scientific and Research Network (USERN), Tehran, Iran

Mitesh Dwivedi C. G. Bhakta Institute of Biotechnology, Uka Tarsadia University, Tarsadi, Surat, Gujarat, India

Mohamed L. Elsaie Dermatology and Venereology, National Research Centre, Cairo, Egypt

Behnaz Esmaeili Immunology Asthma and Allergy Research Institute, Tehran University of Medical Sciences, Tehran, Iran

Alireza Firooz Center for Research & Training in Skin Diseases & Leprosy, Tehran University of Medical Sciences, Tehran, Iran

Navid Jabalameli Network of Dermatology Research (NDR), Universal Scientific Education and Research Network (USERN), Tehran, Iran

Fotini B. Karassa Division of Rheumatology, Department of Medicine, School of Health Sciences, University of Ioannina, Ioannina, Greece

Mansour Nassiri Kashani Center for Research & Training in Skin Diseases & Leprosy, Tehran University of Medical Sciences, Tehran, Iran

Neda Khalili Cancer Immunology Project (CIP), Universal Scientific Education and Research Network (USERN), Tehran, Iran

Alireza Khosravi Mycology Research Center, Faculty of Veterinary Medicine, University of Tehran, Tehran, Iran

Diana Kneiber Department of Dermatology, University of Illinois at Chicago, Chicago, USA

Eric H. Kowalski Department of Dermatology, University of Illinois at Chicago, Chicago, USA

Gizem Filazi Kök Department of Dermatology, Mersin University, Mersin, Turkey

Naresh C. Laddha In Vitro Specialty Lab Pvt. Ltd, Ahmedabad, Gujarat, India

Chaw-Ning Lee Department of Dermatology, National Cheng Kung University Hospital, College of Medicine, Tainan, Taiwan

Parvin Mansouri Research Vice-President of Medical Laser Research Center, Academic Center for Education-Culture and Research, Tehran University of Medical Sciences, Tehran, Iran

Katalin Martits-Chalangari Kasir Dermatology, Dallas, TX, USA

Sabha Mushtaq Department of Dermatology, Venereology, and Leprology, Government Medical College & Associated Hospitals, University of Jammu, Jammu, J&K, India

Nahid Nikkhah Medical Laser Research Centers, Academic Center for Education-Culture and Research, Tehran University of Medical Sciences, Tehran, Iran

Eleftherios Pelechas Division of Rheumatology, Department of Medicine, School of Health Sciences, University of Ioannina, Ioannina, Greece

Fateme Rajabi Network of Dermatology Research (NDR), Universal Scientific Education and Research Network (USERN), Tehran, Iran;
Center for Research & Training in Skin Diseases & Leprosy, Tehran University of Medical Sciences, Tehran, Iran

Zeynab Rajabi Tehran University of Medical Sciences, Tehran, Iran

Nima Rezaei Network of Immunity in Infection, Malignancy and Autoimmunity (NIIMA), Universal Scientific Education and Research Network (USERN), Sheffield, UK;
Research Center for Immunodeficiencies, Children's Medical Center, Tehran University of Medical Sciences, Tehran, Iran;
Department of Immunology, School of Medicine, Tehran University of Medical Sciences, Tehran, Iran

Pietro Rubegni Department of Medical, Surgical and Neurological Science, Dermatology Section, University of Siena, S. Maria Alle Scotte Hospital, Siena, Italy

Emanuele Trovato Department of Medical, Surgical and Neurological Science, Dermatology Section, University of Siena, S. Maria Alle Scotte Hospital, Siena, Italy

Ümit Türsen Department of Dermatology, Mersin University, Mersin, Turkey

Begüm Ünlü Department of Dermatology, Mersin University, Mersin, Turkey

Tak-Wah Wong Department of Dermatology, National Cheng Kung University Hospital, College of Medicine, Tainan, Taiwan;
Department of Biochemistry & Molecular Biology, College of Medicine, Tainan, Taiwan;
Center of Applied Nanomedicine, National Cheng Kung University, Tainan, Taiwan

Mustafa Anıl Yılmaz Department of Dermatology, Mersin University, Mersin, Turkey

Georgios Zouzos Division of Rheumatology, Department of Medicine, School of Health Sciences, University of Ioannina, Ioannina, Greece

Abbreviations

3'UTR	3' untranslated regions
3β-HSD	3β-hydroxysteroid dehydrogenase
5-FU	5-fluorouracil
AA	Alopecia areata
ABC	ATP-binding cassette
ACA	Anti-centromere antibody
ACE	Angiotensin-converting enzyme
ACLE	Acute cutaneous lupus erythematosus
ACOXL	Acyl-coenzyme-A oxidase-like
ACP5	Acid phosphatase 5
ADR	Adverse drug reaction
AEGCG	Annular elastolytic giant cell granuloma
AFND	Allele Frequencies Net Database
AGEP	Acute generalized exanthematous pustulosis
AHS	Abacavir hypersensitivity syndrome
AIBD	Autoimmune blistering disorders
AIF	Allograft inflammatory factor
AIRE	Autoimmune regulator
AJ	Ashkenazi Jewish
AK	Actinic keratosis
ALA	Aminolevulinic acid
AMD	age-related macular degeneration
AMP	Antimicrobial peptide
ANA	Anti-nuclear antibody
ANCA	Antineutrophil cytoplasmic antibodies
AP	Actinic prurigo
APC	Antigen-presenting cell
APECED	Autoimmune polyendocrinopathy-candidiasis-ectodermal dystrophy
AR	Androgen receptor
ARA	Anti-RNA polymerase III autoantibodies antibody
AS	Ankylosing spondylitis
ATA	Anti-topoisomerase antibody
ATG5	Autophagy related 5
BANK1	B cell scaffold protein with ankyrin repeats
BCC	Basal cell carcinoma
BCR	B-cell receptor

BD	Behcet's Disease
BD	Bowen's Disease
BLK	B lymphocyte kinase
BLYS	B-lymphocyte stimulator
BMZ	Basement membrane zone
BP	Bullous pemphigoid
CAD	Chronic actinic dermatitis
cADR	Cutaneous adverse drug reaction
CAH	Congenital adrenal hyperplasia
CAV	Caveolin
ceRNA	ceRNA
CFH	Complement factor H
CFHR	Complement factor H related
CGAS	Candidate gene association study.
CL	Cutaneous leishmaniasis
CLE	Cutaneous lupus erythematosus
CLOXVII	Collagen XVII
CMV	Cytomegalovirus
CNV	Copy number variants
CNVA	Copy number variant analysis.
COX	Cyclooxygenase
CSK	C-Scr kinases
CSNK2B	Casein Kinase 2 subunit Beta
CTGF	Connective tissue growth factor
CTLA4	Cytotoxic T-lymphocyte antigen 4
CXCR	CXC chemokine receptor
DAG	Diacylglycerol
DAMP	Damage associated molecular pattern
DC	Dendritic cell
dcSSC	diffuse cutaneous systemic sclerosis
DDB2	Damage-specific DNA binding protein 2
DDP-4i	Dipeptidyl peptidase 4 inhibitors
DDX6	DEAD-box RNA helicase 6
DEB	Dystrophic epidermolysis bullosa
DEJ	Dermal-epidermal junction
DIF	Direct immunofluorescence
DIHS	Drug-induced hypersensitivity syndrome
DILI	Drug-induced liver disease
DLE	Discoid lupus erythematosus
DNASE	Deoxyribonuclease
DNASE1L3	DNASE1L3: Deoxyribonuclease 1 Like
DNMT	DNA methyltransferase
DRESS	Drug reaction with eosinophilia and systemic symptoms
dsDNA	double-stranded DNA
DSG	Desmoglein
DTH	Delayed-type hypersensitivity
E	Egyptian
EBA	Epidermolysis bullosa acquisita

EBV	Epstien Barr virus
EC	Extracellular
ECM	Patelet derived growth factor
ELISA	Enzyme-linked immunoassay
EMPD	Extramammary Paget's Disease
EMT/EndoMT	Epithelial/Endothelial to mesenchymal transition
eQTL	expression quantitative trait loci
ETC	Electron transport chain
FCAR	Fc fragment of IgA receptor
FcγRs	Fc fragment of IgG receptors
FDE	Fixed drug eruption
FFA	Free fatty acid
FGF	Fibroblast growth factor
FGFR	Fibroblast growth factor receptor
FISH	Fluorescence in situ hybridization
FLOT1	Flotillin-1
FOXP3	Forkhead Protein 3
FS	Fogo selvagem
G	German
GA	Granuloma annulare
GCA	Giant cell arteritis
G-CSF	Granulocyte-colony stimulatory factor
GPA	Granulomatosis with polyangiitis
GST	Glutathione S-transferases
GV	Generalized vitiligo
GWAS	Genome-wide association study
GWAS-MA	Genome-wide association study-Meta Analysis
GWLS	Genome-wide linkage study
HAIR-AN	Hyperandrogenism insulin resistance acanthosis nigricans
HBD	Human beta-defensin
HCV	Hepatitis C virus
HF	Hair follicle
HIF	Hypoxia-inducible factor
HLA	Human leukocyte antigen
HMGB1	High-mobility group box 1
HMME	hematoporphyrin monomethyl ether
HpD	Hematoporphyrin derivative
HRE	Hypoxia response element
HSP	Heat shock protein
HSS	Hypersensitivity syndrome
HV	Hydroa vacciniforme
HVLL	Hydroa vacciniforme-like lymphoma
IA	Indo-Asian
ICAM	Intracellular adhesion molecule
IFIH1	Interferon-induced with helicase C domain 1
IFN	Interferon
IGD	Interstitial granulomatous dermatitis

IGF-1	Insulin-like growth factor 1
IGFBP4	Insulin-like growth factor-binding protein 4
IIF	Indirect immunofluorescence
Ikzf1	IKAROS family zinc finger 1**
IL	interleukin
IL-1RN	IL-1 receptor antagonist
ILP	idiopathic lichen planus
ILT3	Immunoglobulin-like transcript 3
INDEL	Insertion deletion polymorphism
iNKT cells	invariant natural killer T-cells
IP	Immune privilege
IPL	Intense pulse light
IRAK1	Interleukin-1 receptor-associated kinase 1
IRE	IFN regulatory element
IRF	Intron regulatory factor
ISG	Interferon-stimulated genes
ISPI	In Situ Photo-immunotherapy
ISRE	IFN-stimulated response element
ITGAM	Integrin Subunit Alpha M, also known as complement receptor-3 or CD11b
JAZF1	Juxtaposed with another zinc finger protein 1
JNK	Janus kinas
KCNK4	Potassium channel subfamily K member 4
KD	Kawasaki disease
KIR	Killer cell immunoglobulin-like receptors
KLRG1	Killer cell lectin-like subfamily G member 1
LAP	Latency-associated peptide
LCE	Late-cornified envelope
lcSSC	localized cutaneous systemic sclerosis
LD	Linkage disequilibrium
LDL	Low-density lipoprotein
LE	Lupus erythematosus
LECNG8	Leukocyte receptor cluster member 8
LFA-1	Lymphocyte function-associated antigen-1
lncRNA	long non-coding RNA
LP	Lichen planus
LSA	Lichen sclerosus et atrophicus
LY9	Lymphocyte antigen 9
LYN	Yamaguchi sarcoma viral oncogene
Lyp	Lymphomatoid papulosis
MAC	Membrane attack complex
MAF	Musculoaponeurotic fibrosarcoma oncogene homologue
MAPK	Mitogen associated protein kinase
MCHR2	Melanin Concentrating Hormone Receptor 2
MDC	Myeloid dendritic cell
MECP2	Methyl CpG binding protein-2
MHC	Major histocompatibility
MHC2TA	Major histocompatibility complex class II transactivator

MICA	MHC class I chain-related A
MICB	MHC class I chain-related B
MIF	Macrophage migration inhibitory factor
miRISC	miRNA-induced silencing complexes
miRNA	Micro-RNA
MLA	Methyl aminolevulinate
MMP	Matrix metalloproteinases 3,9 and 12
MMP	Mucous membrane pemphigoid
MPO	Myeloperoxidase
mRNA	messenger RNA
MS	Multiple sclerosis
MSH5	MSH5: MutS homolog 5
mTORC1	mechanistic target of rapamycin complex 1
MUC21	Mucin 1
MUFA	Monounsaturated fatty acids
ncRNA	non-coding RNA
NET	Neutrophil extracellular traps
NFκB	nuclear factor-kappa B
NGS	Next-generation sequencing
NK cell	Natural killer cell
NL	Necrobiosis lipoidica
NMSC	Non-melanoma skin cancer
NNRTI	None-nucleoside reverse transcriptase inhibitor
NO	Nitric oxide
NO^{3-}	Peroxynitrite
NOS	Nitric oxide synthetase
NOTCH4	Neurogenic locus notch homolog 4
NPV	Negative predictive value
NRP2	Neuropilin 2
NRTI	Nucleoside reverse transcriptase inhibitor
NS	No significant difference
OCP	Ocular cicatricial pemphigoid
OCR	Open chromatin regions
OLP	Oral lichen planus
OP	Oral pemphigoid
P	Protective
PAMS	Paraneoplastic autoimmune multiorgan syndrome
PAN	Polyarteritis nodosa
PAPA	Pyogenic Arthritis, Pyoderma gangrenosum, Acne
PAPASH	Pyogenic arthritis, Acne, Pyoderma gangrenosum, Acne Suppurativa, Hidradenitis
PASH	Pyoderma gangrenosum, Acne Suppurative, Hidradenitis
PBMC	Peripheral blood mononuclear cells
PDC	Plasmacytoid dendritic cell
PDCD1	Programmed cell death 1
PDGF	Platelet-derived growth factor
PDT	Photodynamic therapy

PF	Pemphigus foliaceous
PG	Pemphigus gestationis
P-gp	P-glycoprotein
PMLE	Polymorphous light eruption
PNGD	Palisaded neutrophilic and granulomatous dermatitis
PPARγ	Proliferator-activated receptor γ
PpIX	Protoporphyrin IX
PPV	Positive predictive value
PRDM1	PR domain zinc finger protein 1
PRDX5	Peroxiredoxin 5 (PRDX5)
PRKCB	Protein kinase C, beta
PRR	Pattern recognition receptors
PS	Psoriasis
PSORS1C1	Psoriasis susceptibility 1 candidate 1
PTPN22	Protein tyrosine phosphatase non-receptor 22**
PUVA	Psoralen-ultraviolet A
PV	Pemphigus vulgaris
RA	Rheumatoid arthritis
RASGRP3	Ras guanyl-releasing protein 3
RDEB	Recessive dystrophic epidermolysis bullosa
RHOB	RAS homolog family member b
ROS	Reactive oxygen species
RPP21	Ribonuclease P protein subunit 21
S	Increased susceptibility
SAA	Serum amyloid-A
SAPHO	Synovitis, Acne, Pustulosis, Hyperostosis, Osteitis
SBE	STAT binding element
SCC	Squamous cell carcinoma
SCLE	Subacute cutaneous lupus erythematosus
SHH	Sonic Hedgehog
SJS	Stevens-Johnson syndrome
SLC15A4	SLC15A4: Solute carrier family 15, member 4
SLE	Systemic lupus erythematosus
SLP	Secondary lichen planus
SNP	Single nucleotide polymorphism
SOD	Superoxide dismutase
SPP	Osteopontin
SRE	Sterol regulatory element-1
SREBP1c	Sterol regulatory element-binding protein-1
SSc	Systemic sclerosis
ssRNA	single-stranded RNA
ST18	Suppression of tumorgenicity
STAT	Signal transducer and activator of transcription
STK	Serine/threonine kinase
STR	Short tandem repeat polymorphism
SU	Solar urticaria
T1D	Type 1 diabetes
TA	Takayasu arteritis

TAP	Transporter associated with antigen processing
TCR	T-cell receptor
TEC	Thymic epithelial cells
TEN	Toxic epidermal necrolysis
TfH	Follicular helper T-cell
Th	T helper
TLR	Toll-like receptor
TNF	Tumor necrosis factor
TNFAIP3	Tumor necrosis factor, alpha-induced protein 3
TNFR	Tumor necrosis factor receptor
TNFR-5	Tumor necrosis factor 5
TNFSF4	Tumor necrosis factor superfamily, member 4
TNIP1	TNFAIP3-interacting protein 1
Treg	Regulatory T-cell
TREX1	Three prime repair exonuclease 1
TRIM39	Tripartite motif-containing protein 39
TWAS	Transcriptome-wide association study
TYK	Tyrosine kinase
UBE2L3	Ubiquitin-conjugating enzyme E2L 3
UBV-S	Ultraviolet B sensible
UVB-R	Ultraviolet B resistant
UVR	Ultraviolet radiation
VCAM	Vascular cell adhesion protein 1
VDR	Vitamin D receptor
VEGF	Vascular endothelial growth factor
VNTR	Variable number of tandem repeat polymorphism
WB	White British
WE	White European
WES	Whole-exome sequencing
WGS	Whole-genome sequencing
XP	Xeroderma pigmentosa

The Concept of Immunogenetics

Fateme Rajabi, Navid Jabalameli, and Nima Rezaei

Abstract

Genetics plays a major role in shaping the immune responses in both physiological and pathological states such as psoriasis, alopecia areata, and other immune-mediated dermatological conditions. The genes encoding the elements of the immune system and its regulators are among the most polymorphous loci in the genome. Subtle variations in these genes can thus alter the balanced defensive responses of the immune system and make an individual liable to diseases and environmental triggers. Immunogenetics deals with finding the precise set of liability genes involved in the pathogenesis of specific complex diseases. In this chapter, we will briefly discuss the basic principles of genetic polymorphisms, the methods used in scanning these polymorphisms, and the strategies employed to find the role of these polymorphisms in complex diseases.

Keywords

Gene polymorphisms · Single nucleotide polymorphism · Insertion-deletion · Variable number of tandem repeat · Copy number variation · Immunogenetics · Human leukocyte antigen

1 Introduction

The immune system plays a major role in the pathogenesis of many dermatological conditions. Pemphigus and epidermolysis bollousa acquisita directly result from an immune attack on the self-proteins residing within the skin. Alopecia areata results from a breach in the immune privilege of one of the most preserved skin structures, hair follicles. Dysregulation of the immune system can promote inflammation and cause diseases such as psoriasis and lichen planus. The immune system may show an exaggerated response to subtle environmental triggers and cause allergic dermatitis. The response of the immune system

F. Rajabi · N. Jabalameli
Network of Dermatology Research (NDR), Universal Scientific Education and Research Network (USERN), Tehran, Iran

F. Rajabi
Center for Research & Training in Skin Diseases & Leprosy, Tehran University of Medical Sciences, Tehran, Iran

N. Rezaei (✉)
Network of Immunity in Infection, Malignancy and Autoimmunity (NIIMA), Universal Scientific Education and Research Network (USERN), Sheffield, UK
e-mail: rezaei_nima@tums.ac.ir

Research Center for Immunodeficiencies, Children's Medical Center, Tehran University of Medical Sciences, Tehran, Iran

Department of Immunology, School of Medicine, Tehran University of Medical Sciences, Tehran, Iran

N. Rezaei and F. Rajabi (eds.), *The Immunogenetics of Dermatologic Diseases*, Advances in Experimental Medicine and Biology 1367,
https://doi.org/10.1007/978-3-030-92616-8_1

against bacteria can get derailed from its normal path and give rise to nodulocystic acne.

Even in genetic conditions such as ichthyosis, the disruption of the skin barrier would result in a higher confrontation of the environment and the immune system resulting in inflammatory responses that could worsen the symptoms. On the whole, it seems that the immune system is a major player in almost all dermatological conditions.

Genetics has a major role in shaping these immune responses in both physiological and pathological states. Genetic variations can alter the production and release of cytokines and adhesion molecules, regulate the affinity and function of signaling pathways, and change the rate of apoptosis, phagocytosis, and antigen presentation.

Thus exploring the genetic basis of the immune responses (immunogenetics) in dermatological conditions may work as a shortcut in understanding the disease pathogenesis. In this chapter, we will briefly discuss the basic principles of genetic polymorphisms, the methods used in scanning these polymorphisms, and the strategies employed to find the role of these polymorphisms in complex diseases.

2 Genetic Variations and Polymorphisms

The human nuclear genome as the basis of inheritance is a 3.2 gigabase long DNA sequence containing approximately 25,000 genes that are arranged in overlapping arrays with their promoters, introns, and exons (Stein 2004). The DNA sequence also contains intragenic regions known as junk DNA that are not translated into RNAs. The junk DNAs are different from the non-coding introns located within the genes (intragenic rather than intergenic). The function of these segments is not fully understood but some may have regulatory roles in the transcription of their nearby genes (Turnpenny et al. 2022).

Though about 99.9% of the genome is common among all human beings, there is ~0.1% human-to-human variation in the DNA sequence (Conrad et al. 2011). These variations could occur in both coding and non-coding regions of the genome. Thus, some of the variations may have little to no effect on RNA transcription and protein functions while others are responsible for most of the phenotypical differences among people. In an extreme case, a variation could result in loss-of-function of an encoded protein and gives rise to genetic diseases such as epidermolysis bollousa. Between these extreme two ends of having no effect at all and having devastating disease-causing effects, there are genetic variations with modest effects size that require the help of other inherited and environmental triggers to be able to induce a phenotypical trait.

All variations in the DNA sequence are caused by mutations in the ancestral sequence but it is common (though not correct) to refer to variations with devastating outcomes as "Mutations" and variations with subtle to no obvious effects as "Polymorphisms" (Turnpenny et al. 2022). Consequently, a gene is considered to be polymorphic if more than one variation (allele) has been detected at the gene's locus with a prevalence of more than 1% in the population. Alleles with a prevalence of less than 1% are called "rare variants" or "private polymorphisms" (Neel 1978).

On the molecular scale, the polymorphisms could range from single to few base changes to alterations of segments 10-kilo base-pair (kbp) long. Based on the type and length of the change in the genetic sequence, mutations are categorized as follows: (a) substitutions of single nucleotides (single nucleotide polymorphisms, SNP) (Sachidanandam et al. 2001); (b) insertions and deletions of single to few nucleotide-long arrays (INDEL) (Mills et al. 2006); (c) changes in the number of tandemly repeated sequences with 1–8 bp known as simple tandem repeats (STR) (micro-satellite); (d) variations in the number of tandemly repeated sequences of 8–100 bp known as the variable number of tandem repeats (VNTR) (mini-satellite)

(Weissenbach et al. 1992); and (e) major structural rearrangement of chromosomal segments (>10 kbp) (Ku et al. 2010). Copy number variations (CNVs) are a subtype of structural changes that describes the number of copies of specific long segments of DNA ($\sim$250 kbp long) throughout the genome (McCarroll and Altshuler 2007; Redon et al. 2006). Figure 1 provides a schema of the most common types of polymorphisms.

The SNPs are the most studied genetic variations with their own structured nomenclature (rs#) and multiple human databases (Sherry et al. 2001). SNPs within the intragenic segments have unknown consequences but those located at exons could alter the protein functions (Ng and Henikoff 2002). SNPs located in the promoter/regulatory segments affect the protein production levels (Kim et al. 2008). Intronic SNPs could also have functionally relevant consequences as they can alter the transcriptional process and induce a splice site mutation (Jin et al. 2018; Ok Yang et al. 2009). The 3′ untranslated regions (3′UTRs) SNPs have been linked to the altered expression of micro-RNAs (miRNA), the major players of epigenetic modification (Gong et al. 2012).

The INDELs are the second most common genetic variations but significantly less investigated in comparison to SNPs (Clark et al. 2007; Ratan et al. 2015). INDELs usually result in a

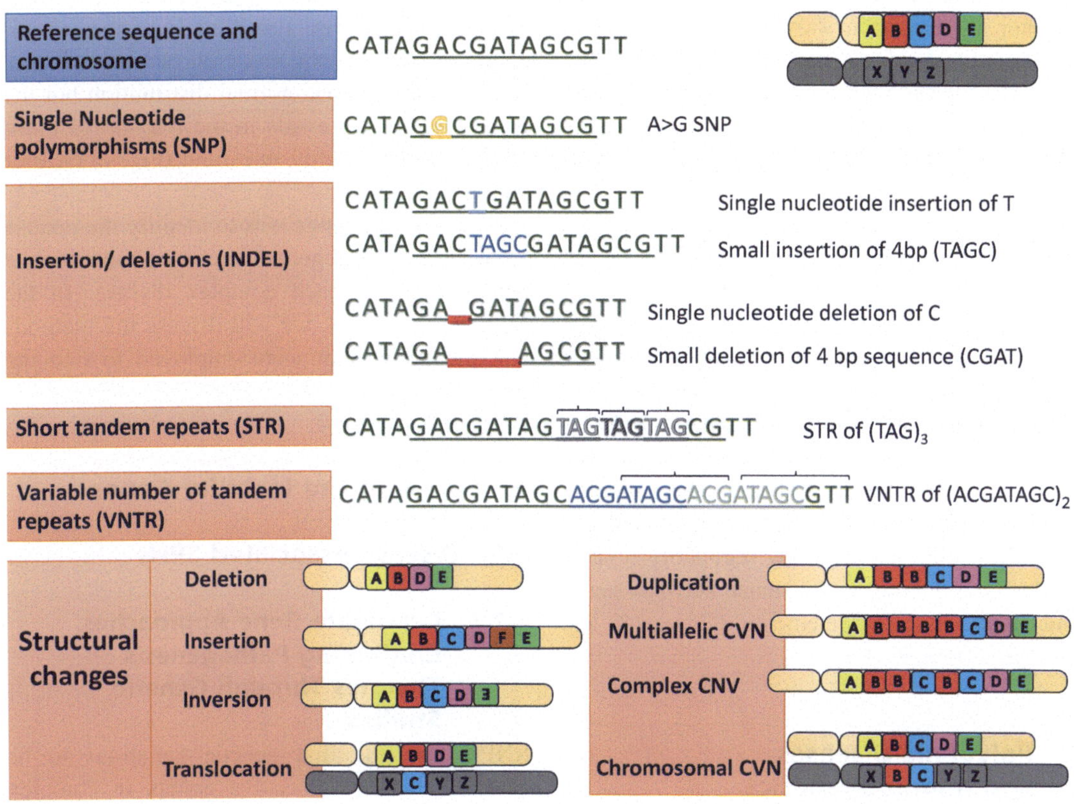

Fig. 1 The main types of genetic polymorphisms. STRs are usually only 1–8 bp long (micro-satellite) while VNTRs are 8–100 bp long (mini-satellite). Structural changes involve segments larger than 10 kbp. CNVs are usually >250 kbp. Another term commonly used for describing a type of genetic variation is the restriction fragment length polymorphism (RFLP). The RFLP denotes variations in the size of DNA fragments after enzymatic ligation. This length variability reflects the locations of restriction sites that are usually 4–8 bps long palindromic sequences that are ligated by restriction enzymes into two overhanging DNA strands. Thus RFLP is not an independent subtype of genetic variation rather it reflects the presence of an SNP or VNTR (Botstein et al. 1980; Saiki et al. 1985)

more significant consequence as they can cause frameshift mutations. The promoter INDELs affect gene expression and intronic INDELs disrupt splicing sites (Lin et al. 2017; Sehn 2015).

The VNTRs and STRs are less common than the other two types of polymorphisms discussed above and are also less investigated (Brookes 2013). Unlike SNPs which are usually biallelic, each STR/ VNTR could have several alleles representing the number of repeats of the tandem sequences. VNTRs and STRs within coding regions often alter the functions of their corresponding proteins by changing the protein length. For instance, a VNTR polymorphism with three major alleles corresponding to 2-, 4-, and 7-repeats at the third exon of the dopamine receptor D4 has been shown to alter receptors response threshold (Asghari et al. 1995). VNTRs and STRs located within the promoter region can affect the functions of the transcriptional machinery and thus alter gene expression levels (Cai et al. 2011). VNTRs located at the 3'UTRs and introns can still have significant effects through alternative splicing (Mignone et al. 2002).

The effects of structural polymorphisms such as CNVs are harder to determine. It has been suggested that the structural variations could make changes to the overall chromatin architecture and thus induce long-range effects on gene expression (Gheldof et al. 2013). The structural variations can affect the expression of multiple genes by adding or removing regulatory regions or changing the physical distance between genes and their regulatory elements (Gamazon and Stranger 2015).

3 Polygenic Diseases and Immunogenetics

Many diseases (including many dermatological conditions) that were initially assigned as acquired conditions with unknown environmental causes, later on, were found to have a clear familial clustering and high concordance rates in twins. Hence a genetic etiology was suspected for these disorders that did not follow the Mendelian model of inheritance. This led to the idea of complex diseases where a network of interactions between environmental factors and multiple genetic variants rather than a single one could be working with and against each other to create a liability toward diseases. This explanation was further drafted into the liability threshold model for polygenic inheritance of complex diseases (Turnpenny et al. 2022). Many polygenic conditions such as dermatology-related traits of skin color, hair color, and hair density are measurable traits that have a continuous normal bell-like distribution among the population. This model is not very well suited for diseases since health vs disease is a dichotomous trait. Thus, it has been suggested that the liability to a specific disease resulting from the combination of both genetic and environmental factors follows a continuous normal distribution but the phenotype only prevails in the fraction of those exceeding the liability threshold (Fig. 2) (Küster and Happle 1984).

The next challenge was to identify the precise environmental and genetic factors involved in the pathogenesis of each complex disease. In the following segment, we will discuss the methods and modalities that were employed to find the causative genes.

4 Pursuing the Liability Genes

4.1 Disease-Associated SPNs

4.1.1 Candidate Gene Approaches, Confirming Pathogenesis Theories Through Genetic Studies

SNPs were the first genetic variations to be evaluated as the causative agents in complex diseases. Candidate gene approaches were and still are the simplest and the most feasible methods to investigate SNPs. Though lately, genome-wide association studies (GWAS) have gained more popularity.

In candidate gene approaches also known as case–control genetic association studies, a gene

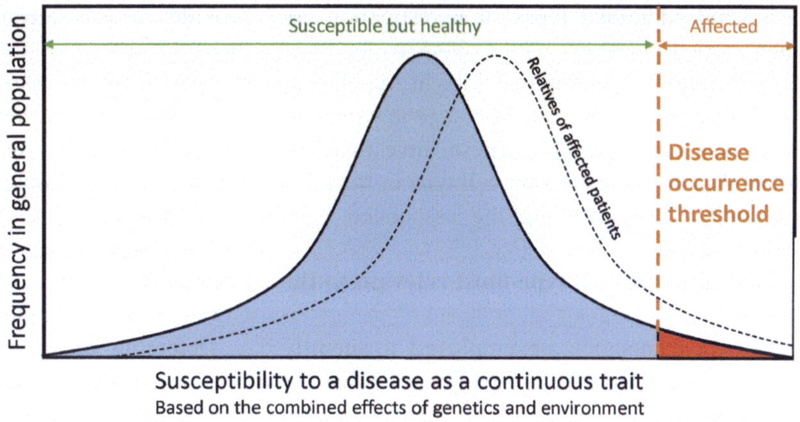

Fig. 2 Liability curve for complex diseases in the general population and in the family members of those affected with diseases who have a higher chance of inheriting multiple susceptibility genes

is selected based on the pathogenic mechanisms. A potentially functional SNP in this gene is chosen using bioinformatic tools and a hypothesis is formed (Conde et al. 2004; Wang et al. 2011). The difference in the incidence of each allele of this specific SNP in the diseased and the control groups are compared. A significant difference provides evidence for the association between the gene and the disease and the odds ratio (OR) implies the direction (causative vs protective) and strength of this association (Turnpenny et al. 2022).

4.1.2 GWAS, from Genes to Probable Mechanisms

With the invention of next-generation sequencing (NGS) techniques, the sequencing of the whole genome became feasible at an individual level (Behjati and Tarpey 2013). The NGS was able to identify numerous types of variants in the human genome that were not reported previously. This gave rise to a new method of exploring the genetics of complex diseases known as genome-wide association studies (GWAS) (Visscher et al. 2012).

The design of GWA studies is the complete opposite of the candidate gene approaches. With no prior assumption or hypothesis, multiple common SNPs (500,000–1,000,000) across the genome are compared between two large groups of cases and controls. A significant difference provides evidence for the association between the previously unknown genes and the disease and thus opens a new path toward investigations on the pathogenesis of that specific condition (Consortium 2007; DeWan et al. 2006; Visscher et al. 2012). Two things should be bared in mind when interpreting GWAS results. First, the P-value of less than 0.5 is not considered significant since we are testing ~1,000,000 hypotheses in a single attempt and it would be likely to have a < 0.5 p-value to only occur by chance. Thus, according to the Bonferroni correction, the p-value of $0.5/10^6 = 5 \times 10^{-8}$ is considered significant. Second, though the GWAS only directly assesses a fraction of all SNPs (1 million in the estimated 10 million SNPs), it is still able to have good coverage of all SNPs with a minor allele frequency of more than 5% in the general population due to the presence of a phenomenon known as linkage disequilibrium (Altshuler et al. 2005; Barrett and Cardon 2006; Zondervan and Cardon 2004). Linkage disequilibrium (LD) refers to the non-random co-occurrence of alleles at different but often near loci due to the higher chance of being co-segregated in the course of meiotic recombination (Slatkin 2008). The inability of GWA studies in detecting rare allele associations is not concerning since it is assumed that common alleles are more likely to give rise to common diseases (Visscher et al. 2012). Further information on GWAS interpretation is beyond the scope of this chapter but we would like to refer our readers to two very well-written articles by Cano-Gamez and Trynka (2020) and Pearson and Manolio (2008).

Several additional types of investigation are often carried out along with GWAS to facilitate the generation of pathophysiological hypotheses and draw a more clear path from a gene variant to functional consequences. These investigations aim to find the most relevant cell type or the most relevant pathways linking the associated gene with the disease.

Detecting the Cell type most relevant to the disease

Statistical methods are employed to identify the most prominent cell type involved in the pathogenesis of specific diseases by integrating GWAS data with gene expression profiles (discussed in detail later in this chapter) in different cells and tissues. Thus, if a disease-associated GWAS locus is overrepresented (enriched) in a certain cell type, that cell type is prioritized for being a causative agent in the pathogenesis of the disease (Hu et al. 2011). For instance, using available data sets on the expression rates of different genes and loci within different cell lines, the expression of the 27 loci (containing 136 genes) associated with lupus by GWAS studies were compared to the expression of other random loci and genes. It was demonstrated that lupus-associated genes had the most significant enrichment in transitional B cells (Hu et al. 2011).

Some recent studies have suggested using data on epigenetic modifications (referred to as chromatin annotations) in different tissue/cell lines instead of gene expression profiling for detecting the important cell line (Chen et al. 2016; Consortium 2012; Kundaje et al. 2015; Maurano et al. 2012). These epigenetic modifications provide indirect evidence of gene transcription rates in different cells. Histone acetylation as a type of epigenetic modification transforms the condensed chromatin into a loose structure that eases DNA access for transcription machinery (Bannister and Kouzarides 2011). Similarly, nucleosome-depleted regions in the DNA known as open chromatin regions (OCRs) are associated with higher transcription rates whereas methylation represses transcription (Boyle et al. 2008; Frommer et al. 1992). Integrating these chromatin marks with GWAS data provides a less erroneous interpretation since there the nature of the variables that are being compared are the same and there could be an actual physical overlap between the two sets of data (Cano-Gamez and Trynka 2020). As an example of employing this method in autoimmune diseases, Onengut-Gumuscu et al. were able to show the enrichment of regulatory loci associated with type 1 diabetes in CD4 + and CD8 + T cells (Onengut-Gumuscu et al. 2015).

Detecting the molecular mechanisms most relevant to the disease

The measurement of molecular traits such as the amount of gene expression (as mRNA levels) can be performed in ancillary to genotyping for common SNPs. When performed in thousands of individuals, this would allow for the detection of associations between SNPs with molecular traits. This process is known as quantitative trait loci (QTL) mapping with eQTL denoting a genomic locus (SNP) that affects the expression levels of a specific mRNA (Rockman and Kruglyak 2006). Expectedly, most eQTLs are located within 1 Mb of the mRNA's reference gene and are thus referred to as cis- or local-eQTLs (Shan et al. 2019; Veyrieras et al. 2008). Nonetheless, many eQTLs, known as trans- or distant-eQTLs, are located far from their mRNA encoding gene, even residing on another chromosome. Most cis-eQTLs are conserved among many cell types but most trans-eQTLs are cell type-specific (Gerrits et al. 2009).

Multiple databases for eQTLs in different cell lines and tissues are available online (Chen et al. 2016; Lonsdale et al. 2013). The process of integrating GWAS data with eQTL maps available through these databases is known as colocalization. The colocalization allows the researchers to have a better understanding of the disease pathogenesis by identifying disease-associated SNPs that are significantly enriched for eQTLs in comparison to frequency-matched control SNPs (Cano-Gamez and Trynka 2020; Dubois et al. 2010). However, nearly half of the common SNPs are eQTLs and thus the overlap of disease-associated SNPs with eQLT maps could occur by chance. The effects of the SNP on the pathogenesis of the disease could also be independent of its role as an eQTL (pleiotropy). Geneticists have come up with strategies to exclude the role of chance but there is no single way to eliminate the second type error and thus the results of the integrated GWAS/eQTL studies should be interpreted with caution (Giambartolomei et al. 2014; He et al. 2013; Hormozdiari et al. 2016; Nica et al. 2010; Wallace et al. 2012).

The strategies used for GWAS-eQTL colocalizations have been employed to interpret data from the integration of GWAS with protein expression mappings (pQTLs), GWAS with DNA methylation mappings (mQTLs), and GWAS with chromatin acetylation mappings (acQTLs). Moreover, these methods have been utilized to integrate data from multiple GWA studies from diseases with shared etiology (e.g., autoimmune diseases) (Alasoo et al. 2018; Bossini-Castillo et al. 2019; Fortune et al. 2015).

4.2 Disease-Associated INDELs

The INDELs as the second most common type of polymorphisms are implicated in the pathogenesis of both Mendelian and polygenic diseases such as cystic fibrosis, hemophilia, and neurofibromatosis (Bakhtiari et al. 2021; Collins et al. 1987; Oldenburg et al. 1998; Ostertag and Kazazian 2001). Specific INDELs have been investigated in the pathogenesis of complex autoimmune and dermatological conditions via candidate gene approaches. For instance, vitiligo has been linked to INDEL polymorphisms in the gene encoding angiotensin-converting enzyme and alopecia areata has been linked to an INDEL at the 3'UTR of the *interleukin-1 alpha* (*IL-1α*) gene (Lu et al. 2013; Patwardhan et al. 2013).

Unlike GWA studies which can directly capture SNPs, INDELs are usually hidden from direct detection by microarray platforms. Consequently, even though the INDEL polymorphisms have greater functional consequences than the SNPs (due to frameshift effect, etc.) they have been less explored on a whole-genome scale (Ratan et al. 2015). Several computational methods have been developed to detect INDELs from data available through next-generation sequencing (NGS) studies such as DINDEL (Albers et al. 2011), piCALL (Bansal and Libiger 2011), SOAP-popINDEL (Shao et al. 2013), PINDEL (Ye et al. 2009), SAMtools (Li et al. 2009), and Platypusand (Hasan et al. 2015; Rimmer et al. 2014). Some of these methods have been employed in the clinical setting to explore the genetic architecture of complex diseases. A recent study has been able to identify 29 INDELs on 17 previously unreported genes to confer susceptibility to psoriasis by utilizing SOAP-PopINDEL as their computational method (Zhen et al. 2019).

As for the SNPs, additional colocalization analyses can also be performed in ancillary to INDEL scanning computational methods to identify insertion/deletion variants that are able to influence the expression of their nearby genes (INDEL specific eQTLs) (Huang et al. 2015). This integration would allow for a better understanding of disease pathogenesis by clarifying the functions of disease-associated variants (Chiang et al. 2017).

4.3 Disease-Associated STRs

The STR variants with three nucleotide repeats (CnG) are responsible for at least several monogenic diseases with an inheritance pattern categorized as "anticipation" where the subsequent generation carrying the mutation will have a more severe phenotype with an earlier age of onset. The intensification happens as a result of CnG repeats being inherently more susceptible to expansion after meiosis (dynamic variants) (Mirkin 2007). The fragile X syndrome and myotonic dystrophy are the prototypes of STR-related monogenic disease where expansion in the number of STRs in each generation is associated with worsening of the diseases. Aside from these mono-variant diseases, hypothetically, STRs can also be associated with complex polygenic diseases. Considering the dynamic nature of STRs, even polymorphisms with a very small effect size can have a considerable effect when expanded through multiple generations. Presumably, this might explain the increasing trends observed in some very common diseases!

Several candidate gene investigations have been able to link individual STRs with dermatological conditions such as alopecia areata and atopic dermatitis using routine PCR methods (Mingorance Gámez et al. 2020; Hersberger et al. 2010).

Since direct genotyping multiple STRs at the whole genome levels is considerably more challenging than the GWA studies for SNPs, the role of the STR polymorphisms in the pathogenesis of complex diseases was largely ignored up until recent years (Lieben 2016).

Aside from direct genotyping by NGS techniques which is not feasible for large cohorts right now, several statistical methods have been invented to call for STRs at a genome-wide level using the already available databases. These methods include lobSTR (Gymrek et al. 2012), HipSTR (Willems et al. 2017), STRViper (Cao et al. 2014), ExpansionHunter (Dolzhenko et al. 2017), TREDPARSE (Tang et al. 2017), and STRetch (Dashnow et al. 2018).

Compared to the methods used for INDEL calling, these computational methods are less popular with clinical investigators and it is still early to determine whether any of these methods can gain the popularity of the GWA studies in clinical settings. However, some of these studies have already gone further with their experiments and have performed colocalization and enrichment analysis. Gymrek et al. identified ~2000 STRs that possessed regulatory effects on expression levels of their nearby genes, known as expression STRs (eSTRs). They also performed colocalization analysis with GWAS studies and were able to identify multiple eSTR-regulated genes enriched in loci significantly associated with autoimmune diseases such as Crohn's disease and rheumatoid arthritis (Gymrek et al. 2016).

4.4 Disease-Associated VNTRs

The VNTR polymorphisms are responsible for several monogenic diseases with Mendelian inheritance and are thought to play a major role in the inheritance of complex diseases (Brookes 2013; Goltsov et al. 1992). Individual VNTR polymorphisms have been investigated in case–control studies (candidate gene approach) on dermatological conditions. For instance, a VNTR polymorphism located at the third intron of the *IL-4* gene has been shown to confer susceptibility to alopecia areata, and an *IL1-receptor antagonist* VNTR polymorphism in intron 2 has been linked to vitiligo (Kalkan et al. 2013; Pehlivan et al. 2009).

Considering the higher length and the greater variability of the VNTR polymorphisms in comparison to STRs, the approaches for imputing these polymorphisms at a genome-wide level are far more complicated and more prone to error (Bakhtiari et al. 2021, 2018; Chiang et al. 2017; Gelfand et al. 2014). Thus for now they account for the missing heritability in complex diseases.

4.5 Disease-Associated Structural Variations

The structural variations including CNVs are abundant in the human genome. Most of these structural variants are thought to have benign consequences resulting in phenotypical traits but some have been linked to well-known syndromes such as Prader-Willi/ Angelman and DiGeorge (McDonald-McGinn et al. 2015; Vogels and Fryns 2002).

The detection of structural variations is perhaps easier due to the sizes of these polymorphisms. They were initially detected by simple methods such as fluorescence in situ hybridization (FISH) in patients assumed to be affected by VNTR-related syndromes. Later on, candidate gene approaches were employed to investigate the association between specific structural variants and complex diseases. As an example of this approach, a case–control study on psoriasis investigated the CNV at the 8p23.1 containing the *beta-defensin* gene cluster and was able to demonstrate a higher risk for developing psoriasis in individuals carrying higher copy numbers of *the beta-defensin* gene (Hollox et al. 2008).

With the advent of techniques that were able to analyze CNVs by using DNA microarrays, genome-wide CNV analyses, studies investigating the contribution of multiple CNVs to the pathogenesis of complex diseases blossomed (Carter 2007; Hollox et al. 2008; Stankiewicz and Lupski 2010). For instance, a 32-kb CNV at 1q21 containing the *late-cornified envelope* (*LCE*) gene cluster was shown to be associated with psoriasis and a cluster containing melanin-related genes on 6q16.3 was linked to alopecia areata by two separate genome-wide CNV analyses (Fischer et al. 2017; Hollox et al. 2008).

4.6 Additional Methods for Finding Disease-Causing Genes

4.6.1 Linkage Studies

In linkage analysis in diseases with familial clustering, the genome of affected and unaffected family members are compared to find causative genes by following the co-segregation of the suspected alleles with diseases trait (Pulst 1999). It was classically reserved for rare variants that were causative for rare monogenic diseases. But with the advent of NGS techniques, linkage analysis coupled with whole-genome sequencing (WGS) is remerging for the identification of rare variants with huge effect sizes in complex diseases (an association that GWA studies were incapable of detecting) (Ott et al. 2015). The *TREX1* gene was identified as the cause of familial lupus through an SNP-based genome-wide linkage analysis (Lee-Kirsch et al. 2006; Yi et al. 2020).

Homozygosity mapping is a subtype of linkage analysis used to identify particular loci at which affected members of a consanguineous family are homozygous. Though this method is usually used for the detection of genes responsible for rare autosomal recessive diseases the concept of regions of homogeneity has been utilized in detecting genes with causative effects in complex diseases (Alkuraya 2010; Ewald et al. 2003; Ku et al. 2011).

4.6.2 Gene Expression Profiling Studies

In gene expression profiling, DNA microarray and RNA sequencing techniques are used to measure the expression levels of several thousands of mRNAs encoded by active genes in a specific tissue/cell in an experimental condition. The data could then be compared to the expression of the genes in a controlled setting to show the effects of the experimental condition on the differential expression of genes (Wang et al. 2000).

Logically they are the next step after genome sequencing since they provide information on the actual genes in effect rather than all the possible events that could be carried out by the whole genome. Nonetheless, they are a step behind proteomic studies that deal with measuring the precise proteins made by a specific cell/ tissue in a specific experimental condition (Mirza and Olivier 2008). The proteomic studies, however, are not feasible right now.

Gene expression profiling has been performed to generate or test hypotheses about the pathogenesis of many dermatological diseases such as alopecia areata and lichen planus (Subramanya et al. 2010; Wenzel et al. 2008). In dermatological conditions where the disease is scattered throughout the skin, the transcriptional profile of the affected tissue, unaffected tissue from a diseased individual, and healthy control skin are often compared to identify the category of genes at play in disease progression (Blumenberg 2012; Rizzo and Maibach 2012).

The profiling studies can also be utilized to evaluate the expression of non-coding micro-RNAs (miRNA) as one of the most important players of epigenetic mechanisms (Glavač and Ravnik-Glavač 2015). The miRNAs are small chains of nucleotides that can bind to messenger-RNA (mRNA) molecules and either repress their translation to proteins or initiate their degradation based on their complementarity to the reference mRNA. Thus by changing protein levels these miRNAs can regulate many intracellular pathways and cause diseases (Jinnin 2014; O'Brien et al. 2018).

5 Human Leukocyte Antigen, the Most Notorious Gene in Complex Diseases

In general, genes that control the response to environmental triggers are more polymorphic than master regulator genes in the control of vital cellular functions. Thus they are more likely to be involved in the pathogenesis of complex diseases. This means that the combined effects of multiple variants of these genes can change how the body responds to environmental triggers and therefore shape the susceptibility to diseases. The immune system is at the frontline of confrontation with the environment. The human leukocyte antigen (HLA) region is the most polymorphous loci in the human genome. It is located at the 6p21.3 and contains more than 300 genes encoding proteins with different functions in the immune system including the two classes of the major histocompatibility complexes (MHC-I and MHC-II) (Ting and Trowsdale 2002).

The MHC-I is composed of a highly variable heavy α subunit with three domains (α_1, α_2, α_3) and a conserved β subunit encoded by a gene on the 15th chromosome. The MHC-II is a heterodimer composed of two polymorphic subunits, α and β each comprising two domains (α_1, α_2, and β_1, β_2) (Fig. 3).

Each pair of the 6th chromosome has three genes coding for the α subunit of the MHC-I gene (HLA-A, HLA-B, and HLA-C). Considering the codominant pattern of expression of these genes, each person possesses six different types of MHC-I (three paternally and three maternally inherited) (Fig. 3). These genes are quite polymorphous with thousands of documented variants (alleles) for each of the three HLA-A, HLA-B, and HLA-C genes (Ting and Trowsdale 2002). For instance, 6766 alleles have been documented as of 2021 for HLA-A coding for 4064 active proteins and 344 null proteins (Table 1).

Each pair of the 6th chromosome has 4–6 clusters of genes that encode for both α and β subunits of MHC-II: (a) DP cluster containing the *HLA-DPA1* encoding for the α subunit and

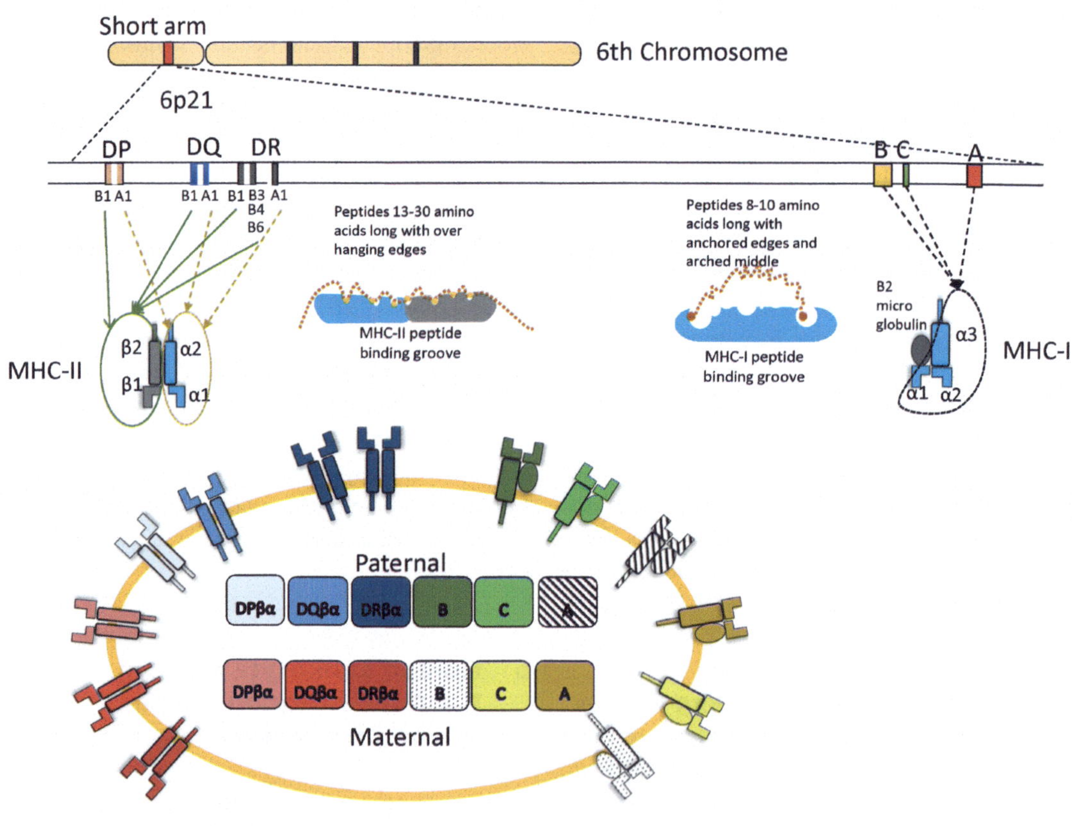

Fig. 3 The major histocompatibility (MHC) encoding genes, the structure of the MHC molecules, and their codominant expression on cell surfaces

Table 1 The number of alleles identified to date for each HLA gene (adapted from Robinson et al. (2015), Marsh et al. (2010))

MHC-I	**Gene**	***A***			***B***			***C***		
	Alleles	6,766			7,967			6,620		
	Proteins	4,064			4,962			3,831		
	Nulls	344			269			286		
MHC-II	**Gene**	***DPA1***	***DPB1***	***DQA1***	***DQB1***	***DRA1***	***DRB1***	***DRB3***	***DRB4***	***DRB5***
	Alleles	258	1,749	306	1,997	29	2,949	390	194	155
	Proteins	107	1,106	143	1,303	2	2,015	293	129	120
	Nulls	7	88	7	86	0	96	18	22	19

HLA-DPB1 encoding for the β subunit; (b) DQ cluster encompassing *HLA-DQA1* and *HLA-DQB1* genes encoding for α and β, respectively; and (c) DR cluster with *HLA-DRA1* encoding for the α subunit and *HLA-DRB1* encoding for the β subunit. Most individuals carry an additional β encoding gene *HLA-DRB3* or *HLA-DRB4* or *HLA-DRB6*. Thus with two pairs of chromosomes, an individual can inherit six to eight functioning class-II alleles. In general, the MHC-II α subunit encoding genes are less polymorphous than the genes encoding for the β subunit (Table 1) (Marsh et al. 2010; Robinson et al. 2015). The HLA alleles have a unanimous nomenclature starting with an HLA prefix followed by the gene name (e.g., HLA-A) and four numeric fields stating the allele group (e.g., HLA-A*02), specific HLA protein (e.g., HLA-A*02:101), the synonymous nucleotide substitutions in the coding region (e.g., HLA-A*02:101:01) and variations in non-coding DNA regions (e.g., HLA-A*02:101:01:02). A suffix is also added at the end to show its expression status at the cell surface (e.g., HLA-A*02:101:01:02 N, N = null) (Mack et al. 2013).

The set of MHC-I and MHC-II alleles on each chromosome forms a haplotype. Thus each individual carries one maternal haplotype and one paternal haplotype. Since the MHC genes are highly polymorphic, the likelihood of two individuals having the same set of haplotypes is extremely rare.

Though HLA molecules bind to antigenic peptides and interact with T-cell receptors (TCR), killer-cell Ig-like receptors (KIR) on Natural killer cells, and leukocyte Ig-like receptor (LIR) on monocytes, it is important to note that the variations in the HLA genes do not result from recombination, in contrast to the immune repertoire of antigen receptors (Shiina et al. 2009). The HLA class I molecules are expressed by all most all cells. They bind with 8–10 amino acids long peptides originated from endogenous antigen processing. Their peptide-binding groove has an adaptable construction and thus peptides with varying sequences can occupy it. The only interactions between the peptide and the HLA-I molecule occur at the two N- and C- ends of the peptide and two specific amino acids at the α1 and α2 domains known as anchor residues. This would allow the central part of the peptide to arch toward the TCR cavity. Since this peptide-binding groove is closed at both ends it can only capture peptides larger than 8–10 amino acids if the central part of the peptide is flexible enough to bend upward (Hsieh 2014; Liao and Arthur 2011).

The HLA class II molecules are only expressed by antigen-presenting cells. They are able to capture 13–18 amino acids long peptides resulting from exogenous antigen processing. Their peptide-binding groove has an adaptable structure and thus peptides with varying sequences can occupy it. Unlike the HLA-I, the binding groove of HLA-II and the peptide touch down in several places along the floor of the binding groove without forming a closed loop. Thus longer peptides, up to 30 amino acids long, could be presented by HLA- II molecules since its end can overhang from the MHC-II groove. However, the multiple hydrogen bindings allow only a particular set of peptides with a specific secondary structure similar to a polyproline chain to be able to fit the HLA-II groove (Hsieh 2014) (Fig. 3).

HLA variants were among the first genetic polymorphisms to be linked to disease susceptibility. Currently, HLA associations are a consistent part of almost all genetic studies concerning complex autoimmune diseases. However, for most parts, it is still unclear how specific HLA alleles could contribute to disease induction or progression. Some have suggested that these variants may show up in GWA studies as a result of linkage disequilibrium with the causative genes. Some have proposed that HLA alleles could be involved in the pathogenesis of autoimmune diseases by affecting the expression and stability of MHC molecules and their peptide-binding abilities. For instance, the immunogenic peptide in celiac diseases, gliadin, has a significantly higher affinity toward *HLA-DQ2* (Dunne et al. 2020). Perhaps a specific HLA variant may be incapable of expressing certain types of pathogenic antigens or it may act as a binding site or an entry receptor for a specific type of disease-provoking pathogen (Ghodke et al. 2005). HLA variants may have certain epitopes that resemble pathogenic antigens and thus could provoke autoimmunity via molecular mimicry. Peptide- HLA complexes could form superantigens (Sheehan 2004). Certain HLA variants may be able to provoke an autoreactive T-cell response by influencing the T-cell repertoire or by presenting self-peptides or altered-self-peptides to T-cells (Howell 2014). Different HLA variants may activate different subcellular signaling pathways upon TCR binding (Crux and Elahi 2017).

It should be noted that even in cases of significant association such as in ankylosing spondylitis (AS) where 98% of the patients are *HLA-B*27* carriers, not all individuals carrying the risk allele will develop the diseases. In fact, the lifelong incidence of AS in *HLA-B*27* carriers is roughly 2% (Linden et al. 1984). Thus HLA variants on their own are not able to induce diseases and there are no monogenic diseases involving HLA mutations.

6 Conclusion

Our knowledge of the genetic basis of the immune responses, immunogenetics, has been greatly improved in recent years owing to both technological advancements and lower costs of genetic sequencing.

This knowledge may help us better understand the pathogenic mechanisms involved in diseases and give us a better perspective on disease outcomes. It can also revolutionize treatment strategies by allowing us to get closer to designing personalized treatment approaches based on specific genetic backgrounds.

The field of immunogenetics holds promises for relatively common dermatological conditions with devastating psychological impacts such as vitiligo and alopecia areata where the precise pathogenesis is still under debate and the curative treatments are far out of sight.

References

Alasoo K, Rodrigues J, Mukhopadhyay S, Knights AJ, Mann AL, Kundu K, Hale C, Dougan G, Gaffney DJ (2018) Shared genetic effects on chromatin and gene expression indicate a role for enhancer priming in immune response. Nat Genet 50:424–431

Albers CA, Lunter G, MacArthur DG, McVean G, Ouwehand WH, Durbin R (2011) Dindel: accurate indel calls from short-read data. Genome Res 21:961–973

Alkuraya FS (2010) Homozygosity mapping: one more tool in the clinical geneticist's toolbox. Genet Med 12:236–239

Altshuler D, Donnelly P, Consortium IH (2005) A haplotype map of the human genome. Nature 437:nature04226

Asghari V, Sanyal S, Buchwaldt S, Paterson A, Jovanovic V, Van Tol HH (1995) Modulation of intracellular cyclic AMP levels by different human dopamine D4 receptor variants. J Neurochem 65:1157–1165

Bakhtiari M, Park J, Ding Y-C, Shleizer-Burko S, Neuhausen SL, Halldórsson BV, Stefánsson K,

Gymrek M, Bafna V (2021) Variable Number Tandem Repeats mediate the expression of proximal genes. Nat Commun 12:1–12

Bakhtiari M, Shleizer-Burko S, Gymrek M, Bansal V, Bafna V (2018) Targeted genotyping of variable number tandem repeats with adVNTR. Genome Res 28:1709–1719

Bannister AJ, Kouzarides T (2011) Regulation of chromatin by histone modifications. Cell Res 21:381–395

Bansal V, Libiger O (2011) A probabilistic method for the detection and genotyping of small indels from population-scale sequence data. Bioinf 27:2047–2053

Barrett JC, Cardon LR (2006) Evaluating coverage of genome-wide association studies. Nat Genet 38:659–662

Behjati S, Tarpey PS (2013) What is next generation sequencing? Arch Dis Child-Educ Pract 98:236–238

Blumenberg M (2012) SKINOMICS: transcriptional profiling in dermatology and skin biology. Curr Genom 13:363–368

Bossini-Castillo L, Glinos DA, Kunowska N, Golda G, Lamikanra A, Spitzer M, Soskic B, Cano-Gamez E, Smyth DJ, Cattermole C (2019) Immune disease variants modulate gene expression in regulatory CD4+ T cells and inform drug targets. BioRxiv:654632

Botstein D, White RL, Skolnick M, Davis RW (1980) Construction of a genetic linkage map in man using restriction fragment length polymorphisms. Am J Hum Genet 32:314

Boyle AP, Davis S, Shulha HP, Meltzer P, Margulies EH, Weng Z, Furey TS, Crawford GE (2008) High-resolution mapping and characterization of open chromatin across the genome. Cell 132:311–322

Brookes K (2013) The VNTR in complex disorders: the forgotten polymorphisms? A functional way forward? Genomics 101:273–281

Cai CQ, Zhang T, Breslin MB, Giraud M, Lan MS (2011) Both polymorphic variable number of tandem repeats and autoimmune regulator modulate differential expression of insulin in human thymic epithelial cells. Diabetes 60:336–344

Cano-Gamez E, Trynka G (2020) From GWAS to function: using functional genomics to identify the mechanisms underlying complex diseases. Front Genet 11

Cao MD, Tasker E, Willadsen K, Imelfort M, Vishwanathan S, Sureshkumar S, Balasubramanian S, Boden M (2014) Inferring short tandem repeat variation from paired-end short reads. Nucleic Acids Res 42:e16–e16

Carter NP (2007) Methods and strategies for analyzing copy number variation using DNA microarrays. Nat Genet 39:S16–S21

Mingorance Gámez CG, Martínez Chamorro A, Moreno Casares AM, Tercedor Sánchez J, Arias-Santiago S, García-Lora E, López-Nevot MA(2020) Joint study of the associations of HLA-B and the transmembrane STR polymorphism of MICA with alopecia areata shows independent associations of both of them with the disease. Clin Exp Dermatol

Chen L, Ge B, Casale FP, Vasquez L, Kwan T, Garrido-Martín D, Watt S, Yan Y, Kundu K, Ecker S (2016) Genetic drivers of epigenetic and transcriptional variation in human immune cells. Cell 167:1398–1414. e1324

Chiang C, Scott AJ, Davis JR, Tsang EK, Li X, Kim Y, Hadzic T, Damani FN, Ganel L, Montgomery SB (2017) The impact of structural variation on human gene expression. Nat Genet 49:692–699

Clark TG, Andrew T, Cooper GM, Margulies EH, Mullikin JC, Balding DJ (2007) Functional constraint and small insertions and deletions in the ENCODE regions of the human genome. Genome Biol 8:1–14

Collins FS, Drumm ML, Cole JL, Lockwood WK, Woude GV, Iannuzzi MC (1987) Construction of a general human chromosome jumping library, with application to cystic fibrosis. Science 235:1046–1049

Conde L, Vaquerizas JM, Santoyo J, Al-Shahrour F, Ruiz-Llorente S, Robledo M, Dopazo J (2004) PupaSNP Finder: a web tool for finding SNPs with putative effect at transcriptional level. Nucleic Acids Res 32:W242–W248

Conrad DF, Keebler JE, DePristo MA, Lindsay SJ, Zhang Y, Casals F, Idaghdour Y, Hartl CL, Torroja C, Garimella KV (2011) Variation in genome-wide mutation rates within and between human families. Nat Genet 43:712

Consortium EP (2012) An integrated encyclopedia of DNA elements in the human genome. Nature 489:57

Consortium WTCC (2007) Genome-wide association study of 14,000 cases of seven common diseases and 3,000 shared controls. Nature 447:661

Crux NB, Elahi S (2017) Human leukocyte antigen (HLA) and immune regulation: how do classical and non-classical HLA alleles modulate immune response to human immunodeficiency virus and hepatitis C virus infections? Front Immunol 8:832

Dashnow H, Lek M, Phipson B, Halman A, Sadedin S, Lonsdale A, Davis M, Lamont P, Clayton JS, Laing NG (2018) STRetch: detecting and discovering pathogenic short tandem repeat expansions. Genome Biol 19:1–13

DeWan A, Liu M, Hartman S, Zhang SS-M, Liu DT, Zhao C, Tam PO, Chan WM, Lam DS, Snyder M (2006) HTRA1 promoter polymorphism in wet age-related macular degeneration. Science 314:989–992

Dolzhenko E, van Vugt JJ, Shaw RJ, Bekritsky MA, van Blitterswijk M, Narzisi G, Ajay SS, Rajan V, Lajoie BR, Johnson NH (2017) Detection of long repeat expansions from PCR-free whole-genome sequence data. Genome Res 27:1895–1903

Dubois PC, Trynka G, Franke L, Hunt KA, Romanos J, Curtotti A, Zhernakova A, Heap GA, Ádány R, Aromaa A (2010) Multiple common variants for celiac disease influencing immune gene expression. Nat Genet 42:295–302

Dunne MR, Byrne G, Chirdo FG, Feighery C (2020) Coeliac disease pathogenesis: the uncertainties of a well-known immune mediated disorder. Front Immunol 11:1374

Ewald H, Kruse TA, Mors O (2003) Genome wide scan using homozygosity mapping and linkage analyses of a single pedigree with affective disorder suggests oligogenic inheritance. Am J Med Genet B Neuropsychiatr Genet 120:63–71

Fischer J, Degenhardt F, Hofmann A, Redler S, Basmanav FB, Heilmann-Heimbach S, Hanneken S, Giehl KA, Wolff H, Moebus S (2017) Genomewide analysis of copy number variants in alopecia areata in a Central European cohort reveals association with MCHR 2. Exp Dermatol 26:536–541

Fortune MD, Guo H, Burren O, Schofield E, Walker NM, Ban M, Sawcer SJ, Bowes J, Worthington J, Barton A (2015) Statistical colocalization of genetic risk variants for related autoimmune diseases in the context of common controls. Nat Genet 47:839–846

Frommer M, McDonald LE, Millar DS, Collis CM, Watt F, Grigg GW, Molloy PL, Paul CL (1992) A genomic sequencing protocol that yields a positive display of 5-methylcytosine residues in individual DNA strands. Proc Natl Acad Sci 89:1827–1831

Gamazon ER, Stranger BE (2015) The impact of human copy number variation on gene expression. Brief Funct Genom 14:352–357

Gelfand Y, Hernandez Y, Loving J, Benson G (2014) VNTRseek—a computational tool to detect tandem repeat variants in high-throughput sequencing data. Nucleic Acids Res 42:8884–8894

Gerrits A, Li Y, Tesson BM, Bystrykh LV, Weersing E, Ausema A, Dontje B, Wang X, Breitling R, Jansen RC (2009) Expression quantitative trait loci are highly sensitive to cellular differentiation state. PLoS Genet 5:e1000692

Gheldof N, Witwicki RM, Migliavacca E, Leleu M, Didelot G, Harewood L, Rougemont J, Reymond A (2013) Structural variation-associated expression changes are paralleled by chromatin architecture modifications. PloS One 8:e79973

Ghodke Y, Joshi K, Chopra A, Patwardhan B (2005) HLA and disease. Eur J Epidemiol 20:475–488

Giambartolomei C, Vukcevic D, Schadt EE, Franke L, Hingorani AD, Wallace C, Plagnol V (2014) Bayesian test for colocalisation between pairs of genetic association studies using summary statistics. PLoS Genet 10:e1004383

Glavač D, Ravnik-Glavač M (2015) Essential role of microRNA in skin physiology and disease. In: microRNA: medical evidence. Springer, pp 307–330

Goltsov AA, Eisensmith RC, Konecki D, Lichter-Konecki U, Woo S (1992) Associations between mutations and a VNTR in the human phenylalanine hydroxylase gene. Am J Hum Genet 51:627

Gong J, Tong Y, Zhang HM, Wang K, Hu T, Shan G, Sun J, Guo AY (2012) Genome-wide identification of SNPs in microRNA genes and the SNP effects on microRNA target binding and biogenesis. Hum Mutat 33:254–263

Gymrek M, Golan D, Rosset S, Erlich Y (2012) lobSTR: a short tandem repeat profiler for personal genomes. Genome Res 22:1154–1162

Gymrek M, Willems T, Guilmatre A, Zeng H, Markus B, Georgiev S, Daly MJ, Price AL, Pritchard JK, Sharp AJ (2016) Abundant contribution of short tandem repeats to gene expression variation in humans. Nat Genet 48:22–29

Hasan MS, Wu X, Zhang L (2015) Performance evaluation of indel calling tools using real short-read data. Hum Genom 9:1–14

He X, Fuller CK, Song Y, Meng Q, Zhang B, Yang X, Li H (2013) Sherlock: detecting gene-disease associations by matching patterns of expression QTL and GWAS. Am J Hum Genet 92:667–680

Hersberger M, Thun G-A, Imboden M, Brandstätter A, Waechter V, Summerer M, Schmid-Grendelmeier P, Bircher A, Rohrer L, Berger W (2010) Association of STR polymorphisms in CMA1 and IL-4 with asthma and atopy: the SAPALDIA cohort. Hum Immunol 71:1154–1160

Hollox EJ, Huffmeier U, Zeeuwen PL, Palla R, Lascorz J, Rodijk-Olthuis D, Van De Kerkhof PC, Traupe H, De Jongh G, Den Heijer M (2008) Psoriasis is associated with increased β-defensin genomic copy number. Nat Genet 40:23–25

Hormozdiari F, Van De Bunt M, Segre AV, Li X, Joo JWJ, Bilow M, Sul JH, Sankararaman S, Pasaniuc B, Eskin E (2016) Colocalization of GWAS and eQTL signals detects target genes. Am J Hum Genet 99:1245–1260

Howell W (2014) HLA and disease: guilt by association. Int J Immunogenet 41:1–12

Hsieh FH (2014) Primer to the immune response. Ann Allergy Asthma Immunol 113:333

Hu X, Kim H, Stahl E, Plenge R, Daly M, Raychaudhuri S (2011) Integrating autoimmune risk loci with gene-expression data identifies specific pathogenic immune cell subsets. Am J Hum Genet 89:496–506

Huang J, Chen J, Esparza J, Ding J, Elder JT, Abecasis GR, Lee Y-A, Lathrop GM, Moffatt MF, Cookson WO (2015) eQTL mapping identifies insertion- and deletion-specific eQTLs in multiple tissues. Nat Commun 6:1–8

Jin Y, Wang J, Bachtiar M, Chong SS, Lee CG (2018) Architecture of polymorphisms in the human genome reveals functionally important and positively selected variants in immune response and drug transporter genes. Hum Genom 12:1–13

Jinnin M (2014) Various applications of microRNAs in skin diseases. J Dermatol Sci 74:3–8

Kalkan G, Karakus N, Baş Y, Takçı Z, Özuğuz P, Ateş Ö, Yigit S (2013) The association between Interleukin (IL)-4 gene intron 3 VNTR polymorphism and alopecia areata (AA) in Turkish population. Gene 527:565–569

Kim B-C, Kim W-Y, Park D, Chung W-H, Shin K-s, Bhak J (2008) SNP@ Promoter: a database of human SNPs (single nucleotide polymorphisms) within the putative promoter regions. In: BMC bioinformatics. Springer, pp 1–5

Ku CS, Loy EY, Salim A, Pawitan Y, Chia KS (2010) The discovery of human genetic variations and their use as disease markers: past, present and future. J Hum Genet 55:403–415

Ku CS, Naidoo N, Teo SM, Pawitan Y (2011) Regions of homozygosity and their impact on complex diseases and traits. Hum Genet 129:1–15

Kundaje A, Meuleman W, Ernst J, Bilenky M, Yen A, Heravi-Moussavi A, Kheradpour P, Zhang Z, Wang J, Ziller MJ (2015) Integrative analysis of 111 reference human epigenomes. Nature 518:317–330

Küster W, Happle R (1984) The inheritance of common baldness: two B or not two B? J Am Acad Dermatol 11:921–926

Lee-Kirsch MA, Gong M, Schulz H, Rüschendorf F, Stein A, Pfeiffer C, Ballarini A, Gahr M, Hubner N, Linné M (2006) Familial chilblain lupus, a monogenic form of cutaneous lupus erythematosus, maps to chromosome 3p. Am J Hum Genet 79:731–737

Li H, Handsaker B, Wysoker A, Fennell T, Ruan J, Homer N, Marth G, Abecasis G, Durbin R (2009) The sequence alignment/map format and SAMtools. Bioinformatics 25:2078–2079

Liao WW, Arthur JW (2011) Predicting peptide binding to major histocompatibility complex molecules. Autoimmun Rev 10:469–473

Lieben L (2016) Repeat, repeat, repeat—gene expression variability explained. Nat Rev Genet 17:69

Lin M, Whitmire S, Chen J, Farrel A, Shi X, Guo J-t (2017) Effects of short indels on protein structure and function in human genomes. Sci Rep 7:1–9

Lonsdale J, Thomas J, Salvatore M, Phillips R, Lo E, Shad S, Hasz R, Walters G, Garcia F, Young N (2013) The genotype-tissue expression (GTEx) project. Nat Genet 45:580–585

Lu D, Chen L, Shi X, Zhang X, Ling X, Chen X, Xie L, Jiang L, Ding L, He Y (2013) A functional polymorphism in interleukin-1α (IL1A) gene is associated with risk of alopecia areata in Chinese populations. Gene 521:282–286

Mack SJ, Cano P, Hollenbach JA, He J, Hurley CK, Middleton D, Moraes ME, Pereira SE, Kempenich JH, Reed EF (2013) Common and well-documented HLA alleles: 2012 update to the CWD catalogue. Tissue Antigens 81:194–203

Marsh SG, Albert E, Bodmer W, Bontrop R, Dupont B, Erlich H, Fernández-Viña M, Geraghty D, Holdsworth R, Hurley C (2010) Nomenclature for factors of the HLA system, 2010. Tissue Antigens 75:291

Maurano MT, Humbert R, Rynes E, Thurman RE, Haugen E, Wang H, Reynolds AP, Sandstrom R, Qu H, Brody J (2012) Systematic localization of common disease-associated variation in regulatory DNA. Science 337:1190–1195

McCarroll SA, Altshuler DM (2007) Copy-number variation and association studies of human disease. Nat Genet 39:S37–S42

McDonald-McGinn DM, Sullivan KE, Marino B, Philip N, Swillen A, Vorstman JA, Zackai EH, Emanuel BS, Vermeesch JR, Morrow BE (2015) 22q11. 2 deletion syndrome. Nat Rev Dis Primers 1:1–19

Mignone F, Gissi C, Liuni S, Pesole G (2002) Untranslated regions of mRNAs. Genome Biol 3:1–10

Mills RE, Luttig CT, Larkins CE, Beauchamp A, Tsui C, Pittard WS, Devine SE (2006) An initial map of insertion and deletion (INDEL) variation in the human genome. Genome Res 16:1182–1190

Mirkin SM (2007) Expandable DNA repeats and human disease. Nature 447:932–940

Mirza SP, Olivier M (2008) Methods and approaches for the comprehensive characterization and quantification of cellular proteomes using mass spectrometry. Physiol Genomics 33:3–11

Neel JV (1978) Rare variants, private polymorphisms, and locus heterozygosity in Amerindian populations. Am J Hum Genet 30:465

Ng PC, Henikoff S (2002) Accounting for human polymorphisms predicted to affect protein function. Genome Res 12:436–446

Nica AC, Montgomery SB, Dimas AS, Stranger BE, Beazley C, Barroso I, Dermitzakis ET (2010) Candidate causal regulatory effects by integration of expression QTLs with complex trait genetic associations. PLoS Genet 6:e1000895

O'Brien J, Hayder H, Zayed Y, Peng C (2018) Overview of microRNA biogenesis, mechanisms of actions, and circulation. Front Endocrinol 9:402

Ok Yang J, Kim WY, Bhak J (2009) ssSNPTarget: genome-wide splice-site single nucleotide polymorphism database. Hum Mutat 30:E1010–E1020

Oldenburg J, Schröder J, Schmitt C, Brackmann H, Schwaab R (1998) Small deletion/insertion mutations within poly-A runs of the factor VIII gene mitigate the severe haemophilia A phenotype. Thromb Haemost 79:452–453

Onengut-Gumuscu S, Chen W-M, Burren O, Cooper NJ, Quinlan AR, Mychaleckyj JC, Farber E, Bonnie JK, Szpak M, Schofield E (2015) Fine mapping of type 1 diabetes susceptibility loci and evidence for colocalization of causal variants with lymphoid gene enhancers. Nat Genet 47:381–386

Ostertag EM, Kazazian HH Jr (2001) Biology of mammalian L1 retrotransposons. Annu Rev Genet 35:501–538

Ott J, Wang J, Leal SM (2015) Genetic linkage analysis in the age of whole-genome sequencing. Nat Rev Genet 16:275–284

Patwardhan M, Pradhan V, Taylor L, Thakkar V, Kharkar V, Khopkar U, Ghosh K, Gawkrodger D, Teare M, Weetman A (2013) The angiotensin-converting enzyme gene insertion/deletion polymorphism in Indian patients with vitiligo: a case–control study and meta-analysis. Br J Dermatol 168:1195–1204

Pearson TA, Manolio TA (2008) How to interpret a genome-wide association study. JAMA 299:1335–1344

Pehlivan S, Ozkinay F, Alper S, Onay H, Yuksel E, Pehlivan M, Ozkinay C (2009) Association between

IL4 (–590), ACE (I)/(D), CCR5 (Δ32), CTLA4 (+ 49) and IL1-RN (VNTR in intron 2) gene polymorphisms and vitiligo. Eur J Dermatol 19:126–128
Pulst SM (1999) Genetic linkage analysis. Arch Neurol 56:667–672
Ratan A, Olson TL, Loughran TP, Miller W (2015) Identification of indels in next-generation sequencing data. BMC Bioinf 16:1–8
Redon R, Ishikawa S, Fitch KR, Feuk L, Perry GH, Andrews TD, Fiegler H, Shapero MH, Carson AR, Chen W (2006) Global variation in copy number in the human genome. Nature 444:444–454
Rimmer A, Phan H, Mathieson I, Iqbal Z, Twigg SR, Wilkie AO, McVean G, Lunter G (2014) Integrating mapping-, assembly-and haplotype-based approaches for calling variants in clinical sequencing applications. Nat Genet 46:912–918
Rizzo AE, Maibach HI (2012) Personalizing dermatology: the future of genomic expression profiling to individualize dermatologic therapy. J Dermatol Treat 23:161–167
Robinson J, Halliwell JA, Hayhurst JD, Flicek P, Parham P, Marsh SG (2015) The IPD and IMGT/HLA database: allele variant databases. Nucleic Acids Res 43:D423–D431
Rockman MV, Kruglyak L (2006) Genetics of global gene expression. Nat Rev Genet 7:862–872
Sachidanandam R, Weissman D, Schmidt SC, Kakol JM, Stein LD, Marth G, Sherry S, Mullikin JC, Mortimore BJ, Willey DL (2001) A map of human genome sequence variation containing 1.42 million single nucleotide polymorphisms. Nature 409:928–934
Saiki RK, Scharf S, Faloona F, Mullis KB, Horn GT, Erlich HA, Arnheim N (1985) Enzymatic amplification of beta-globin genomic sequences and restriction site analysis for diagnosis of sickle cell anemia. Science 230:1350–1354
Sehn JK (2015) Insertions and deletions (indels). In: Clinical genomics. Elsevier, pp 129–150
Shan N, Wang Z, Hou L (2019) Identification of trans-eQTLs using mediation analysis with multiple mediators. BMC Bioinformatics 20:87–97
Shao H, Bellos E, Yin H, Liu X, Zou J, Li Y, Wang J, Coin LJ (2013) A population model for genotyping indels from next-generation sequence data. Nucleic Acids Res 41:e46–e46
Sheehan NJ (2004) The ramifications of HLA-B27. J R Soc Med 97:10–14
Sherry ST, Ward M-H, Kholodov M, Baker J, Phan L, Smigielski EM, Sirotkin K (2001) dbSNP: the NCBI database of genetic variation. Nucleic Acids Res 29:308–311
Shiina T, Hosomichi K, Inoko H, Kulski JK (2009) The HLA genomic loci map: expression, interaction, diversity and disease. J Hum Genet 54:15–39
Slatkin M (2008) Linkage disequilibrium—understanding the evolutionary past and mapping the medical future. Nat Rev Genet 9:477–485
Stankiewicz P, Lupski JR (2010) Structural variation in the human genome and its role in disease. Annu Rev Med 61:437–455
Stein LD (2004) End of the beginning. Nature 431:915–916
Subramanya RD, Coda AB, Sinha AA (2010) Transcriptional profiling in alopecia areata defines immune and cell cycle control related genes within disease-specific signatures. Genomics 96:146–153
Tang H, Kirkness EF, Lippert C, Biggs WH, Fabani M, Guzman E, Ramakrishnan S, Lavrenko V, Kakaradov B, Hou C (2017) Profiling of short-tandem-repeat disease alleles in 12,632 human whole genomes. Am J Hum Genet 101:700–715
Ting JP-Y, Trowsdale J (2002) Genetic control of MHC class II expression. Cell 109:S21–S33
Turnpenny PD, Ellard S, Emery AEH (2022) Emery's elements of medical genetics and genomics
Van der Linden S, Valkenburg H, De Jongh B, Cats A (1984) The risk of developing ankylosing spondylitis in HLA-B27 positive individuals. A comparison of relatives of spondylitis patients with the general population. Arthritis Rheum 27:241–249
Veyrieras J-B, Kudaravalli S, Kim SY, Dermitzakis ET, Gilad Y, Stephens M, Pritchard JK (2008) High-resolution mapping of expression-QTLs yields insight into human gene regulation. PLoS Genet 4:e1000214.
Visscher PM, Brown MA, McCarthy MI, Yang J (2012) Five years of GWAS discovery. Am J Hum Genet 90:7–24
Vogels A, Fryns J-P (2002) The Prader-Willi syndrome and the Angelman syndrome. Genet Couns (geneva, Switzerland) 13:385–396
Wallace C, Rotival M, Cooper JD, Rice CM, Yang JH, McNeill M, Smyth DJ, Niblett D, Cambien F, Consortium C (2012) Statistical colocalization of monocyte gene expression and genetic risk variants for type 1 diabetes. Hum Mol Genet 21:2815–2824
Wang E, Miller LD, Ohnmacht GA, Liu ET, Marincola FM (2000) High-fidelity mRNA amplification for gene profiling. Nat Biotechnol 18:457–459
Wang J, Ronaghi M, Chong SS, Lee CG (2011) pfSNP: an integrated potentially functional SNP resource that facilitates hypotheses generation through knowledge syntheses. Hum Mutat 32:19–24
Weissenbach J, Gyapay G, Dib C, Vignal A, Morissette J, Millasseau P, Vaysseix G, Lathrop M (1992) A second-generation linkage map of the human genome. Nature 359:794–801
Wenzel J, Peters B, Zahn S, Birth M, Hofmann K, Kuesters D, Tomiuk S, Baron JM, Merk HF, Mauch C (2008) Gene expression profiling of lichen planus reflects CXCL9+-mediated inflammation and distinguishes this disease from atopic dermatitis and psoriasis. J Investig Dermatol 128:67–78
Willems T, Zielinski D, Yuan J, Gordon A, Gymrek M, Erlich Y (2017) Genome-wide profiling of heritable and de novo STR variations. Nat Methods 14:590–592

Ye K, Schulz MH, Long Q, Apweiler R, Ning Z (2009) Pindel: a pattern growth approach to detect break points of large deletions and medium sized insertions from paired-end short reads. Bioinformatics 25:2865–2871

Yi C, Li Q, Xiao J (2020) Familial chilblain lupus due to a novel mutation in TREX1 associated with Aicardi–Goutie'res syndrome. Pediatr Rheumatol 18:1–7

Zhen Q, Yang Z, Wang W, Li B, Bai M, Wu J, Ge H, Dong Z, Shen J, Tang H (2019) Genetic study on small insertions and deletions in psoriasis reveals a role in complex human diseases. J Investig Dermatol 139:2302–2312. e2314

Zondervan KT, Cardon LR (2004) The complex interplay among factors that influence allelic association. Nat Rev Genet 5:89–100

The Immunogenetics of Alopecia areata

Fateme Rajabi, Fahimeh Abdollahimajd, Navid Jabalameli, Mansour Nassiri Kashani, and Alireza Firooz

Abstract

Alopecia areata (AA) is an autoimmune disease that targets the hair follicles (HF) and results in non-scarring hair loss. AA results from the collapse of the HF's immune privilege due to a combination of environmental and genetic factors that either change the local HF dynamics or dysregulate the central immune tolerance. Multiple genetic studies have attempted to identify AA susceptibility genes through candidate gene approaches and genome-wide analysis. These studies were able to show an association between AA and multiple immune-related genes such as those encoding cytokines, chemokines, molecules involved in regulatory T-cell functions, and adaptor molecules along with genes involved in autophagy, melanogenesis, and hair cycling pathways. This chapter aims to explore these genes and their contribution to the pathogenesis of the AA.

Keywords

Alopecia areata · Immune privilege · Immunogenetics · Single nucleotide polymorphism · Copy number variants

1 Introduction

Alopecia areata (AA) is an autoimmune disease that targets the hair follicles (HF) and results in non-scarring hair loss. It has an unpredictable course with a wide spectrum of manifestations, ranging from discrete patches of hair loss (patchy AA) to widespread involvement of all hair-bearing areas of the body (alopecia universalis) (Fig. 1). It affects both genders equally with a cumulative lifetime incidence of about two percent and no significant racial predominance (Fricke and Miteva 2015; Mirzoyev et al. 2014; Safavi et al. 1995).

Even though AA is occasionally accounted as a cosmetic issue, the condition is known to have a significant effect on health-related quality of life (HRQoL) (Liu et al. 2016; Rencz et al. 2016; Shi et al. 2013).

The diagnosis of AA can usually be made clinically, but trichogram evaluation, dermoscopy, and histopathological studies are sometimes required (Tosti et al. 2008). The characteristic

F. Rajabi · N. Jabalameli
Network of Dermatology Research (NDR), Universal Scientific Education and Research Network (USERN), Tehran, Iran

F. Rajabi · M. Nassiri Kashani · A. Firooz (✉)
Center for Research & Training in Skin Diseases & Leprosy, Tehran University of Medical Sciences, Tehran, Iran
e-mail: firozali@sina.tums.ac.ir

F. Abdollahimajd
Skin Research Center, Shahid Beheshti University or Medical Sciences, Tehran, Iran

N. Rezaei and F. Rajabi (eds.), *The Immunogenetics of Dermatologic Diseases*, Advances in Experimental Medicine and Biology 1367,
https://doi.org/10.1007/978-3-030-92616-8_2

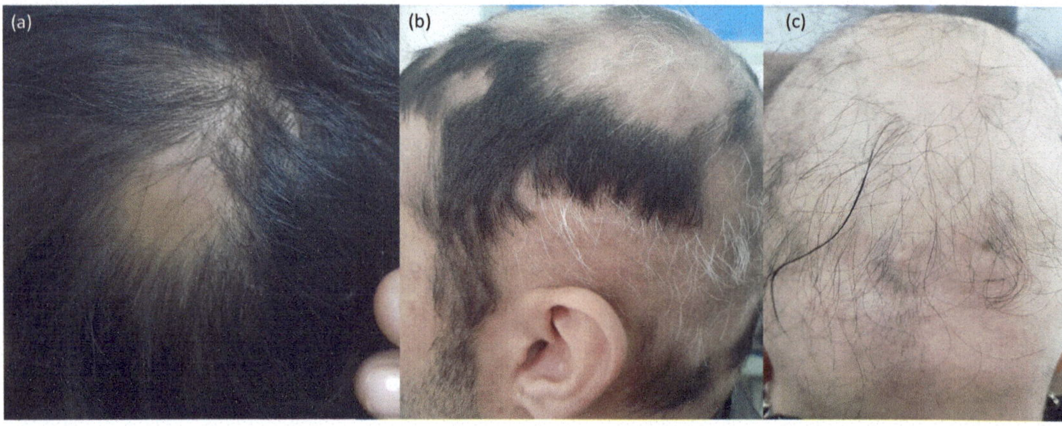

Fig. 1 Clinical features of alopecia areata. **a** Discrete patchy hair loss. **b** Severe patchy alopecia with regrowth of white hair. **c** Alopecia totalis

findings on scalp examination are the "yellow dots" and the "exclamation mark" hairs corresponding to empty follicular ostium and narrowing of the hair shaft near the scalp, respectively. On histopathological examination, lesions reveal peribulbar infiltration of lymphocytes resembling a "swarm of bees." The infiltration mainly consists of CD8+ and CD4+ T-cells (Mounsey and Reed 2009).

Observational studies were the first to hint at a genetic component in AA by demonstrating a higher incidence in the family members of the affected individuals and a higher concordance in twins (Jackow et al. 1998; McDonagh and Tazi-Ahnini 2002a; Steen et al. 1992). Alopecia areata was initially regarded as an autosomal dominant disease with incomplete penetrance but later on, like most autoimmune diseases, it was re-categorized as a complex polygenic disease (Muller 1973).

The first attempts at identifying the AA susceptibility genes were made by candidate gene studies. These included small case–control investigations that compared the frequencies of specific alleles between patients and control subjects and were able to link several human leukocyte antigens (HLAs) and alleles from other immune-related genes to AA susceptibility (Aliagaoglu et al. 2005; Galbraith and Pandey 1995; Kavak et al. 2000; Xiao et al. 2006a, b).

The first study to employ a semi-automated genome-wide scan for AA was a linkage study that compared the genome of 102 affected patients to 118 unaffected individuals from 20 families with multiple AA cases (Martinez-Mir et al. 2007). Shortly after, the first genome-wide association study (GWAS) on 1,054 nonrelated individuals with AA and 3,278 control subjects was conducted yielding some very interesting results (Petukhova et al. 2010). The outcomes of the first GWAS were confirmed through two subsequent large case–control candidate gene studies (Jagielska et al. 2012; Redler et al. 2012). Another large GWAS with twice more participants (2,489 cases and 5,287 controls) was conducted five years later and identified some additional susceptibility loci (Betz et al. 2015a).

Since GWA studies only assess single nucleotide polymorphisms (SNPs), recent investigations have turned their focus to the associations of AA with other types of genetic polymorphisms such as insertion deletions (INDELs), copy number variants (CNVs), variable number of tandem repeats (VNTR), and short tandem repeat (STR) polymorphisms (Fischer et al. 2017; Petukhova et al. 2020).

These large groundbreaking studies along with multiple case–control candidate gene investigations have been able to elucidate many aspects of AA genetics and therefore have been extremely helpful in clarifying the pathogenesis of the disease. Before discussing the finding of these studies a brief review on the pathogenesis of AA might be helpful since they can clarify why some of these genes were selected in candidate gene approaches and how the ones identified in genome screening might contribute to disease progression.

2 The Pathogenesis of AA

The most agreed-upon hypothesis for the pathogenesis of AA is an autoimmune-based scenario (Gilhar and Kalish 2006). However, unlike other autoimmune diseases that occur as a result of loss of tolerance to self-antigens, AA develops due to loss of immune privilege (IP) (McElwee et al. 2013). Immune privilege is an evolutionary adaptation that protects vital organs from destruction by withholding the adaptive and innate immune responses from inciting an inflammation within these tissues. Thus hypothetically, these organs could easily tolerate allografts (Head et al. 1983). The hair follicles (HFs), unlike the eye and the testes, are not fully immune privileged. Rather, only the bulb and the bulge of the HFs enjoy a relative state of IP during the anagen phase (Barker and Billingham 1972; Reynolds et al. 1999).

Several mechanisms are employed to keep the HF out of reach of the immune system. The HF extracellular matrix serves as a physical barrier against inflammation (Paus et al. 2003). The HF cells express Fas ligand and programmed cell death 1 ligand 1 (PD-L1) to induce apoptosis in the infiltrated lymphocytes that have been able to breach the extracellular matrix (Ferguson and Griffith 2006; Kang et al. 2010; Wang et al. 2014). During the anagen phase, HF cells downregulate their major histocompatibility complex I (MHC-I) expression which allows them to keep their intrinsic antigens sequestered and remain out of sight of the immune system. Transforming growth factor-beta (TGF-β), interleukin-10 (IL-10), insulin-like growth factor 1 (IGF-1) and several other proteins known as IP guardians are responsible for the MHC suppression (Ito et al. 2004; Kang et al. 2010). These factors also downregulated MHC-II on antigen-presenting cells (APCs) (Gilhar 2010a; Ito et al. 2004). Since natural killer (NK) cells can detect and attack MHC negative cells (missing self-phenomena), the HF cells are also required to suppress these innate cells in order to preserve their IP. This is mainly achieved by increasing the ratio of inhibitory to excitatory receptors on the surface of NK cells (Ito et al. 2008; Rajabi et al. 2018a).

Alopecia areata occurs when one or more of these IP preservation mechanisms fail. A combination of environmental and genetic factors is responsible for the failure of the IP mechanisms either through changing the local HF dynamics or dysregulating the central immune responses (Paus et al. 1993; Rajabi et al. 2018b).

Environmental stressors coupled with inherent insufficiency in antioxidant clearance mechanisms can increase the amount of intracellular reactive oxygen species (ROS) in HF cells, which promotes the expression of danger molecules such as MHC class I polypeptide-related sequence A (MICA). These danger and damage-associated molecules are recognized and targeted by NK cells, which in turn produce interferon γ (IFNγ) (Bakry et al. 2014; Prie et al. 2015). IFNγ is a master cytokine in AA induction that not only incites inflammation by promoting cytokine and chemokine production but also provokes MHC expression and thus awakens the adaptive immunity (CD8+ T-cells) (Gilhar 2010a; Ito et al. 2008; Yenin et al. 2015). The melanocyte-associated antigens, keratin 16, and trichohyalin are the most prominent sequestered antigens that are targeted in AA (Gilhar et al. 2001a; Leung et al. 2010).

Aside from local disturbances in the HF milieu, dysregulation in the immune system with high levels of IFNγ, IL-15 induced CD8 + NKG2D+ T-cells, IL-2 induced NKG2D+/CD56+ cells, and hypersensitive NK-cells with unbalanced inhibitory to excitatory receptors could also induce IP collapse in the otherwise normal HFs. These cells invade and destruct HFs eventually promoting MHC and MICA expression (McElwee et al. 2005; Wang et al. 2015; Zöller et al. 2002).

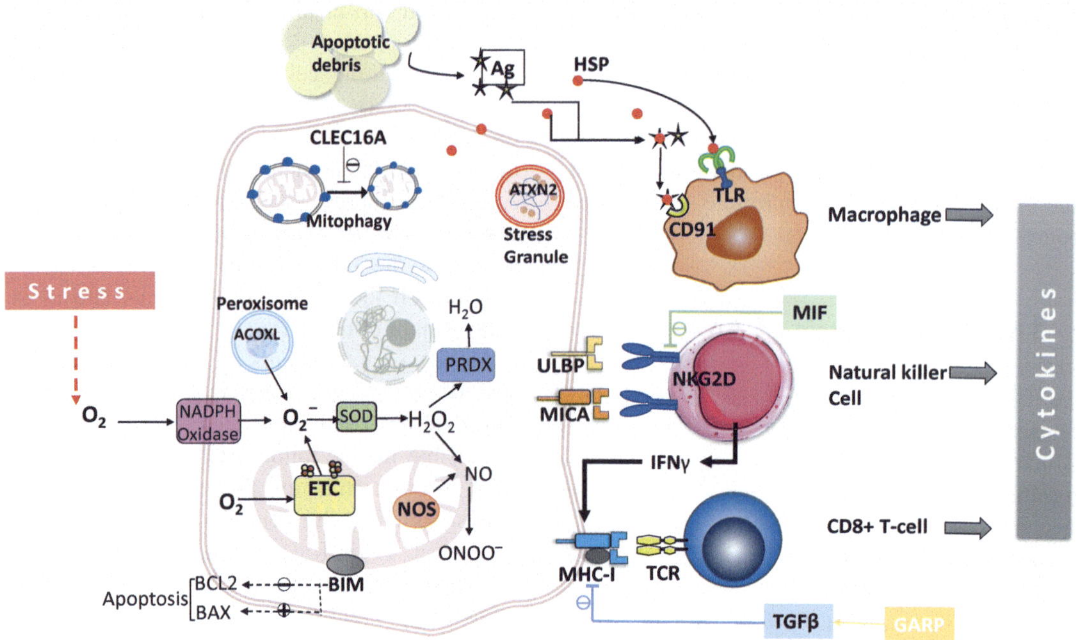

Fig. 2 Local factors involved in immune privilege preservation and collapse. The failure in the mechanisms involved in the clearance of reactive oxygen species (ROS) and the increased production of ROS promote the expression of stress-associated proteins such as MICA, ULBP, and heat shock proteins (HSP). These molecules in turn induce an immune response that could challenge the MHC negativity of hair follicle (HF) cells leading to immune privilege collapse. Ag, antigen; SOD, superoxide dismutase; NOS, nitrite oxide synthase; ETC, electron transport chain

Thus the breach in the IP whether initiated in the HFs or started as immune dysregulation that affects HFs as innocent bystanders proceeds with the infiltration of CD8+ and CD4+ T-cells around anagen hair bulbs and premature induction of catagen (Mounsey and Reed 2009; Rajabi et al. 2018b).

In the following sections, we discuss the AA susceptibility genes and their contribution to the pathogenesis of the diseases in detail (Figs. 2 and 3).

3 The Immunogenetic of AA

3.1 The *HLA* Genes

Multiple HLA alleles have been linked to AA susceptibility by candidate gene approaches in small case–control studies such as *HLA-DQB1*03*, *HLA-DRB1*04*, *HLA-DRB1*16*, and *HLA-DRB1*04* (broad sero name DR4) from the MHC-II, and *HLA-B*15* (broad sero name -B62), *HLA- C*04:01*, and *HLA-C*07:04* from MHC-I (Table 1) (Aliagaoglu et al. 2005; Mingorance Gámez et al. 2020; Haida et al. 2013; Kavak et al. 2000; Kianto et al. 1977; Megiorni et al. 2011a; Xiao et al. 2006a, b). Considering the polymorphous nature of the HLA genes, the variations attributed to ethnicity, and the multiplicity of AA categories (universalis, totalis, patchy, etc.), the results of these small studies though important may not help in explaining the pathogenesis of AA.

The data on GWA studies and meta-analysis, on the other hand, are more reliable on this matter. A meta-analysis of 12 studies with 1283 cases and 32,343 controls was able to demonstrate *HLA-DRB1 ∗ 04* and *HLA-DRB1 ∗ 16* as risk alleles and *HLA-DRB1 ∗ 0301*, *HLA-DRB1 ∗ 09*, and *HLA-DRB1 ∗ 13* as protective alleles for AA (Ji et al. 2018). The second GWAS was able to detect 4 susceptibility loci within the *HLA-DRA* and *HLA-DRB1* genes including (a) an amino-acid substitution at position 37 correspondings to the P9 peptide-binding

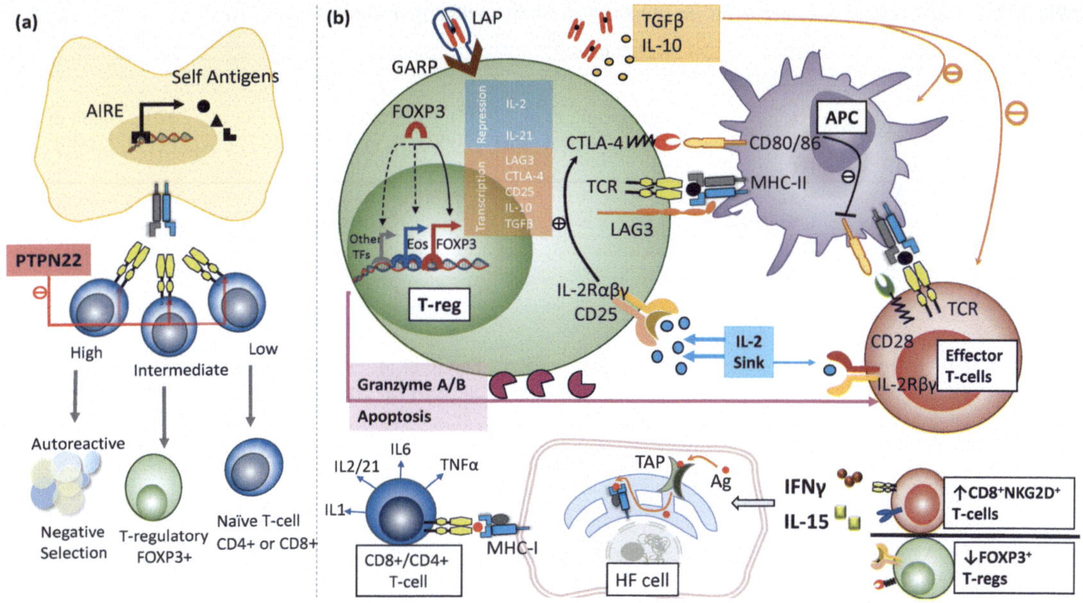

Fig. 3 The role of the central and peripheral immune system in the induction of alopecia areata by immune privilege collapse. **a** T-cell education takes place in the thymus. The naïve T-cells produced in bone marrow enter the thymus in the corticomedullary junction, migrate through the thymic cortex, become double-positive (CD4 + CD8+), undergo positive selection based on their T-cell receptor (TCR) functionality, and differentiate to either CD4+ or CD8+ cells (not shown). The selected cells enter the thymic medulla where they are assessed by their reactivity to self-antigens expressed on medullary thymic epithelial cells (mTEC) under the direction of the AIRE transcription factor. TCRs with high affinity toward self-antigens undergo negative selection, those with intermediated affinity differentiate to FOXP3+ regulatory T-cells (T-regs), and those with low affinity enter the bloodstream as educated T-cells. Failure of these mechanisms in the thymus results in defective T-regs development and leak of autoreactive T-cells. (b) The Tregs maintain the peripheral tolerance via IL-10, TGFβ, CTLA-4, IL-2 receptor αβγ (CD25), LAG3, and granzyme A/B mediated apoptosis. An abnormality in the number and function of Tregs is associated with an increase in proinflammatory cytokines such as interferons that are capable of provoking immune privilege collapse via MHC-I expression. Aside from factors determining T-reg differentiation such as FOXP3 and those crucial for its function such as CTLA4, the genetic polymorphisms in the HLA genes and the transporter associated with antigen processing (TAP) genes could also promote autoimmunity by changing the MHC– TCR affinity in the setting of immune dominance and by affecting peptide selection for antigen presentation, respectively. LAP, latency-associated peptide; APC, antigen-presenting cell

pocket in the HLA-DRβ1 molecule; (b) an amino-acid substitution at position 13 corresponding to the P4 peptide-binding pocket in HLA-DRβ1; (c) an intronic SNP (rs9268657) at *HLA-DRA* gene which is capable of influencing the expression of *HLA-DRB1*; and (d) the well-known *HLA-DRB1*04:01* with shared amino-acid residues at position 70–74 within the peptide-binding groove of the MHC-II molecule (Betz et al. 2015a). Thus three out of four polymorphisms associated with AA according to GWA studies occur at the peptide-binding groove and thus are capable of affecting binding affinities to antigenic peptides. Perhaps this would allow a self-mimicking foreign peptide to be presented via these specific HLA alleles and induce autoimmunity (Arango et al. 2017). Another path through which changes in the affinity of the HLA molecule toward peptide antigens could induce autoimmunity is affecting immune dominance (Wieczorek et al. 2017). This means that although at any given moment multiple combinations of MHC alleles and self and non-self-peptides with the potential of inducing autoimmunity are expressed by APCs, the adaptive immune response is mounted against only a specific HLA-peptide combination that has the most avid connection. Thus

Table 1 HLA association of alopecia areata (underlined HLAs confer protection)

MHC class	Genetic allele	Broad serogroup	References
MHC-I	B*15 C*04:01 C*07:04 C*15:02	A1 B13 B18 B52-CW*0704 B27 B40 B44 (B12) B62, CW3	Aliagaoglu et al. (2005), Mingorance Gámez et al. (2020), Haida et al. (2013), Kavak et al. (2000), Kianto et al. (1977), Xiao et al. (2006a, b)
MHC-II	DPA1*0103 DQB1*0301 DQB1*0303 DQB1*302 DQB1*601 DQB1*603 DQA1*0501 DQA1*0104 DQA1*0606 DQB1*0301 DQB1*0604 DRB1*0401 DRB1*0301 DRB1*1104 DRB1*15	DQ1 DQ3 DQ7 DR1 DR4 DR5 DR6 DR7 DR11 DR16 DR52a DRw52a DPW4	Costa et al. (2006), Duvic et al. (1991), Ji et al. (2018), Kavak et al. (2000), Megiorni et al. (2011a, 2011b), Xiao et al. (2005, 2006c)

autoimmunity can occur as a result of a change in the HLA-peptide affinity rather than the expression of a new HLA-peptide combination (Chicz et al. 1992; Kim and Sadegh-Nasseri 2015; Tsai and Santamaria 2013). The changes in avidity/affinity attributed to HLA polymorphisms could also promote autoimmunity through altering the negative selection of autoreactive T-cells in the thymus (central tolerance). MHC risk alleles with low avidity MHC/T-cell receptor (TCR) interactions reduce the negative selection of autoreactive T-cell and the development of regulatory T-cells (Tsai and Santamaria 2013).

3.2 Genes Linked to Hair Follicle Immune Privilege Preservation and Collapse

The *MICA* and *ULBP* genes

The MICA, MHC class I polypeptide-related sequence B (MICB), and cytomegalovirus UL16-binding protein (ULBP) are three stress-inducible surface proteins that structurally resemble MHC-I (Eleme et al. 2004). MICA and MICB have three α subdomains but no β2-microglobulin and the ULBP consists of only two α subdomains with about 20% sequence homogeneity to the MHC-I (Chalupny et al. 2006; Cosman et al. 2001; Eagle et al. 2009; Groh et al. 1996). These proteins do not express intracellular antigens and they are only conditionally expressed by cells in the setting of major oxidative stress (Groh et al. 1996; Yamamoto et al. 2001). They bind to NKG2D receptors expressed by NK-cells and subsets of T-cells enabling the lysis of the stressed cell via inflammation induced by IFNγ and IL-2 and lysosomal degradation (Zingoni et al. 2018). This mechanism is involved in the pathogenesis of AA where the IP enforces downregulation of MHC-I expression and the buildup of ROS promotes the expression of MICA/ULBP. Since MHC-I molecules can suppress NK-cell activation through binding with inhibitory KIR receptors, the balance is heavily distorted toward the activation of NK cells that subsequently leads to IP collapse and HF destruction (Bauer et al. 1999; Groh et al. 1996; Islam et al. 2015; Yamamoto et al. 2001).

It has been suggested that polymorphisms in genes encoding NKG2D ligands (MICA, MICB, and ULBP) could change the affinity or the expression levels of these proteins in a way that benefits the NK-cell activation (Fernández-Messina et al. 2012; Steinle et al. 2001; Zuo et al. 2017).

The association between AA and the gene encoding for MICA was initially detected by a small genetic linkage study in familial AA that scanned the entire HLA locus (Barahmani et al. 2006). The *MICA* gene is very polymorphous with about 70 SNPs and STR variants. The most studied variant is an STR polymorphism within its transmembrane domain of the gene with five allele groups including A4, A5, A6, and A9 corresponding to the number of (GCT) repeats and A5.1 consisting of five repeats with an extra guanine at the middle ($(GCT)_2G(GCT)_2$) (Bahram et al. 1996; Robinson et al. 2015). This study was able to demonstrate a significantly increased risk of AA associated with carrying the A6 and A5.1 alleles (Barahmani et al. 2006).

A small case–control study in Spanish patients demonstrated an association between *MICA*009* (an SNP within the 4th exon) and AA development (Mingorance Gámez et al. 2020).

The 6p25.1 locus harboring the *cytomegalovirus UL16-binding protein* (*ULBP*) gene cluster was shown to be associated with AA in the first GWAS (Petukhova et al. 2010). Six *ULBP* genes have been identified so far (ULBP1-6) each having several alleles (Antoun et al. 2010; Robinson et al. 2015). A follow-up study was able to confirm this finding by showing an association between *ULBP3/ULBP6* and AA in a large case–control association analysis (Jagielska et al. 2012).

The *HSPA1B* gene

Heat shock proteins (HSPs) are stress-induced proteins that have several functions that help the cell to adapt to stressful environmental conditions. They act as chaperons that help in maintaining the proper folding of proteins, recycling the severely damaged proteins, and forming autophagosomes around protein aggregates (Karademir et al. 2014; Penke et al. 2018; Walter and Buchner 2002). HSPs have an entangled relationship with the immune system. They are involved in MHC-I and MHC-II peptide trafficking and antigen presentation. They facilitate cross-presentation by purging peptides released from lysed cells and act as a medium that binds the peptides to the scavenger receptors such as LOX-1 and LRP1/CD91. The extracellular HPSs can act as damage-associated molecular patterns (DAMPs) and activate Toll-like receptors (TLRs) (Binder 2014; Deffit and Blum 2015; Murshid et al. 2012; Srivastava 2002). The overall outcome of the HSP activities is not unidirectional, rather it can both promote innate/adaptive immune responses along with promoting regulatory pathways (Rajaiah and Moudgil 2009). The HSPs could promote autoimmunity by increasing the expression of sequestered antigens and enhancing the IFN production by activating innate immune responses. HSPs may share homology with pathogenic antigens and thus can become a target for the immune system due to molecular mimicry (Daneri Becerra and Galigniana 2016; Rajaiah and Moudgil 2009; Tukaj and Kaminski 2019). On the other hand, HSPs can downregulate inflammation by attenuating the NFκB and stimulating regulatory T-cell expansion (Tukaj and Kaminski 2019; Wieten et al. 2007). The HSP70 family is the most studied HSP family and encompasses HSPA1A, HSPA1B, and HSPA1L that are encoded by genes in the MHC III region on 6p21.3. Altered expression of HSP70 proteins has been documented in AA lesions compared to normal skin (Thanomkitti et al. 2018; Wikramanayake et al. 2010). Furthermore, anti-inflammatory agents that reduce the tissue levels of HSP70 are found to be effective in the treatment of AA (Wikramanayake et al. 2012).

Based on these observations a candidate gene case–control study in Korean patients investigated the associations between *HSP* genes and AA susceptibility. They found an SNP in the 5'UTR of the *HSPA1B* gene, rs6457452, to be linked to AA with the T allele conferring protection from the disease (Seok et al. 2014a). The association was confirmed in a small study in Jordanian Arabs (Al-Eitan et al. 2019).

The *MIF* gene

The macrophage migration inhibitory factor (MIF) is an immune regulatory protein with a paradoxical set of functions. It promotes the innate and adaptive immune responses by inducing proinflammatory cytokines and increasing the survival and clonal expansion of T-cells (Denkinger et al. 2004; Donn et al. 2004; Illescas et al. 2018; Saeedi et al. 2013), while actively suppressing the NK cells and inhibiting them from attacking MHC-negative cells in IP sites such as HFs (Apte et al. 1998; Ito et al. 2005b; Rajabi et al. 2018b). It is not known whether the lack of effective suppression of NK-cells due to low levels of MIF or the active stimulation of immune response due to high levels of MIF contributes to the pathogenesis of AA.

Multiple studies have argued against the immunosuppressive roles of MIF in AA by demonstrating increased serum levels in AA patients (Eldesouky et al. 2020; Kang et al. 2010; Salem et al. 2016; Shimizu et al. 2002; Younan et al. 2015), while others have suggested that these effects might be reflecting compensatory mechanisms. Moreover, a study was able to show a significantly lower expression of MIF in AA lesions compared to normal skin (Ito et al. 2008).

This argument has also been evaluated from a genetic perspective which could bypass the effect of secondary compensatory mechanisms. The results, however, were contradictory. One study demonstrated the C allele of the rs755622 ($-173G > C$) associated with higher MIF levels to be significantly more common in Japanese AA patients while finding no significant difference between patients and controls in an STR polymorphism within the promoter (-794 [CATT] $_{5-8}$ (Matia-García et al. 2015; Morales-Zambrano et al. 2014; Shimizu et al. 2005). Another study conducted in Iranian patients found the C allele to confer protection from AA (Rajabi et al. 2019a). Nevertheless, a large case–control study of European subjects did not show a significant difference between the patients and controls regarding this polymorphism (Redler et al. 2012). Thus further studies are needed to reach a definite conclusion.

The genes involved in ROS clearance

The increased production of ROS and the insufficiency in the ROS clearance mechanisms could contribute to the pathogenesis of AA by facilitating the buildup of stress (Acharya and Mathur 2020). Polymorphisms in several genes involved in the ROS production and clearance mechanisms have been linked to AA. Some of these genes were identified through the GWA studies including the *PRDX5*, *ATXN2/SH2B3*, and *ACOXL/BCL2L11* while *NOS3* was detected through candidate gene approaches (Betz et al. 2015a, b; Petukhova et al. 2010).

The *nitric oxide synthetase 3* (*NOS3*) is expressed in melanocytes and keratinocytes and produces free radicals in response to pro-inflammatory stimuli. A 27pb VNTR polymorphism within the 4th intron of the *NOS3* gene has been linked to AA susceptibility in a small case–control study (AlFadhli et al. 2008). However subsequent studies were not able to replicate this result (Alzolibani et al. 2015a).

The *peroxiredoxin 5* (*PRDX5*) gene encodes an antioxidant enzyme that catalyzes harmful alkyl peroxides and H_2O_2 into inert products. Surprisingly, the risk allele of the rs694739 SNP has been shown to increase the *PRDX5* expression levels. Perhaps the better clearance of ROS would enable the HF cells to have a longer survival in the setting of oxidative stress, which would allow them to express danger-associated molecules and entangle NK-cells instead of going through simple inflammation-free apoptosis (Abdelaziz 2020). The *PRDX5* polymorphisms are also involved in the pathogenesis of autoimmune diseases such as multiple sclerosis and sarcoidosis (Fischer et al. 2012; Holley et al. 2007). The association between *PRDX5* polymorphisms and AA was replicated by two subsequent case–control studies (Jagielska et al. 2012; Taghiabadi et al. 2018).

The *acyl-coenzyme-A oxidase-like* (*ACOXL*) gene encodes a protein that is involved in the peroxisomal metabolism of lipids. While very little is known about the precise function of this protein, based on the functions of other members of this family, it is likely to operate in the oxidative machinery (Zeng et al. 2017).

The *BCL2-like 11* (*BCL2L11*; *BIM*) is another gene in the locus containing the *ACOXL* to be associated with AA. The BIM is a pro-apoptotic protein that inhibits BCL2 and activates BAX-BAK1. BIM mediates oxidative stress-induced apoptosis in both immune and none immune cells such as melanocytes and keratinocytes (Bouillet et al. 2001; Sinha et al. 2013; Tanaka et al. 2014). Alopecia areata lesions demonstrate increased expression of BIM, confirming its role in HF apoptosis during inflammation. Perhaps the genetic variations in the *BIM* gene could alter the sensitivity of HF keratinocytes and melanocytes to ROS-mediated apoptosis and induction of premature catagen.

BIM-mediated apoptosis of immune cells is involved in the termination of exaggerated long-lasting immune responses and the negative selection of autoreactive T-cells and B-cells. Independent from its pro-apoptotic functions, BIM downregulates autophagy by reducing the formation of autophagosomes (Luo and Rubinsztein 2013). Autophagy is involved in many aspects of the immune response ranging from bacterial killing and antigen presentation to cytokine secretion and thymic selection (Kuballa et al. 2012). Thus expectedly *BIM* mutations and variations have immune consequences as the deletion of BIM has been shown to induce autoimmunity (Chu et al. 2011; Gregersen et al. 2009; Hughes et al. 2006, 2008; Rathmell et al. 2002).

The *Ataxin 2* (*ATXN2*) gene encodes a protein involved in the regulation of cell function under physiologic and stressful conditions (Ostrowski et al. 2017). It controls RNA stability and translation, suppresses the accumulation of the R-loop structures, promotes the formation of stress granules, regulates the circadian rhythm and metabolic pathways, and stimulates antioxidant machinery (Cheung et al. 2003; Meierhofer et al. 2016; Ostrowski et al. 2017). The *ATXN2* variants and mutations have been linked to multiple diseases. Over-expression of *ATXN2* due to an STR mutation (CAG repeat expansion) has been shown to cause a neurodegenerative disorder known as the spinocerebellar ataxia type 2 which is associated with distorted redox balance (Betz et al. 2015b; Cornelius et al. 2017; Dennis et al. 2021). The STR variations also predispose individuals to Parkinson's disease, obesity, amyotrophic lateral sclerosis, and type I diabetes. An SNP within the *ATXN2* gene has been linked to primary open-angle glaucoma (Auburger et al. 2014; Bailey et al. 2016; Elden et al. 2010; Gwinn-Hardy et al. 2000). Since this protein has various functions, it is hard to determine the precise path in which it contributes to the pathogenesis of AA. Thus it is unclear if the AA-associated *ATXN2* SNP is a loss or gain of function variant. The association between *ATNX2/SH2B3* and AA might even reflect linkage disequilibrium with a causative gene.

The Src homology 2-B protein 3 (*SH2B3*), also known as lymphocyte adapter protein (LNK), is a key adaptor protein in the lymphohematopoietic system. It negatively regulates hematopoiesis, B-cell lymphogenesis, TCR and tumor necrosis factor (TNF) signaling, and cell adhesion through interfering with the functions of Janus kinases (JAK2/STAT3-5) and tyrosine kinases (Erk1/2, PI3K/Akt, p38/MAPK) (Devallière and Charreau 2011). The *SH2B3* deletion results in cytokine hypersensitivity and accumulation of B-cells within the spleen and its polymorphisms are associated with increased cytokine production and proliferation of autoreactive T-cells that result in multiple autoimmune diseases such as lupus erythematosus, rheumatoid arthritis, type 1 diabetes, and multiple sclerosis (Devallière and Charreau 2011; Lavrikova et al. 2011; McMullin et al. 2011; Takaki et al. 2000; Velazquez et al. 2002; Zhernakova et al. 2010).

3.3 The Genes Involved in Peripheral and Central Tolerance

The *AIRE* gene

Loss-of-function mutations of the *Autoimmune regulator* (*AIRE*) gene cause an autosomal recessive syndrome known as autoimmune polyendocrinopathy-candidiasis-ectodermal dystrophy (APECED). With AA being a common finding in this syndrome, *AIRE* polymorphisms were interesting candidates to study as a susceptibility gene for AA (Collins et al. 2006; Pforr et al. 2006; Tazi-Ahnini et al. 2002a; Wengraf et al. 2008). AIRE enables self-antigens in thymic epithelial cells (TEC) and is thus involved in T-cell education by negative selection of autoreactive T-cells (Peterson et al. 2008). Decreased AIRE function can alter the expression of self-antigens and brew autoimmunity presumably against HFs by failing to induce energy to random subsets of missed antigens (Liston et al. 2003). Aside from devastating mutations, numerous polymorphisms have been detected in the *AIRE* gene that could perhaps have subtle effects on its functions (Toraih et al. 2020).

The 961G > C polymorphisms associated with amino-acid substitution at the DNA-binding segment have been linked to severe alopecia in young patients (Tazi-Ahnini et al. 2002a). However, further investigations were not able to confirm this association (Pforr et al. 2006; Wengraf et al. 2008). Instead, the C allele of 7215 T > C and the CGCT and CGCC haplotypes of −103C > T, 6528G > A, 7215 T > C, and 11,787 T > C were found to confer susceptibility to AA (Wengraf et al. 2008). The rs2075876 at the intron 5 (A to G substitution) was also linked to AA susceptibility in a more recent study performed in male patients (Toraih et al. 2020). It has been suggested that these polymorphisms either directly result in lower levels of *AIRE* mRNA production or indirectly affect AIRE function by producing stable mRNAs that negatively impact the downstream signaling paths (Toraih et al. 2020; Wengraf et al. 2008).

The *FOXP3* gene

The forkhead box (P3Foxp3) is a regulatory T-cell marker and a key transcriptional factor responsible for the differentiation and functions of regulatory T-cells (T-regs). It does so by establishing a specific gene expression profile through its interaction with other transcription factors (Runx1, CBP/p300, Eos, etc.). It increases the expression of target immunosuppressive cytokines and co-inhibitory molecules such as IL-10, transforming growth factor-β (TGF-β), cytotoxic T lymphocyte antigen 4 (CTLA4), interleukin-2 receptor alpha (CD25), and lymphocyte activation gene 3 protein (LAG3), and decreases the expression of proinflammatory cytokines such as IL-2 and IL-12 (Georgiev et al. 2019; Ono 2020; Rivas and Chatila 2016).

Since the T-regs are one of the main players in preventing autoimmunity, it is plausible for the altered expression and function of FOXP3 to increase the risk of autoimmunity (Bennett et al. 2001; Kim et al. 2009; Lu et al. 2017). Several observations have shown a reduced number of T-regs in the lesions and peripheral blood of patients with AA (Hamed et al. 2019; Han et al. 2015; Speiser et al. 2019).

With the first AA GWAS demonstrating two susceptibility loci within the genes related to the T-reg pathway, *IKZF4* and *GARP* (discussed in detail in the following sections), it seemed rational to investigate the contribution of *FOXP3* polymorphisms in the pathogenesis of AA. More so since multiple studies on autoimmune diseases have been able to draw an association between these polymorphisms and disease susceptibility (He et al. 2013). A study on 120 patients with AA and 84 controls was able to show that the carriers of the A allele of the rs2294020-3675 associated with reduced gene expression were at increased risk for developing AA (Conteduca et al. 2014).

The *IKZF4* gene also known as *Eos*

The region containing the *Ikaros family zinc finger 4* (*IKZF4*) and the *erythroblastic leukemia viral oncogene homolog 3* (*ERBB3*) genes is an AA susceptibility locus identified through GWAS (Petukhova et al. 2010). A follow-up case–control study found a significant association between AA and *IKZF4* rs1701704 but not the *ERBB3* rs705708 (Jagielska et al. 2012). The *ERBB3* gene was later found to be regulated by an AA-associated microRNA (miRNA) (Tafazzoli et al. 2018).

The IZKF family of transcription factors includes five members, Ikaros, Helios, Aiolos, Eos, and Pegasus, encoded by *IZKF-1* to *-5,* respectively (Kelley et al. 1998; Morgan et al. 1997; Perdomo et al. 2000). The members of this family are involved in T-cell differentiation (Powell et al. 2019). The *IZKF4* (Eos) mediates the FOXP3-dependent differentiation of T-regs by repressing the expression of inflammatory genes such as IL-2 (Pan et al. 2009). The EOS also has a critical role in maintaining the suppressive functions of T-regs with its deletion/knockout resulting in the autoimmunity (Gokhale et al. 2019). Though *IZKF4* polymorphisms have been associated with AA susceptibility, their functional consequences are not fully understood.

Though less appreciated, *ERBB3* is also a plausible candidate for AA susceptibility as it encodes an epidermal growth factor receptor expressed during anagen that is involved in hair development and cycling (Mak and Chan 2003). Furthermore, it has been shown that mutation within the ERBB3 gene could result in a phenotype with sparse hair (Li et al. 2019).

The *GARP* gene

The association between the *glycoprotein A repetitions predominant* (*GARP*) gene and AA was documented by the second GWAS though the precise functional effects of the risk allele are not known (Betz et al. 2015a). The GARP, also known as LRRC32, is expressed on various immune cells including T-regs. It regulates the activation and expression of transforming growth factor-β (TGFβ) on the surface of T-regs. GARP mediates the extracellular storing of TGFβ by keeping it attached to the latency-associated peptide (LAP) and regulates its releases in response to integrin signaling (Metelli et al. 2018). Membrane-bound GARP expressed on T-regs augment TGFβ on the cellular surface and thus provide an easily accessed TGF supply for these cells (Stockis et al. 2009; Tran et al. 2009; Wang et al. 2012). TGFβ is a potent immunomodulatory cytokine that through the TGFβ receptor and Smad signaling pathway can downregulate the expression of inflammatory cytokines by changing the gene transcriptome. It is also involved in the self-perpetuating feedback of regulatory T-cells (Chen and Konkel 2010; Fu et al. 2004). Thus the immunosuppressive functions of T-regs are increased by GARP (Tran et al. 2009; Wang et al. 2009). The downregulation of GARP is associated with an increased risk of autoimmunity (Wallace et al. 2018). TGF-β is one of the main IP guardians that downregulates the expression of MHC molecules on the HF cells (Ito et al. 2004; Kang et al. 2010). TGF- β is found to be lower in AA lesions and perilesional sites (Kang et al. 2010; Subramanya et al. 2010). It is a potential treatment target as it could help in reestablishing the IP (Gilhar 2010b; Paus et al. 2018). Surprisingly, GARP has been also found to be expressed on HFs that further supports its role in IP preservation (Betz et al. 2015a).

The *CTLA4* gene

The *cytotoxic T lymphocyte-associated antigen 4* (*CTLA4*) was first detected as an AA susceptibility gene (rs1024161) through GWAS (Petukhova and Christiano 2016; Petukhova et al. 2010). A large case–control study (1,196 patients and 1,280 controls from Central Europe) was also able to show associations between AA and six SNPs within the locus containing this gene with rs3087243 showing the strongest overall association and rs1427678 demonstrating the top odds ratio in the most severely affected patients (John et al. 2011). However, several small case–control studies in other ethnicities found contradictory results. The rs3087243 showed no association with AA in Mexicans and Iranians but the G alleles of this SNP conferred susceptibility to AA in Italian patients (Megiorni et al. 2013; Moravvej et al. 2018a; Salinas-Santander et al. 2020). The rs3087243 was also associated with AA in Egyptians (Ismail et al. 2020). The CTLA4 (also known as CD152) is an immune checkpoint receptor homologous to CD28 in its binding partners, B7-1/B7-2. Both CD28 and CTLA4 are regulators of the TCR–MHC interaction. While CD28 is a co-stimulatory molecule, CTLA4 acts as an inhibitory receptor adjusting the T-cells' responses following antigen presentation (Jago et al. 2004; Krummel and Allison 1996; Oosterwegel et al. 1999). CTLA4 contributes to the immunosuppressive functions of T-regs (Takahashi et al. 2000). Loss-of-function of CTLA4 promotes the proliferation of autoreactive naïve T-cells capable of tissue destruction (Chambers et al. 1997; Jain et al. 2010; Krummel and Allison 1996; Tivol et al. 1995). It has been suggested that the risk alleles may have an impact on CTLA4 expression and some studies have been able to show decreased levels of CTLA4 in the carriers of risk alleles (Maier et al. 2007; Ueda et al. 2003).

The *IL-2RA* gene

Polymorphisms within the gene encoding IL-2 receptor A chain (IL-2RA; CD25) were found to be linked to AA susceptibility in the first GWAS (Petukhova et al. 2010). This finding was replicated by a case–control candidate gene study of 768 patients and 658 controls for rs706778 and in another case–control study of 427 patients and 430 controls for rs3118470 (Miao et al. 2013; Redler et al. 2012).

IL-2 is one of the main proinflammatory cytokines produced in response to antigenic stimulation. Three main receptors exist for IL-2, IL-2RA (CD25) which is fairly specific for IL-2, IL-2RB (CD122) that also binds to IL-15, and IL-2RG (CD132) that can interact with IL-2, IL-4, IL-7, IL-9, IL-15, and IL-21 (Goudy et al. 2013). The CD25 is consecutively expressed by T-regs and thus these cells are the first cells to sense the presence of IL-2 (O'Gorman et al. 2009). The CD25 on T-regs can contribute to immunosuppression by acting as a scavenger receptor purging IL-2 from the surrounding milieu (cytokine sink) (Gasteiger and Kastenmuller 2012). Furthermore, the IL-2/CD25 interaction can upregulate the expression of co-inhibitory CTLA4 on T-regs slowing antigen presentation and effector T-cell activation (Gasteiger and Kastenmuller 2012; Kastenmuller et al. 2011). Thus expectedly, the deletion/inhibition of IL-4RA would result in both immunosuppression and autoimmunity (Goudy et al. 2013). Both SNPs associated with AA are located within the intronic segments of the *IL-2RA* gene and are suggested to decrease the transcription rate (Roh et al. 2006). An AA-associated mi-RNA, miR-30b/d, also regulates the expression of the *IL-2RA* (Tafazzoli et al. 2018).

The *PTPN22* gene

The *PTPN22* gene encodes a lymphoid protein tyrosine phosphatase (LYP) downstream TCR, B-cell receptor (BCR), and TLR signaling pathways. Like most phosphatases and kinases, it acts as an on/off switch for enzyme activity by adding or removing phosphate groups. This would lead to chains of interactions that would eventually change the cellular behavior (Burn et al. 2011). It positively affects TLR signaling and thus promotes innate immunity and IFN production while negatively regulating the NF-κB and MAPK downstream intracellular pattern recognition receptors (PRRs) and Src family of kinases downstream TCR signaling (Fousteri et al. 2013). Numerous candidate gene association and GWA studies have been able to link *PTPN22* polymorphisms (particularly, rs2476601; c.1858C > T) with autoimmune diseases (Burn et al. 2011). It has been suggested to be the most influential polymorphisms in autoimmune induction outside the HLA region. Thus, it seemed rational to investigate its association with AA. To date, six case–control association studies and a single meta-analysis have been published investigating this association. The meta-analysis included five of the previously published studies gathering data on 1129 patients with AA and 1702 controls. They were able to demonstrate a significantly lower risk of AA in individuals carrying the C allele of the rs2476601 (Lei et al. 2019). The same result was obtained by five out of six studies at individual levels (Betz et al. 2008; Bhanusali et al. 2014; Moravvej et al. 2018a; Salinas-Santander et al. 2015; Shehata et al. 2020). The association was not significant for the development of AA in general but was significant in those with severe AA in the remaining one study (Kemp et al. 2006).

The precise functional consequence of this polymorphism is not clear but it has been suggested that the enhanced kinase activity attributed to the risk allele could stimulate the immune system by altering the thymic negative selection of autoreactive T-cells or reducing the suppressive effects of T-regs in the periphery (Fousteri et al. 2013; Mustelin et al. 2019; Vang et al. 2013, 2007).

The *TAP1* gene

The *transporter associated with antigen processing 1* (*TAP1*) gene encodes a protein that is involved in the transportation of antigenic peptides to the endoplasmic reticulum where they are assembled on the MHC molecule (Trowsdale et al. 1990). Mutations of the *TAP1* gene severely alter antigen presentation and are associated with immune-insufficiency (Hanalioglu et al. 2017). More subtle variations in the *TAP1* gene could affect the substrate specificity and peptide selection processes (Lankat-Buttgereit and Tampé 2002; Powis et al. 1992; Qian et al. 2017). The *TAP1* polymorphisms have been linked to susceptibility to multiple autoimmune diseases such as psoriasis, ankylosing spondylitis, and rheumatoid arthritis (Qian et al. 2017; Witkowska-Toboa et al. 2004; Zhang et al. 2002). An evaluation of *TAP1* polymorphisms in patients with AA demonstrated a significant overexpression of the TT genotype of a promoter SNP (rs2071480) in the patient group (Kim et al. 2015a).

The *TLR* genes

TLRs are a subgroup of pattern recognition receptors (PRRs) that are capable of detecting specific molecular signatures from exogenous and endogenous ligands. They activate innate immune responses and regulate adaptive immunity by triggering different subcellular pathways. Their role in the pathogenesis of AA has not been broadly explored but few gene expression profiling studies have documented differences in the expression of TLRs in affected skin compared to normal controls (Alzolibani et al. 2016; Kang et al. 2020; Lee et al. 2013). A small whole-genome sequencing study on alopecia universalis (AU) identified the *TLR1* rs117033348 SNP as susceptibility loci for the AU in the Korean population (Lee et al. 2013). Another candidate gene case–control study also found the *TLR1* C allele of rs4833095 to be significantly associated with the AA susceptibility (Seok et al. 2014b). It has been suggested that these polymorphisms may affect the molecular dynamics of the TLRs toward a more pronounced immune response.

The *IL-2/IL-21* gene

The region containing the *IL-2/IL-21* genes harbors another GWAS susceptibility loci that was confirmed to associate with AA in one large case–control study but failed to show a significant association in another candidate gene investigation with a smaller but still notable sample size (Jagielska et al. 2012; Petukhova et al. 2010; Redler et al. 2012). The *IL-2* and *IL-21* genes are both mapped at 4q27 located within 180 kb from each other. Thus SNPs within this region could potentially affect the expression and function of both genes (Parrish-Novak et al. 2000). Both interleukins belong to the same γc cytokine family that shares a common cytokine receptor γ chain and possess somewhat similar proinflammatory properties (Lin et al. 1995). They differ in their effect on T-regs and subsets of helper T-cells. While IL-2 promotes the differentiation of Th1, Th2, and Th9 and is pro-T-reg survival and expansion, IL-21 suppresses the T-regs and promotes the differentiation of Th17 cells (Dwyer et al. 2019). Both interleukins are increased in the sera of patients with AA (Atwa et al. 2016; Kasumagić-Halilovic et al. 2018) but only IL-2 rich peripheral blood mononuclear cell cultures (PBMC) have been shown to induce AA like lesion and blockade of IL-2 but not IL-21 can prevent AA development (Decot et al. 2010; Divito and Kupper 2014; Gilhar et al. 2012, 2013; Ito et al. 2008; Xing et al. 2014). Thus, it seems more reasonable to assume that AA-associated polymorphisms at 4q27 have an augmenting effect of IL-2 expression or function.

3.4 The Genes Involved in Disease Progression After Immune Privilege Collapse

The IL-1 family

The IL-1 family consists of 11 members of genetically similar cytokines most of which are encoded by genes located at the 2q14. The most prominent members include pro-inflammatory agonistic cytokines, IL-1α, IL-1β, IL-18, IL-36α, IL-36β, and IL-36γ, and their naturally occurring receptor antagonists, IL-1RA and IL-36RA (Sims et al. 2001). In a physiological state the keratinocytes produce considerable amounts of the IL-1RA and IL-36RA holding the balance against inflammation but with the overflow of immune cells in pathological states, IL-1α and

IL-1β increase in the skin milieu and result in the tilting of the balance toward inflammation (Martin et al. 2021). IL-1 (α and β) is not only capable of inciting an immune attack on HFs by provoking the innate and adaptive response but they can also directly inhibit the hair cycle and induce catagen (Hoffmann et al. 1994; Philpott et al. 1996). Thus the ratio of IL-1 agonists to IL-1RA and IL-36RA is a determining factor in the pathogenesis of AA (Gregoriou et al. 2010). Since genetic polymorphisms can influence this ratio by affecting both the constitutive and the stimulated expression of cytokines they have the tendency to influence the susceptibility to diseases. Candidate gene approaches have investigated the association between AA and IL-1α, IL-β1, IL-1RA, and IL-36RA. The *IL1A* rs17561 (+4845G > T) showed a possible but not statistically significant association with AA in a study conducted in Britain (Tazi-Ahnini et al. 2001). This SNP was found to be associated with AA in a subset of AA patients with a positive family history in a subsequent German study (Redler et al. 2012). A 4-bp INDEL polymorphism located at the 3'UTR of *IL1A* was linked to AA susceptibility especially in those with mild patchy disease. Individuals with ins/ins genotype were at increased risk of developing AA as opposed to those with ins/del and del/del genotypes (Lu et al. 2013). Insertion of the "TTCA" at the 3'UTR increases the interleukin transcription by interrupting the binding site of two inhibitory microRNAs, miRNA-122 and microRNA-378 (Gao et al. 2009).

The C allele of the rs16944 (−511C > T) within the promoter region of *IL-1B* was found to confer susceptibility to AA in severe cases in one study on Arab Kuwaiti patients but was not associated with AA in another study on European patients (AlFadhli and Nanda 2014; Tazi-Ahnini et al. 2001). Though the T allele has been linked to higher levels of interleukin production, a haplotype containing the C allele has also been found to contribute to high levels of IL-1β perhaps due to linkage disequilibrium with another gene with Cis-eQTL effects on IL-1β (Pociot et al. 1992; Wen et al. 2006). The rs1143634 (+3954 T > C) within the 5th exon did not show an association with AA in a European case–control study (Tazi-Ahnini et al. 2001). The minor T allele of another SNP, rs1143634 (+3953C > T), located at the 5th exon was also found to confer liability to AA by increasing the expression of the *IL-1B* (Galbraith et al. 1999).

An SNP in the IL-1RA encoding gene (*IL1RN*), rs419598 (+2018 T > C) was found to be associated with AA susceptibility in a European case–control study with the CC genotype conferring disease liability (Tazi-Ahnini et al. 2002b). A VNTR polymorphism of 2 to 6 repeats of a 86 bp segment has been detected in the intron 2 of the *IL-1RN* gene. The alleles with four and two repeats represent the most common alleles designated as *allele 1* and *allele 2*, respectively. Higher frequencies of the *allele 2* and the allele with 3 repeats were documented in patients with AA as opposed to the frequency of the allele with 5 repeats that was more frequent in control subjects (AlFadhli and Nanda 2014). The *allele 2* was shown to confer susceptibility to severe AA (totalis and universalis) in two other studies (Cork et al. 1995a, 1996; McDonagh and Tazi-Ahnini 2002b; Tarlow et al. 1994). A European-based small case–control study was not able to show an association between *allele 2* and alopecia universalis/totalis but instead demonstrated a significant association between *allele 1* and patchy alopecia (Barahamani et al. 2002b). The *allele 2* carriers have lower levels of IL-1RA production compared to *allele 1* carriers (Dewberry et al. 2000)

An SNP (+4734G > A) within the IL-36RA encoding gene (*IL-36RN*) gene (previously designated as IL-1 like molecule 1 (IL-1L1)) has also been linked to AA with the rare allele conferring susceptibility to disease (Tazi-Ahnini et al. 2002b). The functional consequence of this polymorphism is unknown.

IL-18 (encoded by a gene at 11q23.1) also belongs to this cytokine family and has been implicated in the pathogenesis of AA. This proinflammatory cytokine can increase the production of IFNγ by NK cells and promote adaptive immune responses in both Th1 and Th2 pathways (Dinarello 2007). IL-18 is increased in response to ACTH and thus might be one of the mediators that links psychological stress to the occurrence and exacerbation of AA (Sekiyama et al. 2005). IL-18 is increased in the HF microenvironment in the setting AA (Chodorowska et al. 2007; El-Gayyar et al. 2020; Wang et al. 2013).

The G allele and the GG genotype of the *IL-18* rs187238 SNP (−137G > C) located on the promoter of the gene were shown to confer risk for AA in Korean and Turkish patients (Celik and Ates 2018; Kim et al. 2014). The A allele of the rs549908 (Ser35Ser) within the exon of this gene was associated with AA susceptibility in Koreans and the C allele of the rs1946518 (−607C > A) conferred liability to AA in Turkish patients (Celik and Ates 2018; Kim et al. 2014). Both polymorphisms are thought to increase the expression of the cytokine (Giedraitis et al. 2001).

The *IL-4 and IL-13* genes

IL4 and IL-13 are closely related cytokines encoded by genes located at 5q31 with about 50% sequence homology (Wang and Secombes 2015). IL-4 mainly promotes the differentiation of Th2 cells. It is primarily produced by mast cells, basophils, eosinophils, and fully differentiated Th2 cells as a positive feedback loop mechanism. IL-13 is similar to IL-4 in its production and function but has a more prominent role in allergic reactions and IgE production (Sachin et al. 2012).

The *IL-4/IL-13* genetic locus was identified as susceptibility loci for AA in the first GWAS (nominal significance $10^{-4} < P < 5 \times 10^{-7}$) (Petukhova et al. 2010). The association reached a genome-wide significance level ($P < 5 \times 10^{-8}$) for rs20541 when the data on the GWAS and a large case–control study were pooled (Jagielska et al. 2012). Two subsequent case–control association studies investigated the *IL-4* polymorphisms in AA patients. One study on Arab patients with AA was not able to show any association between AA and the *IL-4* -590 T > C and *IL-4R* rs-1801275 (Q551RA > G) polymorphisms (Alzolibani et al. 2015b). However, another study showed a significant association between a 70 bp functional VNTR polymorphism located at the gene intron in Turkish patients (Kalkan et al. 2013b). The P1 allele that conferred risk for AA in this study was associated with higher levels of IL-4 production (Kalkan et al. 2013b).

The contribution of IL-4 and IL-13 to the pathogenesis of AA is not quite clear. The levels of IL-4, IL-13, and IgE are elevated in severe longstanding AA suggesting a shift from Th1 to Th2 in the chronic stage of the disease (Attia et al. 2010; Tembhre and Sharma 2013). Moreover, a transcriptome study found IL-13 to have the greatest expression difference between lesional and non-lesional skin (Suárez-Fariñas et al. 2015). The well-known association of AA with allergic diseases and Th2-mediated atopic dermatitis further highlights the role of IL-4 and IL-13 in the pathogenesis of AA (Goh et al. 2006; Marks and Senna 2020). Perhaps, the entanglement of the Th2 and its cytokines could take place following the breach in the immune privilege of HF and the infiltration of antigen-presenting cells with their MHC-II molecules that are capable of activating CD4+ T cells (Hull et al. 1991).

The *IL-17* gene

The involvement of Th17 and its cytokine (IL-17) in the pathogenesis of AA has been suggested by multiple studies either demonstrating Th17 cell infiltration around AA affected HFs or showing higher levels of IL-17 in the sera of patients with AA (Atwa et al. 2016; Bain et al. 2020; Han et al. 2015; Loh et al. 2018; Tanemura et al. 2013; Tojo et al. 2013). However, an isolated transcriptome study has failed to demonstrate a significant difference in the expression of Th-17 related genes (except for IL-23) in AA lesions compared to normal unaffected skin (Suárez-Fariñas et al. 2015).

Association studies were conducted to assess the role of Th17 and its cytokines from a genetic perspective. The GG genotype of the rs763780 (7488A > G) of the *IL-17F* gene conferred risk for AA development in Turkish patients (Aytekin et al. 2015). The A to G substitution is suggested to alter the expression and function of the IL-17F (Kawaguchi et al. 2006). The A allele and the AA genotype of the *IL-17A* rs2275913 (197G > A) were shown to confer susceptibility to AA in a small Egyptian study (Seleit et al.

2021). The A allele carrying T-cells produce higher levels of IL-17A compared to those with the G allele (Espinoza et al. 2011). Though IL-17A and IL-17F share 50% sequence homology, are capable of forming heterodimers, and their receptors (IL-17RA and IL-17RC, respectively) also form heterodimers, their role in the pathogenesis of autoimmune diseases is quite different. While IL-17A is indispensable in the induction of autoimmunity, in some instances the presence of IL-17F can even ameliorate the risk of autoimmunity. This is attributed to the fact that IL-17F can decrease the potent IL-17A responses by forming IL-17A/F heterodimers with intermediate potency (Dubin and Kolls 2009). Thus the high IL-17A producing risk alleles are more important to the pathogenesis of AA than the low producing IL-17F risk allele.

The G allele of *IL17RA* rs879577 was associated with AA development in Korean patients. The distribution of the *IL-17 receptor A* (*IL17RA*) rs4819554 alleles was significantly different between patients with early-onset vs those with late-onset AA (Lew et al. 2012). The functional consequences of this polymorphism are not known.

All in all, it seems that the Th17 pathways might work in ancillary to the dominant Th1-mediated responses in the induction of hair loss by providing positive feedback loops for Th1 and working as an independent source for IFNγ production (Ramot et al. 2018).

Other interleukin genes

The regions containing the *IL-6* and *IL-26* gene were identified as susceptibility loci for AA in the first GWAS albeit with a nominal significance ($10^{-4} < P < 5 \times 10^{-7}$) (Petukhova et al. 2010).

Several interleukin SNPs were assessed in a large candidate gene approach including *IL10*, *IL12B*, *IL6*, *IL23*, and *IL4R*. Only nominal significance was detected for the association between the AA and *IL12B* rs3212227 and rs2853694 and *IL-6* rs1800795 in a subgroup of AA patients with a positive family history (Redler et al. 2012).

Aside from these high power studies, several smaller case–control association studies have been able to link other cytokine and cytokine receptor genes with AA liability. The GG genotype of the rs17875491within the promoter of *IL-16* conferred susceptibility to AA in Korean patients and the rs11073001 within the exon of this gene was linked to AA liability in patients with a positive family history under the dominant mode of inheritance (AA+AG vs. GG) (Lew et al. 2014a). The C allele and the CC genotype of the *IL12* rs3212227 (1188A/C) were shown to have a significantly higher frequency in Iranian patients with AA. However, this polymorphism did not influence the gene expression rate (Tabatabaei-Panah et al. 2020). This study also demonstrated a significant over-presentation of the A allele and the AA genotype of *IL23R* rs10889677 (+2199A/C) in Iranian patients with AA (Tabatabaei-Panah et al. 2020).

The TNF family

TNFα is one of the most prominent inflammatory cytokines in autoimmune diseases and one of the main therapeutic targets of biological agents. Along with IFNγ, TNFα is one the first cytokines to rise in the follicular milieu after the invasion of NK cells (Rajabi et al. 2018a). Aside from its ability to exacerbate inflammation, it can also directly affect the hair cycle (Ito et al. 2004, 2005a, 2008; Ljunggren and Kärre 1990; McElwee et al. 2013; Rajabi et al. 2018a). However, unlike diseases such as psoriasis, TNFα is less influential in the induction, progression, and severity of AA as apparent from multiple failed attempts at utilizing TNF blockers in treating AA (Abramovits and Losornio 2006; Bolduc and Bissonnette 2012; Ferran et al. 2011; Gorcey et al. 2014; Hernandez et al. 2009; Strober et al. 2005). Attempts at drawing links between AA and *TNFα* gene polymorphisms have been met with similar misfortune. Two SNPs (rs1041981 and rs1800629) within the *TNFα* locus, at the MHC III region, showed significant association with AA in a large candidate gene study (Redler et al. 2012). The AA+GA genotypes of the TNFα rs1800629 (308G > A) were also found to confer risk for AA in a small case–control study in Jordanian Arabs (Al-Eitan et al. 2019). Several other case–control studies have failed to demonstrate an association between TNF polymorphisms and AA (Abd El-Raheem et al. 2020; Galbraith and Pandey 1995;

Moravvej et al. 2018b). The locus containing the *TNFα* gene also harbors the lymphotoxin alpha (LTA) previously designated as TNFβ. Homologous to TNFα, LTA is also a pro-inflammatory cytokine but has a more essential role in T-cell maturation through induction of *AIRE* expression (Chin et al. 2003).

The *SOCS1* gene

The *suppressor of cytokine signaling-1* (*SOCS1*) gene was suggested to be associated with AA by the first GWAS reaching a nominal significance ($10^{-4} < P < 5 \times 10^{-7}$) (Petukhova et al. 2010). Though the association was not significant in a large case–control study on European patients, the meta-analysis of pooled data of the two studies was nominally significant ($P = 1.68 \times 10^{-5}$) (Jagielska et al. 2012).

The *SOCS* family encodes proteins that negatively regulated the JAK/STAT pathways and thus inhibit cytokine production and inflammation (Jagielska et al. 2012). SNPs and microsatellite repeat polymorphisms in the *SOCS1* gene causing decreased gene expression have been linked to susceptibility to autoimmune diseases (Lamana et al. 2020) and treatment with SOCS3 has shown some efficacy in AA (Lamana et al. 2020).

FAS and FASL

The FAS (CD95)/Fas ligand (FASL) interaction activates caspase-dependent apoptosis pathways in the cells expressing the transmembrane FAS receptor. Similar to MIF, two opposing theories have been suggested for the involvement of FAS/FASL in the pathogenesis of AA. The first theory regards the FASL as an IP preserving factor that is expressed by HF cells to induce apoptosis in immune cells that have been able to breach its physical berries (Cheng et al. 2009; Christoph et al. 2000; Ferguson and Griffith 2006; Guleria et al. 2005; Kang et al. 2010; Paus et al. 2003; Wang et al. 2014). The second theory, on the other hand, postulates that the infiltration of immune cells may induce the expression of FAS in HF cells and promote the destruction of the follicular unit via apoptosis. The resistance of FAS/FASL knocked out mice to AA and the expression of FAS on HF in immunohistochemical studies of AA support the later theory (Bertolini et al. 2020; Bodemer et al. 2000; Freyschmidt-Paul et al. 2003). Moreover, FAS/FASL could contribute to the maintenance of central and peripheral tolerance by participating in the negative selection of autoreactive T-cells (Castro et al. 1996; Green et al. 2003; Volpe et al. 2016).

Genetic polymorphism studies can hypothetically determine the best fit scenario for the involvement of FAS/FASL in the pathogenesis of AA. Thus following the steps of investigators in multiple other autoimmune diseases, researchers in the field of AA have also performed case–control association studies for FAS/FASL polymorphisms. Four studies have been conducted thus far. A study on Chinese patients evaluated the *FAS* rs2234767 (1377G > A), *FAS* rs1800682 (−670A > G), and *FASLG* rs763110 (844 T > C) and found that individuals with the AG genotype of rs1800682 had a lower risk for developing AA compared with those with the AA genotype (Fan et al. 2010). A study on Turkish patients evaluated the contribution of *FAS* rs1800682 (−670 A > G) and *FASLG* 5,030,772 (−124 A > G) and also found the GG genotype of *FAS* rs1800682 polymorphism to confer protection against AA (Kalkan et al. 2013a). The same set of polymorphisms were assessed in Egyptian patients but yielded complete opposite results with the G allele and the GG genotype of *FAS* rs1800682 and the AG genotype of the *FASLG* 5,030,772 being more prevalent in cases rather than controls (Seleit et al. 2018). Lastly, an Iranian study investigating these two SNPs showed the G allele of the *FASLG* rs5030772 to confer susceptibility to AA (Seleit et al. 2018). The *FAS* rs1800682 (−670A > G) polymorphism is located at the promoter and its A to G substitution is associated with reduced expression of FAS due to disruption of transcription binding sites (Sibley et al. 2003; Wu et al. 2003). The association between the reduced expression of FAS and lower risk for AA development can only be explained by the second theory.

The *MX1* gene

The *Myxovirus resistance-1* (*MX1*) gene encodes an interferon-inducible protein known as MxA. The reason this gene was investigated as an AA candidate gene was because of its location mapped to the Down syndrome critical region (DSCR) on chromosome 21 (Alves and Ferrando 2011). Down syndrome results from the complete/partial duplication of the 21st chromosome. In cases of partial duplication, the DSCR segment is the smallest fraction necessary and sufficient to induce most features of Down syndrome. Since individuals with Down syndrome have a four times higher risk of developing AA, the genes in this segment are likely to contribute to predisposition to AA (Pelleri et al. 2019). From this set of genes, the *MX1* was the only one to be highly expressed in the bulb of anagen HFs and was thus chosen for evaluation (McDonagh et al. 1994; Tazi-Ahnini et al. 2000). The *MX1* +9959C > T SNP was found to have a significantly different distribution among AA patients and control subjects (Tazi-Ahnini et al. 2000). The gene product is a guanosine triphosphate (GTP) metabolizing protein induced by interferons that interferes with the replication of RNA and DNA viruses. This gene has been linked to several other diseases including lupus (AlFadhli et al. 2016). As an important effector of IFN responses, it may contribute to the pathogenesis of AA by facilitating IFN-mediated immune privilege breakdown.

The *NOTCH4 gene*

The neurogenic locus notch homolog 4 (NOTCH4) belongs to an evolutionarily conserved family of transmembrane proteins that are involved in developmental processes by regulating cell-to-cell interactions. Because of its role as a major determinant in the differentiation of HF keratinocytes and its location within the MHC class III region, this gene seemed to be a good candidate for investigating the genetic bases of AA (Jeck et al. 2012; Lin et al. 2000; Powell et al. 1998; Tazi-Ahnini et al. 2003). A small case–control study was able to show that individuals homozygous for the *NOTCH4* +1297C variant within the coding region of the gene were at increased risk of developing AA (Tazi-Ahnini et al. 2003). These findings were replicated in another case–control study in Kuwaiti patients (AlFadhli and Nanda 2013). Moreover, the *NOTCH4* gene is located near one of the major susceptibility loci identified through GWAS that could have a cis-eQTL effect on the transcription of *NOTCH4* (AlFadhli and Nanda 2013; Petukhova and Christiano 2016). Interestingly, a GWAS meta-analysis identified the *NOTCH4* gene as one of the most significantly enriched hotspots in autoimmune diseases such as psoriasis, scleroderma, celiac disease, primary biliary cirrhosis, asthma, and type I diabetes (Jeck et al. 2012). Thus the contribution of this gene to the pathogenesis of AA may involve pathways beyond HF development. NOTCH signaling mediates the differentiation of immune cells and NOTCH4 disturbs the suppressive effects of T-regs on adaptive immunity (Harb et al. 2020, 2021; Janghorban et al. 2018).

The *vitamin D receptor* gene

Multiple studies in different autoimmune diseases in various ethnic backgrounds regardless of their sample sizes, patient selection, and environmental factors have drawn an undeniable link between vitamin D deficiency and autoimmunity (Bizzaro et al. 2017). Vitamin D exerts its effects by activating a nuclear receptor, VDR. The VDR forms a heterodimer transcription factor by binding to the retinoid X receptor (RXR) and regulates the expression of genes with specific responsive elements at their promoters (Campbell et al. 2010). Vitamin D/VDR signaling greatly impacts the immune system. It diverts T-cell differentiation from Th1 and Th17 toward Th2 and T-regs. It downregulates the production of IFNγ, TNFα, and other cytokines by immune cells and it suppresses antibody production. The collective effect of these changes drives the immune system toward tolerogenic responses (Dankers et al. 2017). Since genetics play a major role in the overall functions of this pathway, from serum levels of the active form of vitamin D to VDR activity, the polymorphisms are expected to have major consequences. Surprisingly, both downregulation and overexpression of *VDR* are associated with an increased risk of autoimmunity (Lahore et al. 2020; Ruiz-

Ballesteros et al. 2020). Out of the fourteen polymorphisms described to date, four of them are more frequently studied: FokI (rs2228570) corresponding to a T to C substitution in the exon 2 also referred to as f to F substitution that results in a more active form of VDR (Gross et al. 1998; Hasan and Ra'ed OA, Muda WAMBW, Mohamed HJBJ, Samsudin AR, 2017); BsmI referring to a G to A (b to B) substitution within the intron 8 (Mahto et al. 2018); ApaI (rs7975232) denoting a C to A (a to A) substitution also located at the intron 8 (Triantos et al. 2018); and TaqI (rs731236) corresponding to a C to T (T > t) substitution located in the exon 9 (Goswami 2016). The three later SNPs are thought to affect the *VDR* mRNA stability (Mahto et al. 2018).

Multiple studies in autoimmune diseases have been able to link specific *VDR* SNPs with disease susceptibility (Ruiz-Ballesteros et al. 2020). The same methods of candidate gene approaches have been employed to investigate the role of *VDR* polymorphisms in AA but none were able to demonstrate a significant association (Ahmet et al. 2004; Akar et al. 2007; Ates 2017). Patients with AA have significantly lower levels of vitamin D (Lee et al. 2018). Thus the lack of association with genetic polymorphisms does not entirely rule out the involvement of this pathway in the pathogenesis of AA.

The chemokine encoding gene

As for most autoimmune diseases, chemokines are involved in the pathogenesis of AA by facilitating the recruitment of immune cells (Ito and Tokura 2014; Pratt et al. 2017; Zainodini et al. 2013). Hypothetically, polymorphism in the genes encoding chemokines can attenuate the severity and chronicity of inflammation by altering their function and/or expression (Qidwai 2016). Though none of the chemokine genes are linked to AA by GWA studies, several case–control studies have found notable results. A South Korean study showed that the C allele of the *CXCL1* rs3117604 (−429C > T) and the C allele of the *CXCL2* rs3806792 (−264 T > C) genes conferred susceptibility to AA (Kim et al. 2015b). A study on Jordanian Arabs, however, failed to replicate these associations (Al-Eitan et al. 2019).

3.5 The Role of Genes Involved in Pigmentation

Hair pigmentation and melanocytes play a major role in the pathogenesis of AA. Several clinical features such as transient or permanent lack of pigment in the regrown hair and the sparing of white hairs are considered as evidence for this claim (Asz-Sigall et al. 2019). Further histopathological and immunological investigations have suggested that the melanocyte-associated sequestered antigens such as Tyr, TRP2, MART, and GP100 are the main targets in AA (Gilhar et al. 2001a, b; Trautman et al. 2009). Several genes encoding proteins involved in the pigmentation pathways have also been linked to AA susceptibility. The *Melanin Concentrating Hormone Receptor 2* (*MCHR2*) was identified as an AA risk gene through a genome-wide CNV analysis on central European individuals (Fischer et al. 2017). The 342.5-kb risk region contains an *MCHR2* duplication. The *MCHR2* encodes a G-coupled protein receptor for melanin-concentrating hormone but contrary to its role in skin pigmentation in fish, its expression in humans is more pronounced in the brain and testes. In humans, this receptor is mainly known for its role in adjusting emotions, behaviors, and energy hemostasis (Shi 2004). It is involved in obesity and psychological disorders such as depression (Ghoussaini et al. 2007; Oh et al. 2020; Urbanavicius et al. 2018). Thus the hypothesis of investigators of the CNV analysis that suggested the pigmentary antigen effects of gene duplication could predispose individuals to AA might not be the only possible explanation (Fischer et al. 2017). Its involvement in the modulation of the neuroendocrine-immune responses to psychological stressors may also contribute to the pathogenesis of AA (Rajabi et al. 2018b; Zheng and Ren 2017).

The autophagy genes, a dilemma between their role in pigmentation and their effects on immune function

Autophagy refers to the process of forming intracellular double-membrane vesicles encapsulating organelles, nucleic acids, and proteins within the cytoplasm and orchestrating their fusion with the lysosome which leads to degradation of the contents. Autophagy is regulated in response to environmental factors such as nutrition and oxygen supply, concentrations of growth factors, and oxidative stress. It facilitates organelle turnover and type II programmed cell death (type I is apoptosis) which are prerequisites for morphogenesis, growth, and differentiation (Mizushima 2007).

Autophagy is linked to the pathogenesis of AA by taking part in three main processes of autoimmunity, melanogenesis, and hair cycling. It is involved in several aspects of the immune response ranging from bacterial killing and antigen presentation to cytokine secretion and thymic selection (Kuballa et al. 2012). It has an essential role in melanogenesis (melanosome formation, maturation, and degradation) and thus can determine skin and hair color (Kim et al. 2020; Yun et al. 2016). It induces anagen in HFs and regulates hair cycling (Chai et al. 2019; Parodi et al. 2018).

Since autophagy is a general physiological phenomenon involved in multiple processes across different cell lines, it is not rational to pigeonhole its effects to a single category. Thus a polymorphism in a gene encoding an autophagy-related protein may simultaneously affect immune responses, melanogenesis, and hair cycle, making it hard to determine which of these effects are more important in the pathogenesis of the disease.

Several autophagy-related genes have been linked to AA. Some have a more prominent role in pigmentation pathways while others have been investigated mainly in immune responses. These genes include *STX17* (Petukhova et al. 2010), *ATG4B* (Petukhova et al. 2020), and KIAA 0350/CLEC16A (Jagielska et al. 2012)

The association between AA and *syntaxin 17* (*STX17*) was first demonstrated through GWAS and was later confirmed by case–control studies (Jagielska et al. 2012; Petukhova et al. 2010; Taghiabadi et al. 2018).

The *STX17* encodes a protein involved in autophagy that acts as an anchor for membrane-to-membrane fusion between autophagosomes and lysosomes (Cheng et al. 2017; Diao et al. 2015; Itakura et al. 2012). STX17 is involved in pigment synthesis and melanogenesis and its genetic variations and mutations affect hair color and induce premature canities (Erjavec 2020; Kichaev et al. 2019; Pielberg et al. 2008). Erjavec et al. performed an investigation to explore the link between *STX17*, hair color, and the pathogenesis of AA. They were able to demonstrate an increased expression of melanocyte sequestered antigens such as MART1 in melanocytes with lower STX17 levels. They also showed that AA-associated risk haplotypes identified through GWAS were associated with lower *STX17* expression (Petukhova et al. 2010). Thus, they hypothesized that genetic variations of *STX17* could predispose individuals to AA by increasing the expression of immune-privileged melanocytic antigens (Erjavec 2020). Aside from genetic polymorphisms, the AA-associated miR-30b could also affect the levels of STX17 (Tafazzoli et al. 2018).

A CNV involving copy number deletion of the *ATG4B* gene has been linked to AA through genome-wide and linkage analysis studies (Petukhova et al. 2020). Likewise, lesions affected with AA demonstrate reduced expression of *ATG4B* (Hardman et al. 2020). This gene encodes a cysteine protease that enables the attachment of a microtubule-associated protein known as LC3 to autophagosome lipid membranes. The LC3 would then mediate the fusion of autophagosomes and lysozymes (Yang et al. 2015). The *ATG4B* plays a major role in melanosome biogenesis and hair cycling (Chai et al. 2019; Parodi et al. 2018). The lower transcriptional dosage of this CNV could have a similar effect to *ATG4B* knockout which results in premature induction of catagen in HF and accumulation of melanosome organelles within melanocytes (Parodi et al. 2018; Ramkumar et al. 2017). This means that the lower autophagic flux attributed to *ATG4B* polymorphisms could predispose individuals to AA by lessening the threshold of catagen induction by IFNγ and inflammatory cytokines (Hardman et al. 2020). In a similar fashion to *STX17* polymorphisms, melanocytic antigen accumulation due to *ATG4B* polymorphisms could also predispose individuals to AA.

Tumoral cells employ autophagy as a mechanism to reduce MHC-I expression and increase co-inhibitory molecules such as PD-1 and CTLA-4 to avoid immune recognition. The blockade of autophagy machinery thus improves the immunogenicity of tumoral cells (Souza et al. 2020; Yamamoto et al. 2020). Perhaps the same mechanism is involved in the immune-privileged sites such as hair follicles. Though this theory has not been directly evaluated, it has been shown that HF cells in AA have lower expression of autophagy-related proteins such as ATG5 and LC3B compared to non-lesional HFs (Hardman et al. 2020). The lower autophagy flux due to genetic variation is also associated with an increased risk of AA which could suggest that the dysregulation of autophagy could even induce the IP collapse by altering the MHC-I negativity of HF cells (Petukhova et al. 2020).

The association between an SNP on the *C-type lectin domain family 16 member A* (*CLEC16A*) gene and AA was first reported by a large case–control study investigating the replicability of the highly associated SPNs reported by the first GWAS (Jagielska et al. 2012). A different SNP of this gene has been linked to susceptibility to multiple autoimmune diseases such as type I diabetes and multiple sclerosis (Nischwitz et al. 2011; Soleimanpour et al. 2014). The SNP associated with AA is in strong linkage disequilibrium with this common autoimmune SNP suggesting a similar path of involvement in the pathogenesis of AA (Booth et al. 2009).

The *KIAA0350/CLEC16A* gene which is highly expressed in immune cells (B-cells > NK cells > T-cells) is an essential promoter of mitophagy, a type of autophagy that keeps mitochondrial health and quality in check (Soleimanpour et al. 2014; Su et al. 2002; Wu et al. 2009). Damaged mitochondria play a major role in amplifying innate immune responses by influencing the cytoplasmic levels of calcium and ROS. They can also activate TLRs, NLRP, and NF-κB mediated cytokine production by releasing mitochondrial DNA (mtDNA), formyl peptides, and cardiolipin (Gkikas et al. 2018). An increase in the mitochondrial population due to defective removal of damaged organelles can thus cause an exaggerated continuous inflammation (Nakahira et al. 2011; Bruggen et al. 2010).

The deletion/ knockout of *CLEC16A* in NK cells has been shown to result in increased cytotoxicity, IFNγ secretion, and altered receptor expression which subsequently affects the cross-talk between NK cells and antigen-presenting cells (Pandey et al. 2018, 2019). The protective alleles in autoimmune-associated SNPs demonstrate increased expression of *CLEC16A* which can restrain mitochondria by promoting mitophagy (Hakonarson et al. 2007). Presumably, the *CLEC16A* gene variants with lower expression and functions may predispose individuals to AA by weakening the negative control over NK-cells that could single-handedly breach the immune privilege.

3.6 Genes Involved in HF Development, Structure, and Cycling

Several genes associated with AA encode either structural proteins or transcriptional factors and cofactors involved in HF development and cycling.

These include *SMARCA2* (Petukhova et al. 2020), *CCHCR1* (Oka et al. 2020), and *TCF7L2* (Rajabi et al. 2019b).

A CNV involving deletion of the *SMARCA2* gene, encoding a transcriptional activator protein, has been shown to confer susceptibility to AA. Mutations of this gene can cause several syndromes with features of hypo- and hypertrichosis such as Nicolaides-Baraitser and Coffin-Siris (Bramswig et al. 2015; Miyake et al. 2016).

A very interesting study recently has been able to identify another SNP (rs142986308) in the MHC-I region that belongs to a gene encoding a keratin-related protein known as coiled-coil alpha-helical rod protein 1 (CCHCR1) to be associated with AA susceptibility. They were able to show that mice carrying this allele developed a type of hair loss clinically resembling AA but pathologically lacking lymphocyte infiltration (Oka et al. 2020). Two things make this study important: (a) they are able to scan the MHC region for rare disease-associated haplotypes that usually remain obscure due to intensive linkage disequilibrium in this region, and (b) their study identified a genetic polymorphism that was singlehandedly able to induce hair loss (Oka et al. 2020).

The *transcription factor 7-like 2* (*TCF7L2*) gene encodes a transcription factor (TCF-4) downstream the Wnt/β-catenin pathway involved in the HF development of and anagen phase progression (Clevers and Nusse 2012; Lien et al. 2014; Omer et al. 1999; Xiong et al. 2014).

The TCF4 may be relevant to the pathogenesis of AA by increasing the vulnerability of the hair cycle to an immunologic attack which could lead to quiescence and premature transition into the catagen phase (Enshell-Seijffers et al. 2010). A case–control study investigated the *TCF7L2* rs7903146 (C > T) polymorphisms in AA patients and demonstrated an increased expression of the T-allele among patients compared to control subjects (Rajabi et al. 2019b).

3.7 Miscellaneous Genes

ZNF814

A copy number deletion of a chromosomal segment harboring the *Zinc finger protein 814* (*ZNF814*) gene has been linked to AA as a rare disease-associated variant (Petukhova et al. 2020). This gene encodes a protein involved in transcription regulation but its role in the pathogenesis of AA remains unknown.

SPATA5

An SNP (rs304650) on the *Spermatogenesis-associated protein 5* (*SPATA5*) gene has been linked to AA by a GWA study (Forstbauer et al. 2012). This gene encodes an ATPase with low tissue specificity and diverse functions in DNA replication, membrane fusion, and protein degradation. No dermatological symptoms have been documented thus far for genetic mutations within this gene but there are reports on intellectual disability and hearing loss (Buchert et al. 2016; Kurata et al. 2016).

MTHFR

The *Methylenetetrahydrofolate reductase* (*MTHFR*) gene was linked to AA by a small Turkish case–control study, demonstrating increased expression of the *MTHFR* rs1801133 (677C > T) T allele and TT genotype in AA patients compared to control subjects (Kalkan et al. 2013c). This enzyme is involved in folate/homocysteine metabolism and the T allele is associated with reduced enzymatic activity resulting in higher levels of homocysteine and a tendency to be affected more severely by low folate intake (Reilly et al. 2014). It has been postulated that the pro-inflammatory effects of homocysteine on the immune system may be responsible for its association with AA (Schroecksnadel et al. 2004).

4 Conclusion

Genetic studies have been able to confirm many of the theories about the pathogenesis of AA. The association of AA with genes involved in ROS clearance mechanisms, those encoding danger-associated proteins such as MICA, ULBP, and HSPs confirm the local IP collapse theory while the AA's association with genes involved in the differentiation and function of regulatory T-cells authenticate the failure of central and peripheral self-tolerance hypothesis in the pathogenesis of AA (Table 2).

The association of AA with genes involved in hair development and cycling is not surprising since regardless of the way the IP is breached these genes can lower the sensitivity of HFs to inflammation-induced catagen. Besides, the IP breach is not clinically apparent until catagen induction manifests as visible hair loss (Gilhar 2010a; Gilhar et al. 2012; McElwee et al. 2013).

Autophagy-related genes are a new category of genes linked to AA susceptibility. These genes have a broad spectrum of functions in the immune system, melanogenesis, and hair cycling and thus further studies are required to understand their precise role in the pathogenesis of AA.

Future investigation should focus on utilizing new methods to screen for other types of polymorphisms besides SNPs such as INDELS, STRs, VNTRs, and CNVs since they can identify genes that are usually left out by GWA studies and clarifies unanswered questions regarding the pathogenesis of AA.

Table 2 Non-HLA genes associated with alopecia areata

Function		Gene	Location	Study	References
Genes affecting local factors involved in IP preservation and collapse	Stress-induced molecules	*MICA: MHC class I polypeptide-related sequence A* *ULBP: Cytomegalovirus UL16-binding protein*	6p21.33 6q25.1	Linkage study GWAS[a]	Barahmani et al. (2006), Mingorance Gámez et al. (2020), Jagielska et al. (2012), Petukhova et al. (2010)
		HSPA1B: Heat shock protein 1B	6p21.3	CGAS[b]	Seok et al. (2014a)
		MIF (macrophage migration inhibitory factor)	22q11.23	CGAS	Rajabi et al. (2019a), Shimizu et al. (2005)
	ROS clearance mechanisms	*NOS3: Nitric oxide synthetase 3*	7q36.1	CGAS	AlFadhli et al. (2008), Alzolibani et al. (2015a)
		PRDX5: Peroxiredoxin 5	11q13	GWAS	Akar et al. (2002), Karasawa et al. (2005), Petukhova et al. (2010)
		ACOXL: Acyl-coenzyme-A oxidase-like *BCL2L11 (BIM): BCL2-like 11*	2q13	GWAS	Betz et al. (2015b)
		ATXN2: Ataxin 2	12q24	GWAS	Betz et al. (2015b), Cheung et al. (2003), Jagielska et al. (2012), Taghiabadi et al. (2018)
	Autophagy	*KIAA 0350/CLEC16A*	16p13	GWAS	Jagielska et al. (2012), Martinez et al. (2010), Petukhova et al. (2010)
Genes affecting central and peripheral immune tolerance	Genes affecting regulatory T-cells	*AIRE*: Autoimmune regulator gene	21q22.3	CGAS	Collins et al. (2006), Pforr et al. (2006), Tazi-Ahnini et al. (2002a), Wengraf et al. (2008)
		Foxp3: Forkhead box P3	Xp11.23	CGAS	Conteduca et al. (2014)
		IKZF4: Ikaros family zinc finger 4 also known as Eos	12q13	GWAS	Pan et al. (2009), Petukhova et al. (2010)
		GARP: Glycoprotein A repetitions predominant also known as LRRC32	11q13.5	GWAS	Betz et al. (2015b), Wang et al. (2009)
		CTLA4: Cytotoxic T lymphocyte-associated antigen 4	2q33.2	GWAS CGAS	Ismail et al. (2020), Megiorni et al. (2013), Moravvej et al. (2018a),

(continued)

Table 2 (continued)

Function		Gene	Location	Study	References
					Petukhova et al. (2010), Salinas-Santander et al. (2020), Wing et al. (2008)
		IL-2RA: Inetrleukin 2 receptor A (CD25)	10p15.1	GWAS	Petukhova et al. (2010)
		PTPN22: Protein tyrosine phosphatase, non-receptor type 22	1p13.2	CGAS Meta-analysis	Betz et al. (2008), Bhanusali et al. (2014), El-Zawahry et al. (2013), Kemp et al. (2006), Moravvej et al. (2018a), Salinas-Santander et al. (2015), Shehata et al. (2020)
	Other genes	*TAP1: Transporter associated with antigen processing 1*	6p21.3	CGAS	Kim et al. (2015a)
		TLR1: Toll-like receptor 1	4p14	CGAS	Seok et al. (2014b)
		IL-2/IL-21:Interleukin 2 and interleukin 21	4q27	GWAS CGAS	Jagielska et al. (2012), Monteleone et al. (2009), Petukhova et al. (2010), Redler et al. (2012)
Genes involved in disease progression after IP collapse	Cytokines	*IL-1α* *IL-1β* *IL1RN: IL-1 receptor antagonist* *IL-36RN: IL-36 receptor antagonist also known as interleukin-1 like molecule 1 (IL-1L1)*	2q14	CGAS	AlFadhli and Nanda (2014), Barahamani et al. (2002a), Barahamani et al. (2002b), Barahmani et al. (2010), Cork et al. (1996), Cork et al. (1995a), Cork et al. (1995b), Galbraith et al. (1999), Gao et al. (2009), Redler et al. (2012), Tarlow et al. (1994), Tazi-Ahnini et al. (2001), Tazi-Ahnini et al. (2002b), Tazi-Ahnini et al. (2002c)
		IL18 gene	11q23.1	CGAS	Kim et al. (2014)
		IL-4 *IL13*	5q31.1	GWAS CGAS	Jagielska et al. (2012), Lloyd and Hessel (2010),

(continued)

Table 2 (continued)

Function		Gene	Location	Study	References
					Petukhova et al. (2010), Kalkan et al. (2013b)
		IL-17A *IL-17F*	6p12.2	CGAS	Lew et al. (2012), Aytekin et al. (2015, Lew et al. (2012), Seleit et al. (2021)
		IL17RA: IL-17 receptor A	22q11.1		
		IL16 gene	15q26.3	CGAS	Lew et al. (2014b)
		IL-6	7p15.3	GWAS	Petukhova et al. (2010), Redler et al. (2012)
		IL-26	12q15		
		IL-12B	5q33.3	CGAS	Redler et al. (2012), Tabatabaei-Panah et al. (2020)
		IL-23R: IL-23 receptor	1p31.3	CGAS	Tabatabaei-Panah et al. (2020)
		TNFα: Tumor necrosis factor-alpha *LTA: Lymphotoxin alpha also known as TNFβ*	6p21.33	CGAS	Abd El-Raheem et al. (2020), Galbraith and Pandey (1995), Moravvej et al. (2018b), Redler et al. (2012)
	Other immune-related receptors and adaptor molecules	*SOCS1: Suppressor of cytokine signaling-1*	16p13.13	GWAS	Petukhova et al. (2010)
		FAS:FAS receptor *FASLG: FAS ligand*	10q23.31 1q24.3	CGAS	Fan et al. (2010), Kalkan et al. (2013a), Seleit et al. (2018)
		MX1: Myxovirus resistance 1	21q22.3	CGAS	Tazi-Ahnini et al. (2000)
		SH2B3 (LNK): Src homology 2-B protein 3	12q24	GWAS	Betz et al. (2015b), Cheung et al. (2003), Jagielska et al. (2012), Taghiabadi et al. (2018)
		NOTCH4: Neurogenic locus notch homolog 4	6p21.3	GWAS CGAS	AlFadhli and Nanda (2013), Petukhova and Christiano (2016), Petukhova et al. (2010), Tazi-Ahnini et al. (2003)
	Chemokines	*CXCL1* *CXCL2*	4q13.3	CGAS	Al-Eitan et al. (2019), Kim et al. (2015b)

(continued)

Table 2 (continued)

Function		Gene	Location	Study	References
Pigmentation genes	Melanogenesis	*MCHR2:Melanin Concentrating Hormone Receptor 2*	6q16.3	CNVA[c]	Fischer et al. (2017)
	Autophagy	*STX17 (syntaxin 17) is expressed in the hair follicle associated with premature hair graying*	9q31.1	GWAS CGAS	Petukhova et al. (2010), Pielberg et al. (2008), Jagielska et al. (2012), Petukhova et al. (2010), Taghiabadi et al. (2018)
		ATG4B: Autophagy related 4b cysteine peptidase	2q37.3	CNVA	Petukhova et al. (2020)
Hair follicle structural genes		*SMARCA2: SWI/SNF related, matrix associated, actin-dependent regulator of chromatin, subfamily a member 2*	9p24.3	CNVA	Petukhova et al. (2020)
		CCHCR1: Coiled-coil alpha-helical rod protein 1	6q21.33	MHC region analysis	Oka et al. (2020)
		TCF7L2: Transcription factor 7-like 2	10q25.3	CGAS	Rajabi et al. (2019b)
		ERBB3: Erythroblastic leukemia viral oncogene homolog 3	12q13	GWAS	Pan et al. (2009), Petukhova et al. (2010)
Gene with Miscellaneous functions		ZNF814: *Zinc finger protein 814*	19q13.43	CNV analysis	Petukhova et al. (2020)
		SPATA5: *Spermatogenesis-associated protein 5*	4q28.1	GWAS	Forstbauer et al. (2012)
		MTHFR: Methylenetetrahydrofolate reductase	1p36.22	CGAS	Kalkan et al. 2013c)

[a] GWAS, genome-wide association study
[b] CGAS, candidate gene association study
[c] CNVA, copy number variant analysis

References

Abd El-Raheem T, Mahmoud RH, Hefzy EM, Masoud M, Ismail R, Aboraia NM (2020) Tumor necrosis factor (TNF)-α-308 G/A gene polymorphism (rs1800629) in Egyptian patients with alopecia areata and vitiligo, a laboratory and in silico analysis. Plos One 15:e0240221

Abdelaziz AR (2020) Genetic and environmental determinants of Alopecia areata. Columbia University, City

Abramovits W, Losornio M (2006) Failure of two TNF-α blockers to influence the course of Alopecia Areata. SKINmed Dermatol Clin 5:177–183

Acharya P, Mathur MC (2020) Oxidative stress in alopecia areata: a systematic review and meta-analysis. Int J Dermatol 59:434–440

Ahmet A, Orkunoglu FE, Ozata M, Sengul A, Gur AR (2004) Lack of association between Vitamin D receptor FokI polymorphism and alopecia areata. Eur J Dermatol 14:156–158

Akar A, Arca E, Erbil H, Akay C, Sayal A, Gür AR (2002) Antioxidant enzymes and lipid peroxidation in the scalp of patients with alopecia areata. J Dermatol Sci 29:85–90

Akar A, Orkunoglu FE, Tunca M, Taştan HB, Kurumlu Z (2007) Vitamin D receptor gene polymorphisms are not associated with alopecia areata. Int J Dermatol 46:927–929

Al-Eitan LN, Al Momani RO, Al Momani KK, Al Warawrah AM, Aljamal HA, Alghamdi MA, Muhanna AM, Al-Qarqaz FA (2019) Candidate gene analysis of alopecia areata in Jordanian population of Arab Descent: a case-control study. Appl Clin Genet 12:221

AlFadhli S, Al-Mutairi M, Al Tameemi B, Nizam R (2016) Influence of MX1 promoter rs2071430 G/T polymorphism on susceptibility to systemic lupus erythematosus. Clin Rheumatol 35:623–629

AlFadhli S, Nj K, Al-Tememy B, Nanda A, Rebai A (2008) Susceptible and protective endothelial nitric oxide synthase gene polymorphism in alopecia areata in the Kuwaiti population. Autoimmunity 41:522–525

AlFadhli S, Nanda A (2013) Genetic evidence for the involvement of NOTCH4 in rheumatoid arthritis and alopecia areata. Immunol Lett 150:130–133

AlFadhli S, Nanda A (2014) Genetic analysis of interleukin-1 receptor antagonist and interleukin-1β single-nucleotide polymorphisms C− 511T and C+ 3953T in alopecia areata: susceptibility and severity association. Clin Exp Med 14:197–202

Aliagaoglu C, Pirim I, Atasoy M, Egerci N, Aktas A (2005) Association between alopecia areata and HLA class I and II in Turkey. J Dermatol 32:711–714

Alves R, Ferrando J (2011) Alopecia areata and Down's syndrome. Int Med Rev down Syn 15:34–36

Alzolibani A, Al Robaee A, Al Shobaili H, Bin Saif G, Ali A, Settin A (2015a) IL23R R381Q and NOS3 E298D gene polymorphisms in alopecia areata. Drugs Future 40:311–315

Alzolibani AA, Al Robaee AA, Al Shobaili HA, Saif GB, Al-Saif F, Ali A, Settin A (2015b) Interleukin-4− 590 T> C and interleukin-4 receptor Q551R A> G gene polymorphisms in Saudi cases with alopecia areata. J Egypt Public Health Assoc 90:20–23

Alzolibani AA, Rasheed Z, Saif GB, Al-Dhubaibi MS, Al Robaee AA (2016) Altered expression of intracellular Toll-like receptors in peripheral blood mononuclear cells from patients with alopecia areata. BBA Clinical 5:134–142

Antoun A, Jobson S, Cook M, O'Callaghan CA, Moss P, Briggs DC (2010) Single nucleotide polymorphism analysis of the NKG2D ligand cluster on the long arm of chromosome 6: extensive polymorphisms and evidence of diversity between human populations. Hum Immunol 71:610–620

Apte RS, Sinha D, Mayhew E, Wistow G, Niederkorn J (1998) Cutting edge: role of macrophage migration inhibitory factor in inhibiting NK cell activity and preserving immune privilege. J Immunol 160:5693–5696

Arango M-T, Perricone C, Kivity S, Cipriano E, Ceccarelli F, Valesini G, Shoenfeld Y (2017) HLA-DRB1 the notorious gene in the mosaic of autoimmunity. Immunol Res 65:82–98

Asz-Sigall D, Ortega-Springall MF, Smith-Pliego M, Rodríguez-Lobato E, Martinez-Velasco MA, Arenas R, Vincenzi C, Tosti A (2019) White hair in alopecia areata: clinical forms and proposed physiopathological mechanisms. J Am Acad Dermatol

Ates O (2017) Analysis of vitamin D receptor (VDR) gene polymorphisms in alopecia areata

Attia EA, El Shennawy D, Sefin A (2010) Serum interleukin-4 and total immunoglobulin E in nonatopic alopecia areata patients and HLA-DRB1 typing. Dermatol Res Pract

Atwa MA, Youssef N, Bayoumy NM (2016) T-helper 17 cytokines (interleukins 17, 21, 22, and 6, and tumor necrosis factor-α) in patients with alopecia areata: association with clinical type and severity. Int J Dermatol 55:666–672

Auburger G, Gispert S, Lahut S, Ömür Ö, Damrath E, Heck M, Başak N (2014) 12q24 locus association with type 1 diabetes: SH2B3 or ATXN2? World J Diab 5:316

Aytekin N, Akcali C, Pehlivan S, Kirtak N, Inaloz S (2015) Investigation of interleukin-12, interleukin-17 and interleukin-23 receptor gene polymorphisms in alopecia areata. J Int Med Res 43:526–534

Bahram S, Mizuki N, Inoko H, Spies T (1996) Nucleotide sequence of the human MHC class I MICA gene. Immunogenetics 44:80–81

Bailey JNC, Loomis SJ, Kang JH, Allingham RR, Gharahkhani P, Khor CC, Burdon KP, Aschard H, Chasman DI, Igo RP (2016) Genome-wide association analysis identifies TXNRD2, ATXN2 and FOXC1 as susceptibility loci for primary open-angle glaucoma. Nat Genet 48:189–194

Bain K, McDonald E, Moffat F, Tutino M, Castelino M, Barton A, Cavanagh J, Ijaz U, Siebert S, McInnes I (2020) Alopecia areata is characterized by dysregulation in systemic type 17 and type 2 cytokines, which may contribute to disease-associated psychological morbidity. Br J Dermatol 182:130–137

Bakry OA, Elshazly RMA, Shoeib MAM, Gooda A (2014) Oxidative stress in alopecia areata: a case–control study. Am J Clin Dermatol 15:57–64

Barahamani N, De Andrade M, Slusser J, Zhang Q, Duvic M (2002a) Interleukin-1 receptor antagonist allele 2 and familial alopecia areata. J Investig Dermatol 118:335–337

Barahamani N, Duvic M, de Andrade M, Slusser J, Zhang Q (2002b) Interleukin-1 receptor antagonist allele 2 and familial alopecia areata. J Investig Dermatol 118:335–337

Barahmani N, De Andrade M, Slusser JP, Zhang Q, Duvic M (2006) Major histocompatibility complex class I chain-related gene A polymorphisms and extended haplotypes are associated with familial alopecia areata. J Investig Dermatol 126:74–78

Barahmani N, Lopez A, Babu D, Hernandez M, Donley S, Duvic M (2010) Serum T helper 1 cytokine levels are greater in patients with alopecia areata regardless of severity or atopy. Clin Exp Dermatol Exp Dermatol 35:409–416

Barker CF, Billingham R (1972) Analysis of local anatomic factors that influence the survival times of

pure epidermal and full-thickness skin homografts in guinea pigs. Ann Surg 176:597
Bauer S, Groh V, Wu J, Steinle A, Phillips JH, Lanier LL, Spies T (1999) Activation of NK cells and T cells by NKG2D, a receptor for stress-inducible MICA. Science 285:727–729
Bennett CL, Christie J, Ramsdell F, Brunkow ME, Ferguson PJ, Whitesell L, Kelly TE, Saulsbury FT, Chance PF, Ochs HD (2001) The immune dysregulation, polyendocrinopathy, enteropathy, X-linked syndrome (IPEX) is caused by mutations of FOXP3. Nat Genet 27:20–21
Bertolini M, McElwee K, Gilhar A, Bulfone-Paus S, Paus R (2020) Hair follicle immune privilege and its collapse in alopecia areata. Exp Dermatol 29:703–725
Betz R, König K, Flaquer A, Redler S, Eigelshoven S, Kortüm AK, Hanneken S, Hillmer A, Tüting T, Lambert J (2008) The R620W polymorphism in PTPN22 confers general susceptibility for the development of alopecia areata. Br J Dermatol 158:389–391
Betz RC, Petukhova L, Ripke S, Huang H, Menelaou A, Redler S, Becker T, Heilmann S, Yamany T, Duvic M (2015a) Genome-wide meta-analysis in alopecia areata resolves HLA associations and reveals two new susceptibility loci. Nat Commun 6:1–8
Betz RC, Petukhova L, Ripke S, Huang H, Menelaou A, Redler S, Becker T, Heilmann S, Yamany T, Duvic M (2015) Genome-wide meta-analysis in alopecia areata resolves HLA associations and reveals two new susceptibility loci. Nat Commun 6
Bhanusali DG, Sachdev A, Olson MA, Gerlach JA, Sinha AA (2014) PTPN22 profile indicates a novel risk group in alopecia areata. Hum Immunol 75:81–87
Binder RJ (2014) Functions of heat shock proteins in pathways of the innate and adaptive immune system. J Immunol 193:5765–5771
Bizzaro G, Antico A, Fortunato A, Bizzaro N (2017) Vitamin D and autoimmune diseases: is vitamin D receptor (VDR) polymorphism the culprit. Isr Med Assoc J 19:438–443
Bodemer C, de Prost Y, Peuchmaur M, Fraitaig S, Chatenoud L, Brousse N (2000) Role of cytotoxic T cells in chronic alopecia areata. J Investig Dermatol 114:112–116
Bolduc C, Bissonnette R (2012) Safety and efficacy of adalimumab for the treatment of severe alopecia areata: case series of three patients. J Cutan Med Surg 16:257–260
Booth DR, Heard RN, Stewart GJ, Goris A, Dobosi R, Dubois B, Lorentzen ÅR, Celius EG, Harbo HF, Spurkland A (2009) The expanding genetic overlap between multiple sclerosis and type I diabetes. Genes Immun 10:11
Bouillet P, Cory S, Zhang L-C, Strasser A, Adams JM (2001) Degenerative disorders caused by Bcl-2 deficiency prevented by loss of its BH3-only antagonist Bim. Dev Cell 1:645–653
Bramswig NC, Lüdecke H-J, Alanay Y, Albrecht B, Barthelmie A, Boduroglu K, Braunholz D, Caliebe A, Chrzanowska KH, Czeschik JC (2015) Exome sequencing unravels unexpected differential diagnoses in individuals with the tentative diagnosis of Coffin-Siris and Nicolaides-Baraitser syndromes. Hum Genet 134:553–568
Buchert R, Nesbitt AI, Tawamie H, Krantz ID, Medne L, Helbig I, Matalon DR, Reis A, Santani A, Sticht H (2016) SPATA5 mutations cause a distinct autosomal recessive phenotype of intellectual disability, hypotonia and hearing loss. Orphanet J Rare Dis 11:1–7
Burn GL, Svensson L, Sanchez-Blanco C, Saini M, Cope AP (2011) Why is PTPN22 a good candidate susceptibility gene for autoimmune disease? FEBS Lett 585:3689–3698
Campbell F, Xu H, El-Tanani M, Crowe P, Bingham V (2010) The yin and yang of vitamin D receptor (VDR) signaling in neoplastic progression: operational networks and tissue-specific growth control. Biochem Pharmacol 79:1–9
Castro JE, Listman JA, Jacobson BA, Wang Y, Lopez PA, Ju S, Finn PW, Perkins DL (1996) Fas modulation of apoptosis during negative selection of thymocytes. Immunity 5:617–627
Celik SD, Ates O (2018) Genetic analysis of interleukin 18 gene polymorphisms in alopecia areata. J Clin Lab Anal 32:e22386
Mingorance Gámez CG, Martínez Chamorro A, Moreno Casares AM, Tercedor Sánchez J, Arias-Santiago S, García-Lora E, López-Nevot MA (2020) Joint study of the associations of HLA-B and the transmembrane STR polymorphism of MICA with alopecia areata shows independent associations of both of them with the disease. Clin Exp Dermatol
Chai M, Jiang M, Vergnes L, Fu X, de Barros SC, Doan NB, Huang W, Chu J, Jiao J, Herschman H (2019) Stimulation of hair growth by small molecules that activate autophagy. Cell Rep 27:3413–3421. e3413
Chalupny NJ, Rein-Weston A, Dosch S, Cosman D (2006) Down-regulation of the NKG2D ligand MICA by the human cytomegalovirus glycoprotein UL142. Biochem Biophys Res Commun 346:175–181
Chambers CA, Sullivan TJ, Allison JP (1997) Lymphoproliferation in CTLA-4–deficient mice is mediated by costimulation-dependent activation of CD4+ T cells. Immunity 7:885–895
Chen W, Konkel JE (2010) TGF-beta and "adaptive" Foxp3(+) regulatory T cells. J Mol Cell Biol 2:30–36
Cheng X, Dai H, Wan N, Moore Y, Vankayalapati R, Dai Z (2009) Interaction of programmed death-1 and programmed death-1 ligand-1 contributes to testicular immune privilege. Transplantation 87:1778–1786
Cheng X, Ma X, Ding X, Li L, Jiang X, Shen Z, Chen S, Liu W, Gong W, Sun Q (2017) Pacer mediates the function of class III PI3K and HOPS complexes in autophagosome maturation by engaging Stx17. Mol Cell 65:1029–1043. e1025
Cheung C, Davies NG, Hoog J-O, Hotchkiss SA, Pease CKS (2003) Species variations in cutaneous alcohol dehydrogenases and aldehyde dehydrogenases

may impact on toxicological assessments of alcohols and aldehydes. Toxicology 184:97–112
Chicz RM, Urban RG, Lane WS, Gorga JC, Stern LJ, Vignali DA, Strominger JL (1992) Predominant naturally processed peptides bound to HLA-DR1 are derived from MHC-related molecules and are heterogeneous in size. Nature 358:764–768
Chin RK, Lo JC, Kim O, Blink SE, Christiansen PA, Peterson P, Wang Y, Ware C, Fu Y-X (2003) Lymphotoxin pathway directs thymic Aire expression. Nat Immunol 4:1121–1127
Chodorowska G, Dabrowska-Czlonka M, Bartosinska J, Jazienicka I, Wawrzycki B, Kowal M (2007) The level of interleukin 12 and interleukin 18 in alopecia areata patients-a pilot study. Dermatologia Kliniczna 9:207
Christoph T, Müller-Röver S, Audring H, Tobin D, Hermes B, Cotsarelis G, Rückert R, Paus R (2000) The human hair follicle immune system: cellular composition and immune privilege. Br J Dermatol 142:862–873
Chu X, Pan C-M, Zhao S-X, Liang J, Gao G-Q, Zhang X-M, Yuan G-Y, Li C-G, Xue L-Q, Shen M (2011) A genome-wide association study identifies two new risk loci for Graves' disease. Nat Genet 43:897
Clevers H, Nusse R (2012) Wnt/β-catenin signaling and disease. Cell 149:1192–1205
Collins S, Dominguez M, Ilmarinen T, Costigan C, Irvine A (2006) Dermatological manifestations of autoimmune polyendocrinopathy–candidiasis–ectodermal dystrophy syndrome. Br J Dermatol 154:1088–1093
Conteduca G, Rossi A, Megiorni F, Parodi A, Ferrera F, Tardito S, Battaglia F, Kalli F, Negrini S, Pizzuti A (2014) Single nucleotide polymorphisms in the promoter regions of Foxp3 and ICOSLG genes are associated with alopecia areata. Clin Exp Med 14:91–97
Cork MJ, Crane AM, Duff GW (1996) Genetic control of cytokines: cytokine gene polymorphisms in alopecia areata. Dermatol Clin 14:671–678
Cork MJ, Tarlow JK, Clay FE, Crane A, Blakemore A, McDonagh A, Messenger AG, Duff GW (1995a) An allele of the interleukin-1 receptor antagonist as a genetic severity factor in alopecia areata. J Invest Dermatol 104:15S-16S
Cork MJ, Tarlow JK, Clay FE, Crane A, Blakemore AI, McDonagh AJ, Messenger AG, Duff GW (1995) An allele of the interleukin-1 receptor antagonist as a genetic severity factor in alopecia areata. J Invest Dermatol 104
Cornelius N, Wardman JH, Hargreaves IP, Neergheen V, Bie AS, Tümer Z, Nielsen JE, Nielsen TT (2017) Evidence of oxidative stress and mitochondrial dysfunction in spinocerebellar ataxia type 2 (SCA2) patient fibroblasts: effect of coenzyme Q10 supplementation on these parameters. Mitochondrion 34:103–114
Cosman D, Müllberg J, Sutherland CL, Chin W, Armitage R, Fanslow W, Kubin M, Chalupny NJ (2001) ULBPs, novel MHC class I–related molecules, bind to CMV glycoprotein UL16 and stimulate NK cytotoxicity through the NKG2D receptor. Immunity 14:123–133
Da Costa CM, Dupont E, Van der Cruys M, Andrien M, Hidajat M, Song M, Stene J (2006) Earlier occurrence of severe alopecia areata in HLA-DRB1* 11-positive patients. Dermatology 213:12–14
Daneri Becerra CdR, Galigniana MD (2016) Regulatory role of heat-shock proteins in autoimmune and inflammatory diseases
Dankers W, Colin EM, van Hamburg JP, Lubberts E (2017) Vitamin D in autoimmunity: molecular mechanisms and therapeutic potential. Front Immunol 7:697
Decot V, Voillard L, Latger-Cannard V, Aissi-Rothé L, Perrier P, Stoltz JF, Bensoussan D (2010) Natural-killer cell amplification for adoptive leukemia relapse immunotherapy: comparison of three cytokines, IL-2, IL-15, or IL-7 and impact on NKG2D, KIR2DL1, and KIR2DL2 expression. Exp Hematol 38:351–362
Deffit SN, Blum JS (2015) A central role for HSC70 in regulating antigen trafficking and MHC class II presentation. Mol Immunol 68:85–88
Denkinger CM, Metz C, Fingerle-Rowson G, Denkinger MD, Forsthuber T (2004) Macrophage migration inhibitory factor and its role in autoimmune diseases. Arch Immunol Ther Exp (warsz) 52:389–400
Dennis A-G, Almaguer-Mederos LE, Raúl R-A, Roberto R-L, Luis V-P, Dany C-A, Yanetza G-Z, Yaimeé V-M, Annelié E-D, Arnoy P-A (2021) Redox imbalance associates with clinical worsening in spinocerebellar ataxia type 2. Oxidat Med Cellul Longevity
Devallière J, Charreau B (2011) The adaptor Lnk (SH2B3): an emerging regulator in vascular cells and a link between immune and inflammatory signaling. Biochem Pharmacol 82:1391–1402
Dewberry R, Holden H, Crossman D, Francis S (2000) Interleukin-1 receptor antagonist expression in human endothelial cells and atherosclerosis. Arterioscler Thromb Vasc Biol 20:2394–2400
Diao J, Liu R, Rong Y, Zhao M, Zhang J, Lai Y, Zhou Q, Wilz LM, Li J, Vivona S (2015) ATG14 promotes membrane tethering and fusion of autophagosomes to endolysosomes. Nature 520:563–566
Dinarello CA (2007) Interleukin-18 and the pathogenesis of inflammatory diseases. In: (eds) Seminars in nephrology. Elsevier, pp 98–114
Divito SJ, Kupper TS (2014) Inhibiting Janus kinases to treat alopecia areata. Nat Med 20:989–990
Donn RP, Plant D, Jury F, Richards HL, Worthington J, Ray DW, Griffiths CE (2004) Macrophage migration inhibitory factor gene polymorphism is associated with psoriasis. J Investig Dermatol 123:484–487
Dubin PJ, Kolls JK (2009) Interleukin-17A and interleukin-17F: a tale of two cytokines. Immunity 30:9–11
Duvic M, Hordinsky MK, Fiedler VC, O'brien WR, Young R, Reveille JD (1991) HLA-D locus associations in alopecia areata: DRw52a may confer disease resistance. Arch Dermatol 127:64–68

Dwyer CJ, Knochelmann HM, Smith AS, Wyatt MM, Rangel Rivera GO, Arhontoulis DC, Bartee E, Li Z, Rubinstein MP, Paulos CM (2019) Fueling cancer immunotherapy with common gamma chain cytokines. Front Immunol 10:263

Eagle RA, Traherne JA, Hair JR, Jafferji I, Trowsdale J (2009) ULBP6/RAET1L is an additional human NKG2D ligand. Eur J Immunol 39:3207–3216

El-Gayyar MA, Helmy ME, Amer ER, Ibrahim LY, Gaballah MA (2020) Evaluation of interleukin-18 and soluble interleukin-2 receptor serum levels in patients with alopecia areata: an Egyptian study. Egypt J Dermatol Venerol 40:34

El-Zawahry BM, Azzam OA, Zaki NS, Abdel-Raheem HM, Bassiouny DA, Khorshied MM (2013) PTPN22 gene polymorphism in Egyptian alopecia areata patients and its impact on response to diphencyprone immunotherapy. Gene 523:147–151

Elden AC, Kim H-J, Hart MP, Chen-Plotkin AS, Johnson BS, Fang X, Armakola M, Geser F, Greene R, Lu MM (2010) Ataxin-2 intermediate-length polyglutamine expansions are associated with increased risk for ALS. Nature 466:1069–1075

Eldesouky F, Ibrahim A-SM, Sharaf SM (2020) Macrophage migration inhibitory factor in alopecia areata and vitiligo: a case-controlled serological study. J Clin Aesthet Dermatol 13:24

Eleme K, Taner SB, Br Ö, Collinson LM, McCann FE, Chalupny NJ, Cosman D, Hopkins C, Magee AI, Davis DM (2004) Cell surface organization of stress-inducible proteins ULBP and MICA that stimulate human NK cells and T cells via NKG2D. J Exp Med 199:1005–1010

Enshell-Seijffers D, Lindon C, Kashiwagi M, Morgan BA (2010) β-catenin activity in the dermal papilla regulates morphogenesis and regeneration of hair. Dev Cell 18:633–642

Erjavec SOT (2020) Utilizing functional genomics approaches to characterize risk genes in alopecia areata. Columbia University, City

Espinoza JL, Takami A, Nakata K, Onizuka M, Kawase T, Akiyama H, Miyamura K, Morishima Y, Fukuda T, Kodera Y (2011) A genetic variant in the IL-17 promoter is functionally associated with acute graft-versus-host disease after unrelated bone marrow transplantation. PloS One 6:e26229

Fan X, Shangguan L, Li M, Li C, Liu B (2010) Functional polymorphisms of the FAS/FASLG genes are associated with risk of alopecia areata in a Chinese population: a case–control analysis. Br J Dermatol 163:340–344

Ferguson TA, Griffith TS (2006) A vision of cell death: Fas ligand and immune privilege 10 years later. Immunol Rev 213:228–238

Fernández-Messina L, Reyburn HT, Valés-Gómez M (2012) Human NKG2D-ligands: cell biology strategies to ensure immune recognition. Front Immunol 3:299

Ferran M, Calvet J, Almirall M, Pujol R, Maymó J (2011) Alopecia areata as another immune-mediated disease developed in patients treated with tumour necrosis factor-α blocker agents. J Eur Acad Dermatol Venereol 25:479–484

Fischer A, Schmid B, Ellinghaus D, Nothnagel M, Gaede KI, Schürmann M, Lipinski S, Rosenstiel P, Zissel G, Höhne K (2012) A novel sarcoidosis risk locus for Europeans on chromosome 11q13. 1. Am J Respir Crit Care Med 186:877–885

Fischer J, Degenhardt F, Hofmann A, Redler S, Basmanav FB, Heilmann-Heimbach S, Hanneken S, Giehl KA, Wolff H, Moebus S (2017) Genomewide analysis of copy number variants in alopecia areata in a C entral E uropean cohort reveals association with MCHR 2. Exp Dermatol 26:536–541

Forstbauer LM, Brockschmidt FF, Moskvina V, Herold C, Redler S, Herzog A, Hillmer AM, Meesters C, Heilmann S, Albert F (2012) Genome-wide pooling approach identifies SPATA5 as a new susceptibility locus for alopecia areata. Eur J Hum Genet 20:326–332

Fousteri G, Liossis S-NC, Battaglia M (2013) Roles of the protein tyrosine phosphatase PTPN22 in immunity and autoimmunity. Clin Immunol 149:556–565

Freyschmidt-Paul P, McElwee KJ, Botchkarev V, Kissling S, Wenzel E, Sundberg JP, Happle R, Hoffmann R (2003) Fas-deficient C3. MRL-Tnfrsf6lpr mice and fas ligand-deficient C3H/HeJ-Tnfsf6gld mice are relatively resistant to the induction of alopecia areata by grafting of alopecia areata-affected skin from C3H/HeJ Mice. In (eds) Journal of investigative dermatology symposium proceedings. Elsevier, pp 104–108

Fricke ACV, Miteva M (2015) Epidemiology and burden of alopecia areata: a systematic review. Clin Cosmet Investig Dermatol 8:397

Fu S, Zhang N, Yopp AC, Chen D, Mao M, Chen D, Zhang H, Ding Y, Bromberg JS (2004) TGF-beta induces Foxp3 + T-regulatory cells from CD4 + CD25 - precursors. Am J Transplant 4:1614–1627

Galbraith GM, Pandey JP (1995) Tumor necrosis factor alpha (TNF-α) gene polymorphism in alopecia areata. Hum Genet 96:433–436

Galbraith GP, Palesch Y, Gore E, Pandey J (1999) Contribution of interleukin 1β and KM loci to alopecia areata. Hum Hered 49:85–89

Gao Y, He Y, Ding J, Wu K, Hu B, Liu Y, Wu Y, Guo B, Shen Y, Landi D (2009) An insertion/deletion polymorphism at miRNA-122-binding site in the interleukin-1α 3′ untranslated region confers risk for hepatocellular carcinoma. Carcinogenesis 30:2064–2069

Gasteiger G, Kastenmuller W (2012) Foxp3+ regulatory T-cells and IL-2: the Moirai of T-cell fates? Front Immunol 3:179

Georgiev P, Charbonnier L-M, Chatila TA (2019) Regulatory T cells: the many faces of Foxp3. J Clin Immunol 39:623–640

Ghoussaini M, Vatin V, Lecoeur C, Abkevich V, Younus A, Samson C, Wachter C, Heude B, Tauber M, Tounian P (2007) Genetic study of the melanin-concentrating hormone receptor 2 in childhood and adulthood severe obesity. J Clin Endocrinol Metab 92:4403–4409

Giedraitis V, He B, Huang W-X, Hillert J (2001) Cloning and mutation analysis of the human IL-18 promoter: a possible role of polymorphisms in expression regulation. J Neuroimmunol 112:146–152

Gilhar A (2010a) Collapse of immune privilege in alopecia areata: coincidental or substantial & quest. J Investig Dermatol 130:2535–2537

Gilhar A (2010b) Collapse of immune privilege in alopecia areata: coincidental or substantial? J Investig Dermatol 130:2535–2537

Gilhar A, Assy B, Shalaginov R, Serafimovich S, Landau M, Kalish RS (2001a) Melanocyte-associated T cell epitopes can function as autoantigens for transfer of alopecia areata to human scalp explants on Prkdc scid mice. J Investig Dermatol 117:1357–1362

Gilhar A, Assy B, Shalaginov R, Serafimovich S, Landau M, Kalish RS (2001b) Melanocyte-associated T cell epitopes can function as autoantigens for transfer of alopecia areata to human scalp explants on Prkdcscid mice. J Investig Dermatol 117:1357–1362

Gilhar A, Etzioni A, Paus R (2012) Alopecia areata. N Engl J Med 366:1515–1525

Gilhar A, Kalish RS (2006) Alopecia areata: a tissue specific autoimmune disease of the hair follicle. Autoimmun Rev 5:64–69

Gilhar A, Keren A, Shemer A, d'Ovidio R, Ullmann Y, Paus R (2013) Autoimmune disease induction in a healthy human organ: a humanized mouse model of alopecia areata. J Investig Dermatol 133:844–847

Gkikas I, Palikaras K, Tavernarakis N (2018) The role of mitophagy in innate immunity. Front Immunol 9:1283

Goh C, Finkel M, Christos P, Sinha A (2006) Profile of 513 patients with alopecia areata: associations of disease subtypes with atopy, autoimmune disease and positive family history. J Eur Acad Dermatol Venereol 20:1055–1060

Gokhale AS, Gangaplara A, Lopez-Occasio M, Thornton AM, Shevach EM (2019) Selective deletion of Eos (Ikzf4) in T-regulatory cells leads to loss of suppressive function and development of systemic autoimmunity. J Autoimmun 105:102300

Gorcey L, Spratt EAG, Leger MC (2014) Alopecia universalis successfully treated with adalimumab. JAMA Dermatol 150:1341–1344

Goswami R (2016) Primer on the metabolic bone diseases and disorders of mineral metabolism. Indian J Med Res 144:489–490

Goudy K, Aydin D, Barzaghi F, Gambineri E, Vignoli M, Mannurita SC, Doglioni C, Ponzoni M, Cicalese MP, Assanelli A (2013) Human IL2RA null mutation mediates immunodeficiency with lymphoproliferation and autoimmunity. Clin Immunol 146:248–261

Green DR, Droin N, Pinkoski M (2003) Activation-induced cell death in T cells. Immunol Rev 193:70–81

Gregersen PK, Amos CI, Lee AT, Lu Y, Remmers EF, Kastner DL, Seldin MF, Criswell LA, Plenge RM, Holers VM (2009) REL, encoding a member of the NF-κB family of transcription factors, is a newly defined risk locus for rheumatoid arthritis. Nat Genet 41:820

Gregoriou S, Papafragkaki D, Kontochristopoulos G, Rallis E, Kalogeromitros D, Rigopoulos D (2010) Cytokines and other mediators in alopecia areata. Mediat Inflammat

Groh V, Bahram S, Bauer S, Herman A, Beauchamp M, Spies T (1996) Cell stress-regulated human major histocompatibility complex class I gene expressed in gastrointestinal epithelium. Proc Natl Acad Sci 93:12445–12450

Gross C, Krishnan AV, Malloy PJ, Eccleshall TR, Zhao XY, Feldman D (1998) The vitamin D receptor gene start codon polymorphism: a functional analysis of FokI variants. J Bone Miner Res 13:1691–1699

Guleria I, Khosroshahi A, Ansari MJ, Habicht A, Azuma M, Yagita H, Noelle RJ, Coyle A, Mellor AL, Khoury SJ (2005) A critical role for the programmed death ligand 1 in fetomaternal tolerance. J Exp Med 202:231–237

Gwinn-Hardy K, Chen J, Liu H-C, Liu T, Boss M, Seltzer W, Adam A, Singleton A, Koroshetz W, Waters C (2000) Spinocerebellar ataxia type 2 with parkinsonism in ethnic Chinese. Neurology 55:800–805

Haida Y, Ikeda S, Takagi A, Komiyama E, Mabuchi T, Ozawa A, Kulski JK, Inoko H, Oka A (2013) Association analysis of the HLA-C gene in Japanese alopecia areata. Immunogenetics 65:553–557

Hakonarson H, Grant SF, Bradfield JP, Marchand L, Kim CE, Glessner JT, Grabs R, Casalunovo T, Taback SP, Frackelton EC (2007) A genome-wide association study identifies KIAA0350 as a type 1 diabetes gene. Nature 448:591–594

Hamed FN, Åstrand A, Bertolini M, Rossi A, Maleki-Dizaji A, Messenger AG, McDonagh AJ, Tazi-Ahnini R (2019) Alopecia areata patients show deficiency of FOXP3+ CD39+ T regulatory cells and clonotypic restriction of Treg TCRβ-chain, which highlights the immunopathological aspect of the disease. PloS One 14:e0210308

Han YM, Sheng YY, Xu F, Qi SS, Liu XJ, Hu RM, Miao Y, Huang GQ, Yang QP (2015) Imbalance of T-helper 17 and regulatory T cells in patients with alopecia areata. J Dermatol 42:981–988

Hanalioglu D, Ayvaz DC, Ozgur TT, van der Burg M, Sanal O, Tezcan I (2017) A novel mutation in TAP1 gene leading to MHC class I deficiency: report of two cases and review of the literature. Clin Immunol 178:74–78

Harb H, Benamar M, Lai PS, Contini P, Griffith JW, Crestani E, Schmitz-Abe K, Chen Q, Fong J, Marri L (2021) Notch4 signaling limits regulatory T-cell-mediated tissue repair and promotes severe lung inflammation in viral infections. Immunity

Harb H, Stephen-Victor E, Crestani E, Benamar M, Massoud A, Cui Y, Charbonnier L-M, Arbag S, Baris S, Cunnigham A (2020) A regulatory T cell Notch4–GDF15 axis licenses tissue inflammation in asthma. Nat Immunol 21:1359–1370

Hardman JA, Nicu C, Tai C, Harries M, Mironov A, Purba TS, Paus R (2020) Does dysfunctional autophagy contribute to immune privilege collapse and alopecia areata pathogenesis? J Dermatol Sci 100:75–78

Hasan HA, Ra'ed OA, Muda WAMBW, Mohamed HJBJ, Samsudin AR (2017) Association of vitamin D receptor gene polymorphisms with metabolic syndrome and its components among adult Arabs from the United Arab Emirates. Diab Metabol Syndr Clin Res Rev 11:S531–S537

He Y, Na H, Li Y, Qiu Z, Li W (2013) FoxP3 rs3761548 polymorphism predicts autoimmune disease susceptibility: a meta-analysis. Hum Immunol 74:1665–1671

Head JR, Neaves WB, Billingham RE (1983) Immune privilege in the testis. I. Basic parameters of allograft survival. Transplantation 36:423–431

Hernandez M, Nogues S, Ruiz-Esquide V, Alsina M, Canete J, Sanmarti R (2009) Development of alopecia areata after biological therapy with TNF-alpha Blockers: description of a case and review of the literature. Clin Exp Rheumatol 27:892–893

Hoffmann R, Wenzel E, Huth A, van der Steen P, Schäufele M, Henninger H-P, Happle R (1994) Cytokine mRNA levels in alopecia areata before and after treatment with the contact allergen diphenylcyclopropenone. J Investig Dermatol 103:530–533

Holley J, Newcombe J, Winyard P, Gutowski N (2007) Peroxiredoxin V in multiple sclerosis lesions: predominant expression by astrocytes. Mult Scler J 13:955–961

Hughes P, Bouillet P, Strasser A (2006) Role of Bim and other Bcl-2 family members in autoimmune and degenerative diseases. Apoptosis Relevance Autoimmun 9:74–94

Hughes PD, Belz GT, Fortner KA, Budd RC, Strasser A, Bouillet P (2008) Apoptosis regulators Fas and Bim cooperate in shutdown of chronic immune responses and prevention of autoimmunity. Immunity 28:197–205

Hull SM, Nutbrown M, Pepall L, Thornton MJ, Cunliffe WJ, Randall VA (1991) Immunohistologic and ultrastructural comparison of the dermal papilla and hair follicle bulb from "active" and "normal" areas of alopecia areata. J Investig Dermatol 96:673–681

Illescas O, Gomez-Verjan JC, García-Velázquez L, Govezensky T, Rodriguez-Sosa M (2018) Macrophage migration inhibitory factor-173 G/C polymorphism: a global meta-analysis across the disease spectrum. Front Genet 9:55

Islam N, Leung PS, Huntley AC, Gershwin ME (2015) The autoimmune basis of alopecia areata: a comprehensive review. Autoimmun Rev 14:81–89

Ismail NA, Toraih EA, Ameen HM, Gomaa AHA, Marie RE-SM (2020) Association of Rs231775 genetic variant of cytotoxic T-lymphocyte associated protein 4 with alopecia areata disease in males: a case–control study. Immunol Invest 1–10

Itakura E, Kishi-Itakura C, Mizushima N (2012) The hairpin-type tail-anchored SNARE syntaxin 17 targets to autophagosomes for fusion with endosomes/lysosomes. Cell 151:1256–1269

Ito T, Ito N, Bettermann A, Tokura Y, Takigawa M, Paus R (2004) Collapse and restoration of MHC class-I-dependent immune privilege: exploiting the human hair follicle as a model. Am J Pathol 164:623–634

Ito T, Ito N, Saathoff M, Bettermann A, Takigawa M, Paus R (2005a) Interferon-γ is a potent inducer of catagen-like changes in cultured human anagen hair follicles. Br J Dermatol 152:623–631

Ito T, Ito N, Saathoff M, Stampachiacchiere B, Bettermann A, Bulfone-Paus S, Takigawa M, Nickoloff BJ, Paus R (2005b) Immunology of the human nail apparatus: the nail matrix is a site of relative immune privilege. J Investig Dermatol 125:1139–1148

Ito T, Ito N, Saatoff M, Hashizume H, Fukamizu H, Nickoloff BJ, Takigawa M, Paus R (2008) Maintenance of hair follicle immune privilege is linked to prevention of NK cell attack. J Investig Dermatol 128:1196–1206

Ito T, Tokura Y (2014) The role of cytokines and chemokines in the T-cell-mediated autoimmune process in alopecia areata. Exp Dermatol 23:787–791

Jackow C, Puffer N, Hordinsky M, Nelson J, Tarrand J, Duvic M (1998) Alopecia areata and cytomegalovirus infection in twins: genes versus environment? J Am Acad Dermatol 38:418–425

Jagielska D, Redler S, Brockschmidt FF, Herold C, Pasternack SM, Bartels NG, Hanneken S, Eigelshoven S, Refke M, Barth S (2012) Follow-up study of the first genome-wide association scan in alopecia areata: IL13 and KIAA0350 as susceptibility loci supported with genome-wide significance. J Investig Dermatol 132:2192–2197

Jago C, Yates J, Olsen Saraiva Câmara N, Lechler R, Lombardi G (2004) Differential expression of CTLA-4 among T cell subsets. Clin Exp Immunol 136:463–471

Jain N, Nguyen H, Chambers C, Kang J (2010) Dual function of CTLA-4 in regulatory T cells and conventional T cells to prevent multiorgan autoimmunity. Proc Natl Acad Sci 107:1524–1528

Janghorban M, Xin L, Rosen JM, Zhang XH-F (2018) Notch signaling as a regulator of the tumor immune response: to target or not to target? Front Immunol 9:1649

Jeck WR, Siebold AP, Sharpless NE (2012) a meta-analysis of GWAS and age-associated diseases. Aging Cell 11:727–731

Ji C, Liu S, Zhu K, Luo H, Li Q, Zhang Y, Huang S, Chen Q, Cao Y (2018) HLA-DRB1 polymorphisms and alopecia areata disease risk: a systematic review and meta-analysis. Medicine 97

John KK, Brockschmidt FF, Redler S, Herold C, Hanneken S, Eigelshoven S, Giehl KA, De Weert J, Lutz G, Kruse R (2011) Genetic variants in CTLA4 are strongly associated with alopecia areata. J Invest Dermatol 131:1169–1172

Kalkan G, Ateş Ö, Karakuş N, Sezer S (2013a) Functional polymorphisms in cell death pathway genes FAS and

FAS ligand and risk of alopecia areata. Arch Dermatol Res 305:909–915

Kalkan G, Karakus N, Baş Y, Takçı Z, Özuğuz P, Ateş Ö, Yigit S (2013b) The association between Interleukin (IL)-4 gene intron 3 VNTR polymorphism and alopecia areata (AA) in Turkish population. Gene 527:565–569

Kalkan G, Yigit S, Karakuş N, Ateş Ö, Bozkurt N, Özdemir A, Pancar GŞ (2013c) Methylenetetrahydrofolate reductase C677T mutation in patients with alopecia areata in Turkish population. Gene 530:109–112

Kang H, Wu W-Y, Lo BK, Yu M, Leung G, Shapiro J, McElwee KJ (2010) Hair follicles from alopecia areata patients exhibit alterations in immune privilege-associated gene expression in advance of hair loss. J Investig Dermatol 130:2677–2680

Kang H, Wu WY, Yu M, Shapiro J, McElwee KJ (2020) Increased expression of TLR7 and TLR9 in alopecia areata. Exp Dermatol 29:254–258

Karademir B, Bozaykut P, Ozer NK (2014) Heat shock proteins and proteasomal degradation in normal and tumor cells. Free Radical Biol Med 75:S35

Karasawa R, Ozaki S, Nishioka K, Kato T (2005) Autoantibodies to peroxiredoxin I and IV in patients with systemic autoimmune diseases. Microbiol Immunol 49:57–65

Kastenmuller W, Gasteiger G, Subramanian N, Sparwasser T, Busch DH, Belkaid Y, Drexler I, Germain RN (2011) Regulatory T cells selectively control CD8+ T cell effector pool size via IL-2 restriction. J Immunol 187:3186–3197

Kasumagić-Halilovic E, Cavaljuga S, Ovcina-Kurtovic N, Zecevic L (2018) Serum levels of interleukin-2 in patients with alopecia areata: Relationship with clinical type and duration of the disease. Skin Appendage Disord 4:286–290

Kavak A, Baykal C, Özarmağan G, Akar U (2000) HLA in alopecia areata. Int J Dermatol 39:589–592

Kawaguchi M, Takahashi D, Hizawa N, Suzuki S, Matsukura S, Kokubu F, Maeda Y, Fukui Y, Konno S, Huang S-K (2006) IL-17F sequence variant (His161Arg) is associated with protection against asthma and antagonizes wild-type IL-17F activity. J Aller Clin Immunol 117:795–801

Kelley CM, Ikeda T, Koipally J, Avitahl N, Wu L, Georgopoulos K, Morgan BA (1998) Helios, a novel dimerization partner of Ikaros expressed in the earliest hematopoietic progenitors. Curr Biol 8:508-S501

Kemp EH, McDonagh AJ, Wengraf DA, Messenger AG, Gawkrodger DJ, Cork MJ, Tazi-Ahnini R (2006) The non-synonymous C1858T substitution in the PTPN22 gene is associated with susceptibility to the severe forms of alopecia areata. Hum Immunol 67:535–539

Kianto U, Reunala T, Karvonen J, Lassus A, Tiilikainen A (1977) HLA-B12 in alopecia areata. Arch Dermatol 113:1716

Kichaev G, Bhatia G, Loh P-R, Gazal S, Burch K, Freund MK, Schoech A, Pasaniuc B, Price AL (2019) Leveraging polygenic functional enrichment to improve GWAS power. Am J Hum Genet 104:65–75

Kim A, Sadegh-Nasseri S (2015) Determinants of immunodominance for CD4 T cells. Curr Opin Immunol 34:9–15

Kim DY, Lee JW, Whang SH, Park YK, Hann SK, Shin YJ (2009) Quality of life for Korean patients with vitiligo: Skindex-29 and its correlation with clinical profiles. J Dermatol 36:317–322

Kim H, Lee H, Lew B, Sim W, Kim Y, Lee S, Lee S, Cho I, Kwon J, Kim H (2015a) Association between TAP1 gene polymorphisms and alopecia areata in a Korean population. Genet Mol Res 14:18820–18827

Kim JY, Kim J, Ahn Y, Lee EJ, Hwang S, Almurayshid A, Park K, Chung HJ, Kim HJ, Lee SH (2020) Autophagy induction can regulate skin pigmentation by causing melanosome degradation in keratinocytes and melanocytes. Pigment Cell Melanoma Res 33:403–415

Kim S, Chung J, Park H, Kang S, Lim D, Byun S, Baek D, Ko H, Lew B, Baik H (2015b) Polymorphisms in the promoter regions of the CXCL1 and CXCL2 genes contribute to increased risk of alopecia areata in the Korean population. Genet Mol Res 14:9667–9674

Kim SK, Park HJ, Chung J-H, Kim JW, Seok H, Lew B-L, Sim W-Y (2014) Association between interleukin 18 polymorphisms and alopecia areata in Koreans. J Interferon Cytokine Res 34:349–353

Krummel MF, Allison JP (1996) CTLA-4 engagement inhibits IL-2 accumulation and cell cycle progression upon activation of resting T cells. J Exp Med 183:2533–2540

Kuballa P, Nolte WM, Castoreno AB, Xavier RJ (2012) Autophagy and the immune system. Annu Rev Immunol 30:611–646

Kurata H, Terashima H, Nakashima M, Okazaki T, Matsumura W, Ohno K, Saito Y, Maegaki Y, Kubota M, Nanba E (2016) Characterization of SPATA5-related encephalopathy in early childhood. Clin Genet 90:437–444

Lahore GF, Raposo B, Lagerquist M, Ohlsson C, Sabatier P, Xu B, Aoun M, James J, Cai X, Zubarev RA (2020) Vitamin D3 receptor polymorphisms regulate T cells and T cell-dependent inflammatory diseases. Proc Natl Acad Sci 117:24986–24997

Lamana A, Villares R, Seoane IV, Andrés N, Lucas P, Emery P, Vital EM, Triguero-Martínez A, Marquez A, Ortiz AM (2020) Identification of a human SOCS1 polymorphism that predicts rheumatoid arthritis severity. Front Immunol 11:1336

Lankat-Buttgereit B, Tampé R (2002) The transporter associated with antigen processing: function and implications in human diseases. Physiol Rev 82:187–204

Lavrikova EY, Nikitin AG, Kuraeva TL, Peterkova VA, Tsitlidze NM, Chistiakov DA, Nosikov VV (2011) The carriage of the type 1 diabetes-associated R262W

variant of human LNK correlates with increased proliferation of peripheral blood monocytes in diabetic patients. Pediatr Diab 12:127–132
Lee S, Kim B, Lee C, Lee W (2018) Increased prevalence of vitamin D deficiency in patients with alopecia areata: a systematic review and meta-analysis. J Eur Acad Dermatol Venereol 32:1214–1221
Lee S, Paik SH, Kim H-J, Ryu HH, Cha S, Jo SJ, Eun HC, Seo J-S, Kim J-I, Kwon OS (2013) Exomic sequencing of immune-related genes reveals novel candidate variants associated with alopecia universalis. PloS One 8:e53613
Lei Z-X, Chen W-J, Liang J-Q, Wang Y-J, Jin L, Xu C, Kang X-J (2019) The association between rs2476601 polymorphism in PTPN22 gene and risk of alopecia areata: a meta-analysis of case–control studies. Medicine 98
Leung MC, Sutton CW, Fenton DA, Tobin DJ (2010) Trichohyalin is a potential major autoantigen in human alopecia areata. J Proteome Res 9:5153–5163
Lew B-L, Cho H-R, Haw S, Kim H-J, Chung J-H, Sim W-Y (2012) Association between IL17A/IL17RA gene polymorphisms and susceptibility to alopecia areata in the Korean population. Ann Dermatol 24:61–65
Lew BL, Chung JH, Sim WY (2014a) Association between IL16 gene polymorphisms and susceptibility to alopecia areata in the K orean population. Int J Dermatol 53:319–322
Lew BL, Chung JH, Sim WY (2014b) Association between IL16 gene polymorphisms and susceptibility to alopecia areata in the Korean population. Int J Dermatol 53:319–322
Li N, Xu Y, Zhang Y, Li G, Yu T, Yao R, Zhou Y, Shen Y, Yin L, Wang X (2019) Biallelic ERBB3 loss-of-function variants are associated with a novel multisystem syndrome without congenital contracture. Orphanet J Rare Dis 14:1–10
Lien W-H, Polak L, Lin M, Lay K, Zheng D, Fuchs E (2014) In vivo transcriptional governance of hair follicle stem cells by canonical Wnt regulators. Nat Cell Biol 16:179
Lin J-X, Migone T-S, Tseng M, Friedmann M, Weatherbee JA, Zhou L, Yamauchi A, Bloom ET, Mietz J, John S (1995) The role of shared receptor motifs and common Stat proteins in the generation of cytokine pleiotropy and redundancy by IL-2, IL-4, IL-7, IL-13, and IL-15. Immunity 2:331–339
Lin M-H, Leimeister C, Gessler M, Kopan R (2000) Activation of the Notch pathway in the hair cortex leads to aberrant differentiation of the adjacent hair-shaft layers. Development 127:2421–2432
Liston A, Lesage S, Wilson J, Peltonen L, Goodnow CC (2003) Aire regulates negative selection of organ-specific T cells. Nat Immunol 4:350–354
Liu LY, King BA, Craiglow BG (2016) Health-related quality of life (HRQoL) among patients with alopecia areata (AA): a systematic review. J Am Acad Dermatol 75:806–812. e803
Ljunggren H-G, Kärre K (1990) In search of the 'missing self': MHC molecules and NK cell recognition. Immunol Today 11:237–244
Lloyd CM, Hessel EM (2010) Functions of T cells in asthma: more than just TH2 cells. Nat Rev Immunol 10:838–848
Loh SH, Moon HN, Lew BL, Sim WY (2018) Role of T helper 17 cells and T regulatory cells in alopecia areata: comparison of lesion and serum cytokine between controls and patients. J Eur Acad Dermatol Venereol 32:1028–1033
Lu D, Chen L, Shi X, Zhang X, Ling X, Chen X, Xie L, Jiang L, Ding L, He Y (2013) A functional polymorphism in interleukin-1α (IL1A) gene is associated with risk of alopecia areata in Chinese populations. Gene 521:282–286
Lu L, Barbi J, Pan F (2017) The regulation of immune tolerance by FOXP3. Nat Rev Immunol 17:703
Luo S, Rubinsztein DC (2013) BCL2L11/BIM: a novel molecular link between autophagy and apoptosis. Autophagy 9:104–105
Mahto H, Tripathy R, Das BK, Panda AK (2018) Association between vitamin D receptor polymorphisms and systemic lupus erythematosus in an Indian cohort. Int J Rheum Dis 21:468–476
Maier LM, Anderson DE, De Jager PL, Wicker LS, Hafler DA (2007) Allelic variant in CTLA4 alters T cell phosphorylation patterns. Proc Natl Acad Sci 104:18607–18612
Mak KK, Chan SY (2003) Epidermal growth factor as a biologic switch in hair growth cycle. J Biol Chem 278:26120–26126
Marks DH, Senna MM (2020) A potential role for IL-4 and IL-13 in an Alopecia Areata–Like Phenotype: A Clinical Perspective. In: (eds) Journal of investigative dermatology symposium proceedings. Elsevier, pp S58–S59
Martin P, Goldstein JD, Mermoud L, Diaz-Barreiro A, Palmer G (2021) IL-1 family antagonists in mouse and human skin inflammation. Front Immunol 12:695
Martinez-Mir A, Zlotogorski A, Gordon D, Petukhova L, Mo J, Gilliam TC, Londono D, Haynes C, Ott J, Hordinsky M (2007) Genomewide scan for linkage reveals evidence of several susceptibility loci for alopecia areata. Am J Hum Genet 80:316–328
Martinez A, Perdigones N, Cénit MC, Espino L, Varade J, Lamas J, Santiago J, Fernández-Arquero M, De La Calle H, Arroyo R (2010) Chromosomal region 16p13: further evidence of increased predisposition to immune diseases. Ann Rheum Dis 69:309–311
Matia-García I, Salgado-Goytia L, Muñoz-Valle JF, García-Arellano S, Hernández-Bello J, Salgado-Bernabé AB, Parra-Rojas I (2015) Macrophage migration inhibitory factor promoter polymorphisms (− 794 CATT5–8 and− 173 G> C): relationship with mRNA expression and soluble MIF levels in young obese subjects. Disease Markers
McDonagh A, Elliott K, Messenger A (1994) Mx protein: a new marker of type I interferon activity in the skin. Br J Dermatol 132:648
McDonagh A, Tazi-Ahnini R (2002a) Epidemiology and genetics of alopecia areata. Clin Exp Dermatol 27:405–409

McDonagh A, Tazi-Ahnini R (2002b) Epidemiology and genetics of alopecia areata. Clin Exp Dermatol Clin Dermatol 27:405–409

McElwee K, Gilhar A, Tobin D, Ramot Y, Sundberg JP, Nakamura M, Bertolini M, Inui S, Tokura Y, King L (2013) What causes alopecia areata? Exp Dermatol 22:609–626

McElwee KJ, Freyschmidt-Paul P, Hoffmann R, Kissling S, Hummel S, Vitacolonna M, Zöller M (2005) Transfer of CD8+ Cells Induces Localized Hair Loss Whereas CD4+/CD25− Cells Promote Systemic Alopecia Areata and CD4+/CD25+ Cells Blockade Disease Onset in the C3H/HeJ Mouse Model. J Investig Dermatol 124:947–957

McMullin MF, Wu C, Percy MJ, Tong W (2011) A nonsynonymous LNK polymorphism associated with idiopathic erythrocytosis. Am J Hematol 86:962

Megiorni F, Mora B, Maxia C, Gerardi M, Pizzuti A, Rossi A (2013) Cytotoxic T-lymphocyte antigen 4 (CTLA4)+49AG and CT60 gene polymorphisms in Alopecia Areata: a case–control association study in the Italian population. Arch Dermatol Res 305:665–670

Megiorni F, Pizzuti A, Mora B, Rizzuti A, Garelli V, Maxia C, Carlesimo M, Fotruna M, Delle Chiaie R, Cavaggioni G (2011a) Genetic association of HLA-DQB1 and HLA-DRB1 polymorphisms with alopecia areata in the Italian population. Br J Dermatol 165:823–827

Megiorni F, Pizzuti A, Mora B, Rizzuti A, Garelli V, Maxia C, Carlesimo M, Fotruna MC, Delle Chiaie R, Cavaggioni G, Rossi A (2011b) Genetic association of HLA-DQB1 and HLA-DRB1 polymorphisms with alopecia areata in the Italian population. Br J Dermatol 165:823–827

Meierhofer D, Halbach M, Şen NE, Gispert S, Auburger G (2016) Ataxin-2 (Atxn2)-knock-out mice show branched chain amino acids and fatty acids pathway alterations. Mol Cell Proteomics 15:1728–1739

Metelli A, Salem M, Wallace CH, Wu BX, Li A, Li X, Li Z (2018) Immunoregulatory functions and the therapeutic implications of GARP-TGF-β in inflammation and cancer. J Hematol Oncol 11:1–11

Miao Y, Kang Z, Xu F, Qi S, Sheng Y, Han Y, Hu R, Guo X, Yang Q (2013) Association analysis of the IL2RA gene with alopecia areata in a Chinese population. Dermatology 227:299–304

Mirzoyev SA, Schrum AG, Davis MD, Torgerson RR (2014) Lifetime incidence risk of Alopecia Areata estimated at 2.1 percent by Rochester Epidemiology Project, 1990–2009. J Invest Dermatol 134:1141

Miyake N, Abdel-Salam G, Yamagata T, Eid MM, Osaka H, Okamoto N, Mohamed AM, Ikeda T, Afifi HH, Piard J (2016) Clinical features of SMARCA2 duplication overlap with Coffin-Siris syndrome. Am J Med Genet A 170:2662–2670

Mizushima N (2007) Autophagy: process and function. Genes Dev 21:2861–2873

Monteleone G, Pallone F, Macdonald TT (2009) Interleukin-21 as a new therapeutic target for immune-mediated diseases. Trends Pharmacol Sci 30:441–447

Morales-Zambrano R, Bautista-Herrera LA, De la Cruz-Mosso U, Villanueva-Quintero GD, Padilla-Gutiérrez JR, Valle Y, Parra-Rojas I, Rangel-Villalobos H, Gutiérrez-Ureña SR, Muñoz-Valle JF (2014) Macrophage migration inhibitory factor (MIF) promoter polymorphisms (-794 CATT5-8 and-173 G> C): association with MIF and TNFα in psoriatic arthritis. Int J Clin Exp Med 7:2605

Moravvej H, Tabatabaei-Panah P-S, Abgoon R, Khaksar L, Sokhandan M, Tarshaei S, Ghaderian SMH, Ludwig RJ, Akbarzadeh R (2018a) Genetic variant association of PTPN22, CTLA4, IL2RA, as well as HLA frequencies in susceptibility to alopecia areata. Immunol Invest 47:666–679

Moravvej H, Tabatabaei-Panah P-S, Ebrahimi E, Esmaeili N, Ghaderian SMH, Ludwig RJ, Akbarzadeh R (2018b) TNF-α-308G/A gene polymorphism in bullous pemphigoid and alopecia areata. Hum Antibodies 26:201–207

Morgan B, Sun L, Avitahl N, Andrikopoulos K, Ikeda T, Gonzales E, Wu P, Neben S, Georgopoulos K (1997) Aiolos, a lymphoid restricted transcription factor that interacts with Ikaros to regulate lymphocyte differentiation. EMBO J 16:2004–2013

Mounsey AL, Reed SW (2009) Diagnosing and treating hair loss. Am Family Phys 80

Muller SA (1973) Alopecia: syndromes of genetic significance. J Investig Dermatol 60:475–492

Murshid A, Gong J, Calderwood SK (2012) The role of heat shock proteins in antigen cross presentation. Front Immunol 3:63

Mustelin T, Bottini N, Stanford SM (2019) The contribution of PTPN22 to rheumatic disease. Arthritis & Rheum 71:486–495

Nakahira K, Haspel JA, Rathinam VA, Lee S-J, Dolinay T, Lam HC, Englert JA, Rabinovitch M, Cernadas M, Kim HP (2011) Autophagy proteins regulate innate immune responses by inhibiting the release of mitochondrial DNA mediated by the NALP3 inflammasome. Nat Immunol 12:222–230

Nischwitz S, Cepok S, Kroner A, Wolf C, Knop M, Müller-Sarnowski F, Pfister H, Rieckmann P, Hemmer B, Ising M (2011) More CLEC16A gene variants associated with multiple sclerosis. Acta Neurol Scand 123:400–406

O'Gorman WE, Dooms H, Thorne SH, Kuswanto WF, Simonds EF, Krutzik PO, Nolan GP, Abbas AK (2009) The initial phase of an immune response functions to activate regulatory T cells. J Immunol 183:332–339

Oh J-Y, Liu QF, Hua C, Jeong HJ, Jang J-H, Jeon S, Park H-J (2020) Intranasal administration of melanin-concentrating hormone reduces stress-induced anxiety-and depressive-like behaviors in rodents. Exp Neurobiol 29:453

Oka A, Takagi A, Komiyama E, Yoshihara N, Mano S, Hosomichi K, Suzuki S, Haida Y, Motosugi N, Hatanaka T (2020) Alopecia areata susceptibility variant in MHC region impacts expressions of genes contributing to hair keratinization and is involved in hair loss. EBioMedicine 57:102810

Omer CA, Miller PJ, Diehl RE, Kral AM (1999) Identification of Tcf4 residues involved in high-affinity β-catenin binding. Biochem Biophys Res Commun 256:584–590

Ono M (2020) Control of regulatory T-cell differentiation and function by T-cell receptor signalling and Foxp3 transcription factor complexes. Immunology 160:24–37

Oosterwegel MA, Greenwald RJ, Mandelbrot DA, Lorsbach RB, Sharpe AH (1999) CTLA-4 and T cell activation. Curr Opin Immunol 11:294–300

Ostrowski LA, Hall AC, Mekhail K (2017) Ataxin-2: from RNA control to human health and disease. Genes 8:157

Pan F, Yu H, Dang EV, Barbi J, Pan X, Grosso JF, Jinasena D, Sharma SM, McCadden EM, Getnet D (2009) Eos mediates Foxp3-dependent gene silencing in CD4+ regulatory T cells. Science 325:1142–1146

Pandey R, Bakay M, Hain HS, Strenkowski B, Elsaqa BZ, Roizen JD, Kushner JA, Orange JS, Hakonarson H (2018) CLEC16A regulates splenocyte and NK cell function in part through MEK signaling. PLoS One 13:e0203952

Pandey R, Bakay M, Hain HS, Strenkowski B, Yermakova A, Kushner JA, Orange JS, Hakonarson H (2019) The autoimmune disorder susceptibility gene CLEC16A restrains NK Cell function in YTS NK cell line and Clec16a knockout mice. Front Immunol 10:68

Parodi C, Hardman JA, Allavena G, Marotta R, Catelani T, Bertolini M, Paus R, Grimaldi B (2018) Autophagy is essential for maintaining the growth of a human (mini-) organ: Evidence from scalp hair follicle organ culture. PLoS Biol 16:e2002864

Parrish-Novak J, Dillon SR, Nelson A, Hammond A, Sprecher C, Gross JA, Johnston J, Madden K, Xu W, West J (2000) Interleukin 21 and its receptor are involved in NK cell expansion and regulation of lymphocyte function. Nature 408:57–63

Paus R, Bulfone-Paus S, Bertolini M (2018) Hair follicle immune privilege revisited: the key to alopecia areata management. In: (eds) Journal of Investigative Dermatology Symposium Proceedings. Elsevier, pp S12–S17

Paus R, Ito N, Takigawa M, Ito T (2003) The hair follicle and immune privilege. In: (eds) Journal of investigative dermatology symposium proceedings. Elsevier, pp 188–194

Paus R, Slominski A, Czarnetzki B (1993) Is alopecia areata an autoimmune-response against melanogenesis-related proteins, exposed by abnormal MHC class I expression in the anagen hair bulb? Yale J Biol Med 66:541

Pelleri MC, Cicchini E, Petersen MB, Tranebjærg L, Mattina T, Magini P, Antonaros F, Caracausi M, Vitale L, Locatelli C (2019) Partial trisomy 21 map: ten cases further supporting the highly restricted Down syndrome critical region (HR-DSCR) on human chromosome 21. Mol Genet Genom Med 7:e797

Penke B, Bogár F, Crul T, Sántha M, Tóth ME, Vígh L (2018) Heat shock proteins and autophagy pathways in neuroprotection: from molecular bases to pharmacological interventions. Int J Mol Sci 19:325

Perdomo J, Holmes M, Chong B, Crossley M (2000) Eos and pegasus, two members of the Ikaros family of proteins with distinct DNA binding activities. J Biol Chem 275:38347–38354

Peterson P, Org T, Rebane A (2008) Transcriptional regulation by AIRE: molecular mechanisms of central tolerance. Nat Rev Immunol 8:948–957

Petukhova L, Christiano AM (2016) Functional interpretation of genome-wide association study evidence in alopecia areata. J Invest Dermatol 136:314

Petukhova L, Duvic M, Hordinsky M, Norris D, Price V, Shimomura Y, Kim H, Singh P, Lee A, Chen WV (2010) Genome-wide association study in alopecia areata implicates both innate and adaptive immunity. Nature 466:113–117

Petukhova L, Patel AV, Rigo RK, Bian L, Verbitsky M, Sanna-Cherchi S, Erjavec SO, Abdelaziz AR, Cerise JE, Jabbari A (2020) Integrative analysis of rare copy number variants and gene expression data in alopecia areata implicates an aetiological role for autophagy. Exp Dermatol 29:243–253

Pforr J, Blaumeiser B, Becker T, Freudenberg-Hua Y, Hanneken S, Eigelshoven S, Cuyt I, De Weert J, Lambert J, Kruse R (2006) Investigation of the p. Ser278Arg polymorphism of the autoimmune regulator (AIRE) gene in alopecia areata. Tissue Antigens 68:58–61

Philpott M, Sanders D, Bowen J, Kealey T (1996) Effects of interleukins, colony-stimulating factor and tumour necrosis factor on human hair follicle growth in vitro: a possible role for interleukin-1 and tumour necrosis factor-α in alopecia areata. Br J Dermatol 135:942–948

Pielberg GR, Golovko A, Sundström E, Curik I, Lennartsson J, Seltenhammer MH, Druml T, Binns M, Fitzsimmons C, Lindgren G (2008) A cis-acting regulatory mutation causes premature hair graying and susceptibility to melanoma in the horse. Nat Genet 40:1004–1009

Pociot F, Mølvig J, Wogensen L, Worsaae H, Nerup J (1992) A Taql polymorphism in the human interleukin-1β (IL-1β) gene correlates with IL-1β secretion in vitro. Eur J Clin Invest 22:396–402

Powell B, Passmore E, Nesci A, Dunn S (1998) The Notch signalling pathway in hair growth. Mech Dev 78:189–192

Powell MD, Read KA, Sreekumar BK, Oestreich KJ (2019) Ikaros zinc finger transcription factors: regulators of cytokine signaling pathways and CD4+ T helper cell differentiation. Front Immunol 10:1299

Powis SJ, Deverson EV, Coadweil WJ, Ciruela A, Huskisson NS, Smith H, Butcher GW, Howard JC

(1992) Effect of polymorphism of an MHC-linked transporter on the peptides assembled in a class I molecule. Nature 357:211–215

Pratt CH, King LE, Messenger AG, Christiano AM, Sundberg JP (2017) Alopecia areata. Nat Rev Dis Primers 3:1–17

Prie B, Voiculescu V, Ionescu-Bozdog O, Petrutescu B, Iosif L, Gaman L, Clatici V, Stoian I, Giurcaneanu C (2015) Oxidative stress and alopecia areata. J Med Life 8:43

Qian Y, Wang G, Xue F, Chen L, Wang Y, Tang L, Yang H (2017) Genetic association between TAP1 and TAP2 polymorphisms and ankylosing spondylitis: a systematic review and meta-analysis. Inflamm Res 66:653–661

Qidwai T (2016) Chemokine genetic polymorphism in human health and disease. Immunol Lett 176:128–138

Rajabi F, Amoli MM, Robati RM, Almasi-Nasrabadi M, Jabalameli N (2019a) Macrophage migration inhibitory factor polymorphism (rs755622) in alopecia areata: a possible role in disease prevention. Arch Dermatol Res 311:589–594

Rajabi F, Amoli MM, Robati RM, Almasi-Nasrabadi M, Jabalameli N, Moravvej H (2019b) The association between genetic variation in Wnt transcription factor TCF7L2 (TCF4) and alopecia areata. Immunol Invest 48:555–562

Rajabi F, Drake L, Senna M, Rezaei N (2018a) Alopecia areata: a review of disease pathogenesis. Br J Dermatol 179:1033–1048

Rajabi F, Drake L, Senna M, Rezaei N (2018b) Alopecia areata: a review of disease pathogenesis. Br J Dermatol

Rajaiah R, Moudgil KD (2009) Heat-shock proteins can promote as well as regulate autoimmunity. Autoimmun Rev 8:388–393

Ramkumar A, Murthy D, Raja DA, Singh A, Krishnan A, Khanna S, Vats A, Thukral L, Sharma P, Sivasubbu S (2017) Classical autophagy proteins LC3B and ATG4B facilitate melanosome movement on cytoskeletal tracks. Autophagy 13:1331–1347

Ramot Y, Marzani B, Pinto D, Sorbellini E, Rinaldi F (2018) IL-17 inhibition: is it the long-awaited savior for alopecia areata? Arch Dermatol Res 310:383–390

Rathmell JC, Lindsten T, Zong W-X, Cinalli RM, Thompson CB (2002) Deficiency in Bak and Bax perturbs thymic selection and lymphoid homeostasis. Nat Immunol 3:932–939

Redler S, Albert F, Brockschmidt F, Herold C, Hanneken S, Eigelshoven S, Giehl K, Kruse R, Lutz G, Wolff H (2012) Investigation of selected cytokine genes suggests that IL2RA and the TNF/LTA locus are risk factors for severe alopecia areata. Br J Dermatol 167:1360–1365

Reilly R, McNulty H, Pentieva K, Strain J, Ward M (2014) MTHFR 677TT genotype and disease risk: is there a modulating role for B-vitamins? Proc Nutrit Soc 73:47–56

Rencz F, Gulácsi L, Péntek M, Wikonkál N, Baji P, Brodszky V (2016) Alopecia areata and health-related quality of life: a systematic review and meta-analysis. Br J Dermatol 175:561–571

Reynolds AJ, Lawrence C, Cserhalmi-Friedman PB, Christiano AM, Jahoda CA (1999) Trans-gender induction of hair follicles. Nature 402:33–34

Rivas MN, Chatila TA (2016) Regulatory T cells in allergic diseases. J Aller Clin Immunol 138:639–652

Robinson J, Halliwell JA, Hayhurst JD, Flicek P, Parham P, Marsh SG (2015) The IPD and IMGT/HLA database: allele variant databases. Nucleic Acids Res 43:D423–D431

Roh T-Y, Cuddapah S, Cui K, Zhao K (2006) The genomic landscape of histone modifications in human T cells. Proc Natl Acad Sci 103:15782–15787

Ruiz-Ballesteros AI, Meza-Meza MR, Vizmanos-Lamotte B, Parra-Rojas I, de la Cruz-Mosso U (2020) Association of vitamin D metabolism gene polymorphisms with autoimmunity: evidence in population genetic studies. Int J Mol Sci 21:9626

Sachin P, Gadani S, Cronk J, Norris G, Kipnis J (2012) Interleukin-4: a cytokine to remember. J Immunol 189:4213–4421

Saeedi M, Amoli M, Robati R, Sayahpour F, Namazi N, Toossi P (2013) Macrophage migration inhibitory factor gene polymorphism is not associated with pemphigus vulgaris in Iranian patients. J Eur Acad Dermatol Venereol 27:1127–1131

Safavi KH, Muller SA, Suman VJ, Moshell AN, Melton LJ (1995) Incidence of alopecia areata in Olmsted County, Minnesota, 1975 through 1989. In: (eds) Mayo clinic proceedings. Elsevier, pp 628–633

Salem SA, Asaad MK, Elsayed SB, Sehsah HM (2016) Evaluation of macrophage migration inhibitory factor (MIF) levels in serum and lesional skin of patients with alopecia areata. International Journal of Dermatology.

Salinas-Santander MA, Cantu-Salinas CS, Ocampo-Candiani J, Suarez-Valencia VdJ, Ramirez-Guerrero JG, Sanchez-Dominguez CN (2020) CTLA4+ 49AG (rs231775) and CT60 (rs3087243) gene variants are not associated with alopecia areata in a Mexican population from Monterrey Mexico. An Bras Dermatol 95:283–288

Salinas-Santander M, Sánchez-Domínguez C, Cantú-Salinas C, Gonzalez-Cárdenas H, Cepeda-Nieto AC, Cerda-Flores RM, Ortiz-López R, Ocampo-Candiani J (2015) Association between PTPN22 C1858T polymorphism and alopecia areata risk. Exp Ther Med 10:1953–1958

Schroecksnadel K, Frick B, Wirleitner B, Winkler C, Schennach H, Fuchs D (2004) Moderate hyperhomocysteinemia and immune activation. Curr Pharm Biotechnol 5:107–118

Sekiyama A, Ueda H, Kashiwamura S-i, Nishida K, Kawai K, Teshima-kondo S, Rokutan K, Okamura H (2005) IL-18; a cytokine translates a stress into medical science. J Med Invest 52:236–239

Seleit I, Bakry OA, Abd El Gayed E, Gawad AED (2018) Polymorphism of FAS and FAS ligand genes in alopecia areata: a case–control study in Egyptian population. Indian J Dermatol 63:220

Seleit IA, Mohamed OAB, El-Hefnawy SM, Azooz SM (2021) Interleukin 17A gene polymorphism in alopecia areata. Menoufia Medical Journal 34:23

Seok H, Jeon HS, Park HJ, Kim SK, Choi JH, Lew B-L, Chung J-H, Sim W-Y (2014a) Association of HSPA1B SNP rs6457452 with alopecia areata in the Korean population. Immunol Invest 43:212–223

Seok H, Suh DW, Jo B, Lee H-B, Jang HM, Park HK, Lew B-L, Chung J-H, Sim W-Y (2014b) Association between TLR1 polymorphisms and alopecia areata. Autoimmunity 47:372–377

Shehata WA, Maraee A, Kamal H, Tayel N, Azmy R (2020) Protein tyrosine phosphatase nonreceptor type 22 gene polymorphism in alopecia areata: does it have an association with disease severity? J Cosmet Dermatol 19:3138–3144

Shi Q, Duvic M, Osei JS, Hordinsky MK, Norris DA, Price VH, Amos CI, Christiano AM, Mendoza TR (2013) Health-Related Quality of Life (HRQoL) in alopecia areata patients—a secondary analysis of the national alopecia areata registry data. In: (eds) Journal of investigative dermatology symposium proceedings. Nature Publishing Group, pp S49–S50

Shi Y (2004) Beyond skin color: emerging roles of melanin-concentrating hormone in energy homeostasis and other physiological functions. Peptides 25:1605–1611

Shimizu T, Hizawa N, Honda A, Zhao Y, Abe R, Watanabe H, Nishihira J, Nishimura M, Shimizu H (2005) Promoter region polymorphism of macrophage migration inhibitory factor is strong risk factor for young onset of extensive alopecia areata. Genes Immun 6:285–289

Shimizu T, Mizue Y, Abe R, Watanabe H, Shimizu H (2002) Increased macrophage migration inhibitory factor (MIF) in the sera of patients with extensive alopecia areata. J Invest Dermatol 118:555

Sibley K, Rollinson S, Allan JM, Smith AG, Law GR, Roddam PL, Skibola CF, Smith MT, Morgan GJ (2003) Functional FAS promoter polymorphisms are associated with increased risk of acute myeloid leukemia. Can Res 63:4327–4330

Sims JE, Nicklin M, Bazan JF, Barton JL, Busfield SJ, Ford JE, Kastelein RA, Kumar S, Lin H, Mulero JJ (2001) A new nomenclature for IL-1-family genes. Trends Immunol 22:536–537

Sinha K, Das J, Pal PB, Sil PC (2013) Oxidative stress: the mitochondria-dependent and mitochondria-independent pathways of apoptosis. Arch Toxicol 87:1157–1180

Soleimanpour SA, Gupta A, Bakay M, Ferrari AM, Groff DN, Fadista J, Spruce LA, Kushner JA, Groop L, Seeholzer SH (2014) The diabetes susceptibility gene Clec16a regulates mitophagy. Cell 157:1577–1590

Souza ASCd, Gonçalves LB, Lepique AP, Araujo-Souza D, Savio P (2020) The role of autophagy in tumor immunology-complex mechanisms that may be explored therapeutically. Front Oncol 10:2691

Speiser JJ, Mondo D, Mehta V, Marcial SA, Kini A, Hutchens KA (2019) Regulatory T-cells in alopecia areata. J Cutan Pathol 46:653–658

Srivastava P (2002) Roles of heat-shock proteins in innate and adaptive immunity. Nat Rev Immunol 2:185–194

Steinle A, Li P, Morris DL, Groh V, Lanier LL, Strong RK, Spies T (2001) Interactions of human NKG2D with its ligands MICA, MICB, and homologs of the mouse RAE-1 protein family. Immunogenetics 53:279–287

Stockis J, Colau D, Coulie PG, Lucas S (2009) Membrane protein GARP is a receptor for latent TGF-β on the surface of activated human Treg. Eur J Immunol 39:3315–3322

Strober BE, Siu K, Alexis AF, Kim G, Washenik K, Sinha A, Shupack JL (2005) Etanercept does not effectively treat moderate to severe alopecia areata: an open-label study. J Am Acad Dermatol 52:1082–1084

Su AI, Cooke MP, Ching KA, Hakak Y, Walker JR, Wiltshire T, Orth AP, Vega RG, Sapinoso LM, Moqrich A (2002) Large-scale analysis of the human and mouse transcriptomes. Proc Natl Acad Sci 99:4465–4470

Suárez-Fariñas M, Ungar B, Noda S, Shroff A, Mansouri Y, Fuentes-Duculan J, Czernik A, Zheng X, Estrada YD, Xu H (2015) Alopecia areata profiling shows TH1, TH2, and IL-23 cytokine activation without parallel TH17/TH22 skewing. J Aller Clin Immunol 136:1277–1287

Subramanya RD, Coda AB, Sinha AA (2010) Transcriptional profiling in alopecia areata defines immune and cell cycle control related genes within disease-specific signatures. Genomics 96:146–153

Tabatabaei-Panah P-S, Moravvej H, Delpasand S, Jafari M, Sepehri S, Abgoon R, Ludwig RJ, Akbarzadeh R (2020) IL12B and IL23R polymorphisms are associated with alopecia areata. Genes Immun 21:203–210

Tafazzoli A, Forstner AJ, Broadley D, Hofmann A, Redler S, Petukhova L, Giehl KA, Kruse R, Blaumeiser B, Böhm M (2018) Genome-wide microRNA analysis implicates miR-30b/d in the etiology of alopecia areata. J Investig Dermatol 138:549–556

Taghiabadi G, Talebzade T, Altafi D, Hosseini I, Hojatiyan H, Taghizadeh M, Houshmand M, Sadeghi S (2018) Identification of single nucleotide polymorphisms as markers of genetic susceptibility for alopecia areata disease risk. J Inf Mol Biol 6:28–35

Takahashi T, Tagami T, Yamazaki S, Uede T, Shimizu J, Sakaguchi N, Mak TW, Sakaguchi S (2000) Immunologic self-tolerance maintained by CD25+ CD4+ regulatory T cells constitutively expressing cytotoxic T lymphocyte–associated antigen 4. J Exp Med 192:303–310

Takaki S, Sauer K, Iritani BM, Chien S, Ebihara Y, Tsuji K-i, Takatsu K, Perlmutter RM (2000) Control of B cell production by the adaptor protein Lnk: definition of a conserved family of signal-modulating proteins. Immunity 13:599–609

Tanaka Y, Komatsu T, Shigemi H, Yamauchi T, Fujii Y (2014) BIM EL is a key effector molecule in oxidative stress-mediated apoptosis in acute myeloid leukemia cells when combined with arsenic trioxide and buthionine sulfoximine. BMC Cancer 14:1–11

Tanemura A, Oiso N, Nakano M, Itoi S, Kawada A, Katayama I (2013) Alopecia areata: infiltration of Th17 cells in the dermis, particularly around hair follicles. Dermatology 226:333–336

Tarlow JK, Clay FE, Cork MJ, Blakemore AI, McDonagh AJ, Messenger AG, Duff GW (1994) Severity of alopecia areata is associated with a polymorphism in the interleukin-1 receptor antagonist gene. J Investig Dermatol 103:387–390

Tazi-Ahnini R, Cork M, Wengraf D, Wilson A, Gawkrodger D, Birch M, Messenger A, McDonagh A (2003) Notch4, a non-HLA gene in the MHC is strongly associated with the most severe form of alopecia areata. Hum Genet 112:400–403

Tazi-Ahnini R, di Giovine FS, McDonagh AJ, Messenger AG, Amadou C, Cox A, Duff GW, Cork MJ (2000) Structure and polymorphism of the human gene for the interferon-induced p78 protein (MX1): evidence of association with alopecia areata in the Down syndrome region. Hum Genet 106:639–645

Tazi-Ahnini R, McDonagh AJ, Cox A, Messenger AG, Britton JE, Ward SJ, Båvik CO, Duff GW, Cork MJ (2001) Association analysis of IL1A and IL1B variants in alopecia areata. Heredity 87:215–219

Tazi-Ahnini R, Cork M, Gawkrodger D, Birch M, Wengraf D, McDonagh A, Messenger A (2002a) Role of the autoimmune regulator (AIRE) gene in alopecia areata: strong association of a potentially functional AIRE polymorphism with alopecia universalis. Tissue Antigens 60:489–495

Tazi-Ahnini R, Cox A, McDonagh A, Nicklin M, Di Giovine F, Timms J, Messenger A, Dimitropoulou P, Duff G, Cork M (2002b) Genetic analysis of the interleukin-1 receptor antagonist and its homologue IL-1L1 in alopecia areata: strong severity association and possible gene interaction. Eur J Immunogenet 29:25–30

Tazi-Ahnini R, Cox A, McDonagh A, Nicklin M, Di Giovine F, Timms J, Messenger A, Dimitropoulou P, Duff G, Cork M (2002c) Genetic analysis of the interleukin-1 receptor antagonist and its homologue IL-1L1 in alopecia areata: strong severity association and possible gene interaction‡. Eur J Immunogenet 29:25–30

Tembhre M, Sharma V (2013) T-helper and regulatory T-cell cytokines in the peripheral blood of patients with active alopecia areata. Br J Dermatol 169:543–548

Thanomkitti K, Kanlaya R, Fong-Ngern K, Kapincharanon C, Sueksakit K, Chanchaem P, Thuangtong R, Thongboonkerd V (2018) Differential proteomics of lesional vs. non-lesional biopsies revealed non-immune mechanisms of alopecia areata. Sci Rep 8:1–13

Tivol EA, Borriello F, Schweitzer AN, Lynch WP, Bluestone JA, Sharpe AH (1995) Loss of CTLA-4 leads to massive lymphoproliferation and fatal multiorgan tissue destruction, revealing a critical negative regulatory role of CTLA-4. Immunity 3:541–547

Tojo G, Fujimura T, Kawano M, Ogasawara K, Kambayashi Y, Furudate S, Mizuashi M, Aiba S (2013) Comparison of interleukin-17-producing cells in different clinical types of alopecia areata. Dermatology 227:78–82

Toraih EA, Ameen HM, Hussein MH, Youssef Elabd AA, Mohamed AM, Abdel-Gawad AR, Fawzy MS (2020) Association of autoimmune regulator gene Rs2075876 variant, but not gene expression with alopecia areata in males: a case–control study. Immunol Invest 49:146–165

Tosti A, Whiting D, Iorizzo M, Pazzaglia M, Misciali C, Vincenzi C, Micali G (2008) The role of scalp dermoscopy in the diagnosis of alopecia areata incognita. J Am Acad Dermatol 59:64–67

Tran DQ, Andersson J, Wang R, Ramsey H, Unutmaz D, Shevach EM (2009) GARP (LRRC32) is essential for the surface expression of latent TGF-β on platelets and activated FOXP3+ regulatory T cells. Proc Natl Acad Sci 106:13445–13450

Trautman S, Thompson M, Roberts J, Thompson CT (2009) Melanocytes: a possible autoimmune target in alopecia areata. J Am Acad Dermatol 61:529–530

Triantos C, Aggeletopoulou I, Kalafateli M, Spantidea PI, Vourli G, Diamantopoulou G, Tapratzi D, Michalaki M, Manolakopoulos S, Gogos C (2018) Prognostic significance of vitamin D receptor (VDR) gene polymorphisms in liver cirrhosis. Sci Rep 8:1–14

Trowsdale J, Hanson I, Mockridge I, Beck S, Townsendt A, Kelly A (1990) Sequences encoded in the class II region of the MHC related to the 'ABC' superfamily of transporters. Nature 348:741–744

Tsai S, Santamaria P (2013) MHC class II polymorphisms, autoreactive T-cells, and autoimmunity. Front Immunol 4:321

Tukaj S, Kaminski M (2019) Heat shock proteins in the therapy of autoimmune diseases: too simple to be true? Cell Stress Chaperones 24:475–479

Ueda H, Howson JM, Esposito L, Heward J, Chamberlain G, Rainbow DB, Hunter KM, Smith AN, Di Genova G, Herr MH (2003) Association of the T-cell regulatory gene CTLA4 with susceptibility to autoimmune disease. Nature 423:506–511

Urbanavicius J, Lagos P, López X, Torterolo P, Scorza C (2018) MCH and depression. In (eds) Melanin-concentrating hormone and sleep. Springer, pp 195–206

van Bruggen R, Köker MY, Jansen M, van Houdt M, Roos D, Kuijpers TW, van den Berg TK (2010) Human NLRP3 inflammasome activation is Nox1-4 independent. Blood J Am Soc Hematol 115:5398–5400

Van der Steen P, Traupe H, Happle R, Boezeman J, Sträter R, Hamm H (1992) The genetic risk for alopecia areata in first degree relatives of severely affected patients An estimate. Acta Derm Venereol 72:373–375

Vang T, Landskron J, Viken MK, Oberprieler N, Torgersen KM, Mustelin T, Tasken K, Tautz L, Rickert RC, Lie BA (2013) The autoimmune-predisposing variant of lymphoid tyrosine phosphatase favors T helper 1 responses. Hum Immunol 74:574–585

Vang T, Miletic AV, Bottini N, Mustelin T (2007) Protein tyrosine phosphatase PTPN22 in human autoimmunity. Autoimmunity 40:453–461

Velazquez L, Cheng AM, Fleming HE, Furlonger C, Vesely S, Bernstein A, Paige CJ, Pawson T (2002) Cytokine signaling and hematopoietic homeostasis are disrupted in Lnk-deficient mice. J Exp Med 195:1599–1611

Volpe E, Sambucci M, Battistini L, Borsellino G (2016) Fas–fas ligand: checkpoint of t cell functions in multiple sclerosis. Front Immunol 7:382

Wallace CH, Wu BX, Salem M, Ansa-Addo EA, Metelli A, Sun S, Gilkeson G, Shlomchik MJ, Liu B, Li Z (2018) B lymphocytes confer immune tolerance via cell surface GARP-TGF-β complex. JCI Insight 3

Walter S, Buchner J (2002) Molecular chaperones—cellular machines for protein folding. Angew Chem Int Ed 41:1098–1113

Wang E, Chong K, Yu M, Akhoundsadegh N, Granville DJ, Shapiro J, McElwee KJ (2013) Development of autoimmune hair loss disease alopecia areata is associated with cardiac dysfunction in C3H/HeJ mice. PloS One 8:e62935

Wang EH, Khosravi-Maharlooei M, Jalili RB, Yu R, Ghahary A, Shapiro J, McElwee KJ (2015) Transfer of alopecia areata to C3H/HeJ mice using cultured lymph node–derived cells. J Invest Dermatol

Wang R, Kozhaya L, Mercer F, Khaitan A, Fujii H, Unutmaz D (2009) Expression of GARP selectively identifies activated human FOXP3+ regulatory T cells. Proc Natl Acad Sci 106:13439–13444

Wang R, Zhu J, Dong X, Shi M, Lu C, Springer TA (2012) GARP regulates the bioavailability and activation of TGFβ. Mol Biol Cell 23:1129–1139

Wang T, Secombes CJ (2015) The evolution of IL-4 and IL-13 and their receptor subunits. Cytokine 75:8–13

Wang X, Marr AK, Breitkopf T, Leung G, Hao J, Wang E, Kwong N, Akhoundsadegh N, Chen L, Mui A (2014) Hair follicle mesenchyme-associated PD-L1 regulates T-cell activation induced apoptosis: a potential mechanism of immune privilege. J Investig Dermatol 134:736–745

Wen A-q, Wang J, Feng K, Zhu P-f, Wang Z-g, Jiang J-x (2006) Effects of haplotypes in the interleukin 1β promoter on lipopolysaccharide-induced interleukin 1β expression. Shock 26:25–30

Wengraf D, McDonagh A, Lovewell T, Vasilopoulos Y, Macdonald-Hull S, Cork M, Messenger A, Tazi-Ahnini R (2008) Genetic analysis of autoimmune regulator haplotypes in alopecia areata. Tissue Antigens 71:206–212

Wieczorek M, Abualrous ET, Sticht J, Álvaro-Benito M, Stolzenberg S, Noé F, Freund C (2017) Major histocompatibility complex (MHC) class I and MHC class II proteins: conformational plasticity in antigen presentation. Front Immunol 8:292

Wieten L, Broere F, van der Zee R, Koerkamp EK, Wagenaar J, van Eden W (2007) Cell stress induced HSP are targets of regulatory T cells: a role for HSP inducing compounds as anti-inflammatory immunomodulators? FEBS Lett 581:3716–3722

Wikramanayake TC, Alvarez-Connelly E, Simon J, Mauro LM, Guzman J, Elgart G, Schachner LA, Chen J, Plano LR, Jimenez JJ (2010) Heat treatment increases the incidence of alopecia areata in the C3H/HeJ mouse model. Cell Stress Chaperones 15:985–991

Wikramanayake TC, Villasante AC, Mauro LM, Perez CI, Schachner LA, Jimenez JJ (2012) Prevention and treatment of alopecia areata with quercetin in the C3H/HeJ mouse model. Cell Stress Chaperones 17:267–274

Wing K, Onishi Y, Prieto-Martin P, Yamaguchi T, Miyara M, Fehervari Z, Nomura T, Sakaguchi S (2008) CTLA-4 control over Foxp3+ regulatory T cell function. Science 322:271–275

Witkowska-Toboa AM, Szczerkowska-Dobosz A, Nedoszytko B, Roszkiewicz J (2004) Polymorphism of the TAP1 gene in Polish patients with psoriasis vulgaris. J Appl Genet 45:391–393

Wu C, Orozco C, Boyer J, Leglise M, Goodale J, Batalov S, Hodge CL, Haase J, Janes J, Huss JW (2009) BioGPS: an extensible and customizable portal for querying and organizing gene annotation resources. Genome Biol 10:1–8

Wu J, Metz C, Xu X, Abe R, Gibson AW, Edberg JC, Cooke J, Xie F, Cooper GS, Kimberly RP (2003) A novel polymorphic CAAT/enhancer-binding protein β element in the FasL gene promoter alters Fas ligand expression: a candidate background gene in African American systemic lupus erythematosus patients. J Immunol 170:132–138

Xiao F-L, Zhou F-S, Liu J-B, Yan K-L, Cui Y, Gao M, Liang Y-H, Sun L-D, Zhou S-M, Zhu Y-G (2005) Association of HLA-DQA1 and DQB1 alleles with alolpecia areata in Chinese Hans. Arch Dermatol Res 297:201–209

Xiao F-L, Yang S, Yan K-l, Cui Y, Liang Y-H, Zhou F-S, Du W-H, Gao M, Sun L-D, Fan X (2006a) Association of HLA class I alleles with aloplecia areata in Chinese Hans. J Dermatol Sci 41:109–119

Xiao FL, Yang S, Liu JB, He PP, Yang J, Cui Y, Yan KL, Gao M, Liang YH, Zhang XJ (2006b) The epidemiology of childhood alopecia areata in China: a study of 226 patients. Pediatr Dermatol 23:13–18

Xiao FL, Ye DQ, Yang S, Zhou FS, Zhou SM, Zhu YG, Liang YH, Ren YQ, Zhang XJ (2006c) Association of HLA haplotype with alopecia areata in Chinese Hans. J Eur Acad Dermatol Venereol 20:1207–1213

Xing L, Dai Z, Jabbari A, Cerise JE, Higgins CA, Gong W, De Jong A, Harel S, DeStefano GM, Rothman L (2014) Alopecia areata is driven by cytotoxic T lymphocytes and is reversed by JAK inhibition. Nat Med 20:1043–1049

Xiong Y, Liu Y, Song Z, Hao F, Yang X (2014) Identification of Wnt/β-catenin signaling pathway in dermal papilla cells of human scalp hair follicles: TCF 4 regulates the proliferation and secretory activity of dermal papilla cell. J Dermatol 41:84–91

Yamamoto K, Fujiyama Y, Andoh A, Bamba T, Okabe H (2001) Oxidative stress increases MICA and MICB gene expression in the human colon carcinoma cell line (CaCo-2). Biochimica et Biophysica Acta (BBA)-General Subjects 1526:10–12

Yamamoto K, Venida A, Perera RM, Kimmelman AC (2020) Selective autophagy of MHC-I promotes immune evasion of pancreatic cancer. Autophagy 16:1524–1525

Yang Z, Wilkie-Grantham RP, Yanagi T, Shu C-W, Matsuzawa S-i, Reed JC (2015) ATG4B (Autophagin-1) phosphorylation modulates autophagy. J Biol Chem 290:26549–26561

Yenin J, Serarslan G, Yönden Z, Ulutaş K (2015) Investigation of oxidative stress in patients with alopecia areata and its relationship with disease severity, duration, recurrence and pattern. Clin Exp Dermatol 40:617–621

Younan DNA, Agamia N, Elshafei A, Ebeid N (2015) Serum level of macrophage migration inhibitory factor (MIF) in Egyptians with alopecia areata and its relation to the clinical severity of the disease. J Clin Lab Anal 29:74–79

Yun WJ, Kim E-Y, Park J-E, Jo SY, Bang SH, Chang E-J, Chang SE (2016) Microtubule-associated protein light chain 3 is involved in melanogenesis via regulation of MITF expression in melanocytes. Sci Rep 6:1–11

Zainodini N, Hassanshahi G, Kazemi Arababadi M, Khorramdelazad H, Mirzaei A (2013) Differential expression of CXCL1, CXCL9 CXCL10 and CXCL12 chemokines in alopecia areata. Iran J Immunol 10:40–46

Zeng J, Deng S, Wang Y, Li P, Tang L, Pang Y (2017) Specific inhibition of Acyl-CoA oxidase-1 by an acetylenic acid improves hepatic lipid and reactive oxygen species (ROS) metabolism in rats fed a high fat diet. J Biol Chem 292:3800–3809

Zhang SL, Chabod J, Penfornis A, Reviron D, Tiberghien P, Wendling D, Toussirot E (2002) TAP1 and TAP2 gene polymorphism in rheumatoid arthritis in a population in eastern France. Eur J Immunogenet 29:241–249

Zheng M, Ren Y (2017) The genetic basis of pigmentation in alopecia areata. Exp Dermatol 26:542–543

Zhernakova A, Elbers CC, Ferwerda B, Romanos J, Trynka G, Dubois PC, De Kovel CG, Franke L, Oosting M, Barisani D (2010) Evolutionary and functional analysis of celiac risk loci reveals SH2B3 as a protective factor against bacterial infection. Am J Hum Genet 86:970–977

Zingoni A, Molfetta R, Fionda C, Soriani A, Paolini R, Cippitelli M, Cerboni C, Santoni A (2018) NKG2D and its ligands: "one for all, all for one." Front Immunol 9:476

Zöller M, McElwee KJ, Engel P, Hoffmann R (2002) Transient CD44 variant isoform expression and reduction in CD4+/CD25+ regulatory T cells in C3H/HeJ mice with alopecia areata. J Investig Dermatol 118:983–992

Zuo J, Willcox BE, Moss P (2017) ULBPs: regulators of human lymphocyte stress recognition. Oncotarget 8:106157

The Immunogenetics of Vitiligo: An Approach Toward Revealing the Secret of Depigmentation

Mitesh Dwivedi, Naresh C. Laddha, and Rasheedunnisa Begum

Abstract

Vitiligo is a hypomelanotic skin disease and considered to be of autoimmune origin due to breaching of immunological self-tolerance, resulting in inappropriate immune responses against melanocytes. The development of vitiligo includes a strong heritable component. Different strategies ranging from linkage studies to genome-wide association studies are used to explore the genetic factors responsible for the disease. Several vitiligo loci containing the respective genes have been identified which contribute to vitiligo and genetic variants for some of the genes are still unknown. These genes include mainly the proteins that play a role in immune regulation and a few other genes important for apoptosis and regulation of melanocyte functions. Despite the available data on genetic variants and risk alleles which influence the biological processes, only few immunological pathways have been found responsible for all ranges of severity and clinical manifestations of vitiligo. However, studies have concluded that vitiligo is of autoimmune origin and manifests due to complex interactions in immune components and their inappropriate response toward melanocytes. The genes involved in the immune regulation and processing the melanocytes antigen and its presentation can serve as effective immune-therapeutics that can target specific immunological pathways involved in vitiligo. This chapter highlights those immune-regulatory genes involved in vitiligo susceptibility and loci identified to date and their implications in vitiligo pathogenesis.

Keywords

Immunogenetics, vitiligo, autoimmunity · Genome-wide association study (GWAS) · Candidate gene association · Single nucleotide polymorphism (SNP) · Cytokines

M. Dwivedi (✉)
C. G. Bhakta Institute of Biotechnology, Uka Tarsadia University, Tarsadi, Surat 394350, Gujarat, India

N. C. Laddha
In Vitro Specialty Lab Pvt. Ltd, 205-210, Golden Triangle, Navrangpura, Ahmedabad 380009, Gujarat, India

R. Begum
Department of Biochemistry, The Maharaja Sayajirao University of Baroda, Vadodara 390002, Gujarat, India

1 Introduction

Vitiligo is an acquired hypomelanotic depigmenting skin disease resulting due to loss of functional melanocytes in the epidermis (Guerra et al. 2010). The depigmentation extent varies from focal to generalized and disease onset can be gradual or sudden (Glassman 2011). The

N. Rezaei and F. Rajabi (eds.), *The Immunogenetics of Dermatologic Diseases*, Advances in Experimental Medicine and Biology 1367,
https://doi.org/10.1007/978-3-030-92616-8_3

prevalence of vitiligo is 0.5–1% in the world population (Alikhan et al. 2011; Taïeb and Picardo 2007), whereas the worldwide prevalence of vitiligo in children/adolescents and adults is 0.5–2% (Krüger and Schallreuter 2012). The highest prevalence of vitiligo was reported in Gujarat and Rajasthan states of India i.e., ~8.8% (Valia and Dutta 1996). The disease manifests mainly on the face, lips, feet, and arms (Fig. 1), irrespective of age and gender (Nordlund et al. 2007). In 50% of cases, vitiligo manifests before 20 years of age and in 25% of cases, the onset of vitiligo is before 14 years of age (Kakourou 2009). Vitiligo causes less self-esteem, psychological stress, social turmoil, and matrimonial problems in the patients (Kent and Al-Abadie 1996). So far, none of the treatments of vitiligo have been universally effective and safe, especially for active vitiligo, as relapse is common and repigmentation is partially achieved (Ongenae et al. 2005).

Studies from the past few decades have suggested several hypotheses for the pathogenesis of vitiligo including the autoimmune, neurogenic, genetic, auto-cytotoxic, viral, apoptotic, cell adhesion, and multivariate theories (Gavalas et al. 2009; Nath et al. 1994; Taïeb and Picardo 2009; Westerhof and d'Ischia 2007) The auto-cytotoxic theory suggests that the toxic intermediates of melanin synthesis process (Moellmann et al. 1982; Pawelek et al. 1980), reduced antioxidant molecules, (Nordlund and Lerner 1982) and excessive hydrogen peroxide generation in skin (Schallreuter et al. 1991, 1994) lead to self-destruction of melanocytes. In the multivariate hypothesis, it was suggested that vitiligo results from the complex interaction of susceptible genes, the environment, and the immune system (Fig. 2) (Laddha et al. 2013).

For the past few past decades, finding the genetic cause of vitiligo has been the focus of many studies. Some of the earliest attempts only considered a possible genetic basis for vitiligo based on familial clustering of the disease (Lernerab 1959; Stuttgen 1950; Teindel 1950). Later on, the candidate gene studies gained popularity but were followed abruptly by genome-wide association studies (GWAS). The GWAS is superior to the candidate gene approach in studying the genetics of the diseases

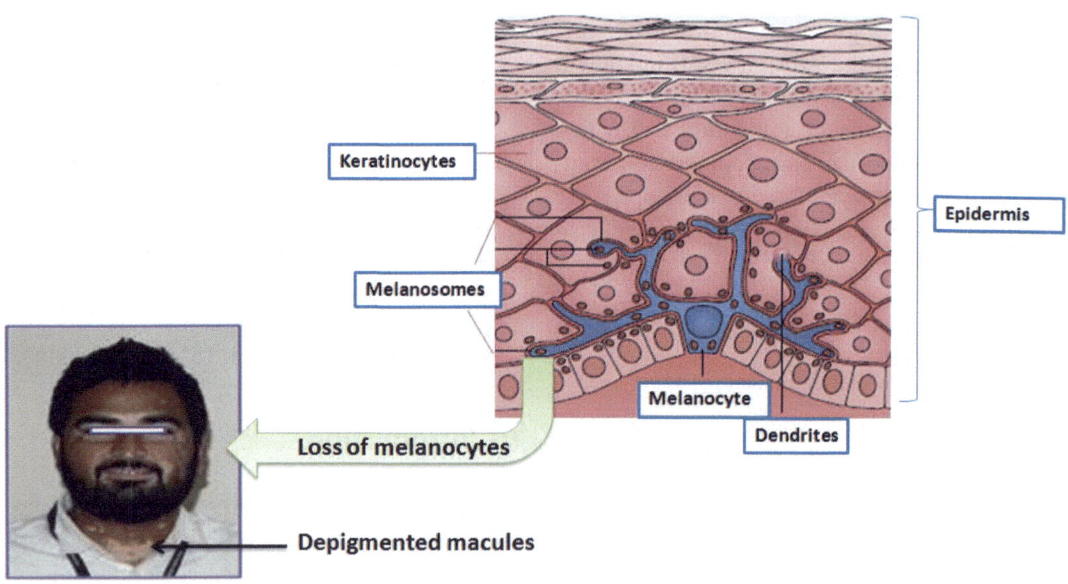

Fig. 1 **The Manifestation of Generalized Vitiligo (GV).** A GV patient with facial depigmentation involving eyes, lips, mouth, and neck regions. The loss of melanocytes residing in the basal layer of epidermis results in depigmented macules. Melanocytes synthesize melanin pigment in specialized compartments known as melanosomes

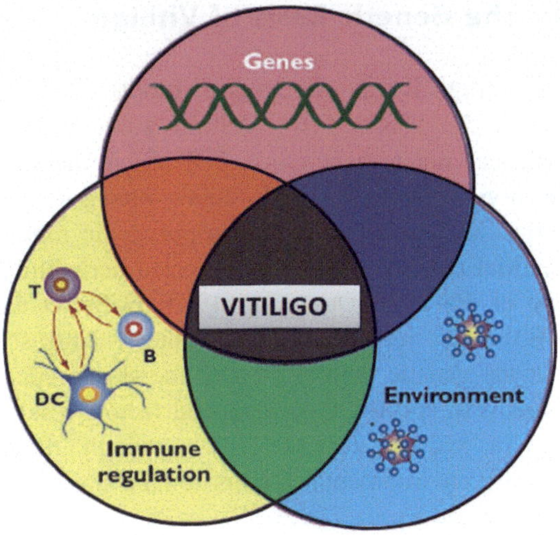

Fig. 2 Interaction of genes, immune system, and environmental factors in vitiligo. The susceptible immune regulatory genes involved in cellular and humoral immune response in conjunction with environmental factors/triggers may lead to the development of Vitiligo

due to its high throughput property to discover novel candidate genes and to reveal specific genetic associations of diseases. The vitiligo susceptibility genes that encode immune components involved in immune-regulatory mechanisms and target the melanocytes for destruction have been identified through GWAS approach (Spritz 2012). Despite being in the GWAS era, the candidate gene association approach for solving the "vitiligo puzzle" has its own importance. Many studies have come up with revealing the functional and genotype–phenotype correlation aspects for the vitiligo candidate genes and tried to solve the "vitiligo puzzle" by adding important pieces. The main purpose of identifying vitiligo genes is that such casual genes provide preliminary evidences for investigating immune-pathomechanisms, identifying the potential targets and designing the treatments. Moreover, several immune-regulatory genes identified for vitligo susceptibility have also been linked with other autoimmune diseases which are associated with vitiligo. The chapter will discuss the genetic basis of vitiligo with a focus on immunogenetic factors involved in vitiligo pathogenesis. Additionally, the advancement made in the genetic approaches to identify vitiligo susceptibility genes, such as linkage studies, GWASs, gene expression, and candidate gene association studies will also be discussed.

2 Autoimmune Pathogenesis of Vitiligo

In many cases, vitiligo has been observed with association of autoimmune diseases such as autoimmune thyroid disease, rheumatoid arthritis, psoriasis, pernicious anemia, systemic lupus erythematosus, Addison's disease, and adult-onset type 1 diabetes mellitus, suggesting its autoimmune etiology (Alkhateeb et al. 2013; Laberge et al. 2005; Macaron et al. 1977; Ochi and DeGroot 1969). Previous studies reported the presence of anti-melanocyte antibodies and melanocyte-specific T cells which target melanocyte antigens in vitiligo patients (Bystryn and Naughton 1985; Naughton et al. 1986). Reports from Indian and Caucasian populations suggested that anti-melanocyte antibodies were found in 75% of vitiligo patients (Laddha et al. 2014; Le Poole and Luiten 2008). Moreover, the study suggested that oxidative stress could be the initial triggering factor which then led to induction of autoimmune factors (Laddha et al. 2013). In support to this, the convergence theory suggests that several factors in synergism can lead to melanocyte destruction (Le Poole and Luiten 2008). The factors such as emotional stress, neural factors, skin physical trauma, hormones can lead to oxidative stress generation in melanocytes resulting in secretion of heat shock protein-70 (HSP-70) and chaperoned melanocyte antigens (Mosenson et al. 2012). The HSP-70 and melanocyte antigens are then taken up by antigen-presenting cells (APCs) such as dendritic cells (DCs), which further activate and recruit anti-melanocyte cytotoxic T cells ($CD8^+$ T-cells) into the skin (Boorn et al. 2009).

The cytotoxic T cells were found to be in increased frequency in vitiligo patients (Jin et al. 2012a; Wańkowicz-Kalińska et al. 2003;

Dwivedi et al. 2013a). Studies have demonstrated that cytotoxic T cells isolated from vitiligo skin are reactive to melanocyte antigens, kill melanocytes effectively (Boorn et al. 2009), and able to induce melanocyte apoptosis by secreting IL-13 and IL-6 (Wu et al. 2013).

The exact mechanisms responsible for inducing and activating anti-melanocyte $CD8^+$ T cells and loss of tolerance to melanocyte autoantigens are not clear; however, functional defects in regulatory T cell (Treg) functions have been suggested (Dwivedi et al. 2013a, 2015; Ben Ahmed et al. 2012; Lili et al. 2012; Giri et al. 2020a, b, 2021). The Tregs maintain the peripheral tolerance by suppressing the self-reactive T-cells. Previous studies showed decreased numbers of Tregs and reduced suppressive function of Tregs in vitiligo patients (Giri et al. 2020a, b, 2021; Dwivedi et al. 2015). These alterations in Tregs might result in increased number of cytotoxic T cells and their activity (Lili et al. 2012; Giri et al. 2020a; Dwivedi et al. 2013b). The importance of Treg cells in the pathogenesis of vitiligo is also evidenced by the recently identified Treg cell-associated susceptibility genes such as *FOXP3*, *TGFβ*, *CTLA4*, and *IL10* (Giri et al. 2020a, b, 2021; Dwivedi et al. 2015). The role of Tissue Resident Memory (TRM) T cells in vitiligo pathogenesis has also been reported (Shah et al. 2021). TRM cells persist within the skin or peripheral tissues with a longer survivability and results into recurrence of skin macules at the same sites where they were observed prior to the treatment. Emerging studies have shown that reactivation of these skin TRMs results in autoreactive TRM cells in various autoimmune diseases including vitiligo (Shah et al. 2021). Increased expression of CXCR3 (a homing receptor of TRM) has been showed in perilesional skin of vitiligo patients with progressive disease (Boniface et al. 2018). Above studies indicate that autoimmunity plays a significant role in vitiligo pathogenesis and the genetic factors which govern the immune response are crucial in the disease pathogenesis, prognosis, and developing effective therapeutics.

3 The Genetic Basis of Vitiligo

The vitiligo is considered as a complex disease and is characterized by multiple susceptibility loci, incomplete penetrance, and genetic heterogeneity (Strömberg et al. 2008; Zhang et al. 2005). Vitiligo is viewed as a polygenic multifactorial condition with an estimated heritability rate of 46–72% (Das et al. 1985; Hafez et al. 1983). The multifactorial hypothesis suggests that the genetic composition of the skin predisposes it to specific environmental factors resulting in vitiligo (Spritz 2011), though these specific environmental factors remain unknown (Boissy and Spritz 2009).

The first evidence of genetic basis for vitiligo was suggested by Stűttgen (1950) and Teindel (1950). They reported that members and relatives of eight families were affected by vitiligo. In particular, Stűttgen reported that in one family, vitiligo exhibited the dominant inheritance due to intermarriage to a family with recessive thyroid disease. Later, studies also reported vitiligo in identical twins (Mohr 1951; Siemens 1953; Vogel 1956) and 11–38% frequency of vitiligo in probands' relatives (Lernerab 1959; Behl 1955; Levai 1958; Sidi and Bourgeois-Gavardin 1953). These early studies formed the genetic basis of vitiligo. More recent data reported that 6–38% of vitiligo patients had family members affected with vitiligo (Dwivedi et al. 2013b; Alkhateeb et al. 2003; Majumder et al. 1993; Ortonne and Bose 1993; Shajil et al. 2006). In first-degree relatives, the relative risk of vitiligo is suggested to be 7–10 folds greater than the normal population (Nath et al. 1994; Bhatia et al. 1992). In addition, early age of onset and larger skin surface involvement was observed in families with multiple relatives affected by vitiligo (Laberge et al. 2005; Alkhateeb et al. 2003). Moreover, it has been observed that vitiligo-associated autoimmune diseases occurred more frequently in the first-degree relatives (not affected by vitiligo) of vitiligo patients, suggestive of sharing of some common genetic factors between the associated autoimmune diseases and vitiligo (Laberge et al. 2005).

4 Identification of Genetic Factors Underlying Vitiligo

Several studies including allelic association of candidate genes, gene expression study, genome-wide linkage study (GWLS), and GWASs are carried out to reveal disease-related genes. The understanding of pathomechanisms involved in vitiligo has been improved by these studies (Spritz 2008). Of these strategies, the GWAS has been considered as the most efficient and robust study to explore the disease-related genetic variants, especially in complex diseases.

Moreover, the Next-generation DNA sequencing and exome sequencing are also used for genetic variants identification in vitiligo (Jin et al. 2012b). Most genes associated with vitiligo are involved in regulation of immune system, some participate in apoptosis and few are involved in melanogenesis (Spritz 2010a). However, the exact mechanisms by which these genes participate in vitiligo induction and progression are yet to be explored (Alkhateeb et al. 2003; Spritz et al. 2004). The following sections describe the immune-related genes identified by different approaches and implicated in vitiligo pathogenesis.

4.1 Genome-Wide Linkage Studies (GWLS)

Through GWLS, identification of genetic loci linked with vitiligo in multiplex families can be carried out that would help in determining the inherited genetic markers' position for the disease. Previously, several GWLS of vitiligo were carried out in diverse populations and multiple linkages to vitiligo were identified (Jin et al. 2010a, 2011a, 2012b; Spritz et al. 2004; Alkhateeb et al. 2002; Birlea et al. 2010; Cheong et al. 2013; Fain et al. 2003; Nath et al. 2001; Quan et al. 2010). For example, linkage signals on chromosomes 7, 8, 9, 11, 13, 17, 19, and 22 were identified in the Caucasian population through GWLSs (Spritz et al. 2004; Fain et al. 2003). The susceptible loci for vitiligo identified by linkage studies are shown in Table 1.

The first GWLS in vitiligo was carried out by Nath et al. (2001) who reported that SLEV1 locus is present on chromosome 17p13 and was linked to SLE affected families that also had relatives affected with vitiligo. Later, another study confirmed the linkage of *SLEV1* by GWLS on families with vitiligo co-occurring with other autoimmune diseases (Spritz et al. 2004). The

Table 1 Susceptibility loci for vitiligo identified by linkage and GWAS studies

Susceptibility loci	Chromosomal region	Protein and function	References
NLRP1 (NALP1; SLEV1)	17p13	NACHT leucine-rich-repeat protein 1; Functions in the innate immune response; Associated with many autoimmune diseases	Spritz et al. (2004), Nath et al. (2001) Jin et al. (2007a, c)
AIS1	1p31.3-p32.2	Autoimmune susceptibility locus 2; Function undefined	Alkhateeb et al. (2002)
AIS2	7p	Autoimmune susceptibility locus 2; Function undefined; Associated with autoimmune disease	Spritz et al. (2004)
FOXP1	3p13	Forkhead box P1; Transcription factor which regulates development of immune cells	Jin et al. (2010b)
MYH15	3q13.13	Myosin heavy chain 15	Jin et al. (2010b)
CCR6	6q27	Cytokine-chemokine receptor for CCL20; Recruits immune cells on binding of ligand; Associated with inflammatory bowel disease	Quan et al. (2010), Jin et al. (2010b)

(continued)

Table 1 (continued)

Susceptibility loci	Chromosomal region	Protein and function	References
C1QTNF6	22q12.3	C1q and tumor necrosis factor-related protein-6; Associated with rheumatoid arthritis and type 1 diabetes mellitus	Jin et al. (2010a)
GZMB	14q12	Granzyme B; Regulates cell-mediated immune responses	Jin et al. (2010a, 2012b)
IL2RA	10p15.1	Interleukin (IL)-2 receptor alpha chain; Receptor for cytokine IL2 which induces T and B cell proliferation. Associated with many autoimmune diseases	Jin et al. (2010a)
LPP	3q27.3-q28	LIM domain-containing preferred translocation partner in lipoma; Function unknown; Associated with celiac disease and rheumatoid arthritis	Jin et al. (2010a)
UBASH3A	21q22.3	Ubiquitin-associated and SH3 domain-containing A gene; Regulates T cell receptor signaling; Associated with type 1 diabetes mellitus	Jin et al. (2010a)
ICA1	7p21.3	Islet cell autoantigen 1; autoantigen in insulin-dependent diabetes mellitus and primary Sjogren's syndrome	Jin et al. (2010b)
TBC1D2	9q22.33	TBC1 domain family member 2; function is unknown	Jin et al. (2010b)
IKZF4	12q13.2	IKAROS family zinc finger 4; transcription factor involved in the control of lymphoid development	Jin et al. (2010b)
SH2B3	12q24.12	SH2B adaptor protein 3; a key negative regulator of cytokine signaling and plays a critical role in hematopoiesis; Associated with celiac disease type 13 and susceptibility to insulin-dependent diabetes mellitus	Jin et al. (2010b)
PTPN22	1p13.2	Lymphoid protein tyrosine phosphatase; Negatively regulates T cell activation; Associated with many autoimmune diseases	Jin et al. (2010a), LaBerge et al. (2008), Laberge et al. (2008), Cantón et al. (2005)
RNASET2	6q27	Ribonuclease T2; novel member of the Rh/T2/S-glycoprotein class of extracellular ribonucleases	Quan et al. (2010)
FGFR1OP	6q27	FGFR1 oncogene partner; a hydrophilic centrosomal protein required for anchoring microtubules to subcellular structures; Associated with Crohn's disease and Graves' disease	Quan et al. (2010)
FOXP3	Xp11.23	Forkhead box P3; Transcription factor which regulates regulatory T cell development; Causes autoimmune IPEX syndrome	Birlea et al. (2011)
TSLP	5q22.1	Thymic stromal lymphopoietin; Cytokine which induces naïve CD4 + T cells to produce T helper cell 2 cytokines	Birlea et al. (2011), Ka et al. (2009)
XBP1	22q12	X-box binding protein 1; Transcription factor which regulates MHC class II gene expression; Associated with inflammatory bowel disease	Birlea et al. (2011), Ren et al. (2009)

(continued)

Table 1 (continued)

Susceptibility loci	Chromosomal region	Protein and function	References
IFIH1	2q24.2	Interferon-induced with helicase C domain 1; involved in alteration of RNA secondary structure such as translation initiation, nuclear and mitochondrial splicing, and ribosome and spliceosome assembly; associated with diabetes mellitus insulin-dependent type 19	Jin et al. (2012b)
CD80	3q13.33	CD80 molecule; induces T-cell proliferation and cytokine production	Jin et al. (2012b)
CLNK	4p16.1	Cytokine-dependent hematopoietic cell linker; regulation of immunoreceptor signaling including PLC-gamma-mediated B cell antigen receptor (BCR) signaling and FC-epsilon R1-mediated mast cell degranulation	Jin et al. (2012b)
BACH2	6q15	BTB domain and CNC homolog 2; a transcriptional activator and regulator of apoptosis	Jin et al. (2012b)
SLA	8q24.22	Src like adaptor; a regulator of T cell antigen receptor signaling	Jin et al. (2012b)
CASP7	10q25.3	Caspase 7; plays a central role in the execution-phase of cell apoptosis	Jin et al. (2012b)
CD44	11p13	CD44 molecule; involved in lymphocyte activation, recirculation and homing, hematopoiesis, and tumor metastasis	Jin et al. (2012b)
TYR	11q21	Tyrosinase; a melanogenic enzyme required for the conversion of tyrosine to melanin	Jin et al. (2012b)
OCA2-HERC2	15q12-13.1	OCA2 melanosomal transmembrane protein which is involved in mammalian pigmentation; HECT and RLD domain containing E3 ubiquitin protein ligase 2; associated with skin/hair/eye pigmentation variability	Jin et al. (2012b)
MC1R	16q24.3	Melanocortin 1 receptor; receptor protein for melanocyte-stimulating hormone (MSH)	Jin et al. (2012b)
TICAM1	19p13.3	Toll-like receptor adaptor molecule 1; involved in native immunity against invading pathogens	Jin et al. (2012b, 2016)
TOB2	22q13.2	Transducer of ERBB2, 2; member of anti-proliferative proteins, which are involved in the regulation of cell cycle progression	Jin et al. (2012b)
PMEL	12q13.2	Premelanosome protein; melanocyte-specific type I transmembrane glycoprotein involved in generating internal matrix fibers of melanosomes	Tang et al. (2013)
FASLG	1q24.3	Fas ligand; induction of apoptosis; essential for immune system regulation through activation-induced cell death (AICD) of T cells and cytotoxic T lymphocyte-induced cell death	Jin et al. (2016)

(continued)

Table 1 (continued)

Susceptibility loci	Chromosomal region	Protein and function	References
PTPRC	1q31.3-q32.1	Protein tyrosine phosphatase receptor type C; essential regulator of T- and B-cell antigen receptor signaling	Jin et al. (2016)
PPP4R3B	2p16.1	Protein phosphatase 4 regulatory subunit 3B	Jin et al. (2016)
BCL2L11	2q13	BCL2 like 11; act as an apoptotic activator and involved in neuronal and lymphocyte apoptosis	Jin et al. (2016)
FARP2-STK25	2q37.3	FERM, ARH/RhoGEF, and pleckstrin domain protein 2; Serine/threonine kinase 25 (plays a role in regulation of cell death)	Jin et al. (2016)
CTLA4	2q33.2	Cytotoxic T-lymphocyte associated protein 4; transmits an inhibitory signal to T cells	Jin et al. (2016)
UBE2E2	3p24.3	Ubiquitin-conjugating enzyme E2 E2; Protein ubiquitination pathway and damage response	Jin et al. (2016)
FBXO45-NRROS	3q29	F-box protein 45 (act as protein-ubiquitin ligases); Negative regulator of reactive oxygen species	Jin et al. (2016), Tang et al. (2019)
PPP3CA	4q24	Protein phosphatase 3 catalytic subunit alpha; T lymphocyte calcium-dependent, calmodulin-stimulated protein phosphatise	Jin et al. (2016)
IRF4	6p25.3	Interferon regulatory factor 4; involved in regulation of interferons in response to infection by virus, and in the regulation of interferon-inducible genes	Jin et al. (2016)
SERPINB9	6p25.2	Serpin family B member 9; member of the serine protease inhibitor family; inhibits the activity of the effector molecule granzyme B	Jin et al. (2016)
CPVL	7p14.3	Carboxypeptidase vitellogenic like; inflammatory protease which trims antigens for presentation	Jin et al. (2016)
NEK6	9q33.3	NIMA related kinase 6; regulator of apoptosis	Jin et al. (2016)
ARID5B	10q21.2	AT-rich interaction domain 5B; involved in cell growth and differentiation of B-lymphocyte progenitors	Jin et al. (2016)
BAD	11q13.1	BCL2 associated agonist of cell death; positively regulates cell apoptosis	Jin et al. (2016)
TNFSF11	13q14.11	TNF superfamily member 11; involved in the regulation of T cell-dependent immune response	Jin et al. (2016)
KAT2AHSPB9-RAB5C	17q21.2	RAB5C, member RAS oncogene family; are small GTPases	Jin et al. (2016)
TNFRSF11A	18q21.33	TNF receptor superfamily member 11a; regulator of the interaction between T cells and dendritic cells	Jin et al. (2016)

(continued)

Table 1 (continued)

Susceptibility loci	Chromosomal region	Protein and function	References
SCAF1-IRF3-BCL2L12	19q13.33	SR-related CTD associated factor 1; Interferon regulatory factor 3 (activates the transcription of interferons alpha and beta); BCL2 like 12 (it is an anti-apoptotic factor that acts as an inhibitor of caspases 3 and 7)	Jin et al. (2016)
PTPN1	20q13.13	Protein tyrosine phosphatase non-receptor type 1; cell growth control, and cell response to interferon stimulation	Jin et al. (2016)
ASIP	20q11.22	Agouti signaling protein; a paracrine signaling molecule that causes hair follicle melanocytes to synthesize pheomelanin	Jin et al. (2016)
IL1RAPL1	Xp21.3-p21.2	Interleukin 1 receptor accessory protein-like 1; plays a role in synapse formation and stabilization	Jin et al. (2016)

NLRP1 gene encoding the inflammasome regulatory protein was also fine-mapped in vitiligo-associated multiple autoimmune diseases (Jin et al. 2007b). In addition, the Autoimmune susceptibility 1 *(AIS1;* chromosome 1p31.3–p32.2) was detected by GWLS in a European-derived White population with vitiligo (Alkhateeb et al. 2002; Fain et al. 2003). Later, *AIS2* (chromosome 7) and *AIS3* (chromosomes 8) were also mapped in European-derived White population with vitiligo (Spritz et al. 2004; Jin et al. 2010a). Further, through GWLS, *AIS4* (chromosome 4q12–q21) (Chen et al. 2005) and two other loci (on chromosome 6p21–p22 and 22q12) were identified in Han Chinese families with vitiligo (Liang et al. 2007).

4.2 Genome-Wide Association Study (GWAS) in Vitiligo

The GWAS through its high efficiency and throughput can identify the disease-causing genes. GWASs have contributed to reveal the important disease-risk variants, frequencies of risk allele, and the relative risks attributed to each allele known as odds ratio (OR). The advancement in the technology through the advent of microarrays, human genome mapping, and inter-individual genetic variation (International HapMap project), the GWASs became possible. GWASs contributed to the identification of >1000 types of complex diseases and their traits. GWASs follow the "common disease–common variant" hypothesis and have screened the >80% of common genetic variations of disease susceptibility (Hirschhorn and Gajdos 2011). In GWAS, the results with P values of $<5 \times 10^{-8}$ are considered as significant with at least 2000 cases and equal number of controls (Craddock et al. 2010). The vitiligo susceptible loci identified by GWASs are shown in Table 1.

The first GWAS for vitiligo reported an association of *SMOC2* SNPs with vitiligo in the Romanian community (Birlea et al. 2010). Three GWASs that followed this study identified 50 additional loci associated with vitiligo (Jin et al. 2010b, 2011b, 2012a, b, 2016; Ben et al. 2018; Spritz and Andersen 2017). These loci include the genes responsible for immune cells regulation, apoptosis, and melanocyte function (Fig. 3). Further, two large-scale GWASs of generalized vitiligo (GV), one in Caucasians (Jin et al. 2010c) and the other in Chinese patients (Quan et al. 2010), identified 16 susceptibility loci for GV. Jin et al. (2010b) through GWAS identified *MYH15, TBC1D2, IKZF4, ICA1, FOXP1, SH2B3,* and *CCR6* genes in association with GV in non-Hispanic White population. In the Chinese population, GWAS identified two of the abovementioned genes and one loci in the MHC for GV (Quan et al. 2010). These genes are responsible for immunoregulatory functions except *TYR* which encodes tyrosinase enzyme which is important for melanin biosynthesis and serve as a major vitiligo autoantigen. It has been suggested that S192Y and R402Q SNPs of *TYR* gene alter the tyrosinase function and render protection from GV and susceptibility to melanoma through modulation of TYR peptide presentation by HLA-A2*01 in melanocytes (Tripathi et al. 1991). In addition, an apoptotic effector protein encoded by *GZMB* (granzyme B; produced by cytotoxic T-cells) contains a vitiligo-associated missense SNP, R55Q, which alters GZMB function (Ferrara et al. 2013). The haplotypes of missense SNPs of *NLRP1* (inflammasome regulatory component) resulted in higher constitutive NLRP1 function and thereby lead to activation of IL1-1β (Levandowski et al. 2013).

Further, the functional analyzes and mapping of these vitiligo loci detected in the European White population revealed that fifty percentage of genetic variants affect the regulatory region of the genes whereas only fifteen percentage variants located in exons cause missense mutations (Spritz and Andersen 2017). The MHC class-I (HLA-A) and MHC class-II (HLA-DRB1/-DQA1) regions have been shown to harbor the SNPs associated with vitiligo, particularly in transciptional enhancer region and lead to increased expression of the respective MHC class genes (Jin et al. 2012a; Hayashi et al. 2016; Cavalli et al. 2016; Fain et al. 2006). The MHC class-II region has also been shown to comprise the quantitative trait locus (QTL) associated with the age of onset of vitiligo (Jin et al. 2011b).

Additionally, Jin et al. (2011b), detected >30 GV susceptibility loci by analyzes of GWAS and genetic linkage data. The study comprised of GWAS of 450 patients and 3182 controls, one

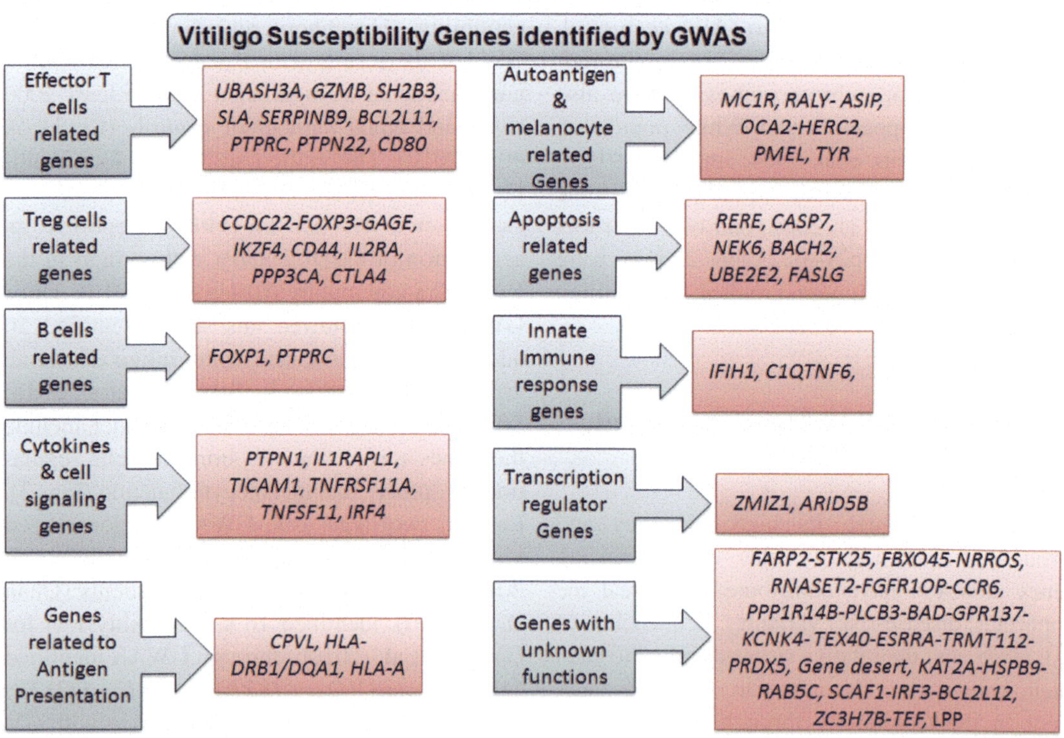

◀ **Fig. 3 Susceptibility genes identified by GWAS.** The large-scale genome-wide association studies in European and Chinese populations have discovered approximately 50 different genetic loci that contribute to vitiligo risk. The majority of these genes are associated with immune system function, for example, **effector T cells related genes** [***UBASH3A*** (ubiquitin-associated and SH3 domain containing protein A) which promotes accumulation of activated T cell receptors on surface, ***GZMB*** (granzyme B) is a apoptosis executioner protein of cytotoxic T lymphocytes, ***SH2B3*** (SH2B adapter protein 3) links T lymphocyte receptor activation signal to phospholipase C-gamma1, GRB2 and phosphatidylinositol 3-kinase, ***SLA*** (Src like adapter) is a regulator of T cell antigen receptor signaling, ***SERPINB9*** (serpin B9) is a endogenous inhibitor of granzyme B, ***BCL2L11*** (BCL2 like 11) is a regulator of apoptosis in thymocyte negative selection, ***PTPRC*** (protein tyrosine phosphatase, receptor type C) is a regulator of T cell antigen receptor signalling, ***PTPN22*** (protein tyrosine phosphatase, non-receptor type 22) is a T cell down regulator molecule which alters responsiveness of T cell receptors, ***CD80*** (T-lymphocyte activation antigen CD80) T-cell co-stimulatory signal], **Treg cells related genes** [***CCDC22-FOXP3-GAGE*** involves in FOXP3 regulatory development and inhibitory function of regulatory Tlymphocytes, ***IKZF4*** (zinc finger protein Eos) is a transcriptional repressor and regulates FOXP3 transcription in regulatory T lymphocytes, ***CD44*** is a regulator of FOXP3 expression, ***IL2RA*** (interleukin-2 receptor subunit alpha) regulates regulator T lymphocytes, ***PPP3CA*** (Serine/threonine-protein phosphatase 2B catalytic subunit alpha isoform) is a T lymphocyte calcium-dependent, calmodulin-stimulated protein phosphatase, ***CTLA4*** (cytotoxic T-lymphocyte-associated protein 4) is a T lymphocyte checkpoint regulator], B cells-related genes [***FOXP1*** (forkhead box protein P1) transcriptional regulator of B-cell development, ***PTPRC*** (protein tyrosine phosphatase, receptor type C) is a regulator of B cell antigen receptor signalling], **cytokines and cell signaling genes** [***PTPN1*** (tyrosine-protein phosphatase non-receptor type 1) dephosphorylates JAK2 and TYK2 kinases and involves in cellular response to interferon, ***IL1RAPL1*** is a Interleukin-1 receptor accessory protein like 1, ***TICAM1*** (TIR domain-containing adapter molecule) is a TLR3/TLR4 adapter which mediates NF kappa-B and interferon-regulatory factor (IRF) activation and induces apoptosis, ***TNFRSF11A*** (tumor necrosis factor receptor superfamily member 11A) regulates interactions between T lymphocytes and dendritic cells, ***TNFSF11*** (tumor necrosis factor ligand superfamily member 11) is a T lymphocyte cytokine which binds to TNFRSF11A and TNFRSF11B, ***IRF4*** (interferon regulatory factor 4) is a transcriptional activator in immune cells and melanocytes], **genes related to antigen presentation** [***CPVL*** *(*probable serine carboxy peptidase CPVL) *is a* inflammatory protease which trims antigens for presentation, ***HLA-DRB1/DQA1*** (HLA MHC class II antigens, DRB1 and DQA1) present peptide antigens to the immune system, ***HLA-A*** (HLA MHC class I antigen, A) presents peptide antigens to the immune system], **autoantigen and melanocyte related genes** [***MC1R*** *(*melanocortin 1 receptor) is melanocyte melanogenic protein acting as vitiligo autoantigen, ***RALY-ASIP*** (agouti signaling protein) is a regulator of melanocytes via MC1R, ***OCA2-HERC2*** (oculocutaneous albinism 2) is melanocyte melanogenic protein acting as vitiligo autoantigen, ***PMEL*** (pre-melanosome protein PMEL) is melanocyte melanosomal type I transmembrane glycoprotein, ***TYR*** (Tyrosinase) is a melanocyte melanogenic enzyme acting as vitiligo autoantigen], **apoptosis related genes** [***RERE*** (Arginine-Glutamic acid dipeptide repeats) is a regulator of apoptosis, ***CASP7*** (caspase-7) is a apoptosis executor protein, ***NEK6*** (NIMA-related serine/threonine-protein kinase Nek6) is regulator of apoptosis, ***BACH2*** (BTB domain and CNC homolog 2) is a transcriptional activator and regulator of apoptosis, ***UBE2E2*** (ubiquitin-conjugating enzyme E2 E2) is involved in protein ubiquitination pathway and damage response, ***FASLG*** (FAS ligand) is a regulator of immune apoptosis], **innate Immune response genes** [***IFIH1*** (interferon induced with helicase C domain 1) is a innate immune receptor, ***C1QTNF6*** is complement C1q tumor necrosis factor related protein 6], transcription regulator genes [***ZMIZ1*** (zinc finger MIZ domain-containing protein 1) is a PIAS-family transcriptional or sumoylation regulator, ***ARID5B*** (AT-rich interactive domain-containing protein 5B) is a transcriptional co-activator]. However, few genes with unknown functions were also found to be associated with vitiligo susceptibility

replication study of 1440 patients and 11,316 controls, and one meta-analysis study of 3187 patients and 6723 controls. The GV susceptibility genes identified by the study include *MC1R, OCA2-HERC2, IFIH1, IKZF4, SH2B3, TOB2, CD44, CD80, BACH2, SLA, CLNK, CASP7*, and a region near *TYR*. Further, one replication study of 6857 patients and 12,025 controls in Chinese Han population detected three important vitiligo susceptibility loci: 12q13.2 (rs10876864), 11q23.3 (rs638893), and 10q22.1 (rs1417210) along with confirmation of three other previously reported loci: 3q28 (rs9851967), 10p15.1 (rs3134883), and 22q12.3 (rs2051582) (Tang et al. 2013). The study suggested that 12q13.2 (rs10876864) was the most significant SNP and found to be present upstream of *PMEL* promoter region. It is worth to note that the *PMEL* gene encodes the major melanocyte-specific antigen and it takes part in vitiligo autoimmunity.

Another GWAS study in Chinese Han and Uygur populations reported an association of MHC class-I, class-II regions, and *RNASET2-FGFR1OP-CCR6* region (chr. 6q24) with vitiligo (Quan et al. 2010). The GWAS study by Tang et al. (2013), reported the association of region comprising *PMEL* gene, 10q22.1 region, a nearby locus containing *ZMIZ1* (Sun et al. 2014), and 11q23.3. Interestingly, GWAS of vitiligo in Japanese patients (Jin et al. 2015), identified association of MHC class-I with HLA-A*02:01 as that of European-derived Caucasians; however, the vitiligo GWAS in Asian Indian and Pakistani patients identified association of MHC class-II as that of European-derived Caucasians (Birlea et al. 2013). Further, a detailed study of MHC in Indians (Singh et al. 2012) found an association of MHC class-II as that of the Chinese population (Quan et al. 2010).

Moreover, the GWAS study by Jin et al. (2016) comprising 4680 patients and 39,586 controls detected twenty-three new loci with genome-wide significance ($P < 5 \times 10^{-8}$) and seven other reported loci. These loci include genes encoding the immune regulatory molecules, apoptotic and melanocyte regulators such as *BCL2L11, UBE2E2, PTPRC, FASLG, FARP2-STK25, IRF4, CPVL, PPP3CA, NEK6, PPP4R3B, SERPINB9, FBXO45-NRROS, ARID5B* (this includes *TNFSF11, BAD, TNFRSF11A, and KAT2AHS PB9-RAB5C*), and *SCAF1-IRF3-BCL2L12*, (this includes *PTPN1, IL1RAPL1, and ASIP*). A potential new locus "PVT1" was also identified with genome-wide significance ($P = 7.74 \times 10^{-9}$); however, it could not be genotyped in the replication study (Jin et al. 2016). Similarly, *LOC1 01060498* and *FLI1* loci were also identified with genome-wide significance ($P = 3.60 \times 10^{-11}$ and $P = 3.76 \times 10^{-8}$); however, these did not replicate successfully.

Recently, the association of rs6583331 "T" allele of the locus within the *FBXO45-NRROS* gene at 3q29 [identified by GWAS by Jin et al. (2016) in the Caucasian population] has been reported with vitiligo in a Chinese Han cohort involving 1472 patients and 1472 controls (Tang et al. 2019). This study suggests that Chinese and Caucasian populations may share a common predisposing genetic factor to the development of vitiligo. Further, seven new loci (*PPARGC1B, PARP12, STAT4, CBFA2T3, C7ORF72, FADS2* and Chr. 7 locus near *AFMID*) attained suggestive significance ($P < 10^{-5}$); however, they failed to obtain the genome-wide significance in the subsequent meta-analysis (Jin et al. 2016). Few of the susceptible genes identified by GWASs have been discussed in the following sections. Though GWASs have identified many susceptible genes and loci, the respective causal genetic variants have been identified for few of the vitiligo susceptibility genes. Hence, further extensive studies involving DNA sequencing of vitiligo patients with large sample size, cautious bioinformatics analyzes, and target-oriented functional studies are needed to elucidate the specific variants and their effects.

4.2.1 Vitiligo Susceptibility Genes with Known Functions as Identified by GWASs

1. *UBASH3A*:

The UBASH3A, a regulator of T-cell–receptor signaling is located on chromosome 21q22.3. Total of nine *UBASH3A* SNPs have been found to associate with GV and the rs2839511 SNP showed the genome-wide significance (Jin et al. 2011b). Also, an association between GV and *UBASH3A* variants have been reported that confer protection from the disease (Jin et al. 2012b).

2. *CLNK*:

CLNK encodes a signal transducer of mast cell receptors and it acts as a positive regulator in receptor signaling (Wu et al. 2004). The GWAS-meta analysis (GWAS-MA) suggested the association of SNPs located at upstream region of *CLNK* (4p16.1; nt 10702156–10729386; rs16872571) including several imputed SNPs (rs11940117) with vitiligo, that was confirmed by the replication study. The "TCATTCTGA" haplotype of *CLNK* has been reported to associate with gout patients (Jin et al. 2015).

3. *GZMB*:

The granzyme B (*GZMB*), a caspase-like serine protease is involved in immune-induced apoptosis of target cells mediated by cytotoxic T cells ($CD8^+$ T cells), NK cells, and Th_2 cells which induce cell death (Devadas et al. 2006; Trapani and Sutton 2003). The GWAS in European-derived Whites reported the association of *GZMB* with vitiligo (Jin et al. 2010b, 2012b). In particular, rs8192917-C-rs11539752-C haplotype (55R-94A) of *GZMB* has been associated with GV pathogenesis (Ferrara et al. 2013). Recently, Xu et al. (2018) has also reported association of *GZMB* rs8192917 SNP with the disease status of vitiligo (OR = 1.39 and $P = 1.92 \times 10^{-8}$). The *GZMB* gene is not a common autoimmunity gene thus it may represent a relatively specific vitiligo susceptibility gene (Rodriguez-Castro et al. 2018).

4. *RERE*:

The *RERE* is located on chromosome 1p36.23 which encodes the arginine–glutamic acid dipeptide repeats protein. RERE is over-expressed in lymphoid cells and as a co-repressor of transcription, it regulates the apoptosis process (Wang and Tsai 2008). Forty SNPs in *RERE* were identified to associate with GV. Particularly, *RERE* rs301819 and rs4908760 SNPs were found to have genome-wide significance and strongly associated with GV (Jin et al. 2010b, 2012b).

5. *CASP7*:

The *CASP7* (Chr. 10q25.3) encodes cysteine-aspartic acid protease (member of caspase family). The caspases through their sequential activation lead to cell apoptosis and inflammation (Lamkanfi and Kanneganti 2010). The association of *CASP7* rs3814231 SNP was shown with vitiligo by GWAS-MA followed by its confirmation through a meta-analysis study and one replication study (Jin et al. 2012b).

6. *SLA*:

The *TG/SLA* loci have been identified by GWAS-MA in the European-derived White (CEU) population (Jin et al. 2012b). The *SLA* encodes Src-like adaptor protein and acts as T-and B-cell receptor signaling inhibitor whereas *TG* encodes thyroglobulin. However, the role of thyroglobulin in the pathogenesis of vitiligo is not clear (Jin et al. 2012b).

7. *BACH2*:

The *BACH2* encodes a B-cell transcriptional repressor (Sasaki et al. 2000). BACH2 regulates the differentiation of $CD4^+$ T-cells and maintains homeostasis between immunity and tolerance.

The GWAS-MA in CEU population showed an association between vitiligo with *BACH2* SNPs (nt 90941239–91915693). In particular, the *BACH2* rs3757247 SNP was later confirmed by replication and meta-analysis studies (Jin et al. 2012b).

8. *IFIH1*:

The *IFIH1* encodes interferon-induced RNA helicase and is essential for providing the antiviral innate immune response (Kato et al. 2006). The GWAS-MA suggested the association of *IFIH1* rs2111485 SNP with vitiligo (Jin et al. 2012b).

9. *TICAM1*:

The *TICAM1* encodes toll-like receptor adaptor molecule 1 and provides antivial innate immune response (Oshiumi et al. 2003). It is also known as TIR domain-containing adaptor-inducing IFN-β (TRIF). The TICAM1 induces type I interferons (IFN-α and IFN-β) and other inflammatory cytokines by activating interferon regulatory factor-3 (IRF-3), NF-κB, AP-1, and other transcription factors (Kumeta et al. 2014). Since, the involvement of viral factors has been suggested in vitiligo pathogensis (Dwivedi et al. 2018), the association of *TICAM1* with vitiligo as confirmed by GWASs may thus be presumable.

10. *IKZF4*:

The *IKZF4* is a regulator of FOXP3-dependent gene silencing in Tregs by directly interacting with FOXP-3 and without affecting the FOXP3 activated genes (Pan et al. 2009), *IKZF4* has been identified as a GV susceptibility gene by two GWASs (Jin et al. 2012b; Tang et al. 2013).

However, the functional analysis and fine mapping are needed to reveal the disease causal variants in *IKZF4*.

11. *BTNL2*:

A GWAS by Jin et al. (2012b), revealed a QTL near *c6orf10-BTNL2* (rs7758128) for age of onset of vitiligo and was suggested to be associated with susceptibility to GV. The BTNL2 is an immunoglobulin superfamily membrane protein and is involved in the activation of T cells.

12. *CXCR5*:

The *CXCR5* encodes a multi-pass membrane protein (member of CXC chemokine receptor family). The CXCR5 by binding to B-lymphocyte chemoattractant (BLC) induces the migration of B-cells into the follicles of spleen and Peyer's patches. The rs638893 (11q23.3) SNP at intergenic region between *CXCR5* and *DDX6* was associated with vitiligo in Chinese Han population (Tang et al. 2013).

13. *CCR6*:

The *CCR6* (6q27) encodes a chemokine receptor 6 and is mainly expressed by immature memory T cells and DCs (Schutyser et al. 2003). The CCR6 binding to CCL20 ligands leads to immune cells' chemo-attraction, thereby playing a crucial in skin and mucosal surface defense mechanisms (Borgne et al. 2006). The GWAS in the Chinese populations identified genome-wide level of significance of *CCR6* rs6902119 SNP with GV (Quan et al. 2010). Furthermore, a significant association of vitiligo with *CCR6* rs6902119 and rs2301436 SNPs was also reported (Jin et al. 2010b).

14. *SH2B3*:

The *SH2B3* encodes a member of the SH2B adaptor family of proteins. The SH2B3 plays a role in cell signaling induced by cytokine and growth factor receptors. In addition, SH2B3 is involved in development and regulation of B and T cells. The GWAS-MA has shown an association of SNPs (nt111708458-112906415; rs3184504, rs4766578) within and near *SH2B3*, located downstream the *ATXN2* gene (Jin et al. 2012b). The *ATXN* encodes Ataxin-2 protein and mutation in *ATXN* gene causes spinocerebellar ataxia type-2.

15. *CD44*:

The *CD44* encodes a cell surface glycoprotein which binds to hyaluronic acid. CD44 is involved in migration and homing of lymphocytes and monocytes (Johnson and Ruffell 2009). CD44 acts as an accessory molecule in TCR mediated signal transduction, and results in T cell proliferation and survival (Föger et al. 2000). The GWAS-MA study has shown association of rs736374 and rs10768122 SNPs (11p13; nt 35242907–35375280; in *CD44* and *SLC1A2* regions) with vitiligo (Jin et al. 2012b). Since, vitiligo is a T cell-mediated autoimmune disease and it has been shown that in vitiligo patients, $CD8^{+}$ T cells express increased levels of CD44, P-selectin, and granzyme-B, thereby lead to melanocyte destruction (Byrne et al. 2014).

16. *CD80*:

The CD80 is present as a surface protein on activated B-cells, DCs, and monocytes that act as co-stimulants when paired with CD28 in T cell priming (Peach et al. 1995). The GWAS-MA study suggested the association of *CD80* SNPs (rs4330287 and rs59374417) with vitiligo and further these SNPs association was confirmed by replication and meta-analysis studies (Jin et al. 2012b). The presence of increased frequency of $CD80^{+}$ monocytes in vitiligo patients also suggested a possible role of CD80 in vitiligo pathogenesis (Basak et al. 2008).

4.2.2 Vitiligo Susceptibility Genes with Unknown Functions as Identified by GWASs

The GWASs have efficiently identified several key loci for vitiligo susceptibility. Despite the genome-wide significance level, few genes' function remains unclear (Fig. 3) and functional studies are required to investigate their role in vitiligo pathogenesis.

1. *SMOC2*:

The SMOC2 is expressed mainly in the epidermis basal layer during embryogenesis and wound-healing processes (Maier et al. 2008). It stimulates the assembly of extracellular matrix and also promotes keratinocyte and endothelial cell attachment and migration (Maier et al. 2008; Rocnik et al. 2006). The *SMOC2* was identified as a GV risk locus in an isolated European population by GWAS (Birlea et al. 2010). However, *SMOC2* rs13208776 SNP was not associated with vitiligo in Jordanian Arab population (Alkhateeb et al. 2010).

2. *KIAA1005*:

The *KIAA1005* encodes retinitis pigmentosa GTPase regulator-interacting protein 1-like (*RPGRIP1L*) protein. The RPGRIP1L protein is located at basal body-centrosome complex or primary cilia and centrosomes in ciliated cells. The role of RPGRIP1L in pathogenesis of vitiligo is not clear; however, the *KIAA1005* 3854 G > A (1264 Asp > Asn) SNP was significantly associated with vitiligo (Cheong et al. 2009).

3. *SLC29A3* and *CDH23*:

It has been reported that the vitiligo-associated rs1417210 SNP (10q22.1) is in linkage disequilibrium (LD) block containing *SLC29A3* and *CDH23* genes (Tang et al. 2013). The SLC29A3 is a nucleoside transporter protein and is involved in the cellular uptake of nucleobases and nucleosides. Its role in vitiligo pathogenesis is not clear yet; however, mutations in *SLC29A3* gene are associated with H syndrome (Molho-Pessach et al. 2008). The *CDH23* encodes calcium-dependent cellular adhesion glycoprotein (member of cadherin superfamily) and suggests to play a role in hair bundle formation and stereocilia organization. However, its role in vitiligo pathogenesis is not clear. Since, the weakening of the attachment of melanocytes to the surrounding epidermis may result in melanocyte detachment followed by transepidermal elimination, a role of cadherins is likely to be suggested in pathogenesis of vitiligo. This is the presumed mechanism underlying the depigmentation seen after chronic mechanical friction in patients with vitiligo (Gauthier et al. 2003). This claim has been backed up with evidence from studies demonstrating decreased levels of Epidermal-cadherin and Discoidin Domain Receptor Tyrosine kinase-1 (DDR-1) in the epidermal layer of vitiligo patients (Kim and Lee 2010; Ricard et al. 2012). Moreover, one recent SNP association study also confirmed the association between the polymorphisms in the *E-cadherin* (*CDH1* rs10431924, C/T) and *DDR1* (rs 2267641, A/C) genes with vitiligo (Almasi-Nasrabadi et al. 2019).

4. *LPP*, *DDX6*, and *C1QTNF6*:

The *LPP* (3q28) encodes a member of LIM domain subfamily proteins. The LPP contains an N-terminal proline-rich region and three C-terminal LIM domains. Previously, *LPP* was reported as vitiligo susceptibility loci in Caucasians (Jin et al. 2012b), and further its association was confirmed in Chinese Han population as well (Tang et al. 2013); however, its role in vitiligo is not known.

The *DDX6* encodes a member of DEAD-box protein family. DDX6 is an RNA helicase found in stress granules and P-bodies and is involved in suppression of translation and degradation of mRNA (Weston and Sommerville 2006). The association of rs638893 SNP (in an intergenic region between *DDX6* and *CXCR5)* has been reported with vitiligo (Tang et al. 2013). The *C1QTNF6* represents C1q and tumor necrosis factor-related protein six genes. The *C1QTNF6* rs229527 SNP was reported to be associated with GV (Jin et al. 2010b).

5. *TOB2*:

The *TOB2* (22q13.2) encodes a cell-cycle progression regulator and is involved in tolerance of T cells (Jia and Meng 2007). Though GWAS-MA showed association with rs79008 SNP upstream of *TOB2* (Jin et al. 2012b); its role in vitiligo pathogenesis is not clear.

4.3 Gene Expression Studies

Based on the differential genes expression in cells or skin from vitiligo patients, the gene expression study identifies the vitiligo susceptibility genes. The main disadvantage of gene expression study is that gene with primary effects and secondary effects on disease causation cannot be differentiated. Hence, gene expression study is not considered strongly for identification of susceptibility genes of vitiligo. The below are few vitiligo-associated genes revealed through gene expression studies.

1. *VIT1* and *MYG1*:

The gene expression studies identified *VIT1* (*FBXO11*) and *MYG1* genes for vitiligo; however, GWLSs and GWASs did not find them as potential vitiligo susceptibility genes (Kingo et al. 2006; Le Poole et al. 2001). Nevertheless, two association studies reported that the -119G allele of *MYG1* (rs1465073; in promoter region) is associated with vitiligo (Dwivedi et al. 2013c; Philips et al. 2010). These studies reported increased *MYG1* transcript expression in patients with vitiligo. In particular, the patients harboring GG and CG genotypes exhibited increased *MYG1* transcript expression compared to controls indicating the involvement of -119G allele in increased *MYG1* expression (Dwivedi et al. 2013c). Moreover, Kingo et al. (2006) also showed increased MYG1 expression in lesional and non-lesional skin of active vitiligo patients and lesional skin of stable vitiligo patients (Kingo et al. 2006).

2. *SUOX*:

A recent study by Qi et al. (2018) has found that expression of vitiligo-associated gene *SUOX* (12q13.2) in sun-exposed skin and nerve (tibia) is significantly associated with vitiligo. This study suggests that *SUOX* can be a susceptibility gene for vitiligo; however no genetic association study has been reported for *SUOX* till date.

3. Genes identified by transcriptomics:

A study by Dey-Rao and Sinha (2017), on vitiligo blood transcriptomics has provided novel genes targets (*MYC, PTPN6, FGFR2, STAT1,* and *PRKCD)* for therapeutic purposes in vitiligo as well as given new insights into disease mechanisms. Totally, twelve skin and blood transcriptional "hot spots" were found by the in silico interactome analysis which can be identified as potential disease risk gene targets (Dey-Rao and Sinha 2017). These include *PSMB8, PSMB9,* and *TAP1* blood dysregulated genes which were earlier identified as potential vitiligo susceptibility genes (Dey-Rao and Sinha 2017).

The signal transducer and activator of transcription 1 (STAT1) is a transcription factor that reacts with growth factors and cytokines. The STAT1 activation is crucial for IFN-γ signaling which has been targeted by simvastatin in mouse models (Agarwal et al. 2015). Further, the Protein kinase C-delta (*PRKCD*), a calcium-activated kinase is involved in IFN-γ signaling, B cell signaling, apoptosis, regulation of growth, and differentiation of various cells (Deb et al. 2003).

The protein tyrosine phosphatase non-receptor type 6 (*PTPN6*) is a negative regulator of epithelial-mesenchymal transition (EMT). The involvement of PTPN6 in loss of cell–cell adhesion, increased cell motility, and reorganization of skin has been reported (Fan et al. 2015). The *MYC* is a family of regulator genes and proto-oncogenes that encode transcription factors (such as BHLH). The *MYC* is involved in apoptosis, cell growth, and metabolism.

The fibroblast growth factor receptor 2 (*FGFR2*) encodes highly conserved protein of FGFR family and loss of FGFR2 function results in melanoma (Gartside et al. 2009). However, no genetic association study is carried out till date for these genes in vitiligo.

4.4 Candidate Gene Association Studies in Vitiligo

To detect the common disease causal variants with modest effect size, the candidate gene association study is the best option (Amos et al. 2011). It has been suggested that candidate gene approach has greater statistical power than genome-wide association tests (Amos et al. 2011). Candidate gene association study involves comparison of allele frequencies in cases and controls and is easy to carry out (Spritz 2011). However, these studies lead to false-positive results due to differences in ethnicity of populations involved, insufficient statistical power, insufficient multiple testing correction, and statistical fluctuations (Spritz 2011).

The first polymorphisms investigated for association studies were human leukocyte antigen (HLA) variations that play a crucial role in many autoimmune diseases (Fernando et al. 2008). Candidate gene association studies identified several genes involved in immune regulation such as *PTPN22, XBP1, FOXP1, NALP1, HLA, IL2RA, MBL2, CTLA4, MHC, ACE,* and *ESR* and their association with GV (Spritz 2007, 2010a, b). Subsequently, the *PRO2268* was identified as a novel vitiligo susceptibility locus at chromosome 12q14 harboring immune regulator genes such as *IL22, IL26,* and *IFNG* (Douroudis et al. 2011). Furthermore, comprehensive reanalysis of genome-wide data of 33 biological candidate genes previously implicated in GV (*ACE, AIRE, CAT, CD4, CLEC11A, COMT, CTLA4, C12orf10, DDR1, EDN1, ESR1, FAS, FBXO11, FOXD3, FOXP3, GSTM1, GSTT1, IL1RN, IL10, KITLG, PTGS2, TNF, STAT4, UVRAG, NFE2L2, MBL2, TGFBR2, TXNDC5, VDR, TSLP, XBP1, PDGFRA-KIT and TAP1-PSMB8*) detected unique association of *FOXP3, TSLP,* and *XBP1* candidate genes with vitiligo (Birlea et al. 2010, 2011; Jin et al. 2010a, c, 2011b; Tang et al. 2013). The below sections describe a few prominent candidate genes studied in vitiligo.

1. Autoimmune Regulator (*AIRE*):

Disruptive mutations in *AIRE* gene lead to autoimmune polyendocrinopathy-candidiasis-ectodermal dystrophy syndrome (APECED). Vitiligo appears as a common feature in APECED. The *AIRE* gene (21q22.3) encodes a transcription factor (Tazi-Ahnini et al. 2008) which is responsible for the transcription of peripheral tissue antigens in the thymus and thus educating T-cells on self-tolerance via negative selection of autoreactive ones (Liston et al. 2003; Peterson et al. 2008). AIRE dysfunction increases the chance for autoimmunity as a consequence of inadequate expression of peripheral self-antigens (Tazi-Ahnini et al. 2008).

In non-Hispanic White GV families, the linkage study detected a minor linkage peak in chromosome 21q that harbors *AIRE* (Fain et al. 2003). However, reanalyzes in these families did not find association of 7 SNPs of *AIRE* gene with GV (Jin et al. 2007b). Further, a UK non-Hispanic White population showed association of *AIRE* rs1800521 (7215C; synonymous; $P = 1.4E-05$) SNP with vitiligo (Tazi-Ahnini et al. 2008). This *AIRE* SNP was not found in the earlier linkage study and HapMap. Further, the study found an association between "CGCC" haplotype with vitiligo using C-103 T, G6528A, T7215C, and T11787C as tag SNPs ($P = 0.003$, OR 2.49, 95% CI 1.45–4.26). However, Birlea et al. (2011) reported that none of the 29 SNPs in the *AIRE* region, including the seven genes studied by Jin et al. (2007b) were associated with vitiligo.

2. NACHT Leucine rich Repeat Protein 1 (*NLRP1*):

The *NLRP1* [also known as *NALP1, CARD7, DEFCAP, NAC,* or NLR Family Pyrin Domain Containing 1 (NLRP1) gene] is located at 17p. It encodes NACHT leucine-rich repeat protein 1, an innate immune system regulator (Jin et al. 2007c). NLRP1 plays an important role in inflammation, apoptosis (Martinon et al. 2002; Tschopp et al. 2003), and active assembly of inflammasomes (Martinon et al. 2002). It leads to secretion of pro-inflammatory cytokines such as TNF-α, IL-1β, and IFN-γ. In addition, studies on melanoma reported for NLRP1 role in preventing apoptosis in melanocytes (Zhai et al. 2017). Since, in vitiligo the melanocyte death has been suggested due to apoptosis with minimal inflammation (Norris et al. 1994), the association between the polymorphisms of this gene and vitiligo may be comprehendible.

Several *NLRP1* SNPs have been studied in vitiligo (Table 2); however, only few SNPs attained a significant association with the disease (Jin et al. 2007a, c; Alkhateeb et al. 2010). The

Table 2 Genetic polymorphisms of candidate genes studied in vitiligo

Gene	Polymorphism	Association	Population	References
AIRE	rs1800521 (7215C)	Yes	Non-Hispanic White	Tazi-Ahnini et al. (2008)
NLRP1 (NALP1)	rs2670660 (A/G promoter)	Yes	Gujarati population, White patients from the UK, USA, and Romania	Jin et al. (2007a), Dwivedi et al. (2013f)
	rs8182352	Yes	White patients from the UK, the USA, and Romania	Jin et al. (2007a)
	rs1008588 (Promoter)	Yes	Jordanian Arab	Alkhateeb and Qarqaz (2010)
	rs6502867 (T/C Intron)	Yes	Gujarati population, White patients from the UK, USA, and Romania	Jin et al. (2007a), Dwivedi et al. (2013f)
	rs12150220 (A/T Exon)	Yes	Gujarati	Dwivedi et al. (2013f)
XBP1	rs2269577	Yes	Han Chinese	Ren et al. 2009)
FAS	rs2234767 (−1377 G > A)	Yes	Han Chinese	Li et al. (2008)
		No	Turkish	Türsen et al. (2014)
	rs1800682 (−670 G > A)	No	Han Chinese	Li et al. (2008)
		Yes	Turkish	Türsen et al. (2014)
	rs763110 (*FASL*-844 T/C)	No	Turkish	Türsen et al. (2014)
	rs5030772 (FASL-IVS2nt −124 A/G)	No	Turkish	Türsen et al. (2014)
PTPN22	rs2476601 (C/T; Exon)	Yes	Caucasians cohort (UK)	Cantón et al. (2005)
		Yes	Romanian	LaBerge et al. (2008)
		Yes	Mexican	Garcia-Melendez et al. (2014)
		Yes	South Indian (Tamil)	Rajendiran et al. (2018)
		Yes	European	Jin et al. (2010a)
		Yes	Saudi Arabians	Huraib et al. (2020)
		No	Egyptian	Elmongy and Khalil (2013)
		No	Jordanian Arab	Alkhateeb et al. (2013)
		No	Gujarati	Laddha et al. (2008)
		No	Turkish	Akbas et al. (2014)
ACE	rs1799752 (I/D; Intron)	Yes	Korean	Jin et al. (2004b)
		Yes	South Indian	Deeba et al. (2009)
		Yes	Egyptian	Badran et al. (2015), Rashed et al. (2015)
		Yes	Indian	Patwardhan et al. (2013)
		No	English	Akhtar et al. (2005)
		No	Gujarati	Dwivedi et al. (2008)
		No	Turkish	Pehlivan et al. (2009)

(continued)

Table 2 (continued)

Gene	Polymorphism	Association	Population	References
MBL2	rs5030737, codon 52 (allele D)	No	Indian	Dwivedi et al. (2009)
	rs1800450, codon 54 (allele B)	Yes	Turkish	Onay et al. (2007)
		No	Indian	Dwivedi et al. (2009)
		No	Non-Hispanic White	Birlea et al. (2011)
		No	Turkish	Karkucak et al. (2015)
	rs1800451, codon 57 (allele C)	No	Indian	Dwivedi et al. (2009)
	rs7096206 (X/Y)	No	Indian	Dwivedi et al. (2009)
PSMB8 (LMP7)	rs2071543 (A/C exon 2; Q49K)	No	Caucasian	Casp et al. (2003)
		Yes	North Indian	Dani et al. (2018)
	rs2071627	No	Western	Birlea et al. (2013)
	rs2071464 (intron 6 G/T)	No	Caucasian	Casp et al. (2003)
		No	Egyptian	Eldin et al (2006)
		No	Saudi	Babalghith (2014)
		Yes	Gujarati (Indian)	Jadeja et al. (2017)
		No	North Indian	Dani et al. (2018)
PSMB9 (LMP2)	rs17587 (G/A exon 3, p.60R > H)	Yes	Saudi	Elhawary et al. (2014)
		No	North Indian	Dani et al. (2018)
		No	Caucasian	Casp et al. (2003)
TAP1	rs1800453(G/A exon 10; D637G)	Yes	Caucasian	Casp et al. (2003)
		Yes	Saudi	Babalghith (2014)
	rs735883 (C/T intron 7)	No	Caucasian	Casp et al. (2003)
	rs1135216 (p.637D > G)	Yes	Saudi	Elhawary et al. (2014)
		No	Gujarati (Indian)	Jadeja et al. (2017)
		No	Western	Birlea et al. (2011)
CD4	VNTR (CD4-1188)	Yes	Iranian	Zamani et al. (2010)
	rs2855534	No	Western	Birlea et al. (2011)
FOXP3	rs2232365 (A/G promoter)	Yes	Han Chinese	Song et al. (2013)
		No	Indian (Gujarati)	Giri et al. (2021)
	rs3761548 (A/C promoter)	Yes	Han Chinese, Indian	Jahan et al. (2013), Song et al. (2013)
		No	Indian (Gujarati)	Giri et al. (2021)
	rs3761547 (A/G promoter)	Yes	Non-Hispanic White, Indian (Gujarati)	Giri et al. (2021), Birlea et al. (2011)
	rs11798415 (*GAGE10*A/T promoter)	Yes	Non-Hispanic White, Indian (Gujarati)	Giri et al. (2021), Birlea et al. (2011)

(continued)

Table 2 (continued)

Gene	Polymorphism	Association	Population	References
CTLA4	rs3087243 (CT60A/G 3'UTR)	Yes	Gujarati, European, Caucasian	Song et al. (2013), Dwivedi et al. (2011), Blomhoff et al. (2005)
	rs231775 (+49A/G Exon1)	No	Gujarati, South Indian, Romanian, European; Iranian, Turkish	Birlea et al. (2010), Song et al. (2013), Dwivedi et al. (2011), Deeba et al. (2010), Yildiz et al. (2016), Ala et al. (2015), Fatahi et al. (2005)
	rs231777 (C/T Intron 1), rs231779 (T/C Intron 1)	No	Korean	Shin et al. (2011)
	Microsatellite $(AT)_n$ polymorphisms (96-bp allele; Exon 3)	Yes	Turkish, Non-Hispanic White cases	Pehlivan et al. (2009), Itirli et al. (2005), Kemp et al. (1998)
	rs12992492 (Promoter)	Yes	Non-Hispanic White cases	Birlea et al. (2011)
	rs11571317 (C > T), rs5742909 (C > T)	Yes	South Indian	Ala et al. (2015)
IFNG	rs2430561 (+874 T/A; Intron 1)	Yes	Egyptian	Karam et al. (2017)
		No	Gujarati, Iranian	Namian et al. (2009), Dwivedi et al. (2013d)
	rs1861494 (+2109A/G)	No	Egyptian	Karam et al. (2017)
	rs1861494 (CA Repeats; Intron 1)	Yes	Gujarati	Dwivedi et al. (2013d)
TNFA	rs361525 (−238; G/A Promoter)	Yes	Gujarati	Laddha et al. (2012)
		Yes	Jordanian	Odeh et al. (2019)
		No	South Indian Tamils	Rajendiran et al. (2020)
	rs1800629 (−308; G/A)	Yes	Gujarati, Maxican, Saudi Arabia, Iranian, Middle Eastern populations, South Indian Tamils, Egyptian Females	Namian et al. (2009), Laddha et al. (2012), Al-Harthi et al. (2013), Rajendiran et al. (2020), Saleh et al. (2014), Lee and Bae (2015), Salinas-Santander et al. (2012)
		No	Turkish	Ac et al. (2006)
		No	Jordanian	Odeh et al. (2019)
	rs1799724 (−857; C/T)	Yes	Gujarati	Laddha et al. (2012)
		No	Chinese Uyghur	Wu et al. (2015)
		No	South Indian Tamils	Rajendiran et al. (2020)
	rs1800630 (−863; C/A)	Yes	Gujarati	Laddha et al. (2012)
		No	South Indian Tamils	Rajendiran et al. (2020)
		No	Chinese Uyghur	Wu et al. (2015)
	rs1799964 (−1031; T/C)	Yes	Gujarati	Laddha et al. (2012)
		No	South Indian Tamils	Rajendiran et al. (2020)
		No	Chinese Uyghur	Wu et al. (2015)

(continued)

Table 2 (continued)

Gene	Polymorphism	Association	Population	References
IL10	rs1800896 (−1082G/A; Promoter)	Yes	Saudi, Turkish	Abanmi et al. (2008), Ie et al. (2015)
	(−592C/A; Promoter)	Yes	Saudi	Abanmi et al. (2008)
	(−819C/T; Promoter)	No	Saudi	Abanmi et al. (2008)
	rs1800871	No	Non-Hispanic White subjects	Birlea et al. (2011)
	rs1800872	No	Non-Hispanic White subjects	Birlea et al. (2011)
TGFBR2	rs2005061	Yes	Korean	Yun et al. (2010)
	rs3773645	Yes	Korean	Yun et al. (2010)
	rs3773649	Yes	Korean	Yun et al. (2010)
IL2RA	rs706779	Yes	Caucasian	Jin et al. (2010a)
	rs7090530	Yes	Caucasian	Jin et al. (2010a)
	rs4750005, rs3920615, rs4747887, rs4750012, rs7099083	Yes	Chinese Mongolian	Rina (2016)
IL4	rs2243250 (−590 C/T)	No	Turkish	Pehlivan et al. (2009)
		Yes	Indian	Imran et al. (2012)
		No	Saudi Arab	Al-Shobaili et al. (2013)
	VNTR (IVS; Intron 3)	Yes	Indian	Imran et al. (2012)
IL1RN	rs2234663 (Intron 2 VNTR)	Yes	Gujarati (Indian)	Singh et al. (2018)
	rs2234663 (Intron 2 VNTR)	Yes	Turkish	Pehlivan et al. (2009)
	rs419598	No	European non-Hispanic White	Birlea et al. (2011)

functional aspects of these SNPs are not known, but they have been suggested to exert regulatory effects on *NLRP1* expression. The *NLRP1* SNPs including rs6502867, rs2670660, and rs8182352 were associated with GV in UK, USA, and Romanian populations (Jin et al. 2007a, c). Moreover, in a family-based study, the *NLRP1* rs6502867 SNP showed significant interactions with rs734930 (7q11), rs6960920 (7p13), and rs4744411 (9q22) SNPs which were associated with GV and other autoimmunity diseases as well (Jin et al. 2010a).

Two promoter SNPs: rs1008588 and rs2670660 in *NLRP1* were also associated with GV in Arab population (Alkhateeb et al. 2010). Further, Laddha et al. (2013) reported a significant association between GV with *NLRP1* rs2670660 and rs6502867 polymorphisms and a marginal association with the rs12150220 polymorphism. This study also suggested for association of "GCT" haplotype with two-fold increased risk of vitiligo. Further analysis suggested that SNP rs6502867-minor allele ("C") was associated with GV in Gujarat vitiligo patients (Laddha et al. 2013) whereas SNP rs6502867-major allele ("T") was associated in White subjects (Jin et al. 2007c). This difference indicates a recombination event which can be correlated with the ethnicity differences and the SNP might not be a causal variant of GV, rather can be tightly linked to the causal variant.

Furthermore, genotype–phenotype correlation of rs2670660 (A/G) and rs6502867 (T/C) in *NLRP1* gene showed an increase in *NLRP1* mRNA with susceptible genotypes of these SNPs in GV patients (Laddha et al. 2013). In addition, the functional analysis of *NLRP1* haplotypes associated with vitiligo demonstrated increased IL-1β processing. Nevertheless, there was no effect of the haplotypes on transcript and protein levels of *NLRP1*, indicating that altered NLRP1 function predisposed to autoimmune disease by inducing the NLRP1 inflammasome (Levandowski et al. 2013). The abovementioned studies indicate that *NLRP1* may serve as a vitiligo candidate gene; however, extensive investigations of the *NLRP1* SNPs with larger sample sizes in different ethnic populations are needed.

3. X box-binding protein 1 (*XBP1*):

The *XBP1* gene (22q12) encodes a transcription factor that binds with X2 promoter on human HLA DP-B and DR-A (Liou et al. 1990). By interacting with *HLA-DR*, *XBP1* has been suggested to involve in vitiligo pathogenesis (Ren et al. 2009). A previous study identified a significant linkage of microsatellites (22q12) with GV in non-Hispanic Whites (Spritz 2007) and these results were later confirmed in the Chinese population (Ren et al. 2009; Liang et al. 2007) also showed significant association of vitiligo with a putative regulatory polymorphism rs2269577 in *XBP1* gene (P = 0.007; OR = 1.36; 95% CI = 1.09–1.71). The rs2269577 SNP was associated with vitiligo in 3 independent Han Chinese cohorts and the study suggested an epistatic effect between *HLA-DRB1*07* allele and rs2269577 SNP (p = 0.033) on vitiligo development. In addition, the SNP's functional analysis suggested for a stronger promoter activity with "C"-risk allele and increased XBP1 expression was also observed in lesional skin of patients harboring the "C"-risk allele. Thus, the study indicated that the germline regulatory polymorphism of *XBP1* affects vitiligo development through *XBP1* transcriptional modulation (Ren et al. 2009). Further, Birlea et al. (2011), observed an association between rs2269577 SNP (P = 7.5E^{-04}, OR = 1.17) and twenty one additional SNPs spanning the *XBP1* region (chr22:29,154,237–29,219,122) with GV. Moreover, the meta-analysis study involving 3 Chinese cohorts and study by Birlea et al. (2011), revealed a high-risk causal allele and showed strong association with GV (P = 9.5E^{-09}; OR = 1.21). However, further *XBP1* SNP replication studies are needed in other populations to elucidate its association with GV.

4. *FAS*:

The *FAS* (or TNFSF6/CD95L; at Chr.10q24.1) encodes a member of TNF superfamily and it comprises of 9 exons and 8 introns (Arcos-Burgos et al. 2002). It plays a role in apoptotic signaling pathway through FAS-Ligand (Sharma et al. 2000; Kavurma and Khachigian 2003). The *FAS* promoter -1377(G > A) SNP was reported to increase the vitiligo risk (OR: 1.49; 95% CI: 1.07–2.08); however, -670(G > A) SNP did not associate with vitiligo in Han Chinese populations (Li et al. 2008). Another study suggested an association of *FAS* -670(G > A) with vitilgo in Turkish population (OR: 2.87; 95% CI: 1.37–6.03) and was suggested as a risk factor (Türsen et al. 2014). However, the study did not find evident vitiligo risk associated with *FAS* -1377, *FASL*-844, and *FASL*-124 SNPs (Türsen et al. 2014). These studies are suggestive of *FAS* gene's role in vitiligo pathogenesis; however, further investigations in different ethnic populations are needed to confirm its association with vitiligo.

5. Protein tyrosine phosphatase non-receptor 22 (*PTPN22*):

The *PTPN22* locus serves as the second strongest genetic predictor for autoimmune disease after the MHC. The *PTPN22* (Chr. 1p13) encodes lymphoid protein tyrosine phosphatase that expresses exclusively in immune cells. PTPN22 is a down regulator of T cell activation

(Siminovitch 2004). The *PTPN22* rs2476601 (1858C/T) SNP is present in the coding region which results in substitution of arginine to tryptophan and is associated with several autoimmune diseases (Burn et al. 2011). The association studies of *PTPN22* rs2476601 SNP in vitiligo are shown in Table 2.

Previously, case–control studies in Caucasians from the UK, (Cantón et al. 2005), and Romania (LaBerge et al. 2008; Laberge et al. 2008) showed a significant association of *PTPN22* rs2476601 (1858C/T) SNP with vitiligo. Moreover, odds ratio of 2.05 was reported for individuals harboring 1858 "T" allele suggesting an expanded autoimmunity phenotype (LaBerge et al. 2008; Laberge et al. 2008). Another European population also showed a significant association of rs2476601 (1858C/T) SNP with GV susceptibility (Jin et al. 2010c).

In the Mexican population, the *PTPN22* rs2476601 (1858C/T) SNP had significant association with active vitiligo (AV) (Garcia-Melendez et al. 2014). Nevertheless, in Indian Gujarati population, the *PTPN22* rs2476601 (1858C/T) SNP was not associated with vitiligo (Laddha et al. 2008), a recent study in a South Indian (Tamil) population reported a significant association between this allele and vitiligo (Rajendiran et al. 2018). Furthermore, two studies in the Egyptians (females) and Jordanian Arabs were unable to show an association between rs2476601 SNP of *PTPN22* and non-segmental vitiligo (Alkhateeb et al. 2010; Elmongy and Khalil 2013); however, these studies were limited by small sample sizes. Recently, one study in Saudi Arabians suggested that the "CT" genotype frequency of *PTPN22* rs2476601 SNP was increased in vitiligo patients ($p < 0.0001$) (Huraib et al. 2020). Moreover, a meta-analysis study reported association of *PTPN22* rs2476601 SNP with vitiligo in European population ($P < 0.001$; OR: 1.53; 95% CI: 1.34–1.75); however, Asian population did not show the association ($P = 0.2$; OR: 0.59; 95% CI: 0.26–1.32) (Agarwal and Changotra 2017).

6. Angiotensin-converting enzyme (*ACE*):

The ACE plays a crucial role in inflammation, vasculature, blood pressure and has been implicated in pathogenesis of several autoimmune diseases (Papadopoulos et al. 2000; Scholzen et al. 2003). The insertion-deletion (I/D) polymorphism is present in intron 16 of *ACE* gene (Rigat et al. 1990). This polymorphism is responsible for variability in ACE activity in serum and particularly, increased ACE activity was detected with D/D genotype whereas decreased ACE activity was associated with I/I genotypes (Rigat et al. 1990). The vitiligo association studies of *ACE* rs2476601 (I/D) polymorphism are shown in Table 2.

Previously, most studies reported significant association of *ACE* rs2476601 (I/D) polymorphism with vitiligo; however, few studies showed marginal significance and few studies did not find the association. These studies were conducted in Korean (Jin et al. 2004a, b), Egyptian (Badran et al. 2015; Rashed et al. 2015), and South Indian populations (Deeba et al. 2009; Tippisetty et al. 2011). In another Indian study, the D allele was found to be the vitiligo susceptibility allele (Patwardhan et al. 2013). However, Indian Gujarati population (Dwivedi et al. 2008), non-Hispanic White patients from UK (Akhtar et al. 2005), and Turkish population (Pehlivan et al. 2009) did not show association of the rs2476601 (I/D) polymorphism. Furthermore, study by Birlea et al. (2010) did not find association of 24 SNPs spanning the *ACE* region (chr17:61; 544, 434–61, 579, 979) with vitiligo. The *ACE* rs2476601 (I/D) polymorphism's meta-analysis reported that in pooled population "D" allele and "DD" genotype were strongly associated with vitiligo risk and suggested that the polymorphism can be used as biomarker for predicting the vitiligo risk (Lv et al. 2013). However, a further South Asian ethnicity-specific meta-analysis of "D" allele did not find association of *ACE* rs2476601 (I/D) polymorphism with vitiligo (Song et al. 2015).

7. Mannose Binding Lectin-2 (*MBL2*):

The MBL2 is an important molecule of innate immune system that activates the lectin pathway of complement system, involves apoptotic cell's clearance and hence, its role in autoimmune diseases is implicated. The *MBL2* gene is located on chromosome 10 (q11.2-q21) with four exons. The studies on *MBL2* gene polymorphisms in vitiligo are shown in Table 2. The exon 1 rs1800450 (codon 54) SNP was significantly associated with GV in Turkish population (Onay et al. 2007); however, in the subsequent study, the SNP was not associated with vitiligo in the Turkish population (Karkucak et al. 2015). It was observed that the sample sizes of these studies were too low to conclude a significant association. Moreover, in an Indian population the rs1800450 (codon 54) SNP as well as other SNPs in exon 1 and promoter region of *MBL2* (rs5030737, rs1800451, and rs7096206) were not associated with vitiligo (Dwivedi et al. 2009). Furthermore, Birlea et al. (2010) also found that the rs1800450 and 15 other SNPs spanning the *MBL2* region were not associated with GV. The abovementioned studies suggest that the *MBL2* polymorphisms may not be a risk factor for vitiligo; however, further studies in this regard can be carried out in other ethnic populations with larger sample size.

8. *TAP1-PSMB8*:

TAP1 and TAP2 molecules are responsible for antigenic peptide transfer from cytosol to the rough endoplasmic reticulum (RER) membrane. The *PSMB8* encodes LMP7 subunit of immunoproteasome and is induced by IFN-γ. The LMP7 degrades the ubiquitinated cytoplasmic proteins into small peptides which are then presented by MHC Class-I molecule of the cell surface (Basler et al. 2013). The PSMB8 (LMP7) or TAP1 proteins alterations can influence the antigen processing, its presentation and thereby lead to altered peripheral tolerance (Groettrup et al. 2001).

Vitiligo patients exhibited a reduced 26S proteasome in skin lesions (Xu et al. 2013). The GWAS also suggested that *TAP1-PSMB8* association with GV derived from linkage disequilibrium (LD) in MHC class-I and class-II regions (Birlea et al. 2011). *TAP1* and *PSMB8* SNPs have been studied for their association with vitiligo in different populations (Table 2).

Casp et al. (2003) reported significant association of *TAP1* rs1800453 (G/A; exon 10) SNP with susceptibility to vitiligo in Caucasian population. The association of *PSMB8* rs2071464 (G/T; intron 6) and rs2071543 (A/C; exon 2) SNPs were also reported with susceptibility to vitiligo in Indian populations (Dani et al. 2018; Jadeja et al. 2017). Previously, a study also showed association of *PSMB9* rs17587 (G/A; exon 3) SNP with vitiligo in Saudi population (Elhawary et al. 2014).

Furthermore, Birlea et al. (2009a) and Jadeja et al. (2017) did not find significant association of *TAP1* rs1135216 SNP; however, Elhawary et al. (2014) reported a significant association of the SNP with vitiligo susceptibility in Saudi population. Another study in Saudi population found significant association of *TAP1* rs1800453 (G/A; D637G; exon 10) SNP with vitiligo susceptibility (Babalghith 2014). In addition, Birlea et al. (2011) further investigated 34 SNPs in *TAP1-PSMB8* region (chr6:32; 807, 987–32, 831, 748) and reported significant association of two SNPs: rs6924102 ($P = 9.4E^{-05}$) and rs3819721 ($P = 5.2E^{-06}$). Moreover, this study suggested that *TAP1-PSMB8* rs6924102 and rs3819721 SNPs showed LD with MHC class-I and class-II association signals.

9. CD4:

Previously, European non-Hispanic white population showed that the *CD4*-1188 variable number of tandem repeats (VNTR) polymorphism was in strong LD with rs2855534 SNP (Kristiansen et al. 2004). Another study in Iranian population showed significant association of the VNTR polymorphism (*CD4*-1188) with vitiligo (Zamani et al.). However, the *CD4* rs2855534 SNP and 28 other SNPs in *CD4* region were not associated with vitiligo in a later study by Birlea et al. (2011).

10. Forkhead box P3 (*FOXP3*):

The FOXP3 is a transcription factor and a specific intracellular marker for Treg cells. FOXP3 plays a crucial role in growth, development and function of Treg cells (Yagi et al. 2004). FOXP3 suppresses the *IL2* and *IL4* genes' transcription and up regulates the expression of *CD25* and *CTLA4* and thereby down regulates the T cell activation (Zheng and Rudensky 2007). *FOXP3* mutations can alter the FOXP3 expression and affects Treg cell function that can lead to autoimmunity (Theos et al. 2005). Moreover, decreased $FOXP3^+$ cells have been suggested to contribute autoimmune diseases (Kim et al. 2009).

Previous studies reported the FOXP3 expression defects in $CD4^+CD25^{high}$ Tregs isolated from vitiligo patients (Dwivedi et al. 2013a; Giri et al. 2020a). In particular, significantly decreased *FOXP3* mRNA levels were observed in both lesional and perilesional skin compared to healthy skin (Hegazy et al. 2014). The *FOXP3* polymorphisms associated with vitiligo predisposition are shown in Table 2.

A meta-analysis study of 37 SNPs in *FOXP3* gene found significant association of promoter rs3761547 (A > G) SNP with vitiligo (Birlea et al. 2011). Moreover, the study also reported a strong LD between rs5906843 (*GAGE1*) and rs11798415 (*GAGE10*) blocks. Studies in Non-Hispanic Whites and Indian population suggested for association of the *GAGE10* rs11798415 (A > T) promoter SNP with vitiligo and the *GAGE10* SNP was in strong LD with the *FOXP3* rs3761547 (A > G) SNP (Giri et al. 2021; Birlea et al. 2011). The presence of these *GAGE10* and *FOXP3* SNPs on same chromosome (Xp11.23) suggests that these SNPs in combination can affect the *FOXP3* expression (Giri et al. 2021). Recently, in Indian population significant association of *FOXP3* promoter rs3761547 (A > G) SNP has been reported with GV (Giri et al. 2021). The study through DNA–protein docking analysis suggested that rs3761547 'G' allele leads to reduced binding of C/EBP transcription factor which in turn affects the *FOXP3* expression (Giri et al. 2021). Moreover, the genotype–phenotype correlation for *FOXP3* rs3761547 (A > G) suggested that patients harboring 'GG' genotypes exhibited reduced FOXP3 mRNA and protein (Giri et al. 2021). Two more *FOXP3* promoter SNPs (rs3761548 and rs2232365) were found to be associated with vitiligo in Indian and Chinese populations (Jahan et al. 2013; Song et al. 2013). The *FOXP3* rs3761548 'AA' genotype affects the c-Myb and E-47 transcription factors and thereby leads to altered FOXP3 levels (Xiao et al. 2008). Moreover, the rs2232365 'GG' genotype has been suggested to regulate the *FOXP3* expression due to the presence of the SNP in the GATA-3 binding site and can promote pro-inflammatory autoimmune diseases (Song et al. 2012).

11. Cytotoxic T lymphocyte antigen-4 (*CTLA4*):

The *CTLA4* gene encodes T cell surface molecule (CD152) and regulates activation of T cells. The knock-out mouse study has suggested that CTLA4 in crucial in maintaining the self-tolerance (Chen et al. 2006). The abnormalities in function and levels of CTLA-4 have been implicated in the etiology of vitiligo (Dwivedi et al. 2011). Studies have reported that vitiligo patients exhibit significantly decreased levels of soluble *CTLA4* (*sCTLA*4) and full-length *CTLA4* (*flCTLA*4) transcripts and proteins which in turn lead to decreased suppressive capacity of Treg (Dwivedi et al. 2011, 2013a; Giri et al. 2020a, b, 2021). The association studies of *CTLA4* polymorphisms in vitiligo are shown in Table 2.

The *CTLA4* 3' UTR rs3087243 (CT60GG) polymorphism was associated with isolated vitiligo (vitiligo without associated autoimmune diseases) and also correlated with decreased *CTLA4* transcripts (Dwivedi et al. 2011). However, study in Caucasian population showed significant association of *CTLA4* rs3087243 polymorphism in vitiligo patients who also had other autoimmune diseases (Blomhoff et al. 2005). Later, the *CTLA4* rs3087243 polymorphism was not found to be associated with vitiligo in Caucasian and Romanian populations (LaBerge et al. 2008; Laberge et al. 2008; Birlea et al. 2009b). Previous study in non-Hispanic whites reported an association of *CTLA4* intragenic microsatellite with strong LD with rs231775 SNP in vitiligo who also had other autoimmune diseases (Kemp et al.). Further, in Turkish population the *CTLA4* microsatellite polymorphism [$(AT)_n$ 96-bp allele; exon 3] was associated with vitiligo patients who did not have associated autoimmune diseases (Pehlivan et al. 2009; Itirli et al. 2005). In another *CTLA4* rs231775 (+49A/G) SNP, the 'G' allele has been suggested to alter the CTLA-4 availability on the cell surface by affecting its intracellular transportation (Kouki et al. 2000). However, the Gujarati (Indian), South Indian, Romanian, European, Iranian and Turkish populations did not find the association of *CTLA4* rs231775 SNP with vitiligo (Dwivedi et al. 2011; Deeba et al. 2010; Yildiz et al. 2016).

Further, the GWAS by Jin et al. (2011b) also reported the maximum association for *CTLA4* rs12992492 promoter SNP. However, the study suggested that these associations with GV are secondary to the *CTLA4* genetic association with other autoimmune diseases associated with vitiligo (Birlea et al. 2011). The *CTLA4* rs231777 and rs231779 *SNPs* (intron 1) were not associated with non-segmental vitiligo in Korean population (Shin et al. 2011). Moreover, a meta-analysis did not find association of *CTLA4* rs231775 (+49A/G) SNP with vitiligo; but was able to demonstrate association of *CTLA4* rs3087243 (CT60GG) polymorphism with vitiligo susceptibility in Europeans (Song et al. 2013). Recently, two more SNPs (rs11571317 and rs5742909) in the *CTLA4* gene have been reported to be associated with vitiligo in the South Indian population (Ala et al. 2015). The above-mentioned studies suggest that CTLA-4 may serve as an important candidate gene for vitiligo susceptibility in certain ethnic populations; however, the functional characterization of the SNPs and larger sample size based studies are needed in different ethnic populations.

12. Interferon-γ (*IFNG*):

The IFN-γ (type II interferon) is a pleiotropic cytokine and key regulator of immune system. *IFNG* gene (chr. 12q24) comprised of four exons and three introns (Naylor et al. 1983). *IFNG* contains two well reported polymorphisms: rs2430561 (+ 874A/T; intron 1) and rs1861494 (CA microsatellite). The association studies of *IFNG* polymorphisms in vitiligo are shown in Table 2.

Study by Pravica et al. (1999) reported that *IFNG* rs2430561 (+ 874A/T) SNP alters the IFN-γ levels and particularly, the 'A' allele led to decreased IFN-γ levels. However, the 'T' allele was suggested to create a putative binding site for NF-kB leading to increased production of IFN-γ (Pravica et al. 2000). In one Indian population, the genotype–phenotype analysis of *IFNG* rs2430561 (+ 874A/T) SNP revealed an increased *IFNG* transcript and protein levels in vitiligo patients harboring 'TT' genotype suggesting the involvement of 'T' allele in increased IFN-γ production (Dwivedi et al.). Moreover, Karam et al. (2017) found that rs2430561 'TT' genotype and 'T' allele frequencies were significantly higher in active vitiligo (AV) patients as compared to stable vitiligo (SV) patients, suggesting the role of the SNP in vitiligo progression. However, the *IFNG* rs2430561 (+874A/T) SNP was not significantly associated with GV in Indian (Gujarati) and Iranian populations (Dwivedi et al.; Namian et al. 2009).

Furthermore, individuals with 12 CA repeats [*IFNG* $(CA)_n$ repeat in intron 1; rs1861494] and a 'T' allele at the polymorphic site has been considered as for normal IFN-γ producers (Pravica et al. 1999, 2000); whereas, individuals with 13 repeats and 'A' allele were suggested as lower IFN-γ producers (Miyake et al. 2002). Interestingly, Dwivedi et al. showed significant association of *IFNG* 12 CA repeats with GV and demonstrated that the serum IFN-γ was higher in individuals harboring this polymorphism. Since few studies have reported association of *IFNG* polymorphisms specifically, rs2430561 (+874A/T) and rs1861494 (CA Repeats; intron 1); their findings must be confirmed by other replicative studies. Nonetheless, the genotype–phenotype study demonstrated by Dwivedi et al. supports the involvement of *IFNG* CA repeats in pathogenesis of vitiligo.

13. Tumor Necrosis Factor-α (*TNFA*):

TNF-α is a pleiotropic cytokine secreted mainly by macrophages, T cells, fibroblasts and keratinocytes. It has been suggested that TNF-α inhibits the melanogenesis by inhibiting tyrosinase and tyrosinase-related proteins (Martínez-Esparza et al. 1998) and also induces apoptosis in melanocytes (Moretti et al. 2002; Laddha et al. 2002). TNF-α also induces the expression of intercellular adhesion molecule-1 (ICAM-1) on melanocytes (Yohn et al. 1990); thereby, making them more vulnerable to killing by Tc cells by enhancing attachment of the melanocyte—Tc cell (Al Badri et al. 1993).

The *TNFA* gene is present within MHC class-III region on Chr. 6p21.31 and contains four exons. The *TNFA* promoter SNPs have been suggested to affect the regulatory regions leading to its altered production. Genetic association studies of *TNFA* polymorphisms in vitiligo are shown in Table 2.

Previously, Laddha et al. (2012) showed association of *TNFA* -238, -308, -857, -863, and -1031 promoter SNPs with vitiligo susceptibility in Indian (Gujarati) population. In addition, the study reported that -308 G/A and -238 G/A SNPs could modulate TNF-α levels in vitiligo patients (Laddha et al. 2012). The study also analyzed the combined effects of the *TNFA* haplotypes and found the "AATCC" haplotype to have the highest risk for developing the disease (Laddha et al. 2012). Interestingly, the "AATCC" haplotype comprised of all the susceptible alleles except -863A, which leads to reduced TNF-α. A recent study in the Jordanian population revealed the significant association of *TNFA* -238 SNP with vitiligo (Odeh et al. 2019). Earlier studies in Iranian population reported significant association of *TNFA* -308 G/A SNP with vitiligo (Namian et al. 2009); however, the *TNFA* -308 G/A SNP was not associated with vitiligo in Turkish and Jordanian populations (Yazici et al. 2006). The contradictory results may arise due to ethnic differences of these populations. Further studies in Mexican, Arab, and South Indian (Tamil) populations also reported a significant association of the *TNFA* -308 GA genotype with vitiligo (Al-Harthi et al. 2013; Rajendiran et al. 2020; Salinas-santander et al. 2012). Moreover, in Egyptian (women) the *TNFA* -308 susceptible genotypes were prevalent in female GV patients and were associated with three-fold increased risk of the disease (Saleh et al. 2014). A meta-analysis study by Lee and Bae (2015) suggested that *TNFA* -308 G/A SNP may serve as vitiligo risk factor in Middle Eastern populations ($P = 3.8 \times 10^{-5}$; OR: 1.569, 95% CI: 1.224–2.013). Later, two meta-analyzes that included six (1391 vitiligo cases and 2455 control subjects) and five (1505 cases and 2253 controls) case–control studies respectively suggested for the non-association of the *TNFA* -308 G/A SNP with vitiligo (Nie et al. 2015; Wu et al. 2015).

A recent meta-analysis of *TNFA* -308 G/A SNP with involvement of 11 studies (1993 vitiligo patients and 1732 controls) has suggested significant association of the susceptible "A" allele with: vitiligo susceptibility in overall populations and specifically with Asian, Middle Eastern, and Egyptian populations; vitiligo disease activity in North American population and localized vitiligo in overall populations and specifically in Asian population (Giri and Dwivedi 2021). These studies suggest that *TNFA* -308 G/A SNP may serve as a candidate marker for the vitiligo susceptibility in these populations; however, further studies with a larger sample size in different ethnic populations are needed to confirm the association.

14. Interleukin-10 (*IL10*):

The IL10 is an immune-suppressive cytokine mainly secreted by Treg cells to suppress the T cell activation. Studies have found the crucial role of IL-10 in vitiligo pathogenesis. Vitiligo patients with active disease exhibited reduced levels of IL-10 indicating that the disease progression is affected by IL-10 (Giri et al. 2020a, b; Tembhre et al. 2013). Recent studies have suggested significant reduced *IL10* mRNA and protein levels in GV patients' blood and Treg cells (Giri et al. 2020a, b). Moreover, the topical treatment of tacrolimus also showed increased expression of IL-10 in vitiligo skin lesions, indicating that unchecked Th1 pathway triggers the inhibition of melanocyte destruction in vitiligo (Taher et al. 2009). Moreover, Type-1 Treg cells are induced by IL-10 that contributes to immunosuppression principally by producing IL-10 (O'Garra et al. 2004).

The *IL10* gene (Chr. 1q31-q32) consists of five exons (Spits and Waal 1992) which harbor five promoter SNPs (at −3575, −2849, −1082, −819, and −592 positions) in the positive and negative regulatory regions of *IL10* (Eskdale et al. 1997). The association studies of *IL10* polymorphisms in vitiligo are shown in Table 2.

The two *IL10* promoters G-1082A and C-592A SNPs are mostly studied. The *IL10* −592 SNP is caused due to single base-pair substitution of cytosine to adenine and *IL10*-1082 polymorphism results from the guanine to adenine. These two SNPs are in strong LD and the haplotypes of these SNPs were demonstrated to associate with decreased IL-10 production by lymphocytes, in vitro (Turner et al. 1997). The *IL10* -592A allele has been suggested to create transcription factor (ETS family) binding site (Shin et al. 2000). In Saudi population, the *IL10* GG (−1082) genotype, CC (−592 and +819) genotype frequencies were significantly higher in vitiligo patients (Abanmi et al. 2008).

Moreover, the *IL10* GG (−1082) genotype frequency was also increased in Turkish vitiligo patients (Ie et al. 2015). However, there is no direct evidence on whether these polymorphisms are accompanied by altered IL-10 expression or not. Study by Birlea et al. (2011) did not find any association between GV and other *IL10* SNPs (rs1800871 or rs1800872) and the meta-analysis was also non-significant. Further analysis of these *IL10* polymorphisms in various populations can provide better information on their role in the etiology of vitiligo.

15. Transforming growth factor-β (*TGFB*):

The regulatory phenotype of the Treg cells is exerted by TGF-β (Joetham et al. 2007), since by inducing CD25 expression on $CD4^+CD25^-$ T cells, the TGF-β transforms these cells into $CD4^+CD25^+$ regulatory T cells, in vitro (Fu et al. 2004). Additionally, TGF-β also induces the expression of FoxP3 in Treg cells (Chen and Konkel 2010). Previous studies demonstrated a decrease in TGF-β levels in serum and lesional skin of vitiligo patients, indicating a defective Treg cell function in the patients (Moretti et al. 2002; Khan et al. 2012). In addition, *TGFB* mRNA and protein levels were also decreased in AV patients as compared to SV patients suggesting that TGF-β is also involved in the disease progression (Giri et al. 2020b; Tembhre et al. 2013). Moreover, the early onset patients (1–20 years) demonstrated decreased *TGFB* transcripts as compared to late-onset patients (41–60 *years*) suggesting the role of *TGFB* in early onset of GV (Giri et al. 2020b; Tembhre et al. 2013). Further, the Treg cells were found to be defective in GV patients due to decreased production of TGF-β and these Treg cells could not suppress the $CD8^+$ and $CD4^+$ T cells, in vitro co-culture assay (Giri et al. 2020b; Tembhre et al. 2013).

Though the role of TGF-β in Tregs suppressive capacity and in vitiligo pathogenesis is evident by previous studies, the *TGFB* genetic polymorphisms studies are lacking in vitiligo. A study in Korean population reported the association of *TGFBR2* rs2005061, rs3773645, and rs3773649 SNPs with vitiligo (Yun et al. 2010); however, the study could not reveal the effects of these SNPs on TGF-β expression.

16. Interleukin 2 Receptor Subunit Alpha (*IL2RA*):

The *IL2RA* gene is located on chromosome 10p15.1 and encodes the interleukin 2 (IL2) receptor alpha (IL2RA) chain. Eight out of known 25 SNP in *IL2RA* gene were significantly associated with GV and achieved the genome-wide significance level. The study suggested the strongest association of *IL2RA* rs7090530 and rs706779 SNPs with GV (Jin et al. 2010b). Individuals with GV were reported to have elevated serum IL2RA levels indicative of T-cell activation (Honda et al. 1997). Additionally, study in Chinese Mongolian population reported association of five SNPs (rs4750005, rs3920615, rs4747887, rs4750012, and rs7099083) in *IL2RA-RBM17* region with vitiligo (Han et al. 2016). However, more studies in different ethnic populations are needed to confirm the role of *IL2RA* SNPs in vitiligo.

17. Interleukin-4 (*IL4*):

The IL-4 cytokine stimulates antibody class switching in B-cell. The *IL4* gene polymorphisms are involved in altered IL-4 levels and hence their role has been suggested in autoimmune diseases including vitiligo (Imran et al. 2012). The *IL4* rs2243250 (−590 C/T) promoter SNP has been suggested to associate with increased IgE levels (Imran et al. 2012). The three tandem repeat allele VNTR (IVS; intron 3) in *IL4* gene has also been reported to associate with increased IL-4 levels (Nakashima et al. 2002). The association studies of *IL4* polymorphisms in vitiligo are shown in Table 2. Study by Imran et al. (2012) showed significant association of *IL4* rs2243250 (−590 C/T) and VNTR polymorphisms with susceptibility to vitiligo in the Gujarati (Indian) population. However, the *IL4* rs2243250 SNP was not associated with vitiligo in Turkish and Saudi Arab populations (Pehlivan et al. 2009; Al-Shobaili et al. 2013). Therefore, more studies are needed in different ethnic populations for confirming the role of *IL4* and its polymorphisms.

18. Interleukin 1 Receptor Antagonist (*IL1RN*):

The *IL1RN* gene encodes a protein which inhibit IL-1A and IL-1B activities and modulates IL-1-related responses. There is 86 bp VNTR in intron 2 of *IL1RN* gene with 6 alleles (1–6 repeats) (Tarlow et al. 1993). A Turkish population study claimed association of *IL1RN* rs2234663 (intron 2 VNTR) polymorphism with vitiligo (Pehlivan et al. 2009); however, the result was not found to be significant upon appropriate multiple-testing correction. Recently, Singh et al. (2018) reported that A2 allele of *IL1RN* rs2234663 (VNTR) polymorphism might be a risk factor for progressive vitiligo. Further, the *IL1RN* rs2234663 (VNTR) was observed in complete LD with *IL1RN* rs419598 (+2018) SNP in vitiligo patients of European non-Hispanic White population (Hutyrová et al. 2002). However, Birlea et al. (2011) did not find association of rs419598 SNP or any of the 54 SNPs of *IL1RN* gene with vitiligo. Hence, further studies are needed for *IL1RN* gene polymorphisms to confirm their role in vitiligo.

4.5 HLA and Its Associations with Vitiligo

The immune regulatory MHC region spans approximately 4 mb and it is the most dense gene region comprising around 250 genes of which 40% genes are related to immune system (The MHC Sequencing Consortium 1999).

The MHC region contains a high degree of polymorphism and LD in the human genome. More than 1000 alleles have been known for *HLA-A* and *HLA-B* genes. The *HLA* gene polymorphisms are involved in genetic susceptibility to several autoimmune diseases including vitiligo, rheumatoid arthritis, multiple sclerosis, celiac disease, type 1 diabetes, and ankylosing spondylitis (Trowsdale 2011).

The alleles of HLA class-I and class-II genes codes for unique amino acid sequences that are necessary for immune response to non-self or self-antigens (autoantigens). It has been seen that alteration in peptide binding efficiency can modulate autoimmune risk in different ways.

For example, increased binding efficiency of sequestered peptides leads to presentation of potentially immunogenic peptides by HLA risk variants; whereas the reduced binding efficiency of particular peptides results in the escape of autoreactive T cell clones from tolerance mechanisms due to the HLA risk variants.

The initial *HLA* association studies in vitiligo reported inconsistent findings due to inadequate statistical power and lack of multiple testing corrections for many different HLA types (Kachru et al. 1978; Metzker et al. 1980; Minev et al. 1985; Nakagawa et al. 1980; Retornaz et al. 1976). Later, one study identified significant association of HLA-DR4 with vitiligo (Foley et al. 1983). Subsequently, many studies found association of other *HLA* genes with vitiligo including *HLA-A*02*, *HLA-A*30*, *HLA-B*13*, *HLA-C*0602*, *HLA-DRB1*04*, *HLA-DRB1*07,* and *HLA-DQB1*03* (Liu et al. 2007; Taştan et al. 2004; Zhang et al. 2004). The *HLA* associations in different populations with vitiligo are shown in Table 3.

Table 3 Association of HLA in different populations with vitiligo

HLA Allele/Polymorphism	Association	Population	References
Bw35	Yes	Yemeni	Metzker et al. (1980)
B13	Yes	Moroccan (Jewish)	Metzker et al. (1980)
DR4	Yes	American (Caucasian)	Foley et al. (1983)
DR4, DQw3	Yes	American (African)	Dunston and Halder (1990)
B07, 15, Bw22	Yes	Asian	Dai (1990)
DR1, B08	Yes	European	Poloy et al. (1991)
A30, B27, Cw6, DQw3	Yes	Italian	Finco et al. (1991)
A3	Yes	Italian (Northern)	Lorini et al. (1992)
A30, Cw6, DQw3	Yes	Italian (Northern)	Orecchia et al. (1992)
DR12, A2	Yes	European	Schallreuter et al. (1993)
B46, A31, Cw4	Yes	Asian	Ando et al. (1993)
DR6	Yes	Dutch	Venneker et al. (1992)
Bw6, DR7	Yes	Asian	Venkataram et al. (1995)
DR6	Yes	European	Valsecchi et al. (1995)
B21, Cw6, DR53	Yes	Asian	AL-Fouzan et al. (1995)
A2, Dw7	Yes	Slovak	Buc et al. (1996)
*DRB1*0701, DQB1*0201, DPB1*1601*	Yes	Slovak	Buc et al. (1998)
A2, A10, A30 + A31, B13, B15	Yes	Asian	Wang et al.
*DRB4*0101, DQB1*0303*	Yes	Dutch	Zamani et al. (2001)
DR3, DR4, DR7	Yes	Asian	Taştan et al. (2004)
DR4, DR53	Yes	Dutch Caucasian	De Vijlder et al. (2004)
*A*2501, A*30, B*13, B*27, Cw*0602*	Yes	Chinese Han	Zhang et al. (2004)
*DQA1*0302,*0601, DQB1*0303,*0503*	Yes	Chinese Han	Yang et al. (2005)
*DRB1*04-DQB1*0301*	Yes	European-American	Fain et al. (2006)

(continued)

Table 3 (continued)

HLA Allele/Polymorphism	Association	Population	References
B05, 07, 15, 35, Bw06	Yes	Asian	Abanmi et al. (2006)
*DRB1*07:01*	Yes	Chinese	Ren et al. (2009)
*HLA-A*3001, HLA-B*1302, HLA-C*0602 and HLA-DRB1*0701* (rs11966200 and rs9468925)	Yes	Chinese Han	Quan et al. (2010)
B63	Yes	Asian	Akay et al. (2010)
HLA-A, HCG9 (rs3823355)	Yes	Caucasian	Jin et al. (2010a)
HLA-DRB1 and HLA-DQA1 (rs532098)	Yes	Caucasian	Jin et al. (2011b)
*HLA-A*02:01*	Yes	Caucasian	Jin et al. (2012b)
*HLA-A*33:01, HLA-A*02:01, HLA-B*44:03, HLA-DRB1*07:01*	Yes	Indian	Singh et al. (2012)
HLA-B and *HLA-C* (rs9468925)	Yes	Chinese Han	Liu et al. (2012)
HLA-DRA (rs3096691, rs3129859)	Yes	European	Birlea et al. (2013)
HLA-DRB1 and *HLA-DQA1* (rs482044)	Yes	European	Birlea et al. (2013)
HLA A2, HLA B49, HLA CW2, HLA CW3 and *HLA CW7*	Yes	Iranian	Nejad et al. (2013)
HLA-DRB1 07:0101* and *DRB1* 11:0101*	Yes	Iraqi Arab	Abdullah et al. (2015)
HLA-A1, A19, B16, CW4, CW 6, DR 4, DR7 and *DQ3*	Yes	Egyptian	Elgendy et al. (2016)
*HLA-A*02, HLA-DRB1*07, HLA-A*32, HLA-DQB1*06*	Yes	Southeast Brazil	Ramire et al. (2016)
*HLA-DRB1*1201/02, DRB1*0701/02, DQA1*0302 and DQB1*0303*	Yes	Chinese Uyghur	Kang et al. (2017)
*DRB1 *0701, *0413*	Yes	Egyptian	Toama et al. (2019)
*HLA-G*01:01:01:01/UTR-1* (rs9380142/G)	Yes	Brazilians	Veiga-Castelli et al. (2019)

HLA association study in Northern Italian patients showed a significant association for HLA-A3, A30, Cw6, and DQw3 (Lorini et al. 1992; Orecchia et al. 1992). A meta-analysis suggested association of *HLA-02, 33, A31* and *HLA-B*13, B*27, Bw*06, Bw*46, Bw*55, Bw*56,* and *Bw*60* with increased vitiligo risk (Li et al. 2016). In a Southeast Brazil study, association of *HLA-A*02*, and *HLA-DRB1*07* was reported with vitiligo whereas, the *HLA-A*32 and HLA-DQB1*06* were associated with both localized and generalized vitiligo (GV) (Ramire et al. 2016). Moreover, *HLA A2, HLA B49, HLA CW2, HLA CW3,* and *HLA CW7* were associated with vitiligo in Iranian population (Nejad et al. 2013).

Furthermore, studies by Birlea et al. (2013) and Singh et al. (2012) in the Indian population, reported association of MHC class-II loci with GV; however, Europian population GWAS showed the association of *HLA-A* in MHC class-I region (Jin et al. 2011b), in addition to multiple signals in MHC class-II region with vitiligo. Birlea et al. (2013) reported that 3 SNPs of MHC class-II (rs3096691, located at upstream of *NOTCH4*; rs3129859, located at upstream of

HLA-DRA, and rs482044, located between *HLA-DRB1* and *HLA-DQA1*) are strongly associated with GV (Birlea et al. 2013). Moreover, significant association of *HLA-A*33:01, HLA-B*44:03,* and *HLA-DRB1*07:01* with vitiligo in North Indian and Gujarati (Indian) populations suggested the common autoimmune link for vitiligo in these cohorts (Singh et al. 2012).

In addition, GWASs in Caucasian and Chinese populations identified strong association signals in *MHC* region (Chr. 6p21.3) for vitiligo and a few of these signals differed between these populations (Quan et al. 2010; Jin et al. 2011b). In particular, Caucasian population showed two major association signals, one signal was in between *HLA-A* and *HCG9* (*MHC Class-I* region) and the other was in between *HLA-DRB1* and *HLA-DQA1* (*MHC Class-II* region) which were in strong LD with *HLA-DRB1*04* (Jin et al. 2011b). The Chinese population showed the major association signal in *MHC Class-III* region, in addition to few independent associations in *MHC class-II* region (Quan et al. 2010). Another study, conducted in the Chinese population suggested for major association in between *HLA-B* and *HLA-C* (*MHC class-I*) region (Liu et al. 2012). The two independent association signals: rs11966200 and rs9468925 SNPs were identified in Chinese population. Further, the rs11966200 SNP showed strong association with vitiligo and suggested that it reflects the association of *HLA-A*3001*, *HLA-B*1302*, *HLA-C*0602,* and *HLA-DRB1*0701* alleles. In addition, the association of rs9468925 SNP with vitiligo suggested the association of *HLA-C/HLA-B* allele (Quan et al. 2010).

Additional studies confirmed the association of rs9468925 SNP with clinical features of GV (Liu et al. 2012) and association of *HLA-C/HLA-B* rs9468925 SNP with psoriasis and vitiligo was also reported (Zhu et al. 2011). This served as the first evidence of sharing common MHC locus between two major autoimmune skin diseases. Moreover, association of rs532098 SNP in vicinity of HLA-DRB1-DQA1 region with the age of onset of GV was also reported, suggesting that this locus may play a role in the onset of the disease (Jin et al. 2011b). Further, an association of *HLA-DRB1*1201/02, DRB1*0701/02, DQA1*0302*, and *DQB1*0303* was reported in Chinese Uygur population with susceptibility to vitiligo (Kang et al. 2017). Recently, *HLA-DRB1 *0701* and **0413* have been found to be associated with good therapeutic response in vitiligo patients, whereas *DRB1*8* and **12* alleles have been reported to be associated with worse therapeutic response among Egyptians (Toama et al. 2019). One recent study has shown the association of allele rs9380142/G (3'UTR, + 3187) at *HLA-G* locus with non-segmental vitiligo ($p = 0.01645$; OR = 2.096) (Veiga-Castelli et al. 2019).

Furthermore, it has been suggested that variations in the *MHC* regulatory regions are more important than *HLA* coding variations in conferring risk for vitiligo and other autoimmune diseases (Jin et al. 2019). The study reported that rs9271597 and rs145954018 SNPs in *MHC Class-II* region are associated with early onset of vitiligo (Jin et al. 2019) and are found within the lymphoid-specific enhancers. In addition, the increased *HLA-DQB1* mRNA and HLA-DQ protein in DCs and monocytes were associated with rs145954018del-rs9271597A haplotype (Jin et al. 2019).

5 Conclusions

The GWASs carried out by various groups in different ethnicities identified several genes for vitiligo susceptibility which encode proteins involved in immune regulation and apoptotic functions and may play an important part in vitiligo pathogenesis. A total of fifty genetic loci have been detected for vitiligo susceptibility, mostly in European-derived Whites. These vitiligo susceptibility genes may serve as novel therapeutic and prophylactic targets for developing effective treatment for vitiligo. Recent candidate gene association studies with genotype–phenotype correlation have also shown that altered functions of immune pathway genes are involved in vitiligo. Although, it is yet difficult to draw a direct line from these causative genes to the development of vitiligo due to the involvement of multiple loci and their interaction with environmental triggers. Moreover, the limited concordance in identical twins suggested that vitiligo development is also influenced by environmental factors.

Therefore, studies linking genetic factors with possible environmental triggers and treatment response are warranted in vitiligo. Nevertheless, collecting large study populations of different ethnicities and detailed clinical follow-ups is a challenge for now. However, further advancements in genetic risk factors of vitiligo and their exact roles in altering the immune pathways and destruction of melanocytes can help in designing the personalized therapy and possible genetic interventions for vitiligo.

Acknowledgements We are grateful to Uka Tarsadia University, Maliba Campus, Tarsadi, Gujarat, India for providing the facilities needed for the preparation of this chapter.

Conflict of Interest The authors declare no conflict of interest.

Funding Sources This work was supported by grant to Dr. Mitesh Dwivedi {ECR/2017/000858} from Science and Engineering Research Board, Department of Science & Technology (SERB-DST), New Delhi.

References

Abanmi A, Al Harthi F, Al Baqami R, Al Assaf S, Zouman A et al (2006) Association of HLA loci alleles and antigens in Saudi patients with vitiligo. Arch Dermatol Res 7:347–352

Abanmi A, Al Harthi F, Zouman A, Kudwah A, Jamal MA et al (2008) Association of interleukin-10 gene promoter polymorphisms in Saudi patients with vitiligo. Dis Markers 1:51–57

Abdullah GA, Yassin M, Alhamamy H, Mahdi BM (2015) The association between human leukocyte antigen-DRB1 and vitiligo

Agarwal S, Changotra H (2017) Association of protein tyrosine phosphatase, non-receptor type 22 +1858C→T polymorphism and susceptibility to vitiligo: systematic review and meta-analysis. Indian J Dermatol Venereol Leprol 2:183–189

Agarwal P, Rashighi M, Essien KI, Richmond JM, Randall L et al (2015) Simvastatin prevents and reverses depigmentation in a mouse model of vitiligo. J Invest Dermatol 4:1080–1088

Akay BN, Bozkir M, Anadolu Y, Gullu S (2010) Epidemiology of vitiligo, associated autoimmune diseases and audiological abnormalities: ankara study of 80 patients in Turkey. J Eur Acad Dermatol Venereol 10:1144–1150

Akbas H, Dertlioglu SB, Dilmec F, Atay AE (2014) Lack of association between PTPN22 Gene +1858 C>T polymorphism and susceptibility to generalized vitiligo in a Turkish population. Ann Dermatol 1:88–91

Akhtar S, Gavalas NG, Gawkrodger DJ, Watson PF, Weetman AP et al (2005) An insertion/deletion polymorphism in the gene encoding angiotensin converting enzyme is not associated with generalised vitiligo in an English population. Arch Dermatol Res 2:94–98

Al Badri AM, Foulis AK, Todd PM, Garioch JJ, Gudgeon JE et al (1993) Abnormal expression of MHC class II and ICAM-1 by melanocytes in vitiligo. J Pathol 2:203–206

Ala Y, Pasha MK, Rao RN, Komaravalli PL, Jahan P (2015) Association of IFN-γ: IL-10 cytokine ratio with nonsegmental vitiligo pathogenesis. Zhou X-J, ed. Autoimmune Dis 423490

AL-Fouzan AA, Al-Arbash M, Fouad F, Kaaba SA, Mousa MA et al (1995) Study of HLA class I/IL and T lymphocyte subsets in Kuwaiti vitiligo patients. Eur J Immunogenet 2:209–213

Al-Harthi F, Zouman A, Arfin M, Tariq M, Al-Asmari A (2013) Tumor necrosis factor-α and -β genetic polymorphisms as a risk factor in Saudi patients with vitiligo. Genet Mol Res 3:2196–2204

Alikhan A, Felsten LM, Daly M, Petronic-Rosic V (2011) Vitiligo: a comprehensive overview Part I. Introduction, epidemiology, quality of life, diagnosis, differential diagnosis, associations, histopathology, etiology, and work-up. J Am Acad Dermatol 3:473–491

Alkhateeb A, Qarqaz F (2010) Genetic association of NALP1 with generalized vitiligo in Jordanian Arabs. Arch Dermatol Res 8:631–634

Alkhateeb A, Stetler GL, Old W, Talbert J, Uhlhorn C et al (2002) Mapping of an autoimmunity susceptibility locus (AIS1) to chromosome 1p31.3-p32.2. Hum Mol Genet 6:661–667

Alkhateeb A, Fain PR, Thody A, Bennett DC, Spritz RA (2003) Epidemiology of vitiligo and associated autoimmune diseases in Caucasian probands and their families. Pigment Cell Res 3:208–214

Alkhateeb A, Al-Dain Marzouka N, Qarqaz F (2010) SMOC2 gene variant and the risk of vitiligo in Jordanian Arabs. Eur J Dermatol 6:701–704

Alkhateeb A, Marzouka NA, Tashtoush R (2013) Variants in PTPN22 and SMOC2 genes and the risk of thyroid disease in the Jordanian Arab population. Endocrine 3:702–709

Almasi-Nasrabadi M, Amoli MM, Robati RM, Rajabi F, Ghalamkarpour F et al (2019) CDH1 and DDR1 common variants confer risk to vitiligo and autoimmune comorbidities. Gene 17–22

Al-Shobaili H, Settin A, Alzolibani A, Al Robaee A, Salem T et al (2013) Interleukin-4 (-590 C>T) and interleukin-4 receptor (Q551R A>G) gene polymorphisms in Saudi patients with vitiligo. Eur J Dermatol 3:402–404

Amos W, Driscoll E, Hoffman JI (2011) Candidate genes versus genome-wide associations: which are better for detecting genetic susceptibility to infectious disease? Proc Biol Sci 1709:1183–1188

Ando I, Chi HI, Nakagawa H, Otsuka F (1993) Difference in clinical features and HLA antigens between familial and non-familial vitiligo of non-segmental type. Br J Dermatol 4:408–410

Arcos-Burgos M, Parodi E, Salgar M, Bedoya E, Builes J et al (2002) Vitiligo: complex segregation and linkage disequilibrium analyses with respect to microsatellite loci spanning the HLA. Hum Genet 4:334–342

Babalghith A (2014) TAP1 and LMP7 gene polymorphisms associated with vitiligo in Saudi community. Int J Curr Microbiol App Sci 4:1–9

Badran DI, Nada H, Hassan R (2015) Association of angiotensin-converting enzyme ACE gene polymorphism with ACE activity and susceptibility to vitiligo in Egyptian population. Genet Test Mol Biomarkers 5:258–263

Basak PY, Adiloglu AK, Koc IG, Tas T, Akkaya VB (2008) Evaluation of activatory and inhibitory natural killer cell receptors in non-segmental vitiligo: a flow cytometric study. J Eur Acad Dermatol Venereol 8:970–976

Basler M, Kirk CJ, Groettrup M (2013) The immunoproteasome in antigen processing and other immunological functions. Curr Opin Immunol 1:74–80

Behl PN (1955) Leucoderma and its treatment with Ammi majus. J Indian Med Assoc 16:615–618

Ben S, Jin Y, Santorico SA, Spritz RA (2018) Genome-Wide Association of PVT1 with Vitiligo. J Invest Dermatol 8:1884–1886

Ben Ahmed M, Zaraa I, Rekik R, Elbeldi-Ferchiou A, Kourda N et al (2012) Functional defects of peripheral regulatory T lymphocytes in patients with progressive vitiligo. Pigment Cell Melanoma Res 1:99–109

Bhatia PS, Mohan L, Pandey ON, Singh KK, Arora SK et al (1992) Genetic nature of vitiligo. J Dermatol Sci 3:180–184

Birlea SA, Costin GE, Norris DA (2009a) New insights on therapy with vitamin D analogs targeting the intracellular pathways that control repigmentation in human vitiligo. Med Res Rev 3:514–546

Birlea SA, LaBerge GS, Procopciuc LM, Fain PR, Spritz RA (2009b) CTLA4 and generalized vitiligo: two genetic association studies and a meta-analysis of published data. Pigment Cell Melanoma Res 2:230–234

Birlea SA, Gowan K, Fain PR, Spritz RA (2010) Genome-wide association study of generalized vitiligo in an isolated European founder population identifies SMOC2, in close proximity to IDDM8. J Invest Dermatol 3:798–803

Birlea SA, Jin Y, Bennett DC, Herbstman DM, Wallace MR B et al (2011) Comprehensive association analysis of candidate genes for generalized vitiligo supports XBP1, FOXP3, and TSLP. J Invest Dermatol 2:371–381

Birlea SA, Ahmad FJ, Uddin RM, Ahmad S, Pal SS et al (2013) Association of generalized vitiligo with MHC class II loci in patients from the Indian subcontinent. J Invest Dermatol 5:1369–1372

Blomhoff A, Kemp EH, Gawkrodger DJ, Weetman AP, Husebye ES et al (2005) CTLA4 polymorphisms are associated with vitiligo, in patients with concomitant autoimmune diseases. Pigment Cell Res 1:55–58

Boissy RE, Spritz RA (2009) Frontiers and controversies in the pathobiology of vitiligo: separating the wheat from the chaff. Exp Dermatol 7:583–585

Boniface K, Jacquemin C, Darrigade A-S, Dessarthe B, Martins C et al (2018) Vitiligo skin is imprinted with resident memory CD8 T cells expressing CXCR3. J Invest Dermatol 2:355–364

Buc M, Busová B, Hegyi E, Kolibásová K (1996) Vitiligo is associated with HLA-A2 and HLA-Dw7 in the Slovak populations. Folia Biol (praha) 1–2:23–25

Buc M, Fazekasová H, Cechová E, Hegyi E, Kolibásová K et al (1998) Occurrence rates of HLA-DRB1, HLA-DQB1, and HLA-DPB1 alleles in patients suffering from vitiligo. Eur J Dermatol 1:13–15

Burn GL, Svensson L, Sanchez-Blanco C, Saini M, Cope AP (2011) Why is PTPN22 a good candidate susceptibility gene for autoimmune disease? FEBS Lett 23:3689–3698

Byrne KT, Zhang P, Steinberg SM, Turk MJ (2014) Autoimmune vitiligo does not require the ongoing priming of naive CD8 T cells for disease progression or associated protection against melanoma. J Immunol 4:1433–1439

Bystryn JC, Naughton GK (1985) The significance of vitiligo antibodies. J Dermatol 1:1–9

Cantón I, Akhtar S, Gavalas NG, Gawkrodger DJ, Blomhoff A et al (2005) A single-nucleotide polymorphism in the gene encoding lymphoid protein tyrosine phosphatase (PTPN22) confers susceptibility to generalised vitiligo. Genes Immun 7:584–587

Casp CB, She JX, McCormack WT (2003) Genes of the LMP/TAP cluster are associated with the human autoimmune disease vitiligo. Genes Immun 7:492–499

Cavalli G, Hayashi M, Jin Y, Yorgov D, Santorico SA et al (2016) MHC class II super-enhancer increases surface expression of HLA-DR and HLA-DQ and affects cytokine production in autoimmune vitiligo. Proc Natl Acad Sci USA 5:1363–1368

Chen W, Konkel JE (2010) TGF-beta and "adaptive" Foxp3(+) regulatory T cells. J Mol Cell Biol 1:30–36

Chen JJ, Huang W, Gui JP, Yang S, Zhou FS et al (2005) A novel linkage to generalized vitiligo on 4q13-q21 identified in a genomewide linkage analysis of Chinese families. Am J Hum Genet 6:1057–1065

Chen Z, Stockton J, Mathis D, Benoist C (2006) Modeling CTLA4-linked autoimmunity with RNA interference in mice. Proc Natl Acad Sci USA 44:16400–16405

Cheong KA, Chae SC, Kim YS, Kwon HB, Chung HT et al (2009) Association of thymic stromal lymphopoietin gene -847C>T polymorphism in generalized vitiligo. Exp Dermatol 12:1073–1075

Cheong KA, Kim NH, Noh M, Lee AY (2013) Three new single nucleotide polymorphisms identified by a genome-wide association study in Korean patients with vitiligo. J Korean Med Sci 5:775–779

Craddock N, Hurles ME, Cardin N, Pearson RD, Plagnol V et al (2010) Genome-wide association study of CNVs in 16,000 cases of eight common diseases and 3,000 shared controls. Nature 7289:713

Dai X (1990) A study on the association of HLA antigens with vitiligo. Chin J Dermatol 31–33

Dani P, Patnaik N, Singh A, Jaiswal A, Agrawal B et al (2018) Association and expression of the antigen-processing gene PSMB8, coding for low-molecular-mass protease 7, with vitiligo in North India: case-control study. Br J Dermatol 2:482–491

Das SK, Majumder PP, Majumdar TK, Haldar B (1985) Studies on vitiligo. II Familial aggregation and genetics. Genet Epidemiol 3:255–262

De Vijlder HC, Westerhof W, Schreuder GMT, De Lange P, Claas FH (2004) Difference in pathogenesis between vitiligo vulgaris and halo nevi associated with vitiligo is supported by an HLA association study. Pigment Cell Res 3:270–274

Deb DK, Sassano A, Lekmine F, Majchrzak B, Verma A et al (2003) Activation of protein kinase C delta by IFN-gamma. J Immunol 1:267–273

Deeba F, Jamil K, Rabbani S, Waheed MA, Rao H (2009) Association of angiotensin converting enzyme gene I/D polymorphism with vitiligo in South Indian population. Int J Med Med Sci 1:9–12

Deeba F, Syed R, Quareen J, Waheed MA, Jamil K et al (2010) CTLA-4 A49G gene polymorphism is not associated with vitiligo in South Indian population. Indian J Dermatol 1:29–32

Devadas S, Das J, Liu C, Zhang L, Roberts AI et al (2006) Granzyme B is critical for T cell receptor-induced cell death of type 2 helper T cells. Immunity 2:237–247

Dey-Rao R, Sinha AA (2017) Vitiligo blood transcriptomics provides new insights into disease mechanisms and identifies potential novel therapeutic targets. BMC Genomics 1:109

Douroudis K, Kingo K, Karelson M, Silm H, Reimann E et al (2011) The PRO2268 gene as a novel susceptibility locus for vitiligo. Acta Derm Venereol 2:189–191

Dunston GM, Halder RM (1990) Vitiligo is associated with HLA-DR4 in black patients. A preliminary report. Arch Dermatol 1:56–60

Dwivedi M, Laddha NC, Shajil EM, Shah BJ, Begum R (2008) The ACE gene I/ D polymorphism is not associated with generalized vitiligo susceptibility in Gujarat population. Pigment Cell Melanoma Res 3:407–408

Dwivedi M, Gupta K, Gulla KC, Laddha NC, Hajela K et al (2009) Lack of genetic association of promoter and structural variants of mannan-binding lectin (MBL2) gene with susceptibility to generalized vitiligo. Br J Dermatol 1:63–69

Dwivedi M, Laddha NC, Imran M, Shah BJ, Begum R (2011) Cytotoxic T-lymphocyte-associated antigen-4 (CTLA-4) in isolated vitiligo: a genotype-phenotype correlation. Pigment Cell Melanoma Res 4:737–740

Dwivedi M, Laddha NC, Arora P, Marfatia YS, Begum R (2013a) Decreased regulatory T-cells and CD4+/CD8 + ratio correlate with disease onset and progression in patients with generalized vitiligo. Pigment Cell Melanoma Res 4:586–591

Dwivedi M, Laddha NC, Imran M, Shah BJ, Begum R et al (2013b) Complete sequence and gene map of a human major histocompatibility complex. The MHC sequencing consortium. Pigment Cell Melanoma Res 1:921–923

Dwivedi M, Laddha NC, Begum R (2013c) Correlation of increased MYG1 expression and its promoter polymorphism with disease progression and higher susceptibility in vitiligo patients. J Dermatol Sci 3:195–202

Dwivedi M, Laddha NC, Shah K, Shah BJ, Begum R (2013d) Involvement of interferon-gamma genetic variants and intercellular adhesion molecule-1 in onset and progression of generalized Vitiligo. J Interf Cytokine Res 11:646–659

Dwivedi M, Laddha NC, Shah K, Shah BJ, Begum R (2013e) Involvement of interferon-gamma genetic variants and intercellular adhesion molecule-1 in onset and progression of generalized vitiligo. J Interferon Cytokine Res 33(11):646–659

Dwivedi M, Laddha NC, Mansuri MS, Marfatia YS, Begum R (2013f) Association of NLRP1 genetic variants and mRNA overexpression with generalized vitiligo and disease activity in a Gujarat population. Br J Dermatol 5:1114–1125

Dwivedi M, Kemp EH, Laddha NC, Mansuri MS Weetman AP et al (2015) Regulatory T cells in vitiligo: implications for pathogenesis and therapeutics. Autoimmun Rev 1:49–56

Dwivedi M, Laddha N, Begum R (2018) Viral causes of vitiligo: a new perspective for vitiligo pathogenesis. Viral Immunol 8:1–4

Eldin N, Teama S, Amro K, Farag H, Eldin SMN et al (2006) Polymorphisms of TAP1/LMP7 loci in Egyptian patients with vitiligo. undefined

Elgendy A, Alshawadfy E, Ali EA, Wadea N, Khalil K et al (2016) Association of HLA Class I and II antigens with vitiligo in Egyptian population

Elhawary NA, Bogari N, Jiffri EH, Rashad M, Fatani A et al (2014) Transporter TAP1–637G and immunoproteasome PSMB9–60H variants influence the risk of developing vitiligo in the Saudi population. Dis Markers 260732

Elmongy NN, Khalil REA (2013) PTPN22 gene polymorphism in Egyptian females with non-segmental vitiligo. Comp Clin Path 5:961–964

Eskdale J, Kube D, Tesch H, Gallagher G (1997) Mapping of the human IL10 gene and further

characterization of the 5' flanking sequence. Immunogenetics 2:120–128
Fain PR, Gowan K, LaBerge GS, Alkhateeb A, Stetler GL et al (2003) A genomewide screen for generalized vitiligo: confirmation of AIS1 on chromosome 1p31 and evidence for additional susceptibility loci. Am J Hum Genet 6:1560–1564
Fain PR, Babu SR, Bennett DC, Spritz RA (2006) HLA class II haplotype DRB1*04-DQB1*0301 contributes to risk of familial generalized vitiligo and early disease onset. Pigment Cell Res 1:51–57
Fan LC, Shiau CW, Tai WT, Hung MH, Chu PY et al (2015) SHP-1 is a negative regulator of epithelial-mesenchymal transition in hepatocellular carcinoma. Oncogene 41:5252–5263
Fatahi MJ, Pezeshki A, Emad M, Lohrasb MH, Shamseddin A et al (2005) Lack of association between CTLA-4 A49G polymorphism and vitiligo. Iran J Immunol 2:97–102
Fernando MMA, Stevens CR, Walsh EC, De Jager PL, Goyette P et al (2008) Defining the role of the MHC in autoimmunity: a review and pooled analysis. PLoS Genet 4:e1000024
Ferrara TM, Jin Y, Gowan K, Fain PR, Spritz RA (2013) Risk of generalized vitiligo is associated with the common 55R–94A-247H variant haplotype of GZMB (encoding granzyme B). J Invest Dermatol 6:1677–1679
Finco O, Cuccia M, Martinetti M, Ruberto G, Orecchia G et al (1991) Age of onset in vitiligo: relationship with HLA supratypes. Clin Genet 1:48–54
Föger N, Marhaba R, Zöller M (2000) CD44 supports T cell proliferation and apoptosis by apposition of protein kinases. Eur J Immunol 10:2888–2899
Foley LM, Lowe NJ, Misheloff E, Tiwari JL (1983) Association of HLA-DR4 with vitiligo. J Am Acad Dermatol 1:39–40
Fu S, Zhang N, Yopp AC, Chen D, Mao M et al (2004) TGF-β induces Foxp3 + T-regulatory cells from CD4 + CD25—precursors. Am J Transplant 10:1614–1627
Garcia-Melendez ME, Salinas-Santander M, Sanchez-Dominguez C, Gonzalez-Cardenas H, Cerda-Flores RM et al (2014) Protein tyrosine phosphatase PTPN22 +1858C/T polymorphism is associated with active vitiligo. Exp Ther Med 5:1433–1437
Gartside MG, Chen H, Ibrahimi OA, Byron SA, Curtis AV et al (2009) Loss-of-function fibroblast growth factor receptor-2 mutations in melanoma. Mol Cancer Res 1:41–54
Gauthier Y, Cario Andre M, Taïeb A (2003) A critical appraisal of vitiligo etiologic theories. Is melanocyte loss a melanocytorrhagy? Pigment Cell Res 4:322–332
Gavalas NG, Gottumukkala RV, Gawkrodger DJ, Watson PF, Weetman AP et al (2009) Mapping of melanin-concentrating hormone receptor 1 B cell epitopes predicts two major binding sites for vitiligo patient autoantibodies. Exp Dermatol 5:454–463
Giri PS, Begum R, Dwivedi M (2022) Meta-analysis for association of TNFA -308 G>A polymorphism with vitiligo susceptibility. Gene 809:146027. https://doi.org/10.1016/j.gene.2021.146027
Giri PS, Dwivedi M, Laddha NC, Begum R, Bharti AH (2020a) Altered expression of nuclear factor of activated T cells, forkhead box P3, and immune-suppressive genes in regulatory T cells of generalized vitiligo patients. Pigment Cell Melanoma Res 4:566–578
Giri PS, Dwivedi M, Begum R (2020b) Decreased suppression of CD8+ and CD4+ T cells by peripheral regulatory T cells in generalized vitiligo due to reduced NFATC1 and FOXP3 proteins. Exp Dermatol 8:759–775
Giri PS, Patel S, Begum R, Dwivedi M (2021) Association of FOXP3 and GAGE10 promoter polymorphisms and decreased FOXP3 expression in regulatory T cells with susceptibility to generalized vitiligo in Gujarat population. Gene 768:145295. https://doi.org/10.1016/j.gene.2020.145295
Glassman SJ (2011) Vitiligo, reactive oxygen species and T-cells. Clin Sci 3:99–120
Groettrup M, Khan S, Schwarz K, Schmidtke G (2001) Interferon-gamma inducible exchanges of 20S proteasome active site subunits: why? Biochimie 3–4:367–372
Guerra L, Dellambra E, Brescia S, Raskovic D (2010) Vitiligo: pathogenetic hypotheses and targets for current therapies. Curr Drug Metab 5:451–467
Hafez M, Sharaf L, Abd el-Nabi SM (1983) The genetics of vitiligo. Acta Derm Venereol 3:249–251
Han J, Liu J, Bai Y (2016) Association of single nucleotide polymorphisms in the IL2RA-RBM17 region with vitiligo in the Chinese Mongolian population. Chinese J Dermatol 6:406–410
Hayashi M, Jin Y, Yorgov D, Santorico SA, Hagman J et al (2016) Autoimmune vitiligo is associated with gain-of-function by a transcriptional regulator that elevates expression of HLA-A*02:01 in vivo. Proc Natl Acad Sci USA 5:1357–1362
Hegazy RA, Fawzy MM, Gawdat HI, Samir N, Rashed LA (2014) T helper 17 and Tregs: a novel proposed mechanism for NB-UVB in vitiligo. Exp Dermatol 4:283–286
Hirschhorn JN, Gajdos ZKZ (2011) Genome-wide association studies: results from the first few years and potential implications for clinical medicine. Annu Rev Med 11–24
Honda Y, Okubo Y, Koga M (1997) Relationship between levels of soluble interleukin-2 receptors and the types and activity of vitiligo. J Dermatol 9:561–563
Huraib GB, Al Harthi F, Arfin M, Aljamal A, Alrawi AS et al (2020) Association of functional polymorphism in protein tyrosine phosphatase nonreceptor 22 (PTPN22) gene with vitiligo. Biomark Insights 1177271920903038
Hutyrová B, Pantelidis P, Drábek J, Zůrková M, Kolek V et al (2002) Interleukin-1 gene cluster polymorphisms in sarcoidosis and idiopathic pulmonary fibrosis. Am J Respir Crit Care Med 2:148–151
Ie A, M K-Ö, A G, P V, S D-A, et al (2015) The combination of tumour necrosis factor-α -308A and interleukin-10-1082G gene polymorphisms and increased serum levels of related cytokines: susceptibility to vitiligo. Clin Exp Dermatol 1:71–77

Imran M, Laddha NC, Dwivedi M, Mansuri MS, Singh J et al (2012) Interleukin-4 genetic variants correlate with its transcript and protein levels in patients with vitiligo. Br J Dermatol 2:314–323

Itirli G, Pehlivan M, Alper S, Yüksel SE, Onay H et al (2005) Exon-3 polymorphism of CTLA-4 gene in Turkish patients with vitiligo. J Dermatol Sci 3:225–227

Jadeja SD, Mansuri MS, Singh M, Dwivedi M, Laddha NC et al (2017) A case-control study on association of proteasome subunit beta 8 (PSMB8) and transporter associated with antigen processing 1 (TAP1) polymorphisms and their transcript levels in vitiligo from Gujarat. PLoS One 7:e0180958

Jahan P, Cheruvu R, Tippisetty S, Komaravalli PL, Valluri V et al (2013) Association of FOXP3 (rs3761548) promoter polymorphism with nondermatomal vitiligo: A study from India. J Am Acad Dermatol 2:262–266

Jia S, Meng A (2007) Tob genes in development and homeostasis. Dev Dyn an off Publ Am Assoc Anat 4:913–921

Jin SY, Park HH, Li GZ, Lee HJ, Hong MS et al (2004a) Association of angiotensin converting enzyme gene I/D polymorphism of vitiligo in Korean population. Pigment Cell Res 1:84–86

Jin SY, Park HH, Li GZ, Lee HJ, Hong MS et al (2004b) Association of estrogen receptor 1 intron 1 C/T polymorphism in Korean vitiligo patients. J Dermatol Sci 3:181–186

Jin Y, Mailloux CM, Gowan K, Riccardi SL, LaBerge G et al (2007a) NALP1 in vitiligo-associated multiple autoimmune disease. N Engl J Med 12:1216–1225

Jin Y, Bennett DC, Amadi-Myers A, Holland P, Riccardi SL et al (2007b) Vitiligo-associated multiple autoimmune disease is not associated with genetic variation in AIRE. Pigment Cell Res 5:402–404

Jin Y, Birlea SA, Fain PR, Spritz RA (2007c) Genetic variations in NALP1 are associated with generalized vitiligo in a Romanian population. J Invest Dermatol 11:2558–2562

Jin Y, Riccardi SL, Gowan K, Fain PR, Spritz RA (2010a) Fine-mapping of vitiligo susceptibility loci on chromosomes 7 and 9 and interactions with NLRP1 (NALP1). J Invest Dermatol 3:774–783

Jin Y, Birlea SA, Fain PR, Mailloux CM, Riccardi SL et al (2010b) Common variants in FOXP1 are associated with generalized vitiligo. Nat Genet 7:576–578

Jin Y, Birlea SA, Fain PR, Gowan K, Riccardi SL et al (2010c) Variant of TYR and autoimmunity susceptibility loci in generalized vitiligo. N Engl J Med 18:1686–1697

Jin Y, Xu A, Wang P, Song X, Liu X (2011a) Long-term follow-up and correlated factors of vitiligo following autologous epidermal transplantation. Cutis 3:137–141

Jin Y, Birlea SA, Fain PR, Gowan K, Riccardi SL et al (2011b) Genome-wide analysis identifies a quantitative trait locus in the MHC class II region associated with generalized vitiligo age of onset. J Invest Dermatol 6:1308–1312

Jin Y, Ferrara T, Gowan K, Holcomb C, Rastrou M et al (2012a) Next-generation DNA re-sequencing identifies common variants of TYR and HLA-A that modulate the risk of generalized vitiligo via antigen presentation. J Invest Dermatol 6:1730–1733

Jin Y, Birlea SA, Fain PR, Ferrara TM, Ben S et al (2012b) Genome-wide association analyses identify 13 new susceptibility loci for generalized vitiligo. Nat Genet 6:676–680

Jin Y, Hayashi M, Fain PR, Suzuki T, Fukai K et al (2015) Major association of vitiligo with HLA-A*02:01 in Japanese. Pigment Cell Melanoma Res 3:360–362

Jin Y, Andersen G, Yorgov D, Ferrara TM, Ben S (2016) Genome-wide association studies of autoimmune vitiligo identify 23 new risk loci and highlight key pathways and regulatory variants. Nat Genet 11: 1418–1424

Jin Y, Roberts GHL, Ferrara TM, Ben S, van Geel N et al (2019) Early-onset autoimmune vitiligo associated with an enhancer variant haplotype that upregulates class II HLA expression. Nat Commun 1:391

Joetham A, Takeda K, Taube C, Miyahara N, Matsubara S et al (2007) Naturally occurring lung CD4(+)CD25(+) T cell regulation of airway allergic responses depends on IL-10 induction of TGF-beta. J Immunol 3:1433–1442

Johnson P, Ruffell B (2009) CD44 and its role in inflammation and inflammatory diseases. Inflamm Allergy Drug Targets 3:208–220

Ka C, Sc C, Ys K, Hb K, Ht C et al (2009) Association of thymic stromal lymphopoietin gene -847C>T polymorphism in generalized vitiligo. Exp Dermatol 12:1073–1075

Kachru RB, Telischi M, Mittal KK (1978) HLA antigens and vitiligo in an American black population. Tissue Antigens 5:396–397

Kakourou T (2009) Vitiligo in children. World J Pediatr 4:265–268

Kang X, Liang J, Chai L, Peng L, Yu S (2017) Association of HLA-DRB1* 1201/02, DRB1* 0701/02, DQA1* 0302 and DQB1* 0303 Alleles with population Uygur patients of vitiligo. Clon Transgen 157:2

Karam RA, Zidan HE, Khater MH (2017) Genetic variants of interferon-gamma and its mRNA expression and inflammatory parameters in the pathogenesis of vitiligo. Biochem Cell Biol 4:474–481

Karkucak M, Solak B, Turan H, Uslu E, Yakut T et al (2015) MBL2 gene polymorphism and risk of vitiligo in Turkish patients. Int J Hum Genet 3:93–96

Kato H, Takeuchi O, Sato S, Yoneyama M, Yamamoto M et al (2006) Differential roles of MDA5 and RIG-I helicases in the recognition of RNA viruses. Nature 7089:101–105

Kavurma MM, Khachigian LM (2003) Signaling and transcriptional control of Fas ligand gene expression. Cell Death Differ 1:36–44

Kemp EH, Gawkrodger DJ, Watson PF, Weetman AP (1998) Autoantibodies to human melanocyte-specific protein Pmel17 in the sera of vitiligo patients: a sensitive and quantitative radioimmunoassay (RIA). Clin Exp Immunol 3:333–338

Kent G, Al-Abadie M (1996) Psychologic effects of vitiligo: a critical incident analysis. J Am Acad Dermatol 6:895–898

Khan R, Gupta S, Sharma A (2012) Circulatory levels of T-cell cytokines (interleukin [IL]-2, IL-4, IL-17, and transforming growth factor-β) in patients with vitiligo. J Am Acad Dermatol 3:510–511

Kim NH, Lee AY (2010) Reduced aquaporin3 expression and survival of keratinocytes in the depigmented epidermis of vitiligo. J Invest Dermatol 9:2231–2239

Kim J, Lahl K, Hori S, Loddenkemper C, Chaudhry A et al (2009) Cutting edge: depletion of Foxp3 + cells leads to induction of autoimmunity by specific ablation of regulatory T cells in genetically targeted mice. J Immunol 12:7631–7634

Kingo K, Philips MA, Aunin E, Luuk H, Karelson M et al (2006) MYG1, novel melanocyte related gene, has elevated expression in vitiligo. J Dermatol Sci 2:119–122

Kouki T, Sawai Y, Gardine CA, Fisfalen ME, Alegre ML et al (2000) CTLA-4 gene polymorphism at position 49 in exon 1 reduces the inhibitory function of CTLA-4 and contributes to the pathogenesis of Graves' disease. J Immunol 11:6606–6611

Kristiansen OP, Karlsen AE, Larsen ZM, Johannesen J, Pociot F et al (2004) Identification of a type 1 diabetes-associated CD4 promoter haplotype with high constitutive activity. Scand J Immunol 6:582–591

Krüger C, Schallreuter KU (2012) A review of the worldwide prevalence of vitiligo in children/adolescents and adults. Int J Dermatol 10:1206–1212

Kumeta H, Sakakibara H, Enokizono Y, Ogura K, Horiuchi M et al (2014) The N-terminal domain of TIR domain-containing adaptor molecule-1, TICAM-1. J Biomol NMR 3:227–230

Laberge G, Mailloux CM, Gowan K, Holland P, Bennett DC et al (2005) Early disease onset and increased risk of other autoimmune diseases in familial generalized vitiligo. Pigment Cell Res 4:300–305

Laberge GS, Birlea SA, Fain PR, Spritz RA (2008) The PTPN22-1858C>T (R620W) functional polymorphism is associated with generalized vitiligo in the Romanian population. Pigment Cell Melanoma Res 2:206–208

LaBerge GS, Bennett DC, Fain PR, Spritz RA (2008) PTPN22 is genetically associated with risk of generalized vitiligo, but CTLA4 is not. J Invest Dermatol 7:1757–1762

Laddha NC, Dwivedi M, Begum R (2002) Vitiligo: a manifestation of apoptosis? Am J Clin Dermatol 5:301–308

Laddha NC, Dwivedi M, Shajil EM, Prajapati H, Marfatia YS et al (2008) Association of PTPN22 1858C/T polymorphism with vitiligo susceptibility in Gujarat population. J Dermatol Sci 3:260–262

Laddha NC, Dwivedi M, Begum R, Shahbaz ANS, Namazi RSM et al (2012) Tumor necrosis factor a promotor polymorphism and nonsegmental vitiligo: a molecular susceptibility marker in Egyptian women. PLoS One 1–17

Laddha NC, Dwivedi M, Mansuri MS, Gani AR, Ansarullah M et al (2013) Vitiligo: Interplay between oxidative stress and immune system. Exp Dermatol 4:245–250

Laddha NC, Dwivedi M, Mansuri MS, Singh M, Patel HH et al (2014) Association of neuropeptide Y (NPY), interleukin-1B (IL1B) genetic variants and correlation of IL1B transcript levels with vitiligo susceptibility. PLoS One 9

Lamkanfi M, Kanneganti T-D (2010) Caspase-7: a protease involved in apoptosis and inflammation. Int J Biochem Cell Biol 1:21–24

Le Borgne M, Etchart N, Goubier A, Lira SA, Sirard JC et al (2006) Dendritic cells rapidly recruited into epithelial tissues via CCR6/CCL20 are responsible for CD8+ T cell crosspriming in vivo. Immunity 2:191–201

Le Poole IC, Luiten RM (2008) Autoimmune etiology of generalized vitiligo. Curr Dir Autoimmun 227–243

Le Poole IC, Sarangarajan R, Zhao Y, Stennett LS, Brown TL et al (2001) "VIT1", a novel gene associated with vitiligo. Pigment Cell Res 6:475–484

Lee YH, Bae SC (2015) Associations between TNF-α polymorphisms and susceptibility to rheumatoid arthritis and vitiligo: a meta-analysis. Genet Mol Res 2:5548–5559

Lernerab AB (1959) Vitiligo. J Invest Dermatol 2. Part 2:285–310

Levai M (1958) A study of certain contributory factors in the development of vitiligo in South Indian patients. AMA Arch Derm 3:364–371

Levandowski CB, Mailloux CM, Ferrara TM, Gowan K, Ben S et al (2013) NLRP1 haplotypes associated with vitiligo and autoimmunity increase interleukin-1β processing via the NLRP1 inflammasome. Proc Natl Acad Sci USA 8:2952–2956

Li M, Sun D, Li C, Zhang Z, Gao L et al (2008) Functional polymorphisms of the FAS gene associated with risk of vitiligo in Chinese populations: a case-control analysis. J Invest Dermatol 12:2820–2824

Li Z, Ren J, Niu X, Xu Q, Wang X et al (2016) Meta-analysis of the association between vitiligo and human leukocyte antigen-A. Biomed Res Int 5412806

Liang Y, Yang S, Zhou Y, Gui J, Ren Y et al (2007) Evidence for two susceptibility loci on chromosomes 22q12 and 6p21-p22 in Chinese generalized vitiligo families. J Invest Dermatol 11:2552–2557

Liou H-C, Boothby MR, Finn PW, Davidon R, Nabavi N et al (1990) A new member of the leucine zipper class of proteins that binds to the HLA DR alpha promoter. Science (80–) 4950:1581–1584

Lili Y, Yi W, Ji Y, Yue S, Weimin S (2012) Global activation of CD8+ cytotoxic T lymphocytes correlates with an impairment in regulatory T cells in patients with generalized vitiligo. PLoS One 5

Liston A, Lesage S, Wilson J, Peltonen L, Goodnow CC (2003) Aire regulates negative selection of organ-specific T cells. Nat Immunol 4:350–354

Liu JB, Li M, Chen H, Zhong SQ, Yang S et al (2007) Association of vitiligo with HLA-A2: a meta-analysis. J Eur Acad Dermatol Venereol 2:205–213

Liu J, Tang H, Zuo X, Liang B, Wang P et al (2012) A single nucleotide polymorphism rs9468925 of MHC region is associated with clinical features of generalized vitiligo in Chinese Han population. J Eur Acad Dermatol Venereol 9:1137–1141

Lorini R, Orecchia G, Martinetti M, Dugoujon JM, Cuccia M (1992) Autoimmunity in vitiligo: relationship with HLA, Gm and Km polymorphisms. Autoimmunity 4:255–260

Lv Y, Lv Y, Li Q, Lei W, Luan Q et al (2013) Association of ACE gene I/D polymorphism with vitiligo: a meta-analysis. Arch Dermatol Res 5:365–370

Macaron C, Winter RJ, Traisman HS, Kahan BD, Lasser AE et al (1977) Vitiligo and juvenile diabetes mellitus. Arch Dermatol 11:1515–1517

Maier S, Paulsson M, Hartmann U (2008) The widely expressed extracellular matrix protein SMOC-2 promotes keratinocyte attachment and migration. Exp Cell Res 13:2477–2487

Majumder PP, Nordlund JJ, Nath SK (1993) Pattern of familial aggregation of vitiligo. Arch Dermatol 8:994–998

Martínez-Esparza M, Jiménez-Cervantes C, Solano F, Lozano JA, García-Borrón JC (1998) Mechanisms of melanogenesis inhibition by tumor necrosis factor-alpha in B16/F10 mouse melanoma cells. Eur J Biochem 1:139–146

Martinon F, Burns K, Tschopp J (2002) The inflammasome: a molecular platform triggering activation of inflammatory caspases and processing of proIL-β. Mol Cell 2:417–426

Metzker A, Zamir R, Gazit E, David M, Feuerman EJ (1980) Vitiligo and the HLA system. Dermatologica 2:100–105

Minev M, Tonkin N, Martinova F (1985) Association of the HLA system with vitiligo. Vestn Dermatol Venerol 5:41–42

Miyake K, Nakashima H, Akahoshi M, Inoue Y, Nagano S et al (2002) Genetically determined interferon-gamma production influences the histological phenotype of lupus nephritis. Rheumatol 5:518–524

Moellmann G, Klein-Angerer S, Scollay DA, Nordlund JJ, Lerner AB (1982) Extracellular granular material and degeneration of keratinocytes in the normally pigmented epidermis of patients with vitiligo. J Invest Dermatol 5:321–330

Mohr J (1951) Vitiligo in a pair of monovular twins. Acta Genet Stat Med 3:252–255

Molho-Pessach V, Lerer I, Abeliovich D, Agha Z, Libdeh AA et al (2008) The H syndrome is caused by mutations in the nucleoside transporter hENT3. Am J Hum Genet 4:529–534

Moretti S, Spallanzani A, Amato L, Hautmann G, Gallerani I et al (2002) Vitiligo and epidermal microenvironment: Possible involvement of keratinocyte-derived cytokines. Arch Dermatol 2:273–274

Mosenson JA, Zloza A, Klarquist J, Barfuss AJ, Guevara-Patino JA et al (2012) HSP70i is a critical component of the immune response leading to vitiligo. Pigment Cell Melanoma Res 1:88–98

Nakagawa H, Otuka F, Kukita A, Mizoguchi M, Ito H et al (1980) Histocompatible antigens in vitiligo vulgaris II (author's transl). Nihon Hifuka Gakkai Zasshi 10:939–941

Nakashima H, Miyake K, Inoue Y, Shimizu S, Akahoshi M et al (2002) Association between IL-4 genotype and IL-4 production in the Japanese population. Genes Immun 2:107–109

Namian AM, Shahbaz S, Salmanpoor R, Namazi MR, Dehghani F et al (2009) Association of interferon-gamma and tumor necrosis factor alpha polymorphisms with susceptibility to vitiligo in Iranian patients. Arch Dermatol Res 1:21–25

Nath SK, Majumder PP, Nordlund JJ (1994) Genetic epidemiology of vitiligo: multilocus recessivity cross-validated. Am J Hum Genet 5:981–990

Nath SK, Kelly JA, Namjou B, Lam T, Bruner GR et al (2001) Evidence for a susceptibility gene, SLEV1, on chromosome 17p13 in families with vitiligo-related systemic lupus erythematosus. Am J Hum Genet 6:1401–1406

Naughton GK, Reggiardo D, Bystryn JC (1986) Correlation between vitiligo antibodies and extent of depigmentation in vitiligo. J Am Acad Dermatol 5 (Pt 1):978–981

Naylor SL, Sakaguchi AY, Shows TB, Law ML, Goeddel DV et al (1983) Human immune interferon gene is located on chromosome 12. J Exp Med 3:1020–1027

Nejad SB, Qadim HH, Nazeman L, Fadaii R, Goldust M (2013) Frequency of autoimmune diseases in those suffering from vitiligo in comparison with normal population. Pak J Biol Sci 12:570–574

Nie G, Qi JH, Huang CW, Yang T, Shi N et al (2015) Meta-analysis of the TNF-α-308G/A polymorphism and vitiligo risk. Genet Mol Res 4:17296–17304

Nordlund JJ, Lerner AB (1982) Vitiligo. It is important. Arch Dermatol 1:5–8

Nordlund JJ, Boissy RE, Hearing VJ, King RA, Oetting WS et al (2007) The pigmentary system: physiology and pathophysiology, 2nd edn. Pigment Syst Physiol Pathophysiol Second Ed 1–1229

Norris DA, Horikawa T, Morelli JG (1994) Melanocyte destruction and repopulation in vitiligo. Pigment Cell Res 4:193–203

O'Garra A, Vieira PL, Vieira P, Goldfeld AE (2004) IL-10-producing and naturally occurring CD4+ Tregs: limiting collateral damage. J Clin Invest 10:1372–1378

Ochi Y, DeGroot LJ (1969) Vitiligo in Graves' disease. Ann Intern Med 5:935–940

Odeh AMA, Bulatova NR, Yousef AF (2019) Genetic Association of TNF-alpha polymorphisms with generalized vitiligo in Jordanian population. J Genet Disord Genet Med 1:1–4

Onay H, Pehlivan M, Alper S, Ozkinay F, Pehlivan S (2007) Might there be a link between mannose binding lectin and vitiligo? Eur J Dermatol 2:146–148

Ongenae K, Dierckxsens L, Brochez L, van Geel N, Naeyaert JM (2005) Quality of life and stigmatization profile in a cohort of vitiligo patients and effect of the use of camouflage. Dermatology 4:279–285

Orecchia G, Perfetti L, Malagoli P, Borghini F, Kipervarg Y (1992) Vitiligo is associated with a significant increase in HLA-A30, Cw6 and DQw3 and a decrease in C4AQ0 in northern Italian patients. Dermatology 2:123–127

Ortonne JP, Bose SK (1993) Vitiligo: where do we stand? Pigment Cell Res 2:61–72

Oshiumi H, Matsumoto M, Funami K, Akazawa T, Seya T (2003) TICAM-1, an adaptor molecule that participates in Toll-like receptor 3–mediated interferon-β induction. Nat Immunol 2:161–167

Pan JY, Theng C, Lee J, Goh BK (2009) Vitiligo as an adverse reaction to topical diphencyprone. Ann Acad Med Singap 3:276–277

Papadopoulos KI, Melander O, Orho-Melander M, Groop LC, Carlsson M et al (2000) Angiotensin converting enzyme (ACE) gene polymorphism in sarcoidosis in relation to associated autoimmune diseases. J Intern Med 1:71–77

Patwardhan M, Pradhan V, Taylor LH, Thakkar V, Kharkar V et al (2013) The angiotensin-converting enzyme gene insertion/deletion polymorphism in Indian patients with vitiligo: a case-control study and meta-analysis. Br J Dermatol 6:1195–1204

Pawelek J, Körner A, Bergstrom A, Bologna J (1980) New regulators of melanin biosynthesis and the autodestruction of melanoma cells. Nature 5773:617–619

Peach RJ, Bajorath J, Naemura J, Leytze G, Greene J et al (1995) Both extracellular immunoglobin-like domains of CD80 contain residues critical for binding T cell surface receptors CTLA-4 and CD28. J Biol Chem 36:21181–21187

Pehlivan S, Ozkinay F, Alper S, Onay H, Yuksel E et al (2009) Association between IL4 (-590), ACE (I)/(D), CCR5 (Delta32), CTLA4 (+49) and IL1-RN (VNTR in intron 2) gene polymorphisms and vitiligo. Eur J Dermatol 2:126–128

Peterson P, Org T, Rebane A (2008) Transcriptional regulation by AIRE: molecular mechanisms of central tolerance. Nat Rev Immunol 12:948–957

Philips MA, Kingo K, Karelson M, Rätsep R, Aunin E et al (2010) Promoter polymorphism-119C/G in MYG1 (C12orf10) gene is related to vitiligo susceptibility and Arg4Gln affects mitochondrial entrance of Myg1. BMC Med Genet 11:56

Poloy A, Tibor L, Kramer J, Anh-Tuan N, Kraszits E et al (1991) HLA-DR1 is associated with vitiligo. Immunol Lett 1:59–62

Pravica V, Asderakis A, Perrey C, Hajeer A, Sinnott PJ et al (1999) In vitro production of IFN-gamma correlates with CA repeat polymorphism in the human IFN-gamma gene. Eur J Immunogenet 1:1–3

Pravica V, Perrey C, Stevens A, Lee JH, Hutchinson IV (2000) A single nucleotide polymorphism in the first intron of the human IFN-gamma gene: absolute correlation with a polymorphic CA microsatellite marker of high IFN-gamma production. Hum Immunol 9:863–866

Qi Z, Xie S, Chen R, Aisa HA, Hon GC et al (2018) Tissue-specific gene expression prediction associates vitiligo with SUOX through an active enhancer. bioRxiv: 337196

Quan C, Ren YQ, Xiang LH, Sun LD, Xu AE et al (2010) Genome-wide association study for vitiligo identifies susceptibility loci at 6q27 and the MHC. Nat Genet 7:614–618

Rajendiran KS, Rajappa M, Chandrashekar L, Thappa DM (2018) Association of PTPN22 gene polymorphism with non-segmental vitiligo in South Indian Tamils. Postep Dermatol Alergol 3:280–285

Rajendiran KS, Rajappa M, Chandrashekar L, Thappa DM, Devaraju P (2020) Association analysis of tumor necrosis factor alpha promoter polymorphisms and vitiligo susceptibility in South Indian Tamils. Dermatology 6:554–564

Ramire LD, Marcos EV, Godoy DA, de Souza-Santana FC (2016) Association of class I and II HLA alleles and haplotypes with susceptibility to vitiligo: a study of patients with vitiligo from southeast Brazil. Int J Dermatol 6:e347–e355

Rashed L, Abdel Hay R, Mahmoud R, Hasan N, Zahra A et al (2015) Association of angiotensin-converting enzyme (ACE) gene polymorphism with inflammation and cellular cytotoxicity in vitiligo patients. PLoS One 7:e0132915

Ren Y, Yang S, Xu S, Gao M, Huang W et al (2009) Genetic variation of promoter sequence modulates XBP1 expression and genetic risk for vitiligo. PLoS Genet 6:e1000523

Retornaz G, Betuel H, Ortonne JP, Thivolet J (1976) HL-A antigens and vitiligo. Br J Dermatol 2:173–175

Ricard AS, Pain C, Daubos A, Ezzedine K, Lamrissi-Garcia I et al (2012) Study of CCN3 (NOV) and DDR1 in normal melanocytes and vitiligo skin. Exp Dermatol 6:411–416

Rigat B, Hubert C, Alhenc-Gelas F, Cambien F, Corvol P et al (1990) An insertion/deletion polymorphism in the angiotensin I-converting enzyme gene accounting for half the variance of serum enzyme levels. J Clin Invest 4:1343–1346

Rina W (2016) Association of single nucleotide polymorphisms in the IL2RA-RBM17 region with vitiligo in the Chinese Mongolian population. Chiense J Dermatol 6:406–410

Rocnik EF, Liu P, Sato K, Walsh K, Vaziri C (2006) The novel SPARC family member SMOC-2 potentiates angiogenic growth factor activity. J Biol Chem 32:22855–22864

Rodriguez-Castro KI, Franceschi M, Miraglia C, Russo M, Nouvenne A et al (2018) Autoimmune diseases in autoimmune atrophic gastritis. Acta Biomed 8-s:100–103

Saleh NF, Nabil N, Bassiouny DA, Khorshied MM (2014) Tumor necrosis factor α promotor polymorphism and nonsegmental vitiligo: a molecular susceptibility marker in Egyptian women. J Egypt Women's Dermatol Soc 2:109–112

Salinas-Santander M, Díaz-García D, Rojas-Martínez A, Cantú-Salinas C, Sánchez-Domínguez C et al (2012) Tumor necrosis factor-α-308G/A polymorphism is associated with active vitiligo vulgaris in a northeastern Mexican population. Exp Ther Med 5:893–897

Sasaki S, Ito E, Toki T, Maekawa T, Kanezaki R et al (2000) Cloning and expression of human B cell-specific transcription factor BACH2 mapped to chromosome 6q15. Oncogene 33:3739–3749

Schallreuter KU, Wood JM, Berger J (1991) Low catalase levels in the epidermis of patients with vitiligo. J Invest Dermatol 6:1081–1085

Schallreuter KU, Levenig C, Kühnl P, Löliger C, Hohl-Tehari M et al (1993) Histocompatibility antigens in vitiligo: Hamburg study on 102 patients from northern Germany. Dermatology 3:186–192

Schallreuter KU, Lemke R, Brandt O, Schwartz R, Westhofen M et al (1994) Vitiligo and other diseases: coexistence or true association? Hamburg study on 321 patients. Dermatology 4:269–275

Scholzen TE, Ständer S, Riemann H, Brzoska T, Luger TA (2003) Modulation of cutaneous inflammation by angiotensin-converting enzyme. J Immunol 7:3866–3873

Schutyser E, Struyf S, Van Damme J (2003) The CC chemokine CCL20 and its receptor CCR6. Cytokine Growth Factor Rev 5:409–426

Shah F, Patel S, Begum R, Dwivedi M (2021) Emerging role of tissue resident memory T cells in vitiligo: from pathogenesis to therapeutics. Autoimmun Rev 8

Shajil EM, Chatterjee S, Agrawal D, Bagchi T, Begum R (2006) Vitiligo: pathomechanisms and genetic polymorphism of susceptible genes. Indian J Exp Biol 7:526–539

Sharma K, Wang RX, Zhang LY, Yin DL, Luo XY et al (2000) Death the Fas way: regulation and pathophysiology of CD95 and its ligand. Pharmacol Ther 3:333–347

Shin HD, Winkler C, Stephens JC, Bream J, Young H et al (2000) Genetic restriction of HIV-1 pathogenesis to AIDS by promoter alleles of IL10. Proc Natl Acad Sci USA 26:14467–14472

Shin MK, Im SH, Park HJ, Kim SK, Yim SV et al (2011) Association study between polymorphisms of CD28, CTLA4 and ICOS and non-segmental vitiligo in a Korean population. Exp Ther Med 6:1145–1149

Sidi E, Bourgeois-Gavardin J (1953) Treatment of vitiligo with Ammi majus. Press Med 21:436–440

Siemens HW (1953) Heredity problem in vitiligo. Ned Tijdschr Geneeskd 38:2449–2450

Siminovitch KA (2004) PTPN22 and autoimmune disease. Nat Genet 12:1248–1249

Singh A, Sharma P, Kar HK, Sharma VK, Tembhre MK et al (2012) HLA alleles and amino-acid signatures of the peptide-binding pockets of HLA molecules in vitiligo. J Invest Dermatol 1:124–134

Singh M, Mansuri MS, Jadeja SD, Marfatia YS, Begum R (2018) Association of interleukin 1 receptor antagonist intron 2 variable number of tandem repeats polymorphism with vitiligo susceptibility in Gujarat population. Indian J Dermatol Venereol Leprol 3:285–291

Song Q-H, Shen Z, Xing X-J, Yin R, Wu Y-Z et al (2012) An association study of single nucleotide polymorphisms of the FOXP3 intron-1 and the risk of Psoriasis vulgaris. Indian J Biochem Biophys 1:25–35

Song P, Wang XW, Li HX, Li K, Liu L et al (2013) Association between FOXP3 polymorphisms and vitiligo in a Han Chinese population. Br J Dermatol 3:571–578

Song GG, Bae SC, Kim JH, Lee YH (2015) The angiotensin-converting enzyme insertion/deletion polymorphism and susceptibility to rheumatoid arthritis, vitiligo and psoriasis: a meta-analysis. J Renin Angiotensin Aldosterone Syst 1:195–202

Spits H, de Waal MR (1992) Functional characterization of human IL-10. Int Arch Allergy Immunol 1:8–15

Spritz RA (2007) The genetics of generalized vitiligo and associated autoimmune diseases. Pigment Cell Res 4:271–278

Spritz RA (2008) The genetics of generalized vitiligo. Curr Dir Autoimmun 244–257

Spritz RA (2010a) Shared genetic relationships underlying generalized vitiligo and autoimmune thyroid disease. Thyroid 7:745–754

Spritz RA (2010b) The genetics of generalized vitiligo: autoimmune pathways and an inverse relationship with malignant melanoma. Genome Med 10.

Spritz RA (2011) Recent progress in the genetics of generalized vitiligo. J Genet Genomics 7:271–278

Spritz RA (2012) Six decades of vitiligo genetics: genome-wide studies provide insights into autoimmune pathogenesis. J Invest Dermatol 2:268–273

Spritz RA, Andersen GHL (2017) Genetics of Vitiligo. Dermatol Clin 2:245–255

Spritz RA, Gowan K, Bennett DC, Fain PR (2004) Novel vitiligo susceptibility loci on chromosomes 7 (AIS2) and 8 (AIS3), confirmation of SLEV1 on chromosome 17, and their roles in an autoimmune diathesis. Am J Hum Genet 1:188–191

Strömberg S, Björklund MG, Asplund A, Rimini R, Lundeberg J et al (2008) Transcriptional profiling of melanocytes from patients with vitiligo vulgaris. Pigment Cell Melanoma Res 2:162–171

Stuttgen G (1950) Hereditary aspects of vitiligo. Z Haut Geschlechtskr 11:451–457

Sun Y, Zuo X, Zheng X, Zhou F, Liang B et al (2014) A comprehensive association analysis confirms ZMIZ1 to be a susceptibility gene for vitiligo in Chinese population. J Med Genet 5:345–353

Taher ZA, Lauzon G, Maguiness S, Dytoc MT (2009) Analysis of interleukin-10 levels in lesions of vitiligo following treatment with topical tacrolimus. Br J Dermatol 3:654–659

Taïeb A, Picardo M (2007) The definition and assessment of vitiligo: a consensus report of the Vitiligo European Task Force. Pigment Cell Res 1:27–35

Taïeb A, Picardo M (2009) Clinical practice. Vitiligo. N Engl J Med 2:160–169

Tang XF, Zhang Z, Hu DY, Xu AE, Zhou HS et al (2013) Association analyses identify three susceptibility Loci for vitiligo in the Chinese Han population. J Invest Dermatol 2:403–410

Tang L, Li J, Fu W, Wu W, Xu J (2019) Suppression of FADS1 induces ROS generation, cell cycle arrest, and apoptosis in melanocytes: implications for vitiligo. Aging (albany NY) 24:11829–11843

Tarlow JK, Blakemore AI, Lennard A, Solari R, Hughes HN et al (1993) Polymorphism in human IL-1 receptor antagonist gene intron 2 is caused by variable numbers of an 86-bp tandem repeat. Hum Genet 4:403–404

Taştan HB, Akar A, Orkunoğlu FE, Arca E, Inal A (2004) Association of HLA class I antigens and HLA class II alleles with vitiligo in a Turkish population. Pigment Cell Res 2:181–184

Taştan HB, Akar A, Orkunoğlu FE, Arca E, İnal A (2004) Association of HLA class I antigens and HLA class II alleles with vitiligo in a Turkish population. Pigment Cell Res 2:181–184

Tazi-Ahnini R, McDonagh AJ, Wengraf DA, Lovewell TR, Vasilopoulos Y et al (2008) The autoimmune regulator gene (AIRE) is strongly associated with vitiligo. Br J Dermatol 3:591–596

Teindel H (1950) Familial vitiligo. Z Haut Geschlechtskr 11:457–462

Tembhre MK, Sharma VK, Sharma A, Chattopadhyay P, Gupta S (2013) T helper and regulatory T cell cytokine profile in active, stable and narrow band ultraviolet B treated generalized vitiligo. Clin Chim Acta 27–32

The MHC Sequencing Consortium (1999) Complete sequence and gene map of a human major histocompatibility complex. Nature 6756:921–923

Theos AC, Truschel ST, Raposo G, Marks MS (2005) The Silver locus product Pmel17/gp100/Silv/ME20: controversial in name and in function. Pigment Cell Res 5:322–336

Tippisetty S, Ishaq M, Komaravalli PL, Jahan P (2011) Angiotensin converting enzyme (ACE) gene polymorphism in vitiligo: protective and predisposing effects of genotypes in disease susceptibility and progression. Eur J Dermatol 2:173–177

Toama MAK, Khattab FM, Marei A (2019) Association of human leukocyte antigen-DRB1 with the response in patients with vitiligo. Egypt J Dermatol Venerol 2:71

Trapani JA, Sutton VR (2003) Granzyme B: pro-apoptotic, antiviral and antitumor functions. Curr Opin Immunol 5:533–543

Tripathi RK, Giebel LB, Strunk KM, Spritz RA (1991) A polymorphism of the human tyrosinase gene is associated with temperature-sensitive enzymatic activity. Gene Expr J Liver Res 2:103–110

Trowsdale J (2011) The MHC, disease and selection. Immunol Lett 1–2:1–8

Tschopp J, Martinon F, Burns K (2003) NALPs: a novel protein family involved in inflammation. Nat Rev Mol Cell Biol 2:95–104

Turner DM, Williams DM, Sankaran D, Lazarus M, Sinnott PJ et al (1997) An investigation of polymorphism in the interleukin-10 gene promoter. Eur J Immunogenet 1:1–8

Türsen Ü, Kaya Tİ, Bulut B, Erdal ME, Ay Öİ et al (2014) Association of FAS gene promoter functional polymorphisms and the risk of vitiligo in Turkish populations. J Turkish Acad Dermatol 3

Valia AK, Dutta PK (1996) IADVL text book and atlas of dermatology, vol-II, and 2

Valsecchi R, Bontempelli M, Cainelli T, Leghissa P, Di Landro A (1995) Vitiligo is associated with a significant increase in HLA-DR6 and a decrease in DQw2 antigens in Northern Italian patients. J Eur Acad Dermatol Venereol 1:9–14

van den Boorn JG, Konijnenberg D, Dellemijn TAM, van der Veen JPW, Bos JD et al (2009) Autoimmune destruction of skin melanocytes by perilesional T cells from vitiligo patients. J Invest Dermatol 9:2220–2232

Veiga-Castelli L, Oliveira ML, Pereira A, Debortoli G, Marcorin L et al (2019) HLA-G polymorphisms are associated with non-segmental vitiligo among Brazilians. Biomolecules 9

Venkataram MN, White AG, Leeny WA, Al Suwaid AR, Daar AS (1995) HLA antigens in Omani patients with vitiligo. Clin Exp Dermatol 1:35–37

Venneker GT, Westerhof W, de Vries IJ, Drayer NM, Wolthers BG et al (1992) Molecular heterogeneity of the fourth component of complement (C4) and its genes in vitiligo. J Invest Dermatol 6:853–858

Vogel F (1956) Dermatological observations on uniovular twins: vitiligo, ichthyosis simplex, psoriasis. Z Haut Geschlechtskr 1:1–4

Wang L, Tsai C-C (2008) Atrophin proteins: an overview of a new class of nuclear receptor corepressors. Nucl Recept Signal 1:nrs. 06009

Wang HN, Qi YM, Gao YF et al. Frequencies of HLA-A2 among patients with tumors, chronic hepatitis C and vitiligo in Henan Province. J Zhengzhou Univ Med Sci 3:349–351

Wańkowicz-Kalińska A, van den Wijngaard RMJGJ, Tigges BJ, Westerhof W, Ogg GS et al (2003) Immunopolarization of CD4+ and CD8+ T cells to Type-1–like is associated with melanocyte loss in human vitiligo. Lab Investig 5:683–695

Westerhof W, d'Ischia M (2007) Vitiligo puzzle: the pieces fall in place. Pigment Cell Res 5:345–359

Weston A, Sommerville J (2006) Xp54 and related (DDX6-like) RNA helicases: roles in messenger RNP assembly, translation regulation and RNA degradation. Nucleic Acids Res 10:3082–3094

Wu CS, Yu CL, Wu CS, Lan CC, Yu HS (2004) Narrow-band ultraviolet-B stimulates proliferation and migration of cultured melanocytes. Exp Dermatol 12:755–763

Wu J, Zhou M, Wan Y, Xu A (2013) CD8+ T cells from vitiligo perilesional margins induce autologous melanocyte apoptosis. Mol Med Rep 1:237–241
Wu D, Shi D, Zhu X (2015) The association between tumor necrosis factor-α-308 G/A polymorphism and risk for vitiligo: a meta-analysis. Int J Dermatol 9:1045–1053
Xiao S, Jin H, Korn T, Liu SM, Oukka M et al (2008) Retinoic acid increases Foxp3+ regulatory T cells and inhibits development of Th17 cells by enhancing TGF-beta-driven Smad3 signaling and inhibiting IL-6 and IL-23 receptor expression. J Immunol 4:2277–2284
Xu W, Lin FQ, Liu JF, Fu LF, Hong WS et al (2013) Impact on tyrosinase expression and export from endoplasmic reticulum by inhibition of 26S proteasome. Zhonghua Yi Xue Za Zhi 2:123–127
Xu M, Liu Y, Liu Y, Li X, Chen G et al (2018) Genetic polymorphisms of GZMB and vitiligo: a genetic association study based on Chinese Han population. Sci Rep 1:13001
Yagi H, Nomura T, Nakamura K, Yamazaki S, Kitawaki T et al (2004) Crucial role of FOXP3 in the development and function of human CD25+ CD4+ regulatory T cells. Int Immunol 11:1643–1656
Yang S, Wang J-Y, Gao M, Liu H-S, Sun L-D et al (2005) Association of HLA-DQA1 and DQB1 genes with vitiligo in Chinese Hans. Int J Dermatol 12:1022–1027
Yazici AC, Erdal ME, Kaya TI, Ikizoglu G, Savasoglu K et al (2006) Lack of association with TNF-alpha-308 promoter polymorphism in patients with vitiligo. Arch Dermatol Res 1:46–49
Yildiz SH, Yildirim A, Özuğuz P, Erdoğan MÖ, Kaçar SD et al (2016) 119C/G in MYG1 gene and 49A/G in CTLA4 gene polymorphisms in Turkish patients with vitiligo. J Adv Intern Med 1:1–5
Yohn JJ, Critelli M, Lyons MB, Norris DA (1990) Modulation of melanocyte intercellular adhesion molecule-1 by immune cytokines. J Invest Dermatol 2:233–237
Yun JY, Uhm YK, Kim HJ, Lim SH, Chung JH et al (2010) Transforming growth factor beta receptor II (TGFBR2) polymorphisms and the association with nonsegmental vitiligo in the Korean population. Int J Immunogenet 4:289–291
Zamani M, Spaepen S, Sghar SS, Huang C, Westerhof W et al (2001) Linkage and association of HLA class II genes with vitiligo in a Dutch population. Br J Dermatol 1:90–94
Zamani M, Tabatabaiefar MA, Mosayyebi S, Mashaghi A, Mansouri P (2010) Possible association of the CD4 gene polymorphism with vitiligo in an Iranian population. Clin Exp Dermatol 5:521–524
Zhai Z, Liu W, Kaur M, Luo Y, Domenico J et al (2017) NLRP1 promotes tumor growth by enhancing inflammasome activation and suppressing apoptosis in metastatic melanoma. Oncogene 27:3820–3830
Zhang XJ, Liu HS, Liang YH, Sun LD, Wang JY et al (2004) Association of HLA class I alleles with vitiligo in Chinese Hans. J Dermatol Sci 2:165–168
Zhang XJ, Chen JJ, Liu JB (2005) The genetic concept of vitiligo. J Dermatol Sci 3:137–146
Zheng Y, Rudensky AY (2007) Foxp3 in control of the regulatory T cell lineage. Nat Immunol 5:457–462
Zhu KJ, Lv YM, Yin XY, Wang ZX, Sun LD et al (2011) Psoriasis regression analysis of MHC loci identifies shared genetic variants with vitiligo. PLoS One 11: e23089

The Immunogenetics of Psoriasis

Emanuele Trovato, Pietro Rubegni,
and Elisa Cinotti

Abstract

Psoriasis vulgaris is a chronic immune-mediated dermatological condition, resulting from an interaction between environmental triggers and genetic susceptibilities. Alteration in the production of the inflammatory mediators plays a pivotal part in the pathogenesis of the disease. Genes encoding the mediators of these inflammatory pathways can dictate susceptibility to psoriasis. These genes have a wide range of functions that involve innate immunity (*IFIH1, TRAF3IP2, CARD14, c-REL, DDX58*), antigen presentation (HLA-Cw6), T-cells development, maturation, and polarization (*RUNX1, RUNX3, STAT3*), cytokine signaling (*IL12Bp40, IL23Ap19, IL23R, JAK2*), and immune regulators (*TNIP1, TNFAIP3, IL36RN, SOCS1, ZC3H12C, NFKBIA*). The risk alleles of these genes can contribute to the overall state of susceptibility to psoriasis by lowering the threshold of the innate immune response that can eventually provoke the pathogenic adaptive immune responses capable of inducing psoriasis. The investigations on genetic associations of psoriasis may allow the discovery of new diseases modifying targets and possibly open a path for the advancement of personalized medicine. They also allow us to discover new aspects of human skin biology.

Keywords

Psoriasis · Immunogenetics · Gene · Immune response · Susceptibility · GWAS

1 Introduction

Psoriasis is a chronic, complex, multifactorial immune-mediated disorder that affects about 3% of the worldwide population (Harden et al. 2015b; Perera et al. 2012). The disease has quite a few clinical subtypes with the most frequent (psoriasis vulgaris) presenting with chronic erythematous plaques with mica-like scales on the extremities, scalp, and the lumbosacral area (Fig. 1). The other subtypes include generalized pustular psoriasis, guttate psoriasis, pustulosis of palms and soles, and erythrodermic psoriasis. The disease can also affect the nails and joints causing psoriatic arthritis.

It is proposed that psoriasis could be related to an interaction between dermal dendritic cells (dDCs), plasmacytoid dendritic cells (pDCs) hyperproliferative keratinocytes, mast cells, neutrophils, and T-cells. In addition, an alteration in immune response may be involved in plaque

E. Trovato · P. Rubegni · E. Cinotti (✉)
Department of Medical, Surgical and Neurological Science, Dermatology Section, University of Siena, S. Maria Alle Scotte Hospital, Siena, Italy

N. Rezaei and F. Rajabi (eds.), *The Immunogenetics of Dermatologic Diseases*, Advances in Experimental Medicine and Biology 1367,
https://doi.org/10.1007/978-3-030-92616-8_4

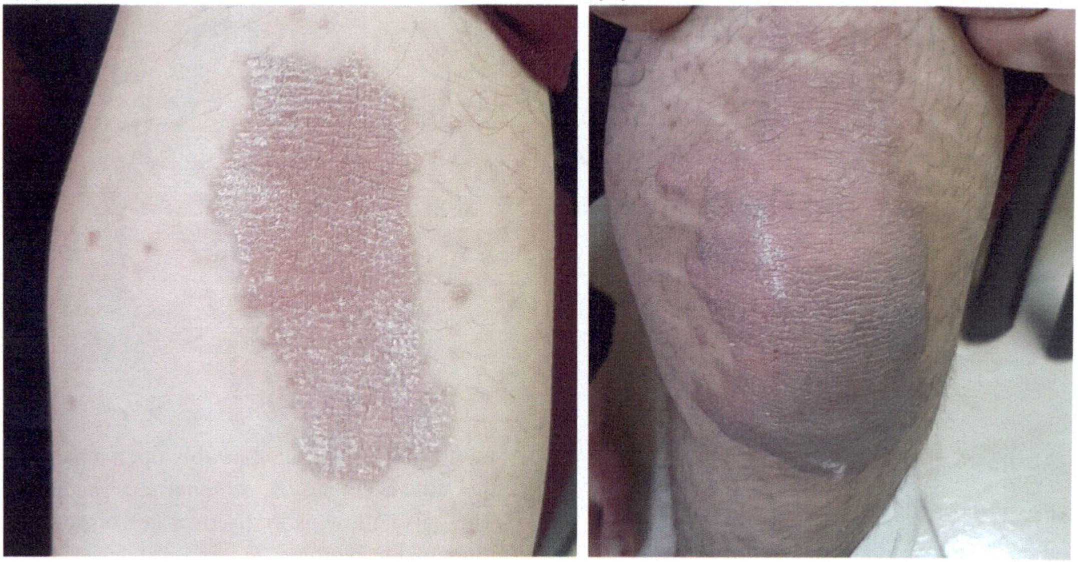

Fig. 1 Clinical presentation of psoriasis **a** mica-like scales. **b** Predominant involvement of extensor surfaces of the limbs

formation (Perera et al. 2012). The importance of the immune response in the etiopathogenesis of psoriasis was revealed when the utilization of immunosuppressive agents, such as methotrexate and cyclosporine proved to be successful in disease amelioration (Chiricozzi et al. 2018; Perera et al. 2012). Initially, the main immunological alteration was believed to be the disproportionally high levels of interferon (IFN)-γ and interleukin (IL)-12, with both CD4+ and CD8+ IFNγ-producing T-cells as key players (Cyclosporin a for Psoriasis 1979; Chiricozzi et al. 2018). Additionally, psoriatic skin was found to be infiltrated by tumor necrosis factor (TNF)-α and inducible nitric oxide synthase (iNOS) producing DCs that polarize T-cells to T helper-1 (Th1) and Th17 pathways (Chiricozzi et al. 2018; Colombo et al. 2013; Perera et al. 2012). More recently, a precise characterization of the immune pathways at play in psoriasis has led to the recognition of the role of specific subclasses of immune cells and their associated cytokines. Thereby, the pathogenic archetype has been completely revised in favor of an IL-23/IL-17 axis (Chiricozzi et al. 2018; Perera et al. 2012) (Fig. 2). Genome-wide association studies (GWAS) have enabled more accurate identification of the genes products involved in the psoriatic inflammation in the nine risk loci, so-called PSOPS (PSORiasis—Susceptibility) (Chiricozzi et al. 2018; Perera et al. 2012). These studies have discovered over fifty chromosomal regions linked to psoriasis susceptibility some of which contain more than one independent susceptibility loci. A substantial proportion of these genes have a role in the immune system. Most susceptibility loci are common between psoriasis vulgaris, psoriatic arthritis, and other autoimmune diseases (Perera et al. 2012). Understanding the pathways through which these genes shape the susceptibility of an individual to psoriasis will not only help us understand the role of autoimmunity in the etiopathogenesis of psoriasis but also elucidate their involvement in the development of psoriasis comorbidities. In addition, this knowledge may also benefit the investigations on other autoimmune diseases. Because most susceptibility loci are common between psoriasis and psoriatic arthritis (Perera et al. 2012), there are not differentially discussed in this chapter.

Although the exact effect of many of the environmental factors that provoke psoriasis is

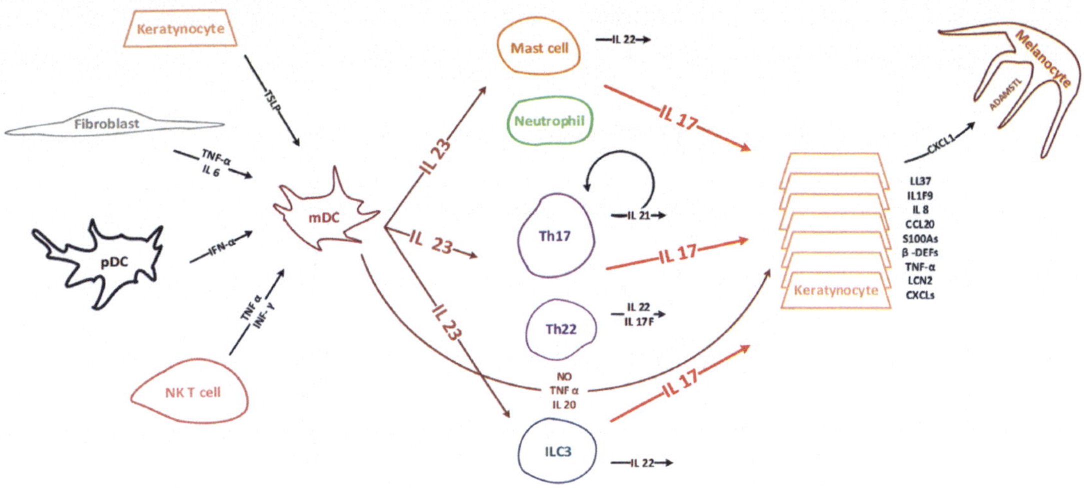

Fig. 2 The pathogenesis of psoriasis. Several factors induce the activation of myeloid dendritic cells (mDCs) including thymic stromal lymphopoietin (TSLP) produced by keratinocytes, interferons (IFNs), tumor necrosis factor α (TNFα), and IL-6 produced by fibroblasts, plasmacytoid dendritic cells (pDCs), and NKT cells. The mDCs in turn release IL-23 which stimulates T-cell subsets, innate lymphoid cells (ILCs), mast cells, and neutrophils, to secrete IL-17. These cytokines in synergism contribute to the development of the clinical features of the disease by affecting the keratinocytes, the endothelial cell, and the melanocytes

not clear, some of these factors such as physical distress are known to stimulate the antimicrobial peptides (AMP) and cathelicidin (LL37) release from keratinocytes. The LL37 can form complexes with self-DNA material that are recognized as foreign by the immune system and thus provoke autoimmunity and breach tolerance to host-nucleic acids (Fig. 3).

Investigations on the immunogenetic pathways involved in psoriasis can greatly enhance planning for individually tailored treatments. Those who suffer from psoriasis elicited by a certain set of polymorphisms may benefit more from a specific treatment compared to others. For instance, those carrying TNF-related gene risk alleles, for instance, *TNFAIP3*, have a better chance of responding to anti-TNFα therapy (Chiricozzi et al. 2018; Perera et al. 2012). Therefore, it is not irrational to think that in the upcoming years, medicine and especially, immunotherapy would be personalized and tailored to each individual based on the specific set of susceptibility genes that they have inherited.

2 Innate Immunity

The skin is one of the major elements of the innate immune system. It offers physical, chemical (via antimicrobial peptides and acidic pH), and immunologic barriers against external pathogens. The innate immune system also sets the tone for further adaptive immune responses.

Innate immune response alterations have been documented in the pathogenesis of psoriasis. On components of this type of immune response are a family of transcription factors known as the NF-kB. These dimeric proteins are made up of different subunits including RelA also known as p65, Rel-B, c-Rel, p50, and p52 that are activated downstream toll-like receptors (TLRs) and cytokine receptors TNFα, IL-1, and IL-17. It also regulates keratinocyte growth and cell cycle progression (Chiricozzi et al. 2018; Perera et al. 2012). Polymorphisms in many genes encoding NF-kB-associated peptides have been linked to psoriasis susceptibility (Chiricozzi et al. 2018; Colombo et al. 2013; Perera et al. 2012).

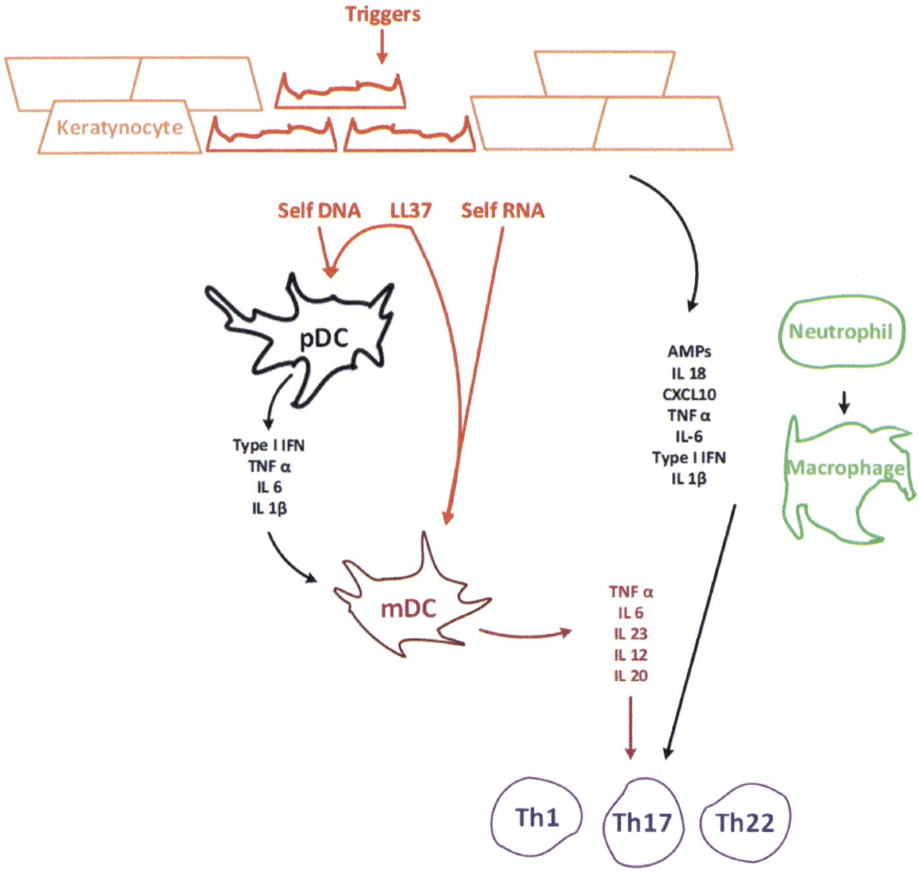

Fig. 3 Induction of psoriasis. The disease triggers including trauma and infectious agents could promote the release of self-nucleic acids which could form autoantigenic complexes with the antimicrobial peptide LL37. This complex is uptaken and presented by plasmacytoid dendritic cells (pDCs) and myeloid dendritic cells (mDCs) to T-cells. pDCs secrete massive amounts of type I interferons (IFN) which could further promote the activation of mDCs. The activated T-cells promote inflammation and release cytokines capable of inducing keratinocyte proliferation

Another psoriasis-associated innate immune gene is *TRAF3 interacting protein 2* (*TRAF3IP2*, also referred to as *Act1*) (Cyclosporin a for Psoriasis 1979; Perera et al. 2012). TRAF3IP2 interacts with TRAF6 and relays signals as a mediator between IL-17 receptor and NF-κB (Perera et al. 2012). It is also involved in CCL20 release from keratinocytes in response to IL-17 (Perera et al. 2012). Altered expression of the *TRAF3IP2* gene has been documented in psoriasis and psoriatic arthritis.

The caspase activation and recruitment domain (CARD) proteins encode scaffolding proteins that play an essential role in the assembly of larger proteins involved in innate inflammation, apoptosis, etc. (Perera et al. 2012). Mutations identified in *CARD14* are responsible for the PSORS2 locus (Chiricozzi et al. 2018; Perera et al. 2012). In the dermis, the *CARD14* is usually expressed by keratinocytes and small vessel endothelial cells. The risk alleles of the *CARD14* gene are associated with amplified NF-κB signaling and thus increase the transcription of chemokine and proinflammatory cytokines (Perera et al. 2012).

Another important gene involved in the innate responses is *IL36RN* that codes the IL36 receptor antagonist protein (IL36Ra). The *IL36RN* mutations are thought to be the cause of generalized pustular psoriasis (Harden et al. 2014).

Genes implicated in the secretion of IFNγ that is involved in the innate antiviral immune pathways have also been involved in the pathogenesis of psoriasis. These genes include the *DDX58* (*DEAD (Asp-Glu-Ala-Asp) box polypeptide 58*) and *IFIH1* that encode two cytosolic pattern recognition receptors (PRRs) capable of sensing RNA and DNA fragments, RIG-I and MDA5, respectively. Both of these PRRs are essential for sensing viral dsRNA and responding via type-I IFN production (Liu et al. 2020; Vabret and Blander 2013). Conversely, the two prominent psoriasis cytokines, TNFα and IFNγ, can stimulate the transcription of *RIG-I* and *MDA5* genes in keratinocytes (Kitamura et al. 2007; Reikine et al. 2014).

3 Adaptive Immunity

The T-cells as one of the main pillars of adaptive immunity have an established role in the development of psoriasis. Both CD4+ helper T cells (Th) and CD8+ cytotoxic T-cells (Tc) are involved in the pathogenesis of psoriasis (Kagami et al. 2010; Rácz et al. 2011; Zhen et al. 2019). Antigen presentation, especially via class I major histocompatibility complex (MHCs), is the first step in the activation and entanglement of T-cells and has been confirmed to be critical in the establishment of the disease as apparent from the linkage between psoriasis and human leukocyte antigens (HLAs). Early onset severe psoriasis (also referred to as type 1 psoriasis) has a very significant correlation with the presence of *HLA-Cw6*. The *HLA-Cw6* explains some of the linkages reported as the PSORS1 association loci at 6p21.3. PSORS1 locus was shown to confer the highest risk for psoriasis (Hijnen et al. 2013; Lowes et al. 2008) and it is found in more than 50% of psoriatic patients (Bowcock 2005). The *HLA-Cw6* is an MHC-I allele thus it is involved in the activation of cytotoxic CD8+ T-cells.

Polymorphisms in the *endoplasmic reticulum aminopeptidase 1* (*ERAP1*) and *ERAP2* genes were also been linked to psoriasis in individuals carrying the *HLA-Cw6* allele by a recent GWA study (Elder 2006; Genetic Analysis of Psoriasis et al. 2010). The ERAP proteins control the processing of peptides that are loaded onto MCHI. So, we may hypothesize that ERAP processed auto-antigens expressed by HLA-Cw6 molecules are capable of triggering autoreactive T-cells into inducing psoriasis (Genetic Analysis of Psoriasis et al. 2010).

Starting from 2014, HLA imputation was used for fine mapping of the MHC associations of psoriasis. *HLA-C*06:02* was found to be one of the strongest susceptibility factors. The *HLA-C*12:03* and variation in the amino acid 67 and 9 of the HLA-B, amino acids 95 of the HLA-A, and amino acid 53 of HLA-DQα1 also had significant associations with psoriasis independently (Genetic Analysis of Psoriasis et al. 2010).

Although more related to the innate rather than the adaptive immune reactions, the *MHC class I polypeptide-related sequence A* (*MICA*) gene is also linked to psoriasis (Yin et al. 2015). MICA is a danger-associated molecule presented on the surfaces of cells in stress. It can bind and activate NKG2D receptors on the surface of natural killer (NK) cells, NKT-cells, and T-cells and result in the recognition and destruction of the stressed cell (Okada et al. 2014). The precise contribution of NK and NKT cells to the pathogenesis of psoriasis has not been completely defined, even though it is known that they are related to the overexpression of a particular set of cytokines (e.g., TNFα, IFNγ, and IL-22) in psoriatic plaques.

3.1 Lymphocyte Populations Involved in Psoriasis

As we know both CD8+ and CD4+ T-cells are present in psoriatic lesions, studies demonstrated that CD4+ Th cells can differentiate into Th1 or Th2, producing IFNγ (antiviral response) or IL-4 and IL-5 (antimicrobial responses), respectively. The already defined Th1/Th2 dichotomy has changed by the complex series of phenotypes for T-cells, such as T-reg (regulatory T-cells), Th17, and Th22 being introduced in recent years. All these subsets contribute to the development of psoriasis. These T-cell subsets are identified through the sets of cytokines they produce. Th1 and Tc1 can express signal transducer and activator of transcription 1 (STAT1) and T-bet (Perera et al. 2012), subsequently causing the release of IFNγ, TNFα, and IL-2 and expression of CXCR3 as a chemokine receptor (González et al. 2008). The Tc17 and Th17 utilize the RAR-related orphan receptor gamma (RORγt) and the STAT3 transcription factors and promote the excretion of IL-17, TNFα, IL-26, IL-21, and IL-22. These cells also possess IL-23 receptors and stimulate cellular differentiation in accordance with the expression of transforming growth factor-beta (TGF-β), IL-1β, and IL-6 (Ono et al. 2007). The differentiation of Tc22 and Th22 is promoted by the presence of TNFα and IL-6. These cells also employ STAT3 to promote the transcription of IL-22 and chemokine receptor CCR10, CCR6, and CCR4 (Andrés et al. 2013).

3.2 Interferon-α

In the setting of psoriasis, IFNα, a type I interferon, is produced and released mainly by DCs and is thought to be one of the main initiators of the inflammatory cascade. It stimulates the production of proinflammatory cytokines upstream the IL-17/IL-23 axis such as IL-15, IL-12, IL-1, IL-18, and IL-23 (Jones 2008). The first hypothesis about its role was based on the induction/exacerbation of psoriatic lesions following IFNα therapy for viral infections (Festen et al. 2011; Lande and Gilliet 2010). Furthermore, IFNα inducible genes have an increased transcription rate in psoriasis-affected skin, compared to non-lesional skin of individuals with psoriasis and normal control subjects. It was also noticed that IFNα neutralization prevented the uninduced occurrence of psoriasis in xenotransplanted mouse models (Funk et al. 1991). Investigations also demonstrated an increased risk of psoriasis in a mouse model deficient in a transcriptional factor that inhibits IFNα/β downstream pathways, IFN regulatory factor-2 (IRF2) (Funk et al. 1991).

3.3 Interferon γ

The IL-12/IFNγ/Th1 axis is another immune pathway that was considered to be involved in psoriasis development. The IFNγ was found to be elevated in the serum and both lesional and normal skin of individuals affected by psoriasis skin. Furthermore, serum IFNγ levels were also found to correlate with the severity of the disease. However, there were no correlations between treatment success and downregulation of IFNγ (Anees et al. 2005; Nestle et al. 2005). Furthermore, a study was able to demonstrate induction of a cellular infiltration pattern similar to that of psoriatic skin following a single intradermal injection of IFNγ (Hida et al. 2000). In ex vivo conditions, through STAT1 mediated pathways, IFNγ stimulates the transcription of over four hundred genes (Johnson-Huang et al. 2010; Lowes et al. 2005). In vitro, IFNγ promotes the transcription of near 1200 genes in a single layer of keratinocytes (Chiricozzi et al. 2014). Recent findings demonstrating the simultaneous production of IL-17 and IFNγ by Th17 cells through IL-12 triggering have been able to reject the prior hypothesis that regards IFNγ as a suppressor of IL-17 (Chiricozzi et al. 2016). Aside from psoriatic plaques, these T-cells capable of producing both IFNγ and IL-17 have also been identified in allergic contact dermatitis (Johnson-Huang et al. 2012). Moreover, it has been shown that IFNγ could be considered as an upstream mediator of the IL-23/IL-17 pathway that drives the DCs to produce IL-23 and IL-1β and the memory T-cells to produce IL-17 (Albanesi et al. 2000; Pennino et al. 2010). Among the upregulated genes, it is possible to detect mediators such as TNFα, iNOS, IL-23p19, CCL19, vascular cell adhesion molecule 1 (VCAM-1), intercellular adhesion molecule-1 (ICAM-1), and TNF-related apoptosis-inducing ligand (TRAIL) which is a death receptor agonist. In addition, IFNγ down-regulates IL-23p19, IL12/23p40, and iNOS (Kryczek et al. 2008). Moreover, the importance of IFNγ in the early stages of the disease, before visible lesions ensue, is supported by investigations showing IFNγ release by autoreactive T-cells and other initiators of the pathological cascade in psoriasis (Harden et al. 2015a). Therefore, an IFNγ signature may be a characteristic feature of the early phases of the disease. Moreover, fontolizumab, an anti-IFNγ antibody, has had limited efficacy in psoriasis. So, compared to the cytokines, such as TNFα and IL-17 that have been used successfully in the treatment of psoriasis, IFNγ may not be relevant from a therapeutic point of view.

3.4 Tumor Necrosis Factor-Alpha (TNFα)

Tumor necrosis factor-alpha (TNFα) is a proinflammatory cytokine that possesses synergistic effects with other inflammatory mediators such as IL-17 (Chiricozzi et al. 2011; Mabuchi et al. 2012). It constitutes a crucial element in psoriasis development as it has been demonstrated by the effectiveness of anti-TNFα monoclonal antibodies in ameliorating psoriasis. Affected skin and serum of individuals with psoriasis demonstrate high levels of TNFα, in comparison to normal and unaffected skin of those with psoriasis (Arican et al. 2005; Lande et al. 2014). T-cells, DCs, and keratinocytes are all capable of producing TNFα (Caldarola et al. 2009; Johnson-Huang et al. 2009).

3.5 Interleukin-12/23

IL-12 is a proinflammatory cytokine composed of two particles, p35 and p40, that are overexpressed in psoriasis. Although a therapy directed at the IL-12/IFNγ/Th1 axis should be logical, a complete response was not achieved in the studies (Harper et al. 2009).

IL-23 is part of the IL-6 cytokine group that was identified in the early 2000s (Oppmann et al. 2000). IL-23 is a heterodimer composed of two particles IL-23p19 and IL-12p40 encoded by the *IL-23A* and *IL-12B* genes, respectively. IL-23p19 is more commonly produced by monocytes, mature DCs, and monocyte-derived DCs present in the papillary dermis. In recent years, it was discovered that IL-23 has a major role in polarizing the differentiation of T-cells into Th17 cells and the production of IL-17A and IL-17F (Corrections to: "Psoriasis and systemic inflammatory diseases: potential mechanistic links between skin disease and co-morbid conditions" 2010; Fiocco et al. 2010). The association between IL-23 and psoriasis is backed up with strong evidence. Independent of IL-17 and Th17, IL-23 is involved in the development of several clinical aspects of psoriasis including erythema and hyperplasia along with features of parakeratotic hyperparakeratosis through interacting with TNFα and IL-20R2 (Hauser 2006). IL-23 can upregulate the expression of human β-defensin-2 (HBD2) and other antimicrobial peptides (AMP) through synergism with IL-1β. The outstanding efficacy of biological agents that target the p19 subunit of IL-23 further demonstrates the importance of this pathway in the pathogenesis of psoriasis.

Several SNPs in genes encoding both subunits of IL-23, IL12Bp40, and IL23Ap19 were identified to be linked with psoriasis susceptibility (Chiricozzi et al. 2015; Li et al. 2007).

The IL-23 receptor (IL-23R) is also a heterodimer composed of two segments encoded by *IL-23R* and *IL-12RB1* genes (Parham et al. 2002). IL-12Rb1 also takes part in the formation of the IL-12 receptor, whereas IL-23R is exclusive to the IL-23 receptor. The IL-23R is present on the surfaces of T-cells (memory cells in particular), NK cells, and DCs. Its expression correlates with the cell's sensitivity to IL23. The IL-23R encoding gene harbors one of the most consistent SNPs linked to psoriasis, a base substitution at 1142 (G > A giving rise to R381Q). The less common Q allele is associated with lower IL-23 activity and could consequently have a protective effect against inflammation and autoimmunity. IL-12RB1 operates through TYK2 while IL-23R relays intracellular signals through JAK2 (Suárez-Fariñas et al. 2012). IL-23 stimulation is associated with the transphosphorylation of JAK molecules bound to the receptor. They phosphorylate tyrosine molecules located in the subcellular domain of the receptor subunits which serve as sites for the STAT molecules. Both IL-12 and IL-23 can activate a similar set of STAT molecules (Gunderson et al. 2013) but their dominant transcription factor defers. While IL-23 often relays signals through STAT3, IL-12 usually utilizes STAT4. Once activated, the STAT molecules form a homodimer that translocates into the cell nucleus and attache to the STAT binding element (SBE) at the promoter of the target genes and induce their transcription. Variants in the coding region of both TYK2 and JAK2 are associated with psoriasis and Crohn's disease (Austin et al. 1999).

3.6 Interleukin-17

The significance of IL-17 signaling in the development of psoriasis is evidenced by the successful targeting of IL-17 (i.e., secukinumab, bimekizumab, and ixekizumab) and its receptor (i.e., broadalumab) (Haider et al. 2008). IL-17-producing T-cells are not the only cells capable of producing IL-17. Other immune cells, including type 3 innate lymphoid cells (ILC3), neutrophils, and mast cells can also produce IL-17 in psoriasis lesions (Kitamura et al. 2007; Reikine et al. 2014; Vabret and Blander 2013). Keratinocytes, fibroblasts, and endothelial cells express IL-17 receptors and in response to IL-17 stimulation produce chemokines such as CXCL1, -3, -5, -8, and CCL20, pro-inflammatory cytokines such as IL-6, and IL-36γ, and AMPs including S100A, LL37, HBD2, and LCN2. The CCL20 binds with further recruits CCR6 positive T-cells including Th17, Tc17, and myeloid DCs (Grützkau 2008). IL-17 maintains neutrophil chemotaxis and activation through the induction of CXCLs, IL-8, and AMPs. Moreover, IL-17 can stimulate autoantigen formation through both direct and indirect pathways. In the direct path, IL-17 induces the expression of LL37 which forms autoantigens by binding to self-DNA particles. Indirectly, IL-17 can promote the release of CXCL-1 and melanocyte-stimulating factor-alpha (αMSH) from keratinocytes which in turn induce ADAMSTL5 in melanocytes (Villanova et al. 2014).

The *runt-related transcription factor-3* (*RUNX3*) is another gene linked to psoriasis. It is upregulated following Th2 differentiation and has an essential role in the further differentiation of CD8+ and Th17 cells (Cai et al. 2011). It is possible that the imbalance between RUNX1 and RUNX3 diverts the naïve T-cells toward the Th17 path in psoriasis patients. These factors can also regulate the functions of NK cells or DCs.

Another important gene in T-cell biology is the *T-cell activation RhoGTPase activating protein* (*TAGAP*). The precise role of TGAP is not completely defined (Perera et al. 2012). The SNPs in the *TAGAP* gene have been linked to multiple autoimmune diseases such as psoriasis, Crohn's disease, and rheumatoid arthritis (Harden et al. 2015b; Hsu et al. 2016).

4 Genes with Unknown Associations

There are several other genes with immunological functions that have a possible association with psoriasis including *nitric oxide synthase-2* (*NOS2A*) and *IL-28 receptor alpha* (*IL28RA*) (Angkasekwinai et al. 2007; Park et al. 2005). The NOS2A is an enzyme induced by IFNγ. It produces nitric oxide in activated immune cells as an agent that can kill pathogens and upregulate inflammation via increasing S100A8, IL-6, and IL-8 (Kleinschek et al. 2007). IL28RA dimerizes with IL-10RB and forms a receptor for IL-28A, IL-28B, and IL-29 (also referred to as type III interferons or IFNλ) (Bissonnette et al. 2013; Reich et al. 2015). The *IL28RA* polymorphisms could increase the susceptibility to psoriasis by increasing the sensitivity of keratinocytes to IFNλ.

Non-coding microRNAs (mRNAs) have been the focus of recent studies in the immunogenetics of psoriasis (Mashiko et al. 2015; Ottaviani et al. 2006). For example, the rs2910164 targets the epidermal growth factor receptor (EGFR) transcript and decreases the ability of miR-146a to suppress EGFR expression (Nickoloff et al. 2000).

Table 1 Genes involved in Psoriasis

Role	Genes associated with psoriasis
Adaptive immune system	Major histocompatibility complexes (*HLA-CW6*)
	T-cells development and polarization *RUNX1, RUNX3, STAT3*
	Th17/IL-23 Axis *IL12Bp40, IL23Ap19, IL23R*, JAK2
Innate immunity	*CARD14,* *c-REL,* *TRAF3IP2,* *DDX58,* *IFIH1*
Negative regulators of immune responses	*TNIP1,* *TNFAIP3,* *NFKBIA,* *ZC3H12C,* *IL36RN,* *SOCS1*
Unknown	*NOS-2*A *IL-28RA* *SH2B3* (*LNK*) *ATXN2*

5 Conclusion

Psoriasis is one of the most studied autoimmune dermatological diseases. Multiple GWAS, immunochip, transcription profiling studies are available for this disease that has paved the way for biological treatments.

Although multiple cell lines and cytokine pathways have been shown to influence the pathogenesis of psoriasis, just a few are essentially crucial for developing psoriasis. Initially, psoriasis was considered to be a Th1 mediated disease with the dominance of the IL-12 pathway. This view has been changed in the light of recent findings showing the importance of IFNγ in activating antigen-presentation as the basis of adaptive immune responses. In the current theory, the IL-23/IL-17 axis is also considered to play an important role. Although many studies have investigated psoriasis susceptibility genes and some have been able to provide theories on how these genetic variants may shape the pathogenesis of psoriasis, still a lot remains to be elucidated especially regarding the contribution of genetic variants residing in intergenic regions.

The data provided by these studies could eventually be used as a guide toward personalizing medicine which can revolutionize the management of these types of chronic diseases. In this way, patients with psoriasis could be regrouped based on their specific genetic profiles and rescice treatments based on their most prominent susceptibility genes. Moreover, genetic subtyping may provide a more accurate prediction of the clinical course of the disease, the response to specific treatments, and the occurrence of adverse drug reactions (Table 1).

References

(1979) Cyclosporin a for psoriasis. N Engl J Med 301:555–555

(2010) Corrections to: "Psoriasis and systemic inflammatory diseases: potential mechanistic links between skin disease and co-morbid conditions". J Invest Dermatol 130:2517

Albanesi C, Scarponi C, Cavani A, Federici M, Nasorri F, Girolomoni G (2000) Interleukin-17 is produced by both Th1 and Th2 lymphocytes, and modulates interferon-γ- and interleukin-4-induced activation of human keratinocytes. J Investig Dermatol 115:81–87

Andrés RM, Hald A, Johansen C, Kragballe K, Iversen L (2013) Studies of Jak/STAT3 expression and signalling in psoriasis identifies STAT3-Ser727 phosphorylation as a modulator of transcriptional activity. Exp Dermatol 22:323–328

Anees MR, Reddymasu S, Bejjanki HR, Caldito G (2005) Pegylated interferon alpha-2a (pegasys) versus pegylated interferon alpha-2b (pegintron) in the treatment of chronic hepatitis C infection. Am J Gastroenterol 100:S142

Angkasekwinai P, Park H, Wang Y-H, Wang Y-H, Chang SH, Corry DB, Liu Y-J, Zhu Z, Dong C (2007) Interleukin 25 promotes the initiation of proallergic type 2 responses. J Exp Med 204:1509–1517

Arican O, Aral M, Sasmaz S, Ciragil P (2005) Serum levels of TNF-alpha, IFN-gamma, IL-6, IL-8, IL-12, IL-17, and IL-18 in patients with active psoriasis and correlation with disease severity. Mediators Inflamm 2005:273–279

Austin LM, Ozawa M, Kikuchi T, Walters IB, Krueger JG (1999) The majority of epidermal T cells in psoriasis vulgaris lesions can produce type 1 cytokines, interferon-γ, interleukin-2, and tumor necrosis factor-α, defining TC1 (cytotoxic T lymphocyte) and TH1 effector populations: 1 a type 1 differentiation bias is also measured in circulating blood T cells in psoriatic patients. J Investig Dermatol 113:752–759

Bissonnette R, Nigen S, Langley RG, Lynde CW, Tan J, Fuentes-Duculan J, Krueger JG (2013) Increased expression of IL-17A and limited involvement of IL-23 in patients with palmo-plantar (PP) pustular psoriasis or PP pustulosis; results from a randomised controlled trial. J Eur Acad Dermatol Venereol 28:1298–1305

Bowcock AM (2005) The genetics of psoriasis and autoimmunity. Annu Rev Genomics Hum Genet 6:93–122

Cai Y, Shen X, Ding C, Qi C, Li K, Li X, Jala VR, Zhang H-g, Wang T, Zheng J, Yan J (2011) Pivotal role of dermal IL-17-producing γδ T cells in skin inflammation. Immunity 35:596–610

Caldarola G, De Simone C, Carbone A, Tulli A, Amerio P, Feliciani C (2009) TNFα and its receptors in psoriatic skin, before and after treatment with etanercept. Int J Immunopathol Pharmacol 22:961–966

Chiricozzi A, Cannizzaro MV, Salandri GA, Marinari B, Pitocco R, Dattola A, Regine F, Saraceno R, Bianchi L, Chimenti S, Costanzo A (2015) Increased levels of IL-17 in tear fluid of moderate-to-severe psoriatic patients is reduced by adalimumab therapy. J Eur Acad Dermatol Venereol 30:e128–e129

Chiricozzi A, Guttman-Yassky E, Suárez-Fariñas M, Nograles KE, Tian S, Cardinale I, Chimenti S, Krueger JG (2011) Integrative responses to IL-17 and TNF-α in human keratinocytes account for key inflammatory pathogenic circuits in psoriasis. J Investig Dermatol 131:677–687

Chiricozzi A, Nograles KE, Johnson-Huang LM, Fuentes-Duculan J, Cardinale I, Bonifacio KM, Gulati N, Mitsui H, Guttman-Yassky E, Suárez-Fariñas M, Krueger JG (2014) IL-17 induces an expanded range of downstream genes in reconstituted human epidermis model. PLoS ONE 9:e90284–e90284

Chiricozzi A, Panduri S, Dini V, Tonini A, Gualtieri B, Romanelli M (2016) Optimizing acitretin use in patients with plaque psoriasis. Dermatol Therapy 30: e12453

Chiricozzi A, Romanelli P, Volpe E, Borsellino G, Romanelli M (2018) Scanning the immunopathogenesis of psoriasis. Int J Mol Sci 19:179

Colombo MD, Cassano N, Bellia G, Vena GA (2013) Cyclosporine regimens in plaque psoriasis: an overview with special emphasis on dose, duration, and old and new treatment approaches. Sci World J 2013:805705–805705

Elder JT (2006) PSORS1: linking genetics and immunology. J Investig Dermatol 126:1205–1206

Festen EAM, Goyette P, Green T, Boucher G, Beauchamp C, Trynka G, Dubois PC, Lagacé C, Stokkers PCF, Hommes DW, Barisani D, Palmieri O, Annese V, van Heel DA, Weersma RK, Daly MJ, Wijmenga C, Rioux JD (2011) A meta-analysis of genome-wide association scans identifies IL18RAP, PTPN2, TAGAP, and PUS10 as shared risk loci for Crohn's disease and celiac disease. PLoS Genet 7: e1001283–e1001283

Fiocco U, Sfriso P, Oliviero F, Roux-Lombard P, Scagliori E, Cozzi L, Lunardi F, Calabrese F, Vezzù M, Dainese S, Molena B, Scanu A, Nardacchione R, Rubaltelli L, Dayer JM, Punzi L (2010) Synovial effusion and synovial fluid biomarkers in psoriatic arthritis to assess intraarticular tumor necrosis factor-α blockade in the knee joint. Arthritis Res Ther 12: R148–R148

Funk J, Langeland T, Schrumpf E, Hanssen LE (1991) Psoriasis induced by interferon-α. Br J Dermatol 125:463–465

Genetic Analysis of Psoriasis C, the Wellcome Trust Case Control C, Strange A, Capon F, Spencer CCA, Knight J, Weale ME, Allen MH, Barton A, Band G, Bellenguez C, Bergboer JGM, Blackwell JM, Bramon E, Bumpstead SJ, Casas JP, Cork MJ, Corvin A, Deloukas P, Dilthey A, Duncanson A, Edkins S, Estivill X, Fitzgerald O, Freeman C, Giardina E, Gray E, Hofer A, Hüffmeier U, Hunt SE, Irvine AD, Jankowski J, Kirby B, Langford C, Lascorz J, Leman J, Leslie S, Mallbris L, Markus HS, Mathew CG, McLean WHI, McManus R, Mössner R, Moutsianas L, Naluai AT, Nestle FO, Novelli G, Onoufriadis A, Palmer CNA, Perricone C, Pirinen M, Plomin R, Potter SC, Pujol RM, Rautanen A, Riveira-Munoz E, Ryan AW, Salmhofer W, Samuelsson L, Sawcer SJ, Schalkwijk J, Smith CH, Ståhle M, Su Z, Tazi-Ahnini R, Traupe H, Viswanathan AC, Warren RB, Weger W, Wolk K, Wood N, Worthington J, Young HS, Zeeuwen PLJM, Hayday A, Burden AD, Griffiths CEM, Kere J, Reis A, McVean G,

Evans DM, Brown MA, Barker JN, Peltonen L, Donnelly P, Trembath RC (2010) A genome-wide association study identifies new psoriasis susceptibility loci and an interaction between HLA-C and ERAP1. Nat Genet 42:985–990

González S, López-Soto A, Suarez-Alvarez B, López-Vázquez A, López-Larrea C (2008) NKG2D ligands: key targets of the immune response. Trends Immunol 29:397–403

Grützkau A (2008) Faculty opinions recommendation of Human interleukin 17-producing cells originate from a CD161+CD4+ T cell precursor. In: Faculty opinions—post-publication peer review of the biomedical literature. Faculty Opinions Ltd

Gunderson AJ, Mohammed J, Horvath FJ, Podolsky MA, Anderson CR, Glick AB (2013) CD8(+) T cells mediate RAS-induced psoriasis-like skin inflammation through IFN-γ. J Invest Dermatol 133:955–963

Haider AS, Lowes MA, Suárez-Fariñas M, Zaba LC, Cardinale I, Khatcherian A, Novitskaya I, Wittkowski KM, Krueger JG (2008) Identification of cellular pathways of "Type 1", Th17 T Cells, and TNF- and inducible nitric oxide synthase-producing dendritic cells in autoimmune inflammation through pharmacogenomic study of cyclosporine A in psoriasis. J Immunol 180:1913–1920

Harden JL, Johnson-Huang LM, Chamian MF, Lee E, Pearce T, Leonardi CL, Haider A, Lowes MA, Krueger JG (2015a) Humanized anti–IFN-γ (HuZAF) in the treatment of psoriasis. J Allergy Clin Immunol 135:553-556.e553

Harden JL, Krueger JG, Bowcock AM (2015b) The immunogenetics of Psoriasis: a comprehensive review. J Autoimmun 64:66–73

Harden JL, Lewis SM, Pierson KC, Suárez-Fariñas M, Lentini T, Ortenzio FS, Zaba LC, Goldbach-Mansky R, Bowcock AM, Lowes MA (2014) CARD14 expression in dermal endothelial cells in psoriasis. PLoS ONE 9:e111255–e111255

Harper EG, Guo C, Rizzo H, Lillis JV, Kurtz SE, Skorcheva I, Purdy D, Fitch E, Iordanov M, Blauvelt A (2009) Th17 cytokines stimulate CCL20 expression in keratinocytes in vitro and in vivo: implications for psoriasis pathogenesis. J Invest Dermatol 129:2175–2183

Hauser C (2006) Faculty opinions recommendation of IL-23 stimulates epidermal hyperplasia via TNF and IL-20R2-dependent mechanisms with implications for psoriasis pathogenesis. In: Faculty opinions—post-publication peer review of the biomedical literature. Faculty Opinions Ltd

Hida S, Ogasawara K, Sato K, Abe M, Takayanagi H, Yokochi T, Sato T, Hirose S, Shirai T, Taki S, Taniguchi T (2000) CD8+ T cell-mediated skin disease in mice lacking IRF-2, the transcriptional attenuator of interferon-α/β signaling. Immunity 13:643–655

Hijnen D, Knol EF, Gent YY, Giovannone B, Beijn SJP, Kupper TS, Bruijnzeel-Koomen CAFM, Clark RA (2013) CD8(+) T cells in the lesional skin of atopic dermatitis and psoriasis patients are an important source of IFN-γ, IL-13, IL-17, and IL-22. J Invest Dermatol 133:973–979

Hsu F-C, Shapiro MJ, Dash B, Chen C-C, Constans MM, Chung JY, Romero Arocha SR, Belmonte PJ, Chen MW, McWilliams DC, Shapiro VS (2016) An essential role for the transcription factor Runx1 in T cell maturation. Sci Rep 6:23533–23533

Johnson-Huang LM, McNutt NS, Krueger JG, Lowes MA (2009) Cytokine-producing dendritic cells in the pathogenesis of inflammatory skin diseases. J Clin Immunol 29:247–256

Johnson-Huang LM, Suárez-Fariñas M, Pierson KC, Fuentes-Duculan J, Cueto I, Lentini T, Sullivan-Whalen M, Gilleaudeau P, Krueger JG, Haider AS, Lowes MA (2012) A single intradermal injection of IFN-γ induces an inflammatory state in both non-lesional psoriatic and healthy skin. J Invest Dermatol 132:1177–1187

Johnson-Huang LM, Suárez-Fariñas M, Sullivan-Whalen M, Gilleaudeau P, Krueger JG, Lowes MA (2010) Effective narrow-band UVB radiation therapy suppresses the IL-23/IL-17 axis in normalized psoriasis plaques. J Invest Dermatol 130:2654–2663

Jones N (2008) Faculty opinions recommendation of newly identified genetic risk variants for celiac disease related to the immune response. In: Faculty opinions—post-publication peer review of the biomedical literature. Faculty Opinions Ltd

Kagami S, Rizzo HL, Lee JJ, Koguchi Y, Blauvelt A (2010) Circulating Th17, Th22, and Th1 cells are increased in psoriasis. J Invest Dermatol 130:1373–1383

Kitamura H, Matsuzaki Y, Kimura K, Nakano H, Imaizumi T, Satoh K, Hanada K (2007) Cytokine modulation of retinoic acid-inducible gene-I (RIG-I) expression in human epidermal keratinocytes. J Dermatol Sci 45:127–134

Kleinschek MA, Owyang AM, Joyce-Shaikh B, Langrish CL, Chen Y, Gorman DM, Blumenschein WM, McClanahan T, Brombacher F, Hurst SD, Kastelein RA, Cua DJ (2007) IL-25 regulates Th17 function in autoimmune inflammation. J Exp Med 204:161–170

Kryczek I, Bruce AT, Gudjonsson JE, Johnston A, Aphale A, Vatan L, Szeliga W, Wang Y, Liu Y, Welling TH, Elder JT, Zou W (2008) Induction of IL-17 + T cell trafficking and development by IFN-gamma: mechanism and pathological relevance in psoriasis. J Immunol (Baltimore, Md. : 1950) 181:4733–4741

Lande R, Botti E, Jandus C, Dojcinovic D, Fanelli G, Conrad C, Chamilos G, Feldmeyer L, Marinari B, Chon S, Vence L, Riccieri V, Guillaume P, Navarini AA, Romero P, Costanzo A, Piccolella E, Gilliet M, Frasca L (2014) The antimicrobial peptide LL37 is a T-cell autoantigen in psoriasis. Nat Commun 5

Lande R, Gilliet M (2010) Plasmacytoid dendritic cells: key players in the initiation and regulation of immune responses. Ann N Y Acad Sci 1183:89–103

Li J, Xe C, Liu Z, Yue Q, Liu H (2007) Expression of Th17 cytokines in skin lesions of patients with psoriasis. J Huazhong Univ Sci Technol 27:330–332

Liu Z-J, Tian Y-T, Shi B-Y, Zhou Y, Jia X-S (2020) Association between mutation of interleukin 36 receptor antagonist and generalized pustular psoriasis: a PRISMA-compliant systematic review and meta-analysis. Medicine 99:e23068–e23068

Lowes MA, Chamian F, Abello MV, Fuentes-Duculan J, Lin S-L, Nussbaum R, Novitskaya I, Carbonaro H, Cardinale I, Kikuchi T, Gilleaudeau P, Sullivan-Whalen M, Wittkowski KM, Papp K, Garovoy M, Dummer W, Steinman RM, Krueger JG (2005) Increase in TNF-alpha and inducible nitric oxide synthase-expressing dendritic cells in psoriasis and reduction with efalizumab (anti-CD11a). Proc Natl Acad Sci USA 102:19057–19062

Lowes MA, Kikuchi T, Fuentes-Duculan J, Cardinale I, Zaba LC, Haider AS, Bowman EP, Krueger JG (2008) psoriasis vulgaris lesions contain discrete populations of Th1 and Th17 T cells. J Investig Dermatol 128:1207–1211

Mabuchi T, Chang TW, Quinter S, Hwang ST (2012) Chemokine receptors in the pathogenesis and therapy of psoriasis. J Dermatol Sci 65:4–11

Mashiko S, Bouguermouh S, Rubio M, Baba N, Bissonnette R, Sarfati M (2015) Human mast cells are major IL-22 producers in patients with psoriasis and atopic dermatitis. J Allergy Clin Immunol 136:351-359.e351

Nestle FO, Conrad C, Tun-Kyi A, Homey B, Gombert M, Boyman O, Burg G, Liu Y-J, Gilliet M (2005) Plasmacytoid predendritic cells initiate psoriasis through interferon-alpha production. J Exp Med 202:135–143

Nickoloff BJ, Bonish B, Huang BB, Porcelli SA (2000) Characterization of a T cell line bearing natural killer receptors and capable of creating psoriasis in a SCID mouse model system. J Dermatol Sci 24:212–225

Okada Y, Han B, Tsoi LC, Stuart PE, Ellinghaus E, Tejasvi T, Chandran V, Pellett F, Pollock R, Bowcock AM, Krueger GG, Weichenthal M, Voorhees JJ, Rahman P, Gregersen PK, Franke A, Nair RP, Abecasis GR, Gladman DD, Elder JT, de Bakker PIW, Raychaudhuri S (2014) Fine mapping major histocompatibility complex associations in psoriasis and its clinical subtypes. Am J Hum Genet 95:162–172

Ono M, Yaguchi H, Ohkura N, Kitabayashi I, Nagamura Y, Nomura T, Miyachi Y, Tsukada T, Sakaguchi S (2007) Foxp3 controls regulatory T-cell function by interacting with AML1/Runx1. Nature 446:685–689

Oppmann B, Lesley R, Blom B, Timans JC, Xu Y, Hunte B, Vega F, Yu N, Wang J, Singh K, Zonin F, Vaisberg E, Churakova T, Liu M-r, Gorman D, Wagner J, Zurawski S, Liu Y-J, Abrams JS, Moore KW, Rennick D, de Waal-Malefyt R, Hannum C, Bazan JF, Kastelein RA (2000) Novel p19 protein engages IL-12p40 to form a cytokine, IL-23, with biological activities similar as well as distinct from IL-12. Immunity 13:715–725

Ottaviani C, Nasorri F, Bedini C, de Pità O, Girolomoni G, Cavani A (2006) CD56brightCD16-NK cells accumulate in psoriatic skin in response to CXCL10 and CCL5 and exacerbate skin inflammation. Eur J Immunol 36:118–128

Parham C, Chirica M, Timans J, Vaisberg E, Travis M, Cheung J, Pflanz S, Zhang R, Singh KP, Vega F, To W, Wagner J, O'Farrell A-M, McClanahan T, Zurawski S, Hannum C, Gorman D, Rennick DM, Kastelein RA, de Waal MR, Moore KW (2002) A receptor for the heterodimeric cytokine IL-23 is composed of IL-12Rβ1 and a novel cytokine receptor subunit, IL-23R. J Immunol 168:5699–5708

Park H, Li Z, Yang XO, Chang SH, Nurieva R, Wang Y-H, Wang Y, Hood L, Zhu Z, Tian Q, Dong C (2005) A distinct lineage of CD4 T cells regulates tissue inflammation by producing interleukin 17. Nat Immunol 6:1133–1141

Pennino D, Eyerich K, Scarponi C, Carbone T, Eyerich S, Nasorri F, Garcovich S, Traidl-Hoffmann C, Albanesi C, Cavani A (2010) IL-17 amplifies human contact hypersensitivity by licensing hapten nonspecific Th1 cells to kill autologous keratinocytes. J Immunol 184:4880–4888

Perera GK, Di Meglio P, Nestle FO (2012) Psoriasis. Annu Rev Pathol 7:385–422

Rácz E, Prens EP, Kant M, Florencia E, Jaspers NG, Laman JD, de Ridder D, van der Fits L (2011) Narrowband ultraviolet B inhibits innate cytosolic double-stranded RNA receptors in psoriatic skin and keratinocytes. Br J Dermatol 164:838–847

Reich K, Papp KA, Matheson RT, Tu JH, Bissonnette R, Bourcier M, Gratton D, Kunynetz RA, Poulin Y, Rosoph LA, Stingl G, Bauer WM, Salter JM, Falk TM, Blödorn-Schlicht NA, Hueber W, Sommer U, Schumacher MM, Peters T, Kriehuber E, Lee DM, Wieczorek GA, Kolbinger F, Bleul CC (2015) Evidence that a neutrophil-keratinocyte crosstalk is an early target of IL-17A inhibition in psoriasis. Exp Dermatol 24:529–535

Reikine S, Nguyen JB, Modis Y (2014) Pattern recognition and signaling mechanisms of RIG-I and MDA5. Front Immunol 5:342–342

Suárez-Fariñas M, Li K, Fuentes-Duculan J, Hayden K, Brodmerkel C, Krueger JG (2012) Expanding the psoriasis disease profile: interrogation of the skin and serum of patients with moderate-to-severe psoriasis. J Invest Dermatol 132:2552–2564

Vabret N, Blander JM (2013) Sensing microbial RNA in the cytosol. Front Immunol 4:468–468

Villanova F, Flutter B, Tosi I, Grys K, Sreeneebus H, Perera GK, Chapman A, Smith CH, Di Meglio P, Nestle FO (2014) Characterization of innate lymphoid cells in human skin and blood demonstrates increase of NKp44+ ILC3 in psoriasis. J Invest Dermatol 134:984–991

Yin X, Low HQ, Wang L, Li Y, Ellinghaus E, Han J, Estivill X, Sun L, Zuo X, Shen C, Zhu C, Zhang A, Sanchez F, Padyukov L, Catanese JJ, Krueger GG, Duffin KC, Mucha S, Weichenthal M, Weidinger S, Lieb W, Foo JN, Li Y, Sim K, Liany H, Irwan I, Teo Y, Theng CTS, Gupta R, Bowcock A, De Jager PL, Qureshi AA, de Bakker PIW, Seielstad M, Liao W, Ståhle M, Franke A, Zhang X, Liu J (2015) Genome-wide meta-analysis identifies multiple novel associations and ethnic heterogeneity of psoriasis susceptibility. Nat Commun 6:6916–6916

Zhen Q, Yang Z, Wang W, Li B, Bai M, Wu J, Ge H, Dong Z, Shen J, Tang H, Sun S, Qiu Y, Xu J, Qu X, Wang Y, Yi M, Hu H, Xu Y, Cheng H, Liang B, Gao J, Shao H, Jiang Z, Gao Q, Sun L (2019) Genetic study on small insertions and deletions in psoriasis reveals a role in complex human diseases. J Investig Dermatol 139:2302–2312.e2314

The Immunogenetics of Lichen Planus

Parvin Mansouri, Nahid Nikkhah, Behnaz Esmaeili, Alireza Khosravi, Reza Chalangari, and Katalin Martits-Chalangari

Abstract

Lichen planus (LP) is a multifaceted autoimmune disease affecting the skin, nails, hair, and mucous membranes, with several clinical subgroups. Cell-mediated immunity plays a key role in its progression. This chapter reviews the known genetic associations of lichen planus including HLA as well as non-HLA genes.

P. Mansouri (✉)
Research Vice-President of Medical Laser Research Center, Academic Center for Education-Culture and Research, Tehran University of Medical Sciences, Tehran, Iran
e-mail: mansorip@sina.tums.ac.ir

N. Nikkhah
Medical Laser Research Centers, Academic Center for Education-Culture and Research, Tehran University of Medical Sciences, Tehran, Iran

B. Esmaeili
Immunology Asthma and Allergy Research Institute, Tehran University of Medical Sciences, Tehran, Iran

A. Khosravi
Mycology Research Center, Faculty of Veterinary Medicine, University of Tehran, Tehran, Iran

R. Chalangari · K. Martits-Chalangari
Kasir Dermatology, Dallas, TX, USA

Keywords

Lichen planus · Immunogenetics of lichen planus · Mucosal lichen plan · Lichen planopilaris · Classic lichen plan · Cutaneous lichen plan · Immunogenetics · Single nucleotide polymorphism · Pathogenesis · GWAS

1 Introduction

Lichen planus (LP) is a chronic inflammatory immune-mediated disease that can affect any ectodermal-derived tissues. The disease was first described in 1869 by William James Erasmus Wilson as leichen planus (Greek leichen, "tree moss"; Latin planus, "flat") (Daoud et al. 2012; Sharma et al. 2012). LP mostly affects individuals in their forties and fifties (between 30 and 70 years old) and has no sexual preference. The prevalence of this disease is approximately 1–2% in the general population and about 2–10% of cases are seen in children (Luis-Montoya et al. 2005; Weston and Payette 2015).

Planar purple, polygonal, pruritic papules and plaques (the six Ps) symmetrically appear on the lateral surfaces of the extremities in classic lichen planus. Lesions may also appear in the site of previous trauma, which reflects the Kobner phenomenon (isomorphic response). Improvement of lichen planus is often accompanied by post-inflammatory hyperpigmentation. Lichen

N. Rezaei and F. Rajabi (eds.), *The Immunogenetics of Dermatologic Diseases*, Advances in Experimental Medicine and Biology 1367,
https://doi.org/10.1007/978-3-030-92616-8_5

planus comes in a variety of forms, depending on the shape of the lesions, their clinical features, and the place of involvement. These types include oral, nail, hypertrophic, palmoplantar, ulcerative, vesiculobullous, actinic, annular, atrophic, linear, follicular LP, lichen planopilaris, LP pemphigoides, LP pigmentosus, and LP pigmentosus-inversus (Bolognia et al. 2018) (Figs. 1, 2, 3, 4, 5, 6, 7, 8).

LP can affect any mucosal surfaces but is mostly seen in the mouth or the genitals (Figs. 9, 10). Inside the oral cavity, LP can cause a burning sensation or painful erosions. Oral lichen plan (OLP) affects 1–2% of the population. It can

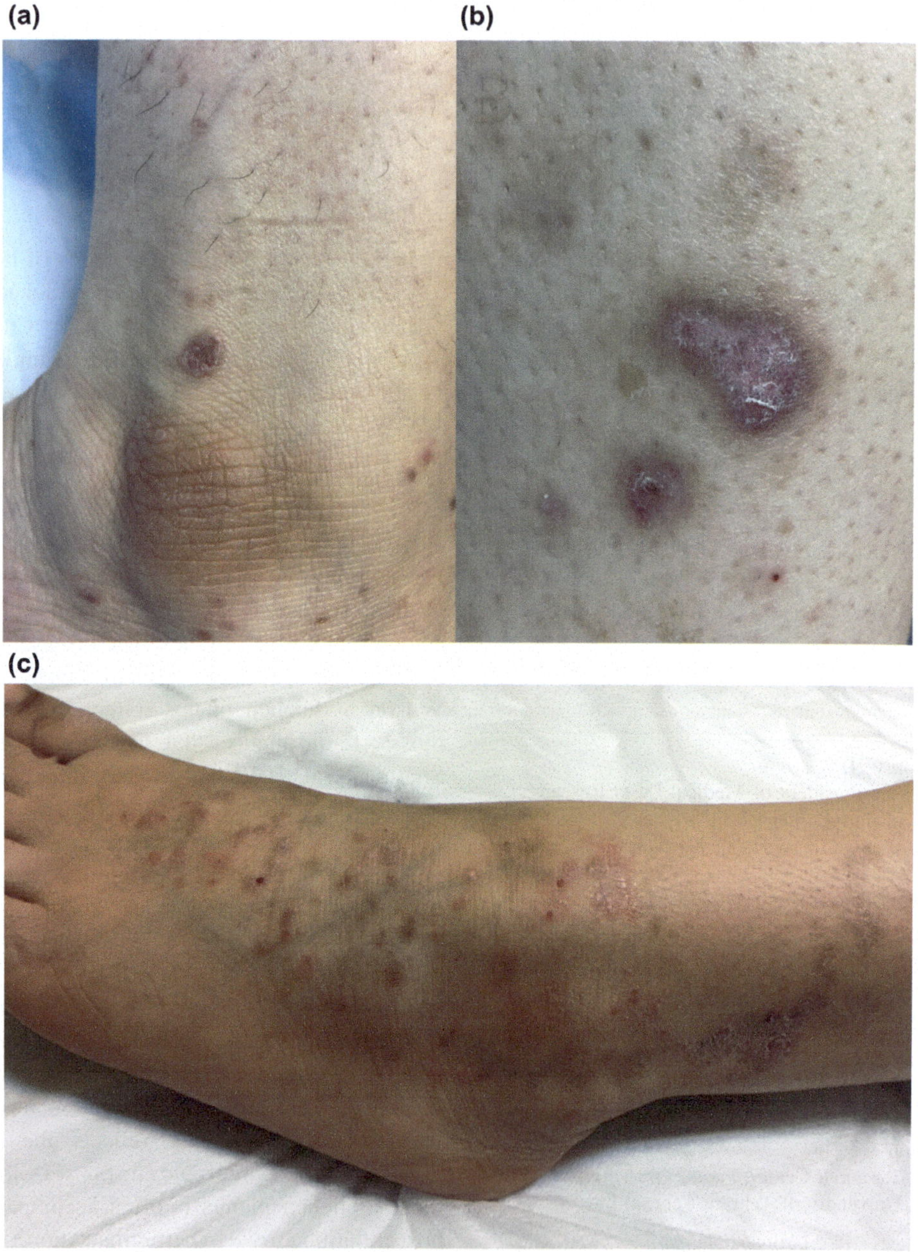

Fig. 1 Violaceous papules and plaques with white scale and Wickham striae on the dorsal foot (**a**, **b**, **c**)

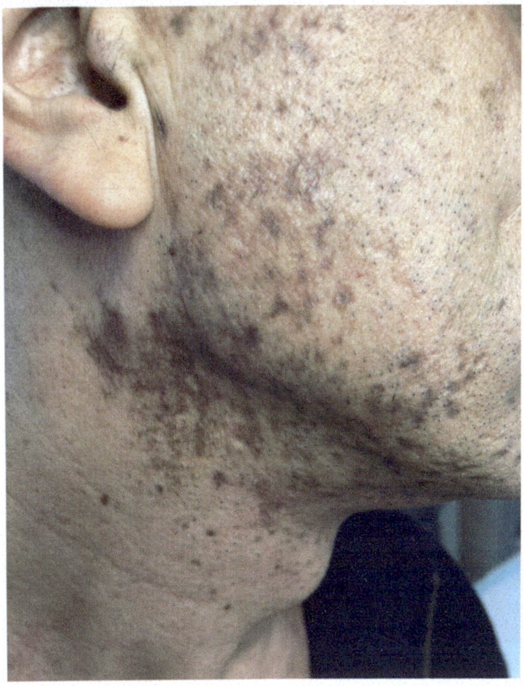

Fig. 2 Lichen planus with post-inflammatory hyperpigmentation

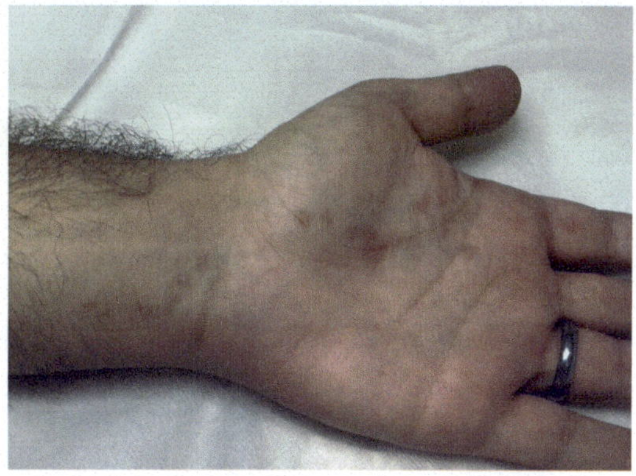

Fig. 4 Linear lichen planus on the wrist and palm

be the only presentation but is often accompanied by cutaneous lesions. Oral lesions have a predilection for middle-aged females (Bombeccari et al. 2011). Morphologically, the OLP can present as reticular, papular, atrophic, erosive, plaque-like, and bullous lesions. The most frequent kind is reticular lesions, which are generally asymptomatic. The erosive and atrophic

(a) (b)

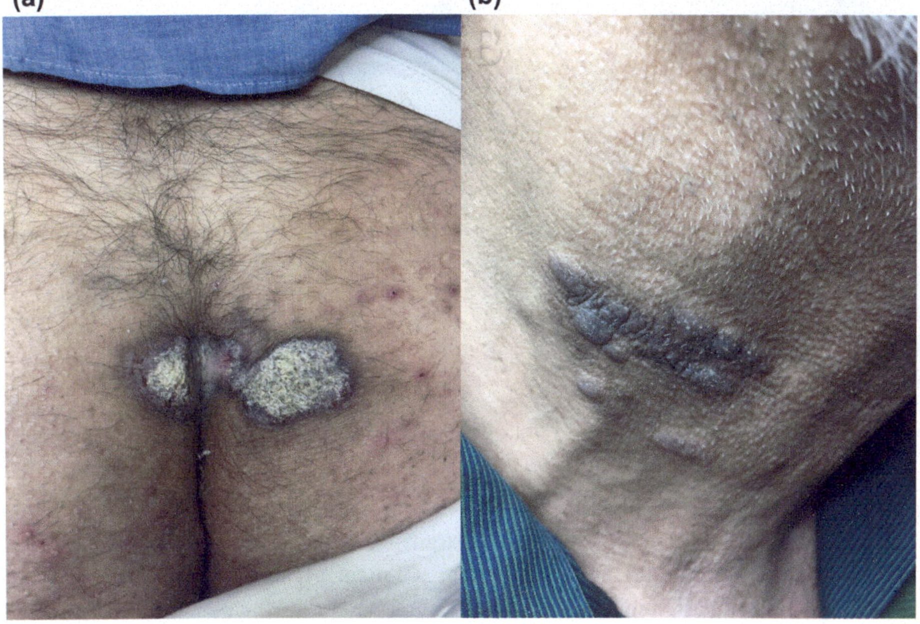

Fig. 3 Hypertrophic lichen planus on the buttocks (**a**) and neck (**b**)

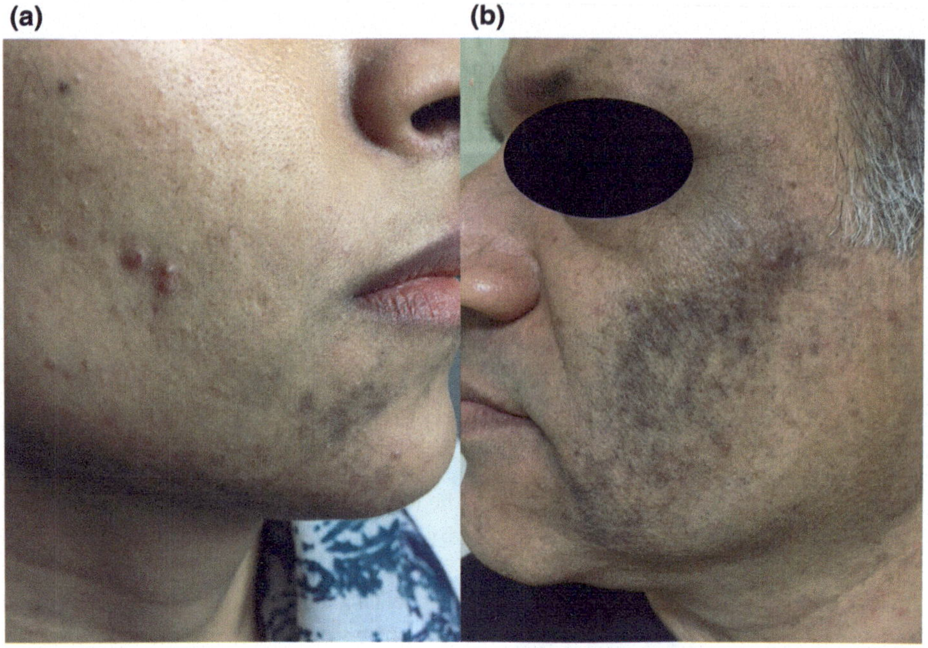

Fig. 5 Lichen planus pigmentosus or actinic on the face (**a**, **b**)

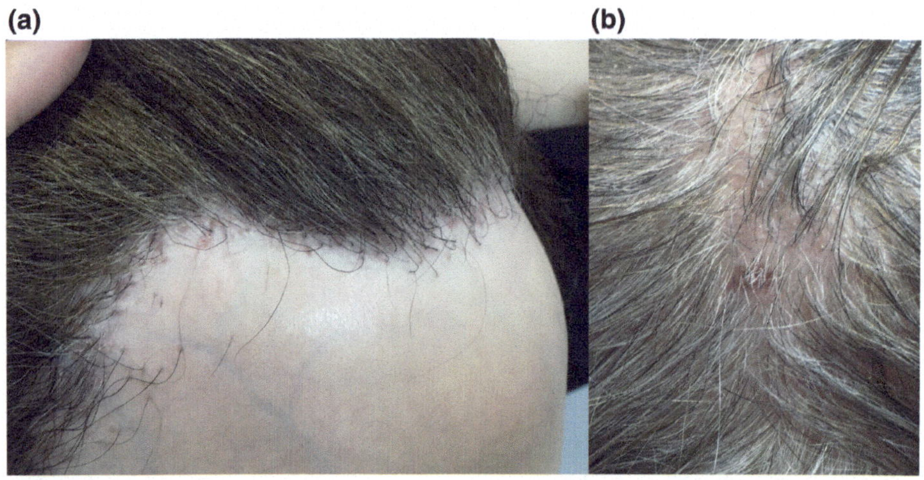

Fig. 6 Lichen planopilaris: cicatricial alopecia with perifollicular inflammation (**a** and **b**)

lesions are often painful (Boorghani et al. 2010). The first case of oral SCC originating from OLP was reported in 1910. Recent systematic reviews have reported the rate of malignant transformation to be 1/1–1/4% (Aghbari et al. 2017; Giuliani et al. 2019). The tongue is the most common location of involvement and the erosive and atrophic lesions are the most common morphological types associated with malignant transformation (Bombeccari et al. 2011).

Clinical features and histopathology are diagnostic in most cases of LP but to differentiate the bullous types from lichen planus pemphigoides, direct and indirect immunofluorescence tests may be needed (Carrozzo et al. 2000; Carrozzo and Thorpe 2009).

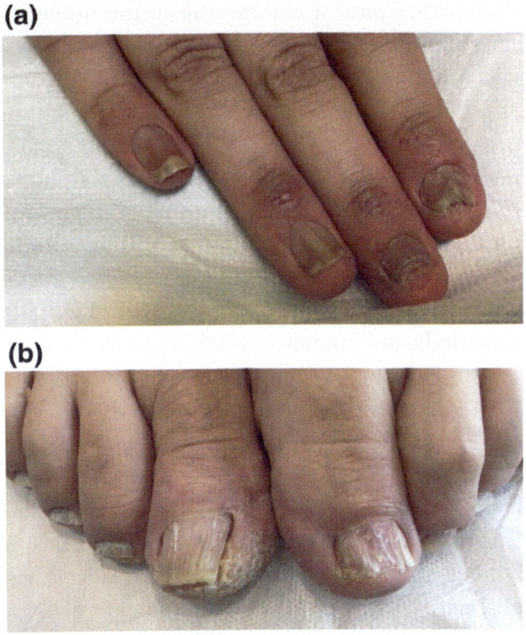

Fig. 7 Nail lichen planus: Thinning of the nail plate, longitudinal ridging and fissuring of nail plates (**a**), Yellow discoloration, onycholysis, subungual hyperkeratosis, and pterygium formation (**b**)

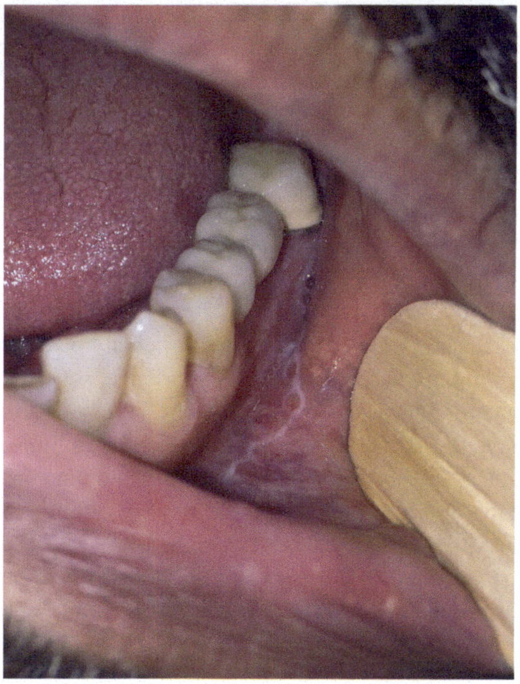

Fig. 9 Oral lichen planus, a white lacy pattern on the buccal mucosa

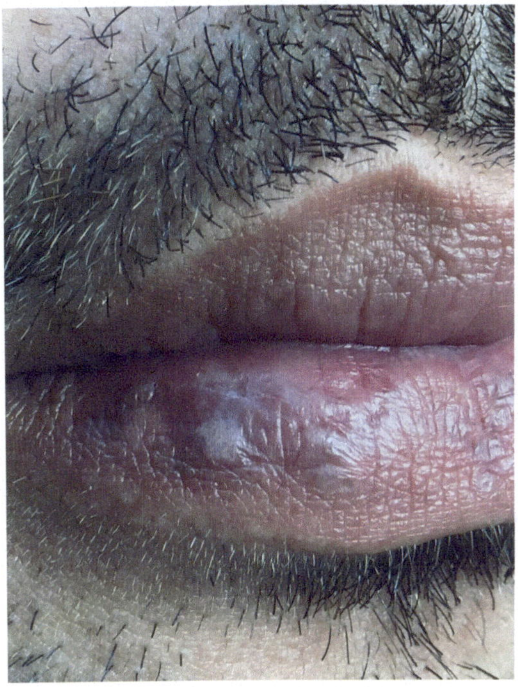

Fig. 8 Lichen planus on the lip with typical Wickham steria

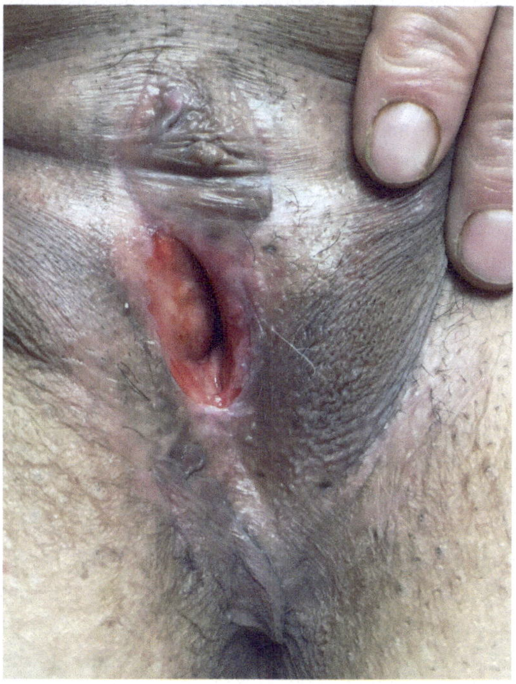

Fig. 10 Erosive genital lichen planus

The histological characteristic of the LP and its variants are somewhat similar. Interface dermatitis with orthokeratosis, hyperkeratosis, lack of parakeratosis, hypergranulosis, and elongation of rete ridges is shown under light microscopy (sawtooth pattern). Additional features are pigmentary incontinence in the superficial dermis, Apoptotic cells, or colloid-hyaline bodies entities at the dermo-epidermal junction. (Gorouhi et al. 2014).

Management of cutaneous lichen plan is commonly based on clinical experience, severity, extent, and site of involvement (Weston and Payette 2015). It may be challenging at times since relapses may occur and spontaneous remission may also be seen in up to two-thirds of the cases with cutaneous LP in the first year. The management of OLP is especially hard since the lesions tend to be more persistent (Usatine and Tinitigan 2011).

2 Pathogenesis of LP

Lichen plan is a complex immune-mediated disease. T helper and T cytotoxic, natural killer (NK) cells, and dendritic cells are Inflammatory cells playing role in this process. T-cell activation and the influx of cytotoxic T-cells into the epithelium, leading to the death of basal keratinocytes, is a crucial component in the pathogenesis of LP. Theoretically, the infiltration of immune cells may be initiated by the expression of CXCR3 and CCR5 on both T-cells and keratinocytes. Although cell-mediated immunity plays a major role, infectious agents (especially hepatitis C, hepatitis B vaccination, and other bacterial and viral antigens), medications, immunodeficiencies, dental materials, stress/anxiety, metabolic abnormalities, and genetic reasons are some of the other intrinsic or extrinsic variables (Alrashdan et al. 2016; Gorouhi et al. 2014; Srinivas et al. 2011). The racial propensity for LP among African, American, and Indian patients, as well as the few occurrences of familial LP point to a hereditary vulnerability to the disease.

Cytokines have a critical role in the initiation and sustaining of inflammatory and immunological responses, as well as intercellular communication. Various cytokines, including interleukin (IL)-2, -4, -6, -8, -10, -12, -17, -22, interferon (IFN)-γ, and tumor necrosis factor (TNF)-α, have been found abnormally expressed in LP mucocutaneous lesions or saliva, serum, and peripheral blood mononuclear cells (PBMCs) specimens from patients with LP. This might indicate immunological dysregulation in these individuals and emphasize the critical role of cytokines in the immune etiology of LP.

IFN-γ, TNF-α, IL-10, IL-17, and IL-22 are the most notable of the numerous cytokines with changed expression levels. TNF-α has a critical function in LP immune modulation. It has a significant role in the activation of Langerhans cells and the death of basal keratinocyte cells.

T helper 1 cells generate IFN-γ, whereas Th2 cells create IL-10. Because LP is characterized by a Th1/Th2 imbalance, the major cytokines IFN-γ and IL-10 have received greater attention in patients with LP than other cytokines. IFN-γ maintains the keratinocyte expression of major histocompatibility complex (MHC) class II molecules, which contributes to disease chronicity. The anti-inflammatory properties of IL-10 are significant.

Much new research is beginning to look at the involvement of IL-17 and IL-22. In general, IL-17 stimulates the production of inflammatory mediators in order to bridge the gap between adaptive and innate responses In LP lesions, T-helper17 cells (IL-17+ CD4 + T cells) have been discovered. The function of IL-22 is to enhance the epithelium's barrier function and may play a role in defense against oral microbiota (Ma et al. 2016).

Elevated levels of MMP9 induced by Th9/IL-9 can aggravate OLP, this may occur directly through increasing Th17 levels or indirectly through a synergistic role with Th17 (Wang et al. 2018).

Recent studies have demonstrated increased expression of IL33 and IL35 in LP lesions; there are more IL33 + cells in the deeper connective tissue region than at the epithelial-connective tissue interface and all the IL35 + cells observed in LP tissues have ovoid/plasmacytoid morphology (Javvadi et al. 2018).

In a recent meta-analysis study, LP patients were demonstrated to have elevated serum and salivary IL-4 levels, this indicates that IL-4 may represent a potential salivary biomarker for the disease (Mozaffari et al. 2019).

Micro-RNAs (mi-RNAs) have also been implicated in the pathogenesis of LP. They can influence the translation of genes to proteins including cytokines. Several mi-RNAs have been found to directly modulate the translation of *TNF-α* and *IL-10* genes (Du et al. 2020; Gassling et al. 2013; Ma et al. 2016). Some other types of miRNAs could indirectly regulate cytokines such as TNF-a, IFN-γ, IL-10, and IL-17 by targeting their downstream proteins and adaptor molecules (Du et al. 2020; Gassling et al. 2013; Ma et al. 2016). A single study has also been able to detect a link between miRNAs and IL-22 (Ma et al. 2016). They found that IL-22 stimulation could result in the upregulation of miR-184 and its precursor in keratinocytes through a signal transducer and activator of transcription 3 (STAT3) dependent manner (Ma et al. 2016).

Most recent investigations on individuals suffering from LP have been able to show the involvement of forkhead box P3, vascular endothelial growth factor (VEGF), matrix metalloproteinase 9 (MMP9), toll-like receptors (TLR) among others in the pathogenesis of the disease. Nonetheless, there are still many gaps in our knowledge regarding the etiopathogenesis of LP (Sinon et al. 2016; Wang et al. 2015; Xie et al. 2014).

Several studies have been able to show an association between polymorphisms in the genes encoding human leukocyte antigens (HLA) and the risk of developing LP lesions (Madalli 2013; Porter et al. 1997b; Weston and Payette 2015). Polymorphisms in genes encoding immune signaling molecules and receptors, matrix metalloproteinases (MMPs) and tissue inhibitors of metalloproteinases (TIMPs), prostaglandin E2 synthesis, transglutaminase pathways, thyroid hormone synthesis, oxidative stress, RANTES (regulated on activation, normal T cell expressed and secreted) and nuclear factor kappa B, as well as epigenetic regulation of genes by some micro-RNAs, are considered to have a role in the pathogenesis of lichen planus (Daoud et al. 2012; Sugerman et al. 2002; Zhou et al. 2001). Unfortunately, there is a substantial shortage in the genetic studies of LP and most of the available studies thus far are focused on OLP (Table 1).

3 Immunogenetic Aspects of LP

3.1 HLA Genes

There is a difference in HLA-associated genetic susceptibility between patients with the idiopathic form of LP (ILP) compared to the patients with secondary form (SLP) caused by drugs or accompanied by other immunological disorders (Nasa et al. 1995). Furthermore, categorizing patients with idiopathic form based on the type of lesions (cutaneous, mucosal, or combined) revealed that they are genetically heterogeneous (Nasa et al. 1995).

3.1.1 HLA Class I Genes

Ethnicity and geographical locations have a major role in the distribution of HLA genes. Thus the association of HLA polymorphisms and diseases may vary between different ethnicities. While Danish studies have shown no significant association between HLA allele frequencies and cutaneous LP, an increase in HLA-A3 frequency was reported in British and French patients with cutaneous LP (Lowe et al. 1976; Saurat et al. 1977; Veien et al. 1979).

Decreased frequency of *HLA-Aw19*, *HLA-A28*, and *HLA-B18* presentation along with increased expression of *HLA-B15* has been observed in Croatian patients with OLP (Ognjenović et al. 1998a, 1998b). There is no significant difference in *HLA-A*, *-B*, and *-C* allele frequencies between Japanese patients with OLP and healthy controls (Watanabe et al. 1986). An increased frequency of *HLA-B27* and *HLA-Bw57* has been documented in British patients with OLP (Porter et al. 1993).

Table 1 Gene implicated in the pathogenesis of lichen planus

Gene		Reference
HLA Class I	*HLA-A3 HLA-A11 HLA-A26 HLA-A*2, HLA-A*69, HLA-A*68, HLA-B2, HLA-B5, HLA-B7, HLA-B8, HLA-B*13, HLA-B15, HLA-B16, HLA-B27, HLA-B*35, HLA-B40, HLA-B51, HLA-Bw57* *HLA-Bw35* and *HLA-Bw57*, HLA-*BX*	Gülsüm et al. (2006), Lowe et al. (1976), Ognjenović et al. (1998a, b), Porter et al. (1993), Saurat et al. (1977), Veien et al. (1979)
HLA class II	*HLA-DR1* (*HLA-DRB1*0101*), *HLA-DQ1, HLA-DR3, HLA-DR5, HLA-DR6, HLA-DRW9, HLA-Te22, HLA-DRw9, HLA-DR10* *HLA-A1-B8-DR3* haplotype *HLA-Bw 61/DRw 9* haplotype	Carrozzo et al. (2001), Jontell et al. (1987), Lin and Sun (1990), Luis-Montoya et al. (2007), Nasa et al. (1995), Powell et al. (1986), Valsecchi et al. (1988), Watanabe et al. (1986), White and Rostom (1994)
Immunity-related genes	*IFNG* *IL4* *TNFα* *TNF receptor 2 (TNFR2)* *IL-1β* *IL-6* *IL-10* *IL-8* *IL-12* *IL-17A* *IL18* *TLR3* *MBL2* *MHC class II transactivator (CIITA)* *P53* *CD24*	Bai et al. (2008), Kimkong et al. (2012) Carrozzo et al. (2004) Carrozzo et al. (2004), Kimkong et al. (2011), Xavier et al. (2007) Fujita et al. (2009) Chauhan et al. (2013) Belluco et al. (2003), Fishman et al. (1998), Xavier et al. (2007) Bai et al. (2009), Xavier et al. (2007) Azab et al. (2018) Jiang et al. (2015) Gueiros et al. (2018) Bai et al. (2007) Stanimirovic et al. (2013) Barkokebas et al. (2011), Polesello et al. (2019) Al-Drobie and Al-Hasnawi (2018), Wu et al. (2013) Ghabanchi et al. (2009), Yanatatsaneeji et al. (2010) Carl et al. (2008), Kaplan et al. (2015)
Genes with miscellaneous functions	DNA methyltransferase 3B (DNMT3B) O6-methylguanine-DNA methyltransferase (MGMT) *High-mobility group box 1* (*HMGB1*) Neuropilin 2 (*NRP2*) Insulin-like growth factor-binding protein 4 (*IGFBP4*). T Hypoxia-inducible factor-1 (HIF-1) Myeloperoxidase (MPO) Cyclooxygenase 2 (COX2) *CYP2D6*4* Vitamin D receptor (VDR)	Fonseca-Silva et al. (2012) Sánchez-Siles et al. (2019) Supic et al. (2015) Nagao et al. (2017) Nagao et al. (2017) Carvalho Fraga et al. (2013) Wu et al. (2015) Abdel Hay et al. (2012) Kragelund et al. (2009), Kujundzic et al. (2016) Kujundzic et al. (2016)

A significant increase in *HLA-A26* and *HLA-B51* frequencies have been observed in British patients with both oral and cutaneous LP lesions (Porter et al. 1993). Irrespective of ethnicity, *HLA-B16* has been reported to have an increased frequency in both cutaneous and mucosal LP and *HLA-Bw35* and *HLA-B8* are related to the cutaneous and the mucosal forms of LP, respectively (Porter et al. 1997a; Simon et al. 1984). A study based on a British population subdivided patients according to the type of their oral lesions into erosive, non-erosive, and mixed and showed that

HLA-B27 and *HLA-Bw57* were increased in the erosive type (Porter et al. 1993). Erosive forms of OLP demonstrate less frequently in *HLA-A11* and *HLA-A26* compared to the plaque form (Ognjenović et al. 1998a). British patients with the mixed type had an increased frequency of *HLA-B51* presentation (Porter et al. 1993). *HLA-A*2*, *HLA-A*69*, *HLA-A*68*, *HLA-B*13*, and *HLA-B*35* alleles are associated with erosive oral LP (without cutaneous lesions) in Turkish patients (Gülsüm et al. 2006). The oral LP patents with carbohydrate disorders show higher frequency in *HLA-B16*, *B2*, and *B40*, and in patients without carbohydrate disorders, *HLA-B5*, *B7* and *BX* frequencies are increased (Ognjenović et al. 1998b).

3.1.2 HLA Class II Genes

Results of a study on 105 patients with Sardinian origin showed an increased frequency of *HLA-DR1* and *HLA-DQ1* and a decreased frequency of *HLA-Q3* in patients with cutaneous LP but not in patients with OLP or SLP (Nasa et al. 1995). Since *HLA-DR1* is associated with the cutaneous and combined forms of idiopathic LP, it has been proposed that this HLA may have a great contribution to the development of the disease (Nasa et al. 1995). Further DNA molecular evaluation on patients with cutaneous form indicated that *HLA-DRB1*0101* is accountable for the genetic susceptibility (Nasa et al. 1995). The *HLA-DRB1*0101* allele increases the risk for LP development in the Mexican Mestizo population (Luis-Montoya et al. 2007). *HLA-DR1* is also found in higher frequency in the generalized form of LP compared to the localized form (Powell et al. 1986). Similar results regarding the association between *HLA-DR1* frequency and increased susceptibility to LP have been reported in American (Powell et al. 1986) and Italian patients (Valsecchi et al. 1988). There is a higher risk of having erosive oral LP in *HLA-DR3* positive individuals (Jontell et al. 1987). The *HLA-A1-B8-DR3* haplotype is more commonly found in both erosive OLP and cutaneous forms of LP than in healthy subjects (Jontell et al. 1987). HLA typing results on 50 Arab patients with cutaneous LP revealed a significant decrease in *HLA-DR5* frequency (White and Rostom 1994). Increased frequency in *HLA-DRW9* and *HLA-Te22* has been observed in Chinese patients with non-erosive OLP (Lin and Sun 1990). In agreement with the findings in the Chinese patients, a significant increase in the frequency of *HLA-DRw9* was reported in Japanese patients with OLP. Moreover, *HLA-Bw 61/DRw 9* haplotype also confers risk for OLP in Japanese patients (Watanabe et al. 1986). In addition to *HLA-DR1*, *HLA-DR10* is another genetic susceptibility locus for cutaneous LP in Arab patients (White and Rostom 1994). The *HLA-DQ1* frequency decreases in non-erosive type of oral LP (Porter et al. 1993). Nonetheless, no association has been observed between frequency of *HLA-DR1* and *HLA-DQ* and susceptibility to oral LP in Chinese patients (Lin and Sun 1990). *HLA-DRB1*01* allele is found at increased frequency in Turkish patients with erosive OLP (without cutaneous lesions). In contrast, *DRB1*11* is a protective allele observed more frequently in healthy controls (Gülsüm et al. 2006).

A reciprocal association exists between LP and hepatitis C virus (HCV) infection. Patients with LP have a higher risk for getting infected with HCV and a higher prevalence of LP is found among HCV-infected patients (Carrozzo et al. 2001; Lodi et al. 2010). In Italy, the *HLA-DR6* allele was found to confer susceptibility to OLP in patients with HCV infection (Carrozzo et al. 2001). No significant difference in *HLA C1/C2* allele frequencies was observed in Italian patients with OLP without hepatitis C virus (HCV) infection compared to those patients with HCV (Carrozzo et al. 2011).

3.1.3 Familial LP

Familial LP refers to the occurrence of LP lesions in two or more members of a single family (Kofoed and Wantzin 1985; Mahood 1983). In comparison to idiopathic non-familial LP, the cases of familial LP are younger and the generalized type of LP is more frequently seen in these patients (Kofoed and Wantzin 1985; Mahood 1983). Studies have been able to demonstrate an increase in the frequency of *HLA-A3* and *HLA-*

B7 in British patients with familial LP (Copeman et al. 1978; Lowe et al. 1976).

3.2 Non-HLA Genes

3.2.1 Gene with Prominent Immunological Functions

Polymorphisms in several non-HLA genes have been linked to LP susceptibility most of which are cytokine encoding genes.

Polymorphisms in the gene encoding IFNγ have been linked to OLP. The T allele and the AT + TT genotypes of the + 874 *IFNG* were associated with OLP in case–control studies in the Chinese and Thai populations (Bai et al. 2008; Kimkong et al. 2012). The TT genotype at position 5644 3'UTR (first intron) on the *IFNG* gene is more frequently presented in Italian patients with OLP (Carrozzo et al. 2004).

In patients with non-erosive OLP, the C allele and CC genotype of the -590 IL4 are considerably greater than in the control group. (Bai et al. 2008). Interestingly the same association has been documented for recurrent aphthous stomatitis (Najafi et al. 2018).

Several single nucleotide polymorphisms (SNPs) in the *TNFα* gene have already been investigated. in patients with OLP from which the −308 (rs1800629) AA genotype was found to confer susceptibility to OLP in the Indian, Thai, and Brazilian populations (Kimkong et al. 2011; Xavier et al. 2007). This genotype is associated with higher cytokine production (Brinkman et al. 1995; Jongeneel and Beutler 1995). The A allele and the AG genotype of this SNP have also been linked to susceptibility to OLP and more so to the additional skin involvement (mucocutaneous LP) in an Italian population (Carrozzo et al. 2004). The gene encoding TNF receptor 2 (TNFR2) has been linked to OLP in a Japanese-based study. The + 587 G allele was shown to confer susceptibility to OLP (Fujita et al. 2009).

An Indian-based study identified the T allele of the 3954 C/T SNP of IL-1β to confer susceptibility to OLP in patients with chronic periodontitis and diabetes were compared to patients with OLP who did not have chronic periodontitis or diabetes mellitus (Chauhan et al. 2013).

Several studies have stated that the high producer G allele and the GG genotype of the *IL-6* −174 SNP confers susceptibility to OLP, while others have opposed this association (Belluco et al. 2003; Fishman et al. 1998; Xavier et al. 2007).

Though the rates of the alleles and genotypes of the *IL-10* SNPs are not different between patients with OLP and control subjects, the frequency of a haplotype consisting of −1082 G/A, −819 C/T, and −592 C/A has been shown to be higher in patients with OLP (Bai et al. 2009; Xavier et al. 2007). This haplotype is associated with lower IL-10 serum levels (Bai et al. 2009).

The IL-8 rs4073 AA and AT genotypes were shown to confer susceptibility to OLP in a study on Egyptian HCV + patients (Azab et al. 2018). While the −251 AA genotype and A allele and the −251 A/+781 C haplotype were found to confer protection against erosive OLP in Chinese patients (Dan et al. 2010). IL-12 rs568408 A allele was linked to OLP and erosive OLP in Chinese patients (Jiang et al. 2015).

The Th17 pathway interleukins have also been evaluated in OLP with the A allele of the *IL-17A* G197A SNP conferring susceptibility to the disease (Gueiros et al. 2018).

The *IL-18* gene has two SNPs, −607C/A and −137G/C, which have been linked to OLP (Bai et al. 2007). The −137 SNP is found in the IL-18 gene's promoter region, and its GG genotype is associated with enhanced gene expression and higher serum levels. The difference in the frequency of this genotype is more pronounced in severe erosive OLP (Bai et al. 2007).

The polymorphisms of the Toll-like receptor (TLR) genes as the main receptors of innate immunity have also been evaluated in LP. The TT genotype of the rs5743312 SNP of TLR3 gene polymorphism has been shown to confer susceptibility to OLP in a European-based study (Stanimirovic et al. 2013). The minor mutated allele of the *TLR2* rs3804099 demonstrated a protective effect in this population (Stanimirovic et al. 2013).

Another innate immunity factor that has been evaluated in the pathogenesis of OLP is mannose-binding lectin from the Lectin complement pathway. It has been hypothesized that the lower activity of the lectin pathway and the innate immune responses may lead to the compensatory hyperresponsiveness of the adaptive immune system and thus provoke autoimmunity (Dean et al. 2011). Two studies have investigated the association of polymorphisms in the MBL encoding gene (*MBL2*) with OLP. One study did not find a significant association between OLP and *MBL* structural mutations and SNPs in the Brazilian population but the other study was able to demonstrate significantly higher expression of low producing X allele (rs7096206) and CT genotype of the D allele (rs5030737) in Italian patients with OLP (Barkokebas et al. 2011; Polesello et al. 2019).

Two very small case–control studies consisting of only 15 and 30 patients with OLP have been able to draw an association between OLP and the rs4774 and rs6498122 polymorphisms within a gene encoding a transcriptional cofactor known as major histocompatibility complex (MHC) CIITA is a class II transactivator that induces the expression of MHCII on the cell surface (Al-Drobie and Al-Hasnawi 2018; Wu et al. 2013). Though this gene has been linked to multiple autoimmune diseases since the sample size of the study linking it to OLP is very small further studies are required to confirm this association with confidence (Eike et al. 2012; Koizumi et al. 2005).

Since cytotoxic T lymphocyte-mediated apoptotic pathways are implicated in the pathogenesis of LP, the genes encoding these pathway particles have also been investigated (Schifter et al. 1998). One of these genes is the *P53* tumor suppressor gene involved in Fas/FasL-induced apoptosis. An SNP at P53 codon 72 has been linked to OLP in Iranian and Tai populations (Ghabanchi et al. 2009; Yanatatsaneeji et al. 2010). The CC genotype which translates to proline/proline is associated with high expression of Fas/FasL and enhanced apoptosis (Schneider-Stock et al. 2004).

Polymorphisms of the gene encoding CD24 have also been evaluated in the pathogenesis of OLP along with multiple other autoimmune diseases (Carl et al. 2008). This cell surface glycoprotein is involved in cell adhesion, proliferation, and survival. It serves as a costimulatory factor for T-cells and is involved in B-cell activation and differentiation (Tan et al. 2016). It is also involved in the clonal deletion of autoreactive thymocytes (Carl et al. 2008). Individuals homozygous for the common allele of the A1626 G (rs1058881) have a higher chance of getting OLP, while carriers of the A1056G SNP's main allele (rs1058818) have a significantly lower risk of developing OLP (Kaplan et al. 2015).

3.2.2 Genes with Miscellaneous Functions

The epigenetic modifications can change the genomic landscape by inducing/suppressing gene expression without affecting the genetic sequence and thus play a key role in the development of immune-mediated illnesses like OLP (Cruz et al. 2018; Dillenburg et al. 2015). DNA methylation and histone acetylation aided are the two most important types of epigenetic modifications (Larsson 2018). The DNA methylation patterns can be inherited or induced by environmental factors. The de novo methylation patterns are mainly carried out by DNA methyltransferase (DNMT) enzymes. A case–control study looked at the prevalence of the DNMT3B C46359T SNP in the promoter region of the gene in Brazilian patients with lichen planus in order to better understand the role of epigenetics in the etiology of the disease. The CT genotype, which was linked to greater enzymatic activity, was shown to be substantially more common in patients than in controls. (Fonseca-Silva et al. 2012).

A subtype of the DNMT family of enzymes known as O6-methylguanine-DNA methyltransferase (MGMT), is a genome correction enzyme that reduces the gene mutation rate by transferring a methyl group to damaged guanine nucleosides (Yu et al. 2020).

Interestingly, the methylation of CpG patterns in the MGMT gene's promoter region increases the chance of carcinogenesis by gene silencing (Bouras et al. 2019). A promoter SNP (rs16906252) has been shown to increase *MGMT* methylation (Hawkins et al. 2009). For carriers of the rs16906252 T allele the chance of having their *MGMT* gene silenced due to hypermethylation is approximately eight times higher and the T allele is more frequent in patients with OLP. This might explain the malignant transformation in longstanding OLP lesions (Sánchez-Siles et al. 2019). Another gene that has been linked to the progression of OLP to squamous cell carcinoma is the *high-mobility group box 1* (*HMGB1*) gene (Supic et al. 2015).

Two SNPs within genes encoding Neuropilin 2 (*NRP2*) and insulin-like growth factor-binding protein 4 (*IGFBP4*) represent susceptibility loci for hepatitis C-driven OLP, rs884000, and rs538399, respectively (Nagao et al. 2017). The IGFBP4 is a growth factor highly expressed by cancerous cells and neuropilin 2 is a transmembrane receptor that is hypothesized to have a play a function in cancer progression and metastasis (Durai et al. 2006; Gray et al. 2008). Both genes may have a role in the malignant transformation of OLP lesions, according to some researchers (Nagao et al. 2017).

Hypoxia-mediated inflammation and angiogenesis is another route implicated in the development of OLP. Cells sense the reduced oxygen content via the alpha subunit of the hypoxia-inducible factor-1 (HIF-1). HIF in turn translocates to the nucleus, forming a dimer with the beta subunit, and acts as a transcription factor. The C1772T and G1790A SNPs of the *HIF-1α* gene have been linked to OLP in a Brazilian study (Carvalho Fraga et al. 2013).

The myeloperoxidase (MPO) enzyme is involved in the formation of reactive oxygen species in polymorphonuclear cells during inflammation and thus can lead to the pathogenesis of autoimmune disorders (Strzepa et al. 2017). Polymorphisms in the gene encoding this enzyme have been linked to the pathogenesis of many immune-mediated diseases.

A study in Chinese patients with OLP identified the *MPO* rs2243828 AA and female patients with OLP have more AA + AG genotypes, while male patients with OLP have more rs2243828 AG + GG and GG genotypes. Thus they suggested that the effects of sex hormones combined with genetic susceptibility could influence the involvement of oxidative stress in the pathogenesis of OLP (Wu et al. 2015).

The prostaglandins contribute to the chronicity of inflammation by promoting cytokine and chemokine production. The conversion of arachidonic to prostaglandin is catalyzed by cyclooxygenase (COX) enzymes, which can impact the pathophysiology of immune-mediated illnesses like OLP. The C allele of the *COX2* G765C SNP was shown to confer susceptibility to erosive OLP in Egyptian patients (Abdel Hay et al. 2012).

Since environmental factors such as drug exposure have been implicated in the pathogenesis of OLP, some studies have investigated the association between drug-metabolizing agents such as the CYP enzymes and OLP. Polymorphisms in the genes encoding CYP2C9, CYP2C19, CYP2D6, CYP27B1, and CYP24A1 have been evaluated in patients with OLP (Kragelund et al. 2009; Kujundzic et al. 2016). It has been demonstrated that individuals heterozygous for the *CYP24A1* rs2296241 had a lower risk for developing OLP and the individuals carrying the common non-functional *CYP2D6*4* alleles were at higher risk for developing OLP (Kragelund et al. 2009; Kujundzic et al. 2016). However, these studies weren't able to draw a direct link between pharmacological effects of these polymorphisms and LP pathogenesis instead it was suggested that molecular mimicry between *CYP2D6**4 and common oral microbial flora such as herpes simplex-1 and candidal antigens may be involved (Kragelund et al. 2009).

Polymorphisms within the vitamin D receptor (VDR) gene have also been linked to OLP. In patients with OLP, the *FokI* (rs2228570), *ApaI* (rs7975232), *EcoRV* (rs4516035), and *TaqI* (rs731236) genes have been studied, however only the heterozygous and mutant genotypes of *VDR FokI* (rs2228570) have been proven to confer vulnerability to OLP (Kujundzic et al. 2016).

3.3 The Role of MicroRNAs in Lichen Planus

MicroRNAs (miRNAs) are epigenetic modifiers that are composed of short (17–24 bases), single-stranded, non-coding RNA molecules. The miRNAs adjust protein expression at the post-transcriptional level by decreasing translation and/or causing degradation of the target messenger RNA (mRNA) through incorrect base pairing with the 3′ untranslated regions (UTR) of the target mRNA (Khosravi and Erle 2016). MiRNAs have been discovered to be critical regulators of cell cycling, differentiation, and apoptosis and thus play a crucial role in modulating immune responses and inflammation. The innate and adaptive immunity against intracellular bacterial infections, for example, have been found to be controlled by miR-29. In addition, miR-155 has been shown to block IFN-γ signaling in helper T cells. Both miRNA-146a and miRNA-155 were shown to be increased in the PBMCs and lesional mucosa of individuals with OLP in investigations (Ahmadi-Motamayel et al. 2017; Arão et al. 2012; Liu et al. 2015). As a result, it's been suggested that the microRNA-messenger RNA (miRNA-mRNA) network is involved in the development of LP through the regulation of cytokine expression (Ma et al. 2016).

A miRNA microarray investigation of mucosal tissues in LP patients and healthy subjects revealed 70 miRNAs that were significantly dysregulated (Tao et al. 2019). Gassling et colleagues discovered 16 miRNAs that were expressed differently in mucosal regions in LP patients and healthy people. Six miRNAs, including miR31, 146a, 155, and 21, were upregulated by more than twofold, whereas miR923 and 30a were downregulated (Gassling et al. 2013). Because miR155 is connected to cytokines linked to LP, it is a good candidate miRNA for participation in the disease's pathophysiology.

The level of miR27b3p has been found to be lower in LP samples (Chen et al. 2019a). Downregulation of miR27b3p prevents epithelial keratinocyte death via upregulating the production of cyclophilin D (Chen et al. 2019a). Furthermore, cyclophilin D directly binds to Bcl2 and enhances its protein stability. Caspase9/3 activation and cytochrome C release are inhibited by Bcl2 (Chen et al. 2019b). MiR-27b and Polo Like Kinase 2 (PLK2) expression in LP tissues was found to be abnormal in another study. In human oral keratinocytes, decreased miR-27b may have stimulated cell proliferation by raising PLK2 levels (Chen et al. 2019a).

Twenty-one miRNAs, including miR-940, 4484, 663a, and 1290, have a two-fold difference in two sets of miRNA microarray profiles between LP and healthy people. 9 miRNAs (miR-121, 137, 146a, 155, 21, 203, 26b, 375, and 4484) were shown to be altered in individuals with LP during additional research (Ma et al. 2016). MiR-122 and miR-199 induce autophagy by targeting the mTOR and AKT pathways, which are important in the pathophysiology of LP. These data imply that miR122 and miR199 could be used as potential LP therapy targets (Wang et al. 2019).

4 Conclusions

Lichen planus (LP) is a chronic inflammatory skin and mucous membrane illness that involves hereditary variables as well as innate and adaptive immune cells. The co-occurrence of LP in two or more members of a single family, the disease's racial predisposition, and its relationship with HLA alleles all point to genetic factors playing a role in LP etiology. The miRNAs are small non-coding RNA molecules that play a fundamental role in the immune response. It has been revealed that lichen planus is accompanied by a change in miRNAs expression levels. Future improvements in therapy will be aided by a better knowledge of the function of genes and the miRNA/mRNA-cytokine interaction in the development of LP. Furthermore, such discoveries could be useful in single-gene treatment.

References

Abdel Hay R, Fawzy M, Metwally D, Kadry D, Ezzat M, Rashwan W, Rashed L (2012) DNA polymorphisms and tissue cyclooxygenase-2 expression in oral lichen planus: a case-control study. J Eur Acad Dermatol Venereol 26:1122–1126

Aghbari SMH, Abushouk AI, Attia A, Elmaraezy A, Menshawy A, Ahmed MS, Elsaadany BA, Ahmed EM (2017) Malignant transformation of oral lichen planus and oral lichenoid lesions: a meta-analysis of 20095 patient data. Oral Oncol 68:92–102

Ahmadi-Motamayel F, Bayat Z, Hajilooi M, Shahryar-Hesami S, Mahdavinezhad A, Samie L, Solgi G (2017) Evaluation of the miRNA-146a and miRNA-155 expression levels in patients with oral lichen planus. Iran J Immunol 14:316–324

Al-Drobie BF, Al-Hasnawi ZA (2018) Assessment of SNPs (rs4774, rs6498122) of CIITA gene in buccal swabs and blood of oral lichen planus patients in Iraq. Int J Med Res Health Sci 7:110–115

Alrashdan M, Cirillo N, McCullough M (2016) Oral lichen planus: a literature review and update. Arch Dermatol Res 308

Arão TC, Guimarães ALS, de Paula AMB, Gomes CC, Gomez RS (2012) Increased miRNA-146a and miRNA-155 expressions in oral lichen planus. Arch Dermatol Res 304:371–375

Azab NA, Abd El Salam L, Ahmed E, El Sharkawy M, ElSharkawy A, El Asheiry SG (2018) Interferon gamma and interleukin 8 gene polymorphisms in patients with hepatitis C virus related oral lichen planus. Arch Oral Biol 96:189–194

Bai J, Zhang Y, Lin M, Zeng X, Wang Z, Shen J, Jiang L, Gao F, Chen Q (2007) Interleukin-18 gene polymorphisms and haplotypes in patients with oral lichen planus: a study in an ethnic Chinese cohort. Tissue Antigens 70:390–397

Bai J, Jiang L, Lin M, Zeng X, Wang Z, Chen Q (2009) Association of polymorphisms in the tumor necrosis factor-α and interleukin-10 genes with oral lichen planus: a study in a Chinese cohort with Han ethnicity. J Interferon Cytokine Res 29:381–388

Bai J, Lin M, Zeng X, Zhang Y, Wang Z, Shen J, Jiang L, Gao F, Chen Q (2008) Association of polymorphisms in the human IFN-γ and IL-4 gene with oral lichen planus: a study in an ethnic Chinese cohort. J Interferon Cytokine Res 28:351–358

Barkokebas A, Alessandra de Albuquerque TC, de Souza PRE, Gomez RS, Xavier GM, Ribeiro CMB, Crovella S, Porter SR, Leão JC (2011) Mannose-binding lectin gene (MBL-2) polymorphism in oral lichen planus. Clin Oral Invest 15:699–704

Belluco C, Olivieri F, Bonafè M, Giovagnetti S, Mammano E, Scalerta R, Ambrosi A, Franceschi C, Nitti D, Lise M (2003) 174 G> C polymorphism of interleukin 6 gene promoter affects interleukin 6 serum level in patients with colorectal cancer. Clin Cancer Res 9:2173–2176

Bolognia J, Schaffer JV, Cerroni L (2018) Dermatology

Bombeccari GP, Guzzi G, Tettamanti M, Gianni AB, Baj A, Pallotti F, Spadari F (2011) Oral lichen planus and malignant transformation: a longitudinal cohort study. Oral Surg Oral Med Oral Pathol Oral Radiol Endod 112:328–334

Boorghani M, Gholizadeh N, Taghavi Zenouz A, Vatankhah M, Mehdipour M (2010) Oral lichen planus: clinical features, etiology, treatment and management; a review of literature. J Dental Res Dental Clin Dental Prospects 4:3–9

Bouras E, Karakioulaki M, Bougioukas KI, Aivaliotis M, Tzimagiorgis G, Chourdakis M (2019) Gene promoter methylation and cancer: An umbrella review. Gene 710:333–340

Brinkman B, Zuijdeest D, Kaijzel EL, Breedveld FC, Verweij CL (1995) Relevance of the tumor necrosis factor alpha (TNF alpha)-308 promoter polymorphism in TNF alpha gene regulation. J Inflamm 46:32–41

Carl JW, Liu J-Q, Joshi PS, El-Omrani HY, Yin L, Zheng X, Whitacre CC, Liu Y, Bai X-F (2008) Autoreactive T cells escape clonal deletion in the thymus by a CD24-dependent pathway. J Immunol 181:320–328

Carrozzo M, Thorpe R (2009) Oral lichen planus: a review. Minerva Stomatol 58:519–537

Carrozzo M, Porter S, Mercadante V, Fedele S (2019) Oral lichen planus: A disease or a spectrum of tissue reactions? Types, causes, diagnostic algorhythms, prognosis, management strategies. Periodontol 80:105–125

Carrozzo M, Francia Di Celle P, Gandolfo S, Carbone M, Conrotto D, Fasano M, Roggero S, Rendine S, Ghisetti V (2001) Increased frequency of HLA-DR6 allele in Italian patients with hepatitis C virus-associated oral lichen planus. Br J Dermatol 144:803–808

Carrozzo M, Dametto E, Fasano ME, Arduino P, Broccoletti R, Vezza D, Rendine S, Curtoni ES, Gandolfo S (2004) Tumor necrosis factor-α and interferon-γ polymorphisms contribute to susceptibility to oral lichen planus. J Investig Dermatol 122:87–94

Carrozzo M, Elia A, Mereu V, Dametto E, Fasano ME, Broccoletti R, Rendine S, Amoroso A (2011) HLA-C/KIR genotypes in oral lichen planus patients infected or non-infected with hepatitis C virus. Oral Dis 17:309–313

Chauhan I, Beena V, Srinivas L, Sathyan S, Banerjee M (2013) Association of cytokine gene polymorphisms with oral lichen planus in Malayalam-speaking ethnicity from South India (Kerala). J Interferon Cytokine Res 33:420–427

Chen J, Du G, Chang Y, Wang Y, Shi L, Mi J, Tang G (2019a) Downregulated miR-27b promotes keratinocyte proliferation by targeting PLK 2 in oral lichen planus. J Oral Pathol Med 48:326–334

Chen J, Wang Y, Du G, Zhang W, Cao T, Shi L, Wang Y, Mi J, Tang G (2019b) Down-regulation of miRNA-27b-3p suppresses keratinocytes apoptosis in oral lichen planus. J Cell Mol Med 23:4326–4337

Copeman P, Tan RH, Timlin D, Samman P (1978) Familial lichen planus another disease or a distinct people? Br J Dermatol 98:573–577

Cruz AF, de Resende RG, de Lacerda JCT, Pereira NB, Melo LA, Diniz MG, Gomes CC, Gomez RS (2018) DNA methylation patterns of genes related to immune response in the different clinical forms of oral lichen planus. J Oral Pathol Med 47:91–95

Dan H, Liu W, Zhou Y, Wang J, Chen Q, Zeng X (2010) Association of interleukin-8 gene polymorphisms and haplotypes with oral lichen planus in a Chinese population. Inflammation 33:76–81

Daoud M, Pittelkow M, Goldsmith L, Katz S, Gilchrest B, Paller A, Leffell D, Wolff KJNYMGHI (2012) Lichen planus. Fitzpatrick's Dermatol Gen Med 296–312

de Carvalho Fraga CA, Alves LR, Marques-Silva L, de Sousa AA, Jorge ASB, de Jesus SF, Vilela DN, Pinheiro UB, Jones KM, de Paula AMB (2013) High HIF-1α expression genotypes in oral lichen planus. Clin Oral Invest 17:2011–2015

Dean MM, Flower RL, Eisen DP, Minchinton RM, Hart DN, Vuckovic S (2011) Mannose-binding lectin deficiency influences innate and antigen-presenting functions of blood myeloid dendritic cells. Immunology 132:296–305

Dillenburg CS, Martins MA, Almeida LO, Meurer L, Squarize CH, Martins MD, Castilho RM (2015) Epigenetic modifications and accumulation of DNA double-strand breaks in oral lichen planus lesions presenting poor response to therapy. Medicine 94

Du J, Gao R, Wang Y, Nguyen T, Yang F, Shi Y, Liu T, Liao W, Li R, Zhang F (2020) MicroRNA-26a/b have protective roles in oral lichen planus. Cell Death Disease 11:1–13

Durai R, Davies M, Yang W, Yang SY, Seifalian A, Goldspink G, Winslet M (2006) Biology of insulin-like growth factor binding protein-4 and its role in cancer. Int J Oncol 28:1317–1325

Eike M, Skinningsrud B, Ronninger M, Stormyr A, Kvien T, Joner G, Njølstad P, Førre Ø, Flatø B, Alfredsson L (2012) CIITA gene variants are associated with rheumatoid arthritis in Scandinavian populations. Genes Immun 13:431–436

Fishman D, Faulds G, Jeffery R, Mohamed-Ali V, Yudkin JS, Humphries S, Woo P (1998) The effect of novel polymorphisms in the interleukin-6 (IL-6) gene on IL-6 transcription and plasma IL-6 levels, and an association with systemic-onset juvenile chronic arthritis. J Clin Investig 102:1369–1376

Fonseca-Silva T, De Oliveira MVM, de Carvalho Fraga CA, Farias LC, Gomes ÉPP, Barros LO, Roy A, Gomez RS, De Paula AMB, Guimarães ALS (2012) DNMT3B (C46359T) polymorphisms and immunoexpression of DNMT3b and DNMT1 proteins in oral lichen planus. Pathobiology 79:18–23

Fujita H, Kobayashi T, Tai H, Nagata M, Hoshina H, Nishizawa R, Takagi R, Yoshie H (2009) Assessment of 14 functional gene polymorphisms in Japanese patients with oral lichen planus: a pilot case-control study. Int J Oral Maxillofac Surg 38:978–983

Gassling V, Hampe J, Açil Y, Braesen JH, Wiltfang J, Häsler R (2013) Disease-associated miRNA-mRNA networks in oral lichen planus. PloS One 8:e63015

Ghabanchi J, Fattahi MJ, Mardani M, Tadbir AA, Paydar AA (2009) Polymorphism of tumor protein P53 codon 72 showed no association with oral lichen planus in Shiraz, Iran. J Craniofacial Surg 20:2168–2170

Giuliani M, Troiano G, Cordaro M, Corsalini M, Gioco G, Lo Muzio L, Pignatelli P, Lajolo C (2019) Rate of malignant transformation of oral lichen planus: a systematic review. Oral Dis 25:693–709

Gorouhi F, Davari P, Fazel N (2014) Cutaneous and mucosal lichen planus: a comprehensive review of clinical subtypes, risk factors, diagnosis, and prognosis. Sci World J 2014:742826

Gray MJ, Van Buren G, Dallas NA, Xia L, Wang X, Yang AD, Somcio RJ, Lin YG, Lim S, Fan F (2008) Therapeutic targeting of neuropilin-2 on colorectal carcinoma cells implanted in the murine liver. J Natl Cancer Inst 100:109–120

Gueiros L, Arão T, Souza T, Vieira C, Gomez R, Almeida O, Lodi G, Leao J (2018) IL 17A polymorphism and elevated IL 17A serum levels are associated with oral lichen planus. Oral Dis 24:377–383

Gülsüm A, Diler S, Koray M, Savran-Oğuz F, Önal E, Ordulu M, Çarin M, Tanyeri H (2006) HLA antigens in erosive oral lichen planus. Balkan J Stomatol 10:7–11

Hawkins NJ, Lee JH, Wong JJ, Kwok C-T, Ward RL, Hitchins MP (2009) MGMT methylation is associated primarily with the germline C> T SNP (rs16906252) in colorectal cancer and normal colonic mucosa. Mod Pathol 22:1588–1599

Javvadi L, Parachuru V, Milne T, Seymour G, Rich AM (2018) Expression of IL33 and IL35 in oral lichen planus. Arch Dermatol Res 310:431–441

Jiang C, Yao H, Cui B, Zhou Y, Wang Y, Tang G (2015) Association of interleukin 12A gene polymorphisms with oral lichen planus in Chinese population. J Oral Pathol Med 44:602–606

Jongeneel CV, Beutler B (1995) Genetic polymorphism in the human TNF region: correlation or causation? J Inflamm 46

Jontell M, Ståhlblad P-Å, Rosdahl I, Lindblom B (1987) HLA-DR3 antigens in erosive oral lichen planus, cutaneous lichen planus, and lichenoid reactions. Acta Odontol Scand 45:309–312

Kaplan I, Nabiochtchikov I, Leshno A, Moshkowitz M, Shlomi B, Kleinman S, Dagan Y, Meshiach Y, Galazan L, Arber N (2015) Association of CD24 and the adenomatous polyposis coli gene polymorphisms with oral lichen planus. Oral Surg Oral Med Oral Pathol Oral Radiol 120:378–385

Khosravi AR, Erle DJ (2016) Chitin-induced airway epithelial cell innate immune responses are inhibited by carvacrol/thymol. PloS One 11:e0159459

Kimkong I, Hirankarn N, Nakkuntod J, Kitkumthorn N (2011) Tumour necrosis factor-alpha gene polymorphisms and susceptibility to oral lichen planus. Oral Dis 17:206–209

Kimkong I, Nakkuntod J, Sodsai P, Hirankarn N, Kitkumthorn N (2012) Association of interferon-gamma gene polymorphisms with susceptibility to oral lichen planus in the Thai population. Arch Oral Biol 57:491–494

Kofoed ML, Wantzin GL (1985) Familial lichen planus: More frequent than previously suggested? J Am Acad Dermatol 13:50–54

Koizumi K, Okamoto H, Iikuni N, Nakamura T, Kawamoto M, Momohara S, Ichikawa N, Furuya T, Kotake S, Taniguchi A (2005) Single nucleotide polymorphisms in the gene encoding the major histocompatibility complex class II transactivator (CIITA) in systemic lupus erythematosus. Ann Rheum Dis 64:947–950

Kragelund C, Hansen C, Reibel J, Nauntofte B, Broesen K, Pedersen A, Smidt D, Eiberg H, Torpet L (2009) Polymorphic drug metabolizing CYP-enzymes–a pathogenic factor in oral lichen planus? J Oral Pathol Med 38:63–71

Kujundzic B, Zeljic K, Supic G, Magic M, Stanimirovic D, Ilic V, Jovanovic B, Magic Z (2016) Association of vdr, cyp27b1, cyp24a1 and mthfr gene polymorphisms with oral lichen planus risk. Clin Oral Invest 20:781–789

Larsson L (2018) Epigenetics in the oral cavity. In: Oral Mucosa in health and disease. Springer, pp 119–125

Lin SC, Sun A (1990) HLA-DR and DQ antigens in Chinese patients with oral lichen planus. J Oral Pathol Med 19:298–300

Liu F, Wu J, Ye F (2015) Expression of miRNA-155 and miRNA-146a in peripheral blood mononuclear cells and plasma of oral lichen planus patients. Zhonghua kou qiang yi xue za zhi= Zhonghua kouqiang yixue zazhi. Chin J Stomatol 50:23–27

Lodi G, Pellicano R, Carrozzo M (2010) Hepatitis C virus infection and lichen planus: a systematic review with meta-analysis. Oral Dis 16:601–612

Lowe N, Cudworth A, Woodrow J (1976) HL-A antigens in lichen planus. Br J Dermatol 95:169–171

Luis-Montoya P, Domínguez-Soto L, Vega-Memije M (2005) Lichen planus in 24 children with review of the literature. Pediat Dermatol 22:295–298

Luis-Montoya P, Yamamoto-Furusho J, Vega-Memije E, Rodríguez-Carreón A, Ruiz-Morales J, Vargas-Alarcón G, Domínguez-Soto L, Granados J (2007) HLA-DRB1* 0101 is associated with the genetic susceptibility to develop lichen planus in the Mexican Mestizo population. Arch Dermatol Res 299:405–407

Ma H, Wu Y, Yang H, Liu J, Dan H, Zeng X, Zhou Y, Jiang L, Chen Q (2016) MicroRNAs in oral lichen planus and potential miRNA–mRNA pathogenesis with essential cytokines: a review. Oral Surg Oral Med Oral Pathol Oral Radiol 122:164–173

Madalli V (2013) Lichen planus-a review. IOSR J Dental Med Sci 12:61–69

Mahood JM (1983) Familial lichen planus: a report of nine cases from four families with a brief review of the literature. Arch Dermatol 119:292–294

Mozaffari HR, Zavattaro E, Saeedi M, Lopez-Jornet P, Sadeghi M, Safaei M, Imani MM, Nourbakhsh R, Moradpoor H, Golshah A (2019) Serum and salivary interleukin-4 levels in patients with oral lichen planus: a systematic review and meta-analysis. Oral Surg Oral Med Oral Pathol Oral Radiol

Nagao Y, Nishida N, Toyo-Oka L, Kawaguchi A, Amoroso A, Carrozzo M, Sata M, Mizokami M, Tokunaga K, Tanaka Y (2017) Genome-wide association study identifies risk variants for lichen planus in patients with hepatitis C virus infection. Clin Gastroenterol Hepatol 15:937–944.e935

Najafi S, Mohammadzadeh M, Rajabi F, Zare Bidoki A, Yousefi H, Farhadi E, Rezaei N (2018) Interleukin-4 and interleukin-4 receptor alpha gene polymorphisms in recurrent aphthous stomatitis. Immunol Invest 47:680–688

Nasa GL, Cottoni F, Mulargia M, Carcassi C, Vacca A, Pizzati A, Ledda A, Montesu M, Cerimele D, Contu L (1995) HLA antigen distribution in different clinical subgroups demonstrates genetic heterogeneity in lichen planus. Br J Dermatol 132:897–900

Ognjenović M, Karelović D, Cindro VV, Tadin I (1998a) Oral lichen planus and HLA A. Coll Antropol 22:89–92

Ognjenović M, Karelović D, Mikelić M, Tadin I, Vrebalov-Cindro V (1998b) Oral lichen planus and HLA B. Coll Antropol 22:93–96

Polesello V, Segat L, Biasotto M, Ottaviani G, Gobbo M, Di Lenarda R, Crovella S, Zupin L (2019) Mannose-Binding Lectin 2 (MBL2) combined genotypes deficiency is associated with susceptibility for Oral Lichen Planus. Genet Mol Biol

Porter K, Klouda P, Scully C, Bidwell J, Porter S (1993) Class I and II HLA antigens in British patients with oral lichen planus. Oral Surg Oral Med Oral Pathol 75:176–180

Porter S, Kirby A, Olsen I, Barrett W (1997a) Immunologic aspects of dermal and oral lichen planus: a review. Oral Surg Oral Med Oral Pathol Oral Radiol Endodontol 83:358–366

Porter SR, Kirby A, Olsen I, Barrett W (1997b) Immunologic aspects of dermal and oral lichen planus: a review. Oral Surg Oral Med Oral Pathol Oral Radiol Endod 83:358–366

Powell F, Rogers R, Dickson E, Moore SB (1986) An association between HLA DR1 and lichen planus. Br J Dermatol 114:473–478

Sánchez-Siles M, Aliaga-Sánchez A, Medina S, Adoamnei E, Fernández-Ruiz JA, Pelegrín-Hernández JP, Corno-Caparrós A, Rosa-Salazar V, Camacho-Alonso F (2019) Genotyping of the C> T allele of rs16906252, predictor of O16-methylguanine-DNA methyltransferase (MGMT) promoter methylation status, in erosive atrophic lesions of oral lichen planus. Int J Dermatol 58:1078–1082

Saurat JH, Lemarchand F, Hors J, Nunez-Roldan A, Gluckman E, Dausset J (1977) HLA markers and lymphocytotoxins in lichen planus. Arch Dermatol 113:1719–1720

Schifter M, Jones AM, Walker DM (1998) Epithelial p53 gene expression and mutational analysis, combined with growth fraction assessment, in oral lichen planus. J Oral Pathol Med 27:318–324

Schneider-Stock R, Mawrin C, Motsch C, Boltze C, Peters B, Hartig R, Buhtz P, Giers A, Rohrbeck A, Freigang B (2004) Retention of the arginine allele in codon 72 of the p53 gene correlates with poor apoptosis in head and neck cancer. Am J Pathol 164:1233–1241

Sharma A, Białynicki-Birula R, Schwartz RA, Janniger CKJC (2012) Lichen planus: an update and review. Cutis 90:17–23

Simon M Jr, Djawari D, Schöunberger A (1984) HLA antigens associated with lichen planus. Clin Exp Dermatol 9:435–435

Sinon SH, Rich AM, Parachuru VP, Firth FA, Milne T, Seymour GJ (2016) Downregulation of toll-like receptor-mediated signalling pathways in oral lichen planus. J Oral Pathol Med 45:28–34

Srinivas K, Konidena A, Ratnakar P, Nigam N, Gupta S (2011) Oral lichen planus—review on etiopathogenesis. Natl J Maxillofacial Surg 2:15–16

Stanimirovic D, Zeljic K, Jankovic L, Magic M, Hadzi-Mihajlovic M, Magic Z (2013) TLR 2, TLR 3, TLR 4 and CD 14 gene polymorphisms associated with oral lichen planus risk. Eur J Oral Sci 121:421–426

Strzepa A, Pritchard KA, Dittel BN (2017) Myeloperoxidase: a new player in autoimmunity. Cell Immunol 317:1–8

Sugerman PB, Savage NW, Walsh LJ, Zhao ZZ, Zhou XJ, Khan A, Seymour GJ, Bigby M (2002) The pathogenesis of oral lichen planus. Crit Rev Oral Biol Med 13:350–365

Supic G, Kozomara R, Zeljic K, Stanimirovic D, Magic M, Surbatovic M, Jovic N, Magic Z (2015) HMGB 1 genetic polymorphisms in oral squamous cell carcinoma and oral lichen planus patients. Oral Dis 21:536–543

Tan Y, Zhao M, Xiang B, Chang C, Lu Q (2016) CD24: from a hematopoietic differentiation antigen to a genetic risk factor for multiple autoimmune diseases. Clin Rev Allergy Immunol 50:70–83

Tao Y, Ai R, Hao Y, Jiang L, Dan H, Ji N, Zeng X, Zhou Y, Chen Q (2019) Role of miR-155 in immune regulation and its relevance in oral lichen planus. Exp Therap Med 17:575–586

Usatine RP, Tinitigan MJAFP (2011) Diagnosis and treatment of lichen planus. Am Family Phys 84

Valsecchi R, Bontempelli M, Rossi A, Bellavita P, Barcella A, Di AL, Cainelli T (1988) HLA-DR and DQ antigens in lichen planus. Acta Dermato-Venereologica 68:77–80

Veien N, Risum G, Jørgensen H, Svejgaard A (1979) HLA antigens in patients with lichen planus. Acta Dermato-Venereologica 59:205–209

Wang H, Guan X, Luo Z, Liu Y, Ren Q, Zhao X (2018) The association and potentially destructive role of Th9/IL-9 is synergistic with Th17 cells by elevating MMP9 production in local lesions of oral lichen planus. J Oral Pathol Med 47:425–433

Wang L, Wu W, Chen J, Li Y, Xu M, Cai Y (2019) miR-122 and miR-199 synergistically promote autophagy in oral lichen planus by targeting the Akt/mTOR pathway. Int J Mol Med 43:1373–1381

Wang X, Tang G, Sun H (2015) Effect of hypoxia on the proliferation and expressions of hypoxia-inducible factor-1α, vascular endothelial growth factor and matrix metalloproteinase-9 in keratinocytes obtained from oral lichen planus lesions. Zhonghua kou qiang yi xue za zhi= Zhonghua kouqiang yixue zazhi. Chin J Stomatol 50:89–94

Watanabe T, Ohishi M, Tanaka K, Sato H (1986) Analysis of HLA antigens in Japanese with oral lichen planus. J Oral Pathol Med 15:529–533

Weston G, Payette M (2015) Update on lichen planus and its clinical variants. Int J Women's Dermatol 1:140–149

White A, Rostom A (1994) HLA antigens in Arabs with lichen planus. Clin Exp Dermatol 19:236–237

Wu D, Wang L, Sun M, Wang G, Fu S, Dong G, Wu Y (2013) CIITA rs4774 and rs6498122 polymorphisms are associated with oral lichen planus in C hinese people: a case–control study. Eur J Oral Sci 121:69–75

Wu D, Chen X, Dong C, Liu Q, Yang Y, He C, Wang J, Sun M, Wu Y (2015) Association of single nucleotide polymorphisms in MPO and COX genes with oral lichen planus. Int J Immunogenet 42:161–167

Xavier GM, Sá AR, Guimarães ALS, Silva TA, Gomez RS (2007) Investigation of functional gene polymorphisms interleukin-1β, interleukin-6, interleukin-10 and tumor necrosis factor in individuals with oral lichen planus. J Oral Pathol Med 36:476–481

Xie S, Feng L, Zhu S, Ding L (2014) Expressions of RORγT; and FOXP3 and clinical significance in patients with oral lichen planus. Shanghai kou qiang yi xue. Shanghai J Stomatol 23:472–476

Yanatatsaneeji P, Kitkumthorn N, Dhammawipark C, Rabalert J, Patel V, Mutirangura A (2010) Codon72 polymorphism in the P53 tumor suppressor gene in oral lichen planus lesions in a Thai population

Yu W, Zhang L, Wei Q, Shao A (2020) O6-methylguanine-DNA methyltransferase (MGMT): challenges and new opportunities in glioma chemotherapy. Front Oncol 9:1547

Zhou XJ, Sugerman PB, Savage NW, Walsh LJ (2001) Matrix metalloproteinases and their inhibitors in oral lichen planus. J Cutan Pathol 28:72–82

The Immunogenetics of Acne

Mohamed L. Elsaie and Dalia G. Aly

Abstract

Acne vulgaris results from a complex interaction between environment and genetic factors. While colonization of the pilosebaceous unit with Propionibacterium was previously considered to be the main cause of acne, the contribution of host-related factors that allow the growth of the bacteria and its immune response against bacterial components are now considered to be more important. Many of these host characteristics have a genetic base that is either involved in the regulation of the immune responses or the steroid hormones metabolisms. This chapter aims to explore the functions of these genes and their role in the pathogenesis of acne.

Keywords

Acne vulgaris · Propionibacterium · Immunogenetics · Single nucleotide polymorphism · Pathogenesis · GWAS

Present Address:
M. L. Elsaie (✉) · D. G. Aly
Dermatology and Venereology, National Research Centre, Cairo, Egypt

1 Introduction

Acne vulgaris is a complex skin disorder that affects a significant fraction of people (Tan et al. 2017). It is considered a common disorder disturbing up to 95% of adolescents, about 50% of young adults older than 25, and 3–12% of middle-aged adults (Cordain et al. 2002). Acne vulgaris affects the pilosebaceous unit in the regions of the body with prominent sebum secretion including the face, the upper trunk, and the upper portion of the arms. Its manifestations range from non-inflammatory pinpoint papules known as comedones to inflammatory papules, pustules, and nodules that can potentially cause scarring. Infantile acne, acne conglobate, and acne fulminans are considered variants of acne. Infantile acne affects 6 weeks to 18-month-old infants and its lesions resemble acne vulgaris but are limited to the cheeks and are more common in males and females (Serna-Tamayo et al. 2014) (Fig. 1). Acne conglobate is a severe type of acne vulgaris with nodulocystic inflammatory lesions, abscesses, and sinus tracts that result in severe scarring. Severe acne complicated by systemic signs and symptoms such as fever, arthritis, and malaise is called acne fulminans (Zaba et al. 2011) (Fig. 2).

Several rare diseases are also associated with severe acne including SAPHO (Synovitis, Acne, Pustulosis, Hyperostosis, and Osteitis), PASH (Pyoderma gangrenosum, Acne Suppurativa, and Hidradenitis suppurativa), PAPA (Pyogenic

N. Rezaei and F. Rajabi (eds.), *The Immunogenetics of Dermatologic Diseases*, Advances in Experimental Medicine and Biology 1367,
https://doi.org/10.1007/978-3-030-92616-8_6

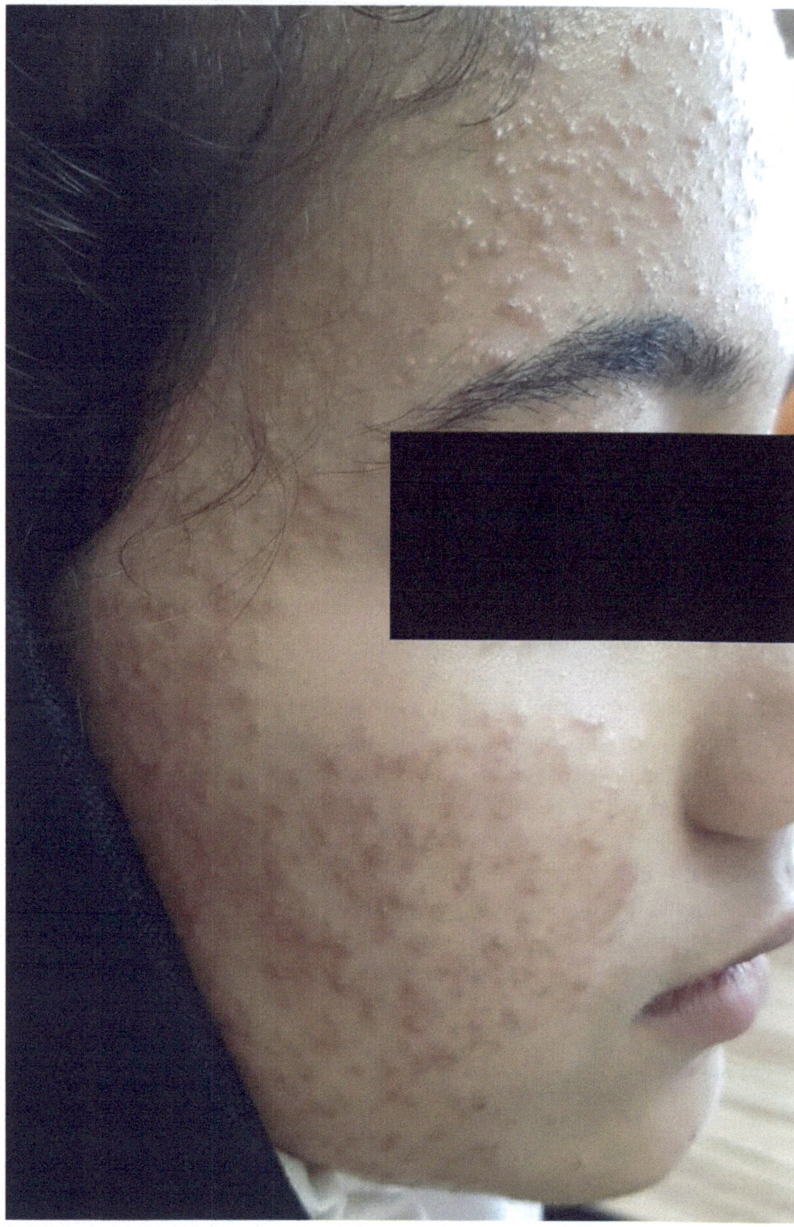

Fig. 1 Papular acne

Arthritis, Pyoderma gangrenosum, and Acne vulgaris), PAPASH (Pyogenic Arthritis, Pyoderma gangrenosum, Acne, and Suppurative Hidradenitis), and Apert syndrome (Cugno et al. 2017). Acne is also a feature of hormonal syndromes such as CAH (congenital adrenal hyperplasia) and HAIR-AN (Hyper Androgenism Insulin Resistance Acanthosis Nigricans) (Chen et al. 2011).

The disease significantly alters the quality of life and a profound financial burden (Layton et al. 2021). Thus in recent years, more studies have aimed at understanding the pathogenesis of the disease and the role of environmental causes (pollution, diet, cosmeceuticals) and genetic factors in triggering acne lesions (Chamaie-Nejad et al. 2018).

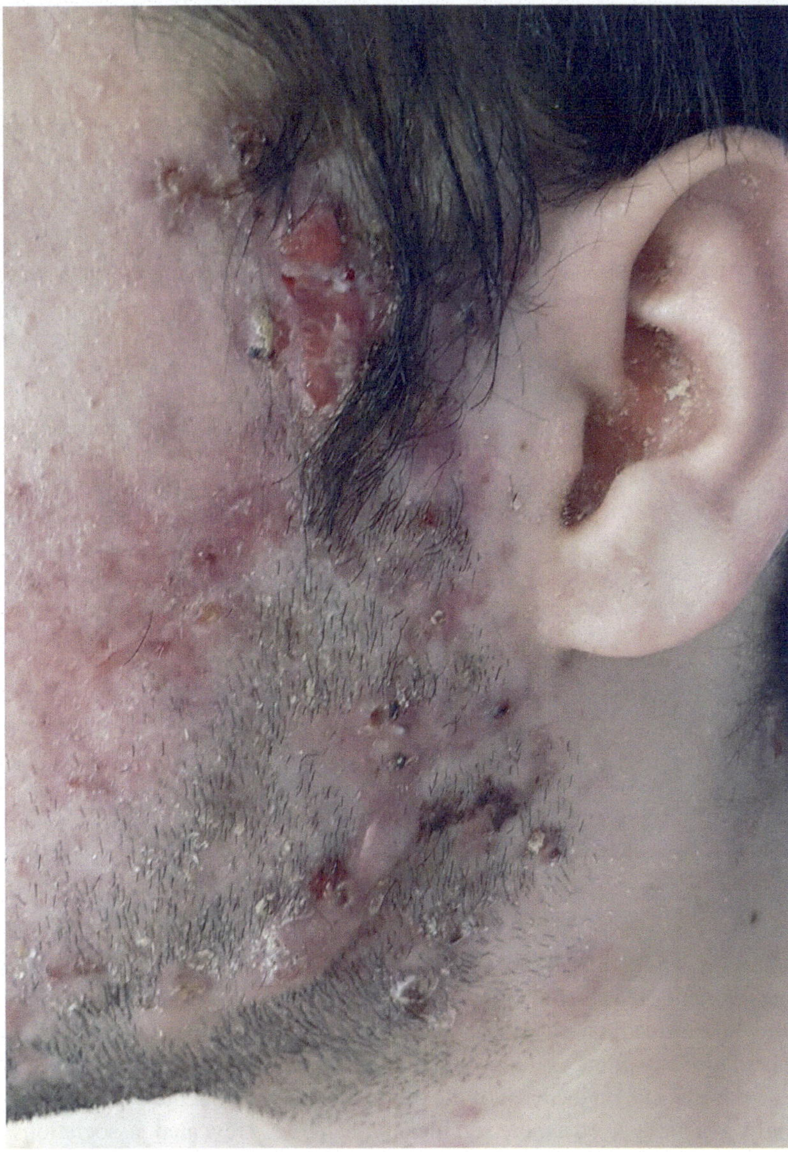

Fig. 2 Nodulocystic acne

Follicular hyperkeratinization, sebum production, Propionibacterium acnes (P. acnes), and immunologic processes leading to inflammation are the main aspects of acne pathogenesis (Xu et al. 2007).

Hecht in 1960 was the first group to investigate the contribution of inheritance in the pathogenesis of acne. Neonatal acne and severe form of the adolescent acne (nodulocystic acne and acne conglobata) were proven to have genetic bases (Herane and Ando 2003). Post-adolescent acne is associated with a 50% chance of an occurrence of the condition in first-degree relatives.

Familial studies were also able to demonstrate clustering of the diseases in certain families (Goulden et al. 1999). High heritability rates have been reported in twin studies. Monozygotic twins showed a higher proportion of sebum excretion when compared to dizygotic twins (Stewart et al. 1986; Walton et al. 1988). Studies showed that such variance could be attributed mostly to genetic

Table 1 Gene associated with increased risk for acne

Candidate gene (gene locus)	Protein	Mutation	Functional abnormality
CYP21A2 6p21.3 excess	Steroid 21-hydroxylase	Various mutations leading to deficiency	Congenital adrenal hyperplasia (CAH) with DHEA
HSD3B2 1p13.1	3β-Hydroxysteroid dehydrogenase II	Mutations leading to deficiency	Late-onset CAH, DHEA excess
CYP11B1 8q21	Steroid 11-β-hydroxylase	Loss-of-function mutation	Late-onset CAH, DHEA excess
CYP1A1 15q22-24	Cytochrome P450 Overexpression of m1-alleles	Accelerated retinoid degradation	modification of sebocyte differentiation
SRD5A1 5p15	Steroid 5α-reductase type I	Haplotypes with PCOS and hirsutism	Increased conversion of testosterone to DHT
AR Xq11-q12	Androgen receptor	CAG repeat polymorphisms (<20) GGN repeat polymorphisms	Increased androgen receptor transcriptional activity
FGFR2 10q26	Fibroblast growth factor receptor 2	Ser252Trp and Pro253Arg mutations in Apert syndrome; Ser252Trp mutation in acneiform nevus	Gain-of-function mutations with decreased FGFR2 degradation and increased PI3K/Akt activation
IL1A 2q14	Interleukin-1α	Interleukin 1A + 4845 (G > T) polymorphism	Increased susceptibility for acne and inflammatory reactions
TNF 6p21.3	Tumor necrosis factor-α	TNFα polymorphism	Increased susceptibility for acne and inflammation
MUC1 1q21	Mucin 1 glycoprotein	A large number of tandem repeats	Association with severe acne, modify cation of β-catenin- and PI3K/Akt/FoxO signaling

influence while only 19% could be related to environmental effects (Bataille et al. 2002). Another study performed on twins showed that genetic inheritance was more common in individuals suffering from acne on the back of the trunk. Surprisingly, genetics played a more significant role in the development of facial acne in boys compared to girls and common environmental elements played a more prominent role in the induction of lesions in females (Evans et al. 2005).

A positive family history of acne predicted an earlier age of onset, a more severe disease, and a higher rate of relapse after isotretinoin therapy (Ballanger et al. 2006).

Despite genetic studies suggesting inheritance as an important mode of disease pathogenesis, yet genetic identification of specific genes only started in the early 1990s (Szabó and Kemény 2011). Though there are a large number of gene polymorphisms implicated in acne development (Table 1), there is still a relative scarcity of research on the genetic causes of acne. Nonetheless, genetic investigations have revealed associations between susceptibility to acne with chromosomal abnormalities and polymorphisms of various genes including HLA phenotypes. These studies will be discussed in detail in this chapter (Elsaie et al., 2016).

2 Pathogenesis of Acne

Elevated levels of sebum, alteration in the composition of sebum, and follicular hyperkeratinization mark the initial step in the development of acne.

Androgens and insulin-like growth factor 1 (IGF-1) promote sebaceous lipogenesis through activating the c isoform of the sterol regulatory element-binding protein-1 (SREBP1c) and to a lesser extent peroxisome proliferator-activated receptor gamma (PPARγ) and androgen receptor (Lai et al. 2012; Plewig et al. 2019; Trivedi et al. 2006a). The SREBP1 is a type of transcription factor that attaches to the sterol regulatory element-1 (SRE1) in the promoter region of genes such as acetyl-CoA carboxylase and desaturase. These enzymes mediate the desaturation of free fatty acids and the synthesis of triacylglycerol and squalene. The SREBP1 activation path involves Akt-mediated phosphorylation deactivation of FOXO1 and AKT-mediated activation of the mechanistic target of rapamycin complex 1 (mTORC1) (Plewig et al. 2019).

The effects of IGF-1 on sebum production are way more prominent than androgens. Moreover, IGF-1 promotes androgen production in several stages including stimulation of adrenal and gonadal synthesis of androgens and induction of 5-alpha reductase (5αR) (Plewig et al. 2019).

The waxy sebum decelerates desquamation of the infundibulum leading to retention of corneocytes and obstruction of the pilosebaceous unit potentially causing comedones.

The anaerobic waxy environment of the pilosebaceous unit is colonized by P. acnes that can produce lipases that break the triacylglycerols to free fatty acids (FFA) and use them as an energy source. The waxy sebum provides the bacteria with a glue-like structure that facilitates their attachment to keratinocytes and other bacteria. This would eventually enable the P.acnes colonization to form a biofilm within the pilosebaceous unit (Jahns and Alexeyev 2014). The concentrations of P.acnes do not show a significant association with disease severity and in commensal conditions, they do not relay danger signals related to inflammation. Thus it has been hypothesized that the formation of microfilms is what changes the benign nature of the bacteria to a pathogenic phenotype (Jahns et al. 2012; Leyden et al. 1975; Lwin et al. 2014; Simonart 2013). The formation of biofilm is associated with increased immunogenicity which explains the progression of the comedones to popular and pustular lesions (Burkhart and Burkhart 2003; Lwin et al. 2014).

P. acnes biofilms catalyze the triacylglycerol more effectively releasing high amounts of diacylglycerol (DAG) and monounsaturated fatty acids (MUFA) like oleic and palmitic acids. DAG activates toll-like receptor 2 (TLR2) and protein kinase C (PKC) in keratinocytes and thus increases the production of interleukin 1 (IL-1) and tumor necrosis factor α (TNFα) (Kolczynska et al. 2020; Plewig et al. 2019). Oleic acids increase the Ca^{++} influx in keratinocytes and thus alter the keratinization of the follicular infundibulum (Choi et al. 1997). MUFAs have a proinflammatory effect on dendritic cells, monocytes, and sebocytes by increasing the reactive oxygen species (ROS) within the mitochondria which in turn stimulates the NLR family pyrin domain containing 3 (NLRP3). The NLRP3 belongs to the family of pattern recognition receptors (PRRs) and upon activation promotes IL-1 release (Brombacher and Everts 2020; Haneklaus et al. 2013; Li et al. 2014). Palmitate can also activate TLR2 by inducing its heterodimerization with TLR1 (Snodgrass et al. 2013). MUFA are more susceptible to ultraviolet (UV) damage and the peroxidized squalene and MUFA can induce a strong immunogenic response (Ottaviani et al. 2005).

In a pathogenic state, P.acnes can directly release neutrophil chemotactic factors and trigger TLRs (TLR2 and 4) on keratinocytes and monocytes to produce IL-1α, IL-1β, IL-6, IL-8, IL-12, TNFα, and antimicrobial peptides (AMP) such as human beta-defensin 2 (HBD2) and LL-37, and matrix metalloproteinases (MMP) including MMP1, 2, 3, 9, and 13 (Jugeau et al. 2005; Kim et al. 2002; Nagy et al. 2005; Platsidaki and Dessinioti 2018). The proteases released by P. acnes also contribute to cytokine and MMP production by activating proteinase-activated receptor-2 (PAR-2) via proteolytic cleavage (Lee et al. 2010). This inflammatory milieu attracts immune cells to the pilosebaceous unit which initially only consists of CD4+ T-cells, macrophages, and dendritic cells. Eventually, neutrophils and later CD8 + T-cells join the infiltration (Kelhälä et al. 2014). P. acnes and the inflammatory cytokine milieu trigger the differentiation of Th1 and Th17 cells. These cells release IL-17 which in turn perpetuates inflammation and comedogenesis by inducing keratinocytes to produce AMPs, chemokines, and granulocyte-colony stimulatory factor (G-CSF) (Kelhälä et al. 2014).

The MMPs and neutrophil proteases provoke follicular rupture releasing antigenic material that could eventually lead to the formation of cysts and nodules with granulomatous reaction (Dessinioti and Katsambas 2010).

3 Genes Implicated in the Pathogenesis of Acne

Combinations of gene polymorphisms with subtle effects can change the function, expression, and configuration of numerous proteins that in combination can cause major changes such as shaping the susceptibility to a complex disease (Hoogendoorn et al. 2003). Thus it is feasible to imagine that genes encoding hormonal receptors and their downstream signaling pathways, the innate immunity-related genes, and their early cytokines, and adaptive immunity genes can alter the tolerance of an individual to environmental triggers. As such genetic polymorphisms could set the threshold for the keratinocytes' reactivity to the skin microbiome with over-reactivity causing inflammatory responses that are more destructive than protective (Chamaie-Nejad et al. 2018).

3.1 Non-immune Genes

The genes involved in lipogenesis in sebaceous glands were among the first to be evaluated in the pathogenesis of acne.

The *Androgen receptor* (*AR*) gene variants with lower numbers of tandem repeats (CAG_n) have been shown to be linked to an increased risk for acne (Yang et al. 2009). The *damage-specific DNA binding protein 2* (*DDB2*) gene located at 11p11.2 is one of the two main susceptibility loci that has been linked to acne in a Chinese genome-wide association study (GWAS) (He et al. 2014). This gene encodes a protein involved in nucleotide excision repair (Stoyanova et al. 2009). It also regulates the AR ubiquitination/degradation and thus can influence the pathogenesis of acne (Chang et al. 2012).

A GWAS on European-American adolescents with severe acne revealed a susceptibility loci at 8q24. The SNP rs4133274 is located near the *MYC* proto-oncogene. Since MYC can upregulate the expression of the *AR* gene, its involvement in the development of acne has been credited to its role in increasing responsiveness to hormones (Zhang et al. 2014).

The type 1 isoform of the 3β-hydroxysteroid dehydrogenase (3β-HSD) which transforms dehydroepiandrosterone to androstenedione, the type 3 isoform of the 17β-HSD 17 which transforms androstenedione to testosterone, and the type 1 isoform of the 11β-HSD1 which transforms inactive cortisone to cortisol are expressed in the skin and the pilosebaceous unit. The genes encoding these enzymes, *HSD3B1* at 1p13, *HSD17B3* at 9q22, and *HSD11B1* at 1q32.2 have been investigated in patients with acne vulgaris (Heng et al. 2021). However, only rs846910 of *HSD11B1* in Egyptian patients and rs6428829 of *HSD3B1* in Chinese patients showed an association with acne (Farag et al. 2019; Lichtenberger et al. 2017; Yang et al. 2013).

Cytochromes P450 family are another group involved in the metabolism of steroids and thus have been investigated in the pathogenesis of acne (Lichtenberger et al. 2017). The *Cytochrome P-450 1A1* (*CYP1A1*), *CYP19A1, and CYP17A1* gene variants are linked to acne susceptibility in patients from different ethnicities. However, only *CYP17A1* rs743572 was significantly linked to acne in meta-analysis (Heng et al. 2021).

The results of case–control studies regarding the IGF-1 coding gene are inconsistent. While studies in the Indian and Turkish populations found a significant difference in polymorphic CA-repeat, a study on the Egyptian population and the pooled meta-analysis was insignificant (El-Tahlawi et al. 2014; Heng et al. 2021; Rahaman et al. 2016; Tasli et al. 2013).

Similarly, though a polymorphism of the *PPARG* gene was linked to acne in the Iranian and Egyptian population the meta-analysis of the results did not confirm the association (Amr et al. 2014; Heng et al. 2021; Saeidi et al. 2018).

A tandem repeats polymorphism in the *MUC1* gene was shown to be linked to severe acne (Ando et al. 1998). The mucin1 protein binds to β-catenin and changes its downstream signaling. β-catenin is involved in the suppression of sebaceous gland differentiation and function (Lo Celso et al. 2008). MUC1 overexpression is linked to increased phosphoinositol-3 kinase (PI3K) activity (Raina et al. 2004). Increased PI3K activity reduces the FOXO levels in the nucleus, a transcription factor with inhibitory effects on sebaceous lipogenesis. Thus *MUC1* polymorphisms might indirectly increase the risk of acne by affecting FFA formation (Melnik 2010). Moreover, the gene encoding phosphoinositide-3-kinase regulatory subunit-1 (PIK3R1), has been linked to acne by an Australian GWAS on twins (Mina-Vargas et al. 2017).

A recent GWAS study has been able to identify five acne susceptibility loci involved in the morphogenesis of the pilosebaceous unit (Petridis et al. 2018). These genetic variations could alter the structure and function of the pilosebaceous unit in a way that makes it more susceptible to occlusion, inflammation, and bacterial colonization. These genes include the *WNT10A*, *SEMA4B*, *LGR6*, *LAMC2*, and *GLI2* (Tripathi et al. 2020).

The A-allele of *WNT10A* rs121908120 confers protection from acne with a genome-wide level of significance (Petridis et al. 2018). WNT10 A is a signaling protein that regulates the cell fate in developmental processes. WNT10A loss of function mutations causes ectodermal dysplasia syndromes with loss of pilosebaceous unit (Xu et al. 2017). Thus the reduced expression of sebum production associated with the missense A-allele is thought to be responsible for the prevention of acne in the carriers of this allele. Another locus involved in the morphogenesis of the pilosebaceous unit also demonstrates association with acne on a genome-wide level of significance in the 15q26.1. The rs34560261 is located within the biding site of the TP63 transcription factor at the intron of the *SEMA4B* gene. The TP63 plays a significant role in cutaneous morphogenesis and is linked to ectodermal dysplasia (Romano et al. 2010; Bokhoven et al. 2001).

The rs788790 at 1q32.1 linked to the *LGR6* gene and the rs10911268 located at 1q25.3 linked to the *LAMC2* gene are also associated with acne. The *LAMC2* gene encodes Laminin subunit gamma-2, an extracellular matrix protein (Huang et al. 2017). The *LRG6* gene encodes a Wnt signaling pathway mediator (Huang et al. 2017).

The C-allele of the rs109247 near *GLI2* (2q14.2) confers susceptibility to acne. GLI2 mediates the effects of sonic hedgehog on hair follicle morphogenesis and the constitutively active forms of *GLI2* can compensate for the loss of function of the sonic hedgehog gene rescuing the follicular development (Mill et al. 2003).

The *fibroblast growth factor-2* (*FGF2*) gene, also harbors a susceptibility loci for acne (Petridis et al. 2018). The FGF2 is a mitogenic protein involved in wound healing (Ortega et al. 1998). Apert and Crouzon syndromes which are associated with severe acne and comedogenesis are caused by a mutation in the *FGF receptor 2* (*FGFR2*) gene. These mutations enhance the FGF2-FGFR2 binding affinity (Ibrahimi et al. 2001; Rice 2008). The FGFR2, in turn, increases sebocyte differentiation and lipogenesis through activating the sonic hedgehog, MAPK, and PI3K pathways and upregulating the expression of *SREBP1* (Melnik 2009).

The functions of some genes that have been linked to acne susceptibility are not quite clear. These genes include *BCL11A* which encodes a transcriptional factor involved in hematopoiesis (Liu et al. 2006) and *SPECC1L* which encodes a cytoskeleton cross-linking protein (Petridis et al. 2018; Saadi et al. 2011).

3.2 Immune-Related Genes

Polymorphisms of genes encoding inflammatory cytokines such as IL-1α and TNFα and their receptors can also play a role in predisposing individuals to acne or defining the course and phenotype of the disorder and its sensitivity to treatment (Pang et al. 2008; Szabó et al. 2011).

A gene expression profiling study has identified 211 genes that were differentially expressed in acneic skin. Most of these genes, as anticipated, were immune-related. The β-defensin 4, matrix metalloproteinase, IL-8, and granulysin encoding genes were among the most highly expressed genes in acneic compared to normal skin. Conversely, a much smaller set of genes (18 genes in total) showed a lower expression in acne-affected skin compared to normal. Among these genes, the secretoglobin family was the most prominent category (Trivedi et al. 2006c).

These immune-related genes will be discussed in further detail in the following segments.

The *Tumor Necrosis Factor* (*TNF*) gene

TNF is a cardinal chemokine that exerts an influence in regulating the inflammatory response in acne (Grech et al. 2014; Yang et al. 2014). Increased expression of the *TNFα* gene has been reported in acneic skin lesions. The *TNFα* gene resides at 6p21.3 within the major histocompatibility complex III gene cluster (Al-Shobaili et al. 2012b). The *TNF* gene promoter region polymorphisms at −1031, −238, −308, −857, and −863 are known to influence the transcription rate (Heng et al. 2021; Yang et al. 2014). Some of these SNP predispose individuals to acne vulgaris and some offer protection from this skin disorder (Grech et al. 2014; Heng et al. 2021). The *TNF-α* rs1800629 (308 G/A) is the most studied SNP in this regard. A significantly higher frequency of the GA genotype and A-allele of the *TNFα* rs1800629 has been documented in Caucasians (Greece, Hungry, and Romania) and Asians (Turkey, Saudi Arabia, Singapore, and Pakistan) acne patients compared with healthy controls (Aisha et al. 2016; Al-Shobaili et al. 2012a; Baz et al. 2008; Szabó et al. 2011). Most of these studies were not able to detect a meaningful difference between the male and the female patients and there was a weak correlation between the TNFα genotypes and acne severity (Heng et al. 2021). Two studies in polish and Hungarian populations reported a lack of association between the *TNFα* rs1800629 and acne vulgaris (Sobjanek et al. 2009) (Szabó et al. 2011).

A metanalysis on TNF polymorphisms associated with acne showed that the 308 G/A SNP conferred susceptibility to acne under the recessive inheritance model with the AA genotype being more common in patients with acne vulgaris than the sum of AG and GG genotypes. An ethnicity-based analysis also showed that the 308G/A SNP confers susceptibility to acne vulgaris in both Caucasian and Asian populations. Compared to the more frequent G allele, the TNF 308 A-allele is associated with a higher transcription level. Thus as expected, patients with the *TNF* GA genotype have higher TNF levels (Yang et al. 2014).

In a study (Escobar-Morreale et al. 2001), comparing sixty females with hyperandrogenism with 24 healthy subjects, the incidence of the 308 *TNF* SNP GA genotype was reported to be 29.8% in cases and 20.8% in the healthy controls. The significant difference between the frequency of genotypes in the two groups led the authors to assume that the association between TNFα levels and acne may be beyond inflammatory mechanisms and may also involve androgen production.

The *TNFα* -238 G/A SNP (rs361525) was associated with acne in a single study in the Pakistani population (Aisha et al. 2016). However other case–control studies on other ethnicities and meta-analyses failed to link this SNP with acne (Heng et al. 2021).

The -857 C/T SNP (rs1799724) showed an association with acne in the Hungarian and Romanian populations (Szabó et al. 2011). This was not confirmed in a study based on the American population (Zhang et al. 2014).

A relatively newer study examined the *TNFα* 238, 376, and 308 SNPs of the gene in a Caucasian population. The study established that the GAG haplotype corresponding to G at location

376, A at location 308, and G at location 238 conferred risk for acne (Grech et al. 2014).

Tian et al. were able to document a significant association between a *TNF Receptor 2* (*TNFR2*) polymorphism (M196R) and acne in patients with Chinese ancestry (Tian et al. 2010). This finding was not replicated in the Caucasian population (Zhang et al. 2014).

The *Interleukin* genes

Interleukin-1α (IL-1α) was intensely studied in inflammatory processes and its polymorphism was linked to acne vulgaris. Moreover, a significant correlation between the *IL-1α* 4845 (G/T) gene and *IL-1α* 889 (C/T) gene polymorphisms and acne have been reported (Younis and Javed 2015).

The IL-1α transcription rate depends on genetic variation at position 889. The T/T genotype is associated with higher *IL-1α* gene expression than the C/C genotype. Enhanced cytokines synthesis increases the risk of inflammatory disorders.

Sobjanek et al. (Sobjanek et al. 2013) investigated the frequency of the *IL-1α* rs1800587 (889 C/T) SNP in 115 patients with acne and 100 healthy controls and were able to show a link between this SNP and susceptibility to acne vulgaris. The TT genotype was a conferred risk for acne in a Polish study. Dominici et al. (Dominici et al. 2002) showed that the individuals with the TT genotype had five-folds higher IL-1a levels than those with the CC genotype and about two-fold higher levels than individuals with the CT genotype. A study by Younis and Javed (Younis and Javed 2015) indicated that the *IL-1α* 889 C/T variants conferred risk for acne Pakistani patients. The association between rs1800587 and acne was significant in a meta-analysis of four studies conducted in Pakistan, Singapore, Greece, and Poland (Heng et al. 2021).

Szabo et al. (Szabó et al. 2010) analyzed polymorphisms in the *IL-1α* gene in the Hungarian and Romanian populations. They witnessed that the uncommon T allele of the *IL-1α* 4845 (G/T) polymorphisms coffered risk for acne. Moreover, the presence of the TT genotype predicted a more severe phenotype. IL-1α is produced in a precursor form known as pre-IL-1A confined to the nucleus. In an inflammatory state and presence of appropriate stimuli, it is cleaved by caspases and transformed into the mature IL-1 which can leave the nucleus. The 4845 SNP results in the substitution of serine for alanine in position 114 and is associated with enhanced proteolytic cleavage (Kobayashi et al. 1990; Szabó and Kemény 2011). This increased cleavage can alter the homeostasis of cytokines in the epidermal milieu and thus exacerbate the acne symptoms.

IL-6 is another pleiotropic cytokine that has been extensively studied in immune-mediated conditions. This cytokine is involved in host defense mechanisms and promotes hematopoiesis and inflammation. IL-6 produced by keratinocytes is involved in the progression of both local and systemic inflammation in the acneic setting (Yamamoto et al. 1994). Several immune-mediated diseases have been linked to *IL-6* polymorphisms, however, there is a relative scarcity in studies on the association of acne with *IL-6* gene polymorphisms (Younis and Javed 2015).

SNPs at the promoter region of IL-6 including 597 G/A, 373A/T, 572 G/C, and 174 G/C are thought to influence gene transcription rates and can thus affect the susceptibility to diseases (Brull et al. 2001) (Phillips et al. 2003; Younis and Javed 2015). The -572 G/C SNP at the promoter region of *IL-6* influences cytokine expression and the C allele is associated with enhanced cytokine production (Brull et al. 2001; Mälarstig et al. 2007).

The C allele of the *IL-6* 572 G/C was shown to confer risk for acne by a Pakistani study (Younis and Javed 2015). Furthermore, this study demonstrated a significant association between the *IL-6* 572 and *IL-1α* 889 haplotypes and susceptibility to acne. These findings were not replicated in studies on other ethnicities (Heng et al. 2021; Ragab et al. 2019).

In an immunohistochemical analysis of acne lesions, the investigators were able to find increased expression of IL-8 in the follicular and perifollicular sites compared to normal skin where IL-8 expression is minimal (Tanghetti 2013). The IL-8 levels were 3,000 times higher in lesional skin when compared to the adjacent normal skin. In comparison, IL-10 levels were only 46 times higher in the acneic skin (Kang et al. 2005). IL-8 is a potent neutrophil attractant. The release of lysosomal enzymes by these neutrophils can rupture the follicular epithelium and exacerbate inflammation.

The gene encoding IL-8 resides at 4q12-q21. Increased levels of plasma IL-8, as well as association with *IL-8* 251 T/A polymorphism, were discovered in Pakistani acne patients (Hussain et al. 2015b). In contrast to such findings, Sobjanek et al. showed no significant linkage between *IL-8* gene variants and acne in polish patients. These conflicting results may reflect the difference in ethnicity of examined individuals or dissimilarities in gene-environment relations (Sobjanek et al. 2013). A meta-analysis of the data provided by these studies did not detect an association between *IL-8* 251 T/A and susceptibility to acne (Heng et al. 2021).

An investigation that was able to draw an association between TNF-α and IL-10 levels and acne also demonstrated increased expression of pro-inflammatory IL-8 and TNF-α in peripheral blood mononuclear cells (PBMCs) of patients suffering from acne upon stimulation with P. acnes. Conversely, P. acnes stimulation resulted in a significant decline in the expression of immunomodulatory IL-10 (Caillon et al. 2010).

The Interleukin-10 gene resides at 1q31–q32 and its promoter region contains several common SNPs including 1082 (G/A), 819 (C/T), 592 (C/A), and 1082 (G/A) that have been linked to susceptibility to multiple immune-mediated disorders (Al-Shobaili et al. 2012a). Alshobaili et al. investigated the *IL-10* 1082 (G/A) SNP in patients with acne and was not able to draw an association between the two (Al-Shobaili et al. 2012b).

IL-4 and its receptor (IL-4R) are involved in the development of multiple immune-mediated diseases. It promotes Th2 and innate immune responses (Najafi et al. 2018). Though not directly implicated in the development of acne, a single case–control study in Saudi Arabia was able to document a significant association between IL-4R A/G (rs1801275) polymorphisms and acne (Al Robaee et al. 2012).

Multiple case–control studies conducted on genes encoding other interleukins and interleukin receptors such as IL-1 receptor antagonist (IL-1RN), IL-4, IL-17, IL-17R, and IL-23R were not able to find an association with acne (Akoglu et al. 2019; Ehm et al. 2017; Szabó et al. 2010).

The *Toll-like receptor* genes

Since TLR2 and TLR4 play a significant role in detecting P. acnes and stimulating an immune response against it, there have been speculations on the effects of genetic polymorphisms of these two PRRs and their role in susceptibility to acne. The results from case–control studies, however, are controversial on this matter with only one study on the Chinese population linking *TLR2* + 2258 G/A to acne susceptibility (Tian et al. 2010). The risk allele of this SNP has been found to significantly influence the function of TLR2 and its downstream signaling pathway (Brown et al. 2009).

A genome-wide association study based in Singapore also found an association between acne vulgaris and fifteen SNPs within the 3′ UTR region of TLR4 (Heng et al. 2021).

The *Resistin* (*RETN*) gene

Among proinflammatory cytokine genes associated with acne, the *resistin* (*RETN*) gene is relatively novel. Resistin which was initially thought to be an adipocyte-specific hormone has recently been identified as the hormone that links obesity to insulin resistance (Al-Shobaili et al. 2012a). Apart from its role in insulin resistance, it also possesses a major regulatory role in inflammation. Resistin promotes the expression of TLR-2, IL-1β, IL-6, IL-8, IL-12, TNFα, and monocyte chemotactic protein-1 (MCP-1) through activating the NF-κB and Janus kinase pathways (JNK) pathways (Pang and Le 2006; Tripathi et al. 2020). Increased levels of resistin have also been documented in inflammatory diseases such as psoriasis (Johnston et al. 2008).

The gene encoding resistin (*RETN*) is located on chromosome 9p13.3 and its 420C/G and 299 G/A polymorphisms confer susceptibility to acne (Younis et al. 2016). These SNPs are associated with higher transcriptional activity and enhanced expression rate (Osawa et al. 2005).

Since resistin is expressed in basal sebocytes it may be implicated in the development of acne by increasing the expression of TLR-2 and increasing its chance of interaction with P. acnes (Hussain et al. 2015a; Younis et al. 2016).

The genes encoding antimicrobial peptides

As a part of the innate defense system, human skin express a number of peptides known as antimicrobial peptides, namely the β defensin family which are present in all epithelial tissues. Thus far, only human β-defensin-1, -2, and -3 (hBD1, hBD2, and hBD3) have been shown to take part in the skin defense mechanisms (Raj and Dentino 2002).

As a result of inflammatory stimuli by TNF and TLRs, such peptides are upregulated, namely the hBD2 that represents the most important defense molecule (Jugeau et al. 2005; Nagy et al. 2005). Though there is still a substantial lack of knowledge regarding the contribution of hBD2 to the innate defense mechanisms, a dual role of hBD2 has been suggested. It can directly take part in the non-oxidative killing of Gram-negative bacteria by destabilizing their membranes (Mukherjee and Hooper 2015). It can also indirectly mediate the stimulation of host-adaptive immunity by recruiting macrophages, neutrophils, dendritic cells, and CD45RO memory T-cells (Lehrer 2004).

Chronell et al. found a higher expression of HBD2 (and to a lesser extent HBD1) in acneic skin and proposed that this higher expression is most likely secondary to the inflammation present in acne lesions (Chronnell et al. 2001). A study by Trivedi et al. also showed increased expression of HBD2 in the acne-affected epidermis but not in healthy skin (Trivedi et al. 2006b). The keratinocytes are a chief source of HBD2 in acne and the HBD2 induction by P. acnes in keratinocyte cultures are isolate specific. However, not all P. acnes strains could upregulate the HBD2 mRNA expression (Nagy et al. 2005). TLR2 and 4 mediate the induction of HBD2 by P. acnes and HBD, in turn, restricts bacterial growth (Jugeau et al. 2005; Nagy et al. 2005). The finding by Nagy et al. highlighted the important role of HBD2 in acne development through the regulation of adaptive immune responses (Harder et al. 2013; Nagy et al. 2005).

HBD2 is encoded by a *DEFB4* gene of the β-defensin gene cluster (DEFB) located at 8p.23.1. Polymorphisms in the gene copy number correlate with mRNA transcriptions (Hollox et al. 2008).

Consistent with its role in inducing inflammation, individuals with hidradenitis suppurativa have a higher copy number of the gene (Giamarellos-Bourboulis et al. 2016). Moreover, the 8p23.1 was found to harbor a susceptibility loci for acne in a recent GWAS (Petridis et al. 2018).

Surprisingly, a case–control study found polymorphisms in another gene in this cluster, *DEFB1* (encoding HBD1), to confer susceptibility to acne in the Han Chinese population. The *DEFB1* -44 GG and -20 AA genotypes resulted in enhanced gene transcription and were associated with a reduced risk for acne development (Tian and Ke 2021).

A type of the alpha defensin, Human neutrophil peptide (HNP)-1-3, was found to have an increased expression in neutrophils present in inflammatory pustular acne (Adışen et al. 2010). This AMP is a very powerful chemoattractant that also contributes to bacterial killing (Harder et al. 2007; Presicce et al. 2009). HNP1-3 is considered to take a major part in the progression to severe pustular acne (Harder et al. 2013).

Granulysin is another type of antimicrobial peptide with increased expression in acne lesions. Granulysin is involved in the cell-mediated cytotoxicity of pathogenic bacteria and can also act as a chemoattractant (Harder et al. 2013). As with the efficacy of antibiotics in acne management, the higher expression of antimicrobial peptides such as granulysin could be beneficial in reducing acne lesions. Recent investigations have not been able to show a change in the levels of IL-8 with the addition of granulysin peptides although other chemokines might be reduced (Trivedi et al. 2006a).

LL-37 is another AMP induced by P.acnes (Lee et al. 2008). It limits bacterial growth by dissolving its membrane through the formation of micelles (Hans and Madaan Hans 2014). LL-37 possesses both anti-inflammatory and pro-inflammatory properties. It reduces TNFα release by macrophages, neutralizes lipopolysaccharide, and promotes the recruitment of inflammatory cells (Brown et al. 2011; Reinholz et al. 2012; Scott et al. 2011).

Psoriasin, RNase-7, and Adrenomedullin are three highly expressed AMPs in acneic skin that only reduce bacterial load (Ganceviciene et al. 2006; Harder and Schröder 2002; Müller et al. 2003).

There have been no reports linking the genetic polymorphisms of these AMPs and susceptibility to acne.

The *NOD-like receptor protein 3 (NLRP3)* gene

NLRP3 belongs to the nucleotide-binding oligomerization domain and leucine-rich repeat-containing receptors (NLR) family of pattern recognition receptors (PRRs). It senses cytosolic danger signals associated with cellular stress and pathogenic motifs and in response stimulates the secretion of inflammatory cytokines including IL-1β and IL-18 (Swanson et al. 2019). P. acnes can induce monocytes to secrete IL-1β through the activation of NLRP3 (Qin et al. 2014). The *NLRP3* polymorphisms can affect the gene expression rate and mRNA stability (Zhang et al. 2011). The G-allele of the *NLRP3* SNP rs10754558 was found to have an increased presentation in Chinese patients with acne vulgaris (Shen et al. 2019).

The *selectin L* (*SELL*) gene

The *SELL* is located at 1q24.2 near other selectin encoding genes (selectin P and E). A GWAS based on the Chinese population demonstrated that the A-allele of the rs7531806 SNP located within the selectin encoding region confers susceptibility to acne (He et al. 2014). This association was not replicated in European-based GWAS studies (Navarini et al. 2014; Petridis et al. 2018). L-selectin is an adhesion molecule expressed on the surface of immune cells. Its ligands are present on the surface of endothelial cells and lymphoid tissue. It facilitates the migration of immune cells toward inflammation (Ivetic et al. 2019). The L-selectin mRNA is highly expressed in acne lesions and is believed to be involved in the regulation of inflammation and scar formation (He et al. 2014; Trivedi et al. 2006b).

The transforming growth factor β (TGFβ) related genes

TGFβ is involved in the pathogenesis of acne through multiple pathways. It reduces sebum production through inhibiting desaturase, PPARγ, and other genes involved in sebaceous differentiation and lipogenesis (McNairn et al. 2013). It reduces keratinocyte proliferation which is involved in obstruction of the pilosebaceous unit and comedone formation (Knaggs et al. 1994; Plewig et al. 1971). It also possesses immunomodulatory effects on innate and adaptive immune responses (Sanjabi et al. 2017). TGFβ has a prominent role in wound healing with high levels of TGFβ1 and TGFβ2 increasing the risk of scarring and high levels of TGFβ3 contributing to scarless wound healing (Liu et al. 2016; Wu et al. 1997).

Thus genetic polymorphisms altering the TGFβ mediated pathways can hypothetically promote acne. Moreover, altered levels of TGFβ and its downstream signaling molecules have been documented in acneic lesions (Yang et al. 2018).

The *OVOL1* gene encodes a transcriptional factor downstream of TGFβ signaling pathways. There is a delicate balance between the two main types of OVOL in normal skin (Tsuji et al. 2018). OVOL1 promotes keratinocyte differentiation and up-regulates the expression of filaggrin and loricrin whereas OVOL2 promotes keratinocyte proliferation (Furue et al. 2019; Koster and Roop 2007; Nair et al. 2006). OVOL1 deletion causes epidermal thickening, barrier disturbance, and increased infiltration of immune cells in murine models (Sun et al. 2020). Dysregulation of OVOL1 and 2 have been documented in atopic dermatitis, psoriasis, and skin cancers (Tsuji et al. 2018).

Follistatin is a soluble neutralizing agent that binds with the members of the TGF-β superfamily, precisely activin (Ham et al. 2020). Follistatin reduces the expression of connective tissue growth factor (CTGF), fibronectin, and collagens and thus delays wound healing in favor of reduced scars (Antsiferova et al. 2009; Ham et al. 2020). A recent study has been able to demonstrate lower levels of Follistatin in patients with severe scarring acne compared to normal individuals (El-Taweel et al. 2021).

Two large GWASs based on a European population have been able to identify three separate susceptibility loci for acne all of which are related to the TGFβ pathway (Navarini et al. 2014; Petridis et al. 2018). These genes include the *Ovo Like Transcriptional Repressor-1* (*OVOL1*) (rs478304 located at 11q13.1), *Follistatin* (*FST*) (rs38055 located at 5q11.2), and *transforming growth factor beta-2* (*TGFB2*) (rs1159268 at 1q41) (Navarini et al. 2014). The *OVOL1* and *TGFB2* genes also demonstrate reduced expression within acneic lesions compared to normal skin.

4 Conclusion

Though the role of inheritance has long been documented in acne vulgaris, the precise genes involved have only been investigated in recent years. A hand full of GWAS and case–control studies have been able to demonstrate the effects of common alleles of genes related to metabolic and immunologic and developmental pathways in conferring susceptibility to acne. There is still a substantial shortage in genetic studies of acne.

References

Adışen E, Yüksek J, Erdem O, Aksakal F, Aksakal A (2010) Expression of human neutrophil proteins in acne vulgaris. J Eur Acad Dermatol Venereol 24:32–37

Aisha N, Haroon J, Hussain S, Tahir C, Ikramullah M, Rahim H, Kishwar N, Younis S, Hassan M, Javed Q (2016) Association between tumour necrosis-α gene polymorphisms and acne vulgaris in a P akistani population. Clin Exp Dermatol 41:297–301

Akoglu G, Tan C, Ayvaz DC, Tezcan I (2019) Tumor necrosis factor α-308 G/A and interleukin 1 β-511 C/T gene polymorphisms in patients with scarring acne. Journal of Cosmetic Dermatology 18:395–400

Al-Shobaili HA, Salem TA, Alzolibani AA, Al Robaee A, Settin AA (2012a) Tumor necrosis factor-α– 308 G/A and interleukin 10–1082 A/G gene polymorphisms in patients with acne vulgaris. J Dermatol Sci 68:52–55

Al-Shobaili HA, Salem TA, Alzolibani AA, Robaee AA, Settin AA (2012b) Tumor necrosis factor-α -308 G/A and interleukin 10–1082 A/G gene polymorphisms in patients with acne vulgaris. J Dermatol Sci 68:52–55

Al Robaee AA, AlZolibani A, Al Shobaili H, Settin A (2012) Association of interleukin 4 (-590 T/C) and interleukin 4 receptor (Q551R A/G) gene polymorphisms with acne vulgaris. Ann Saudi Med 32:349–354

Amr K, Abdel-Hameed M, Sayed K, Nour-Edin F, Abdel Hay R (2014) The Pro12Ala polymorphism of the gene for peroxisome proliferator activated receptor-gamma is associated with a lower Global Acne Grading System score in patients with acne vulgaris. Clin Exp Dermatol 39:741–745

Ando I, Kukita A, Soma G, Hino H (1998) A large number of tandem repeats in the polymorphic epithelial mucin gene is associated with severe acne. J Dermatol 25:150–152

Antsiferova M, Klatte JE, Bodó E, Paus R, Jorcano JL, Matzuk MM, Werner S, Kögel H (2009) Keratinocyte-derived follistatin regulates epidermal homeostasis and wound repair. Lab Invest 89:131–141

Ballanger F, Baudry P, N'Guyen JM, Khammari A, Dréno B (2006) Heredity: a prognostic factor for acne. Dermatology 212:145–149

Bataille V, Snieder H, MacGregor AJ, Sasieni P, Spector TD (2002) The influence of genetics and environmental factors in the pathogenesis of acne: a twin study of acne in women. J Invest Dermatol 119:1317–1322

Baz K, Erdal ME, Söylemez F, Güvenç U, Taşdelen B, Ikizoğlu G (2008) Association between tumor necrosis factor-alpha gene promoter polymorphism at position-308 and acne in Turkish patients. Arch Dermatol Res 300:371

Brombacher EC, Everts B (2020) Shaping of dendritic cell function by the metabolic micro-environment. Front Endocrinol 11:555

Brown KL, Poon GF, Birkenhead D, Pena OM, Falsafi R, Dahlgren C, Karlsson A, Bylund J, Hancock RE, Johnson P (2011) Host defense peptide LL-37 selectively reduces proinflammatory macrophage responses. J Immunol 186:5497–5505

Brown RA, Gralewski JH, Razonable RR (2009) The R753Q polymorphism abrogates toll-like receptor 2 signaling in response to human cytomegalovirus. Clin Infect Dis 49:e96–e99

Brull DJ, Montgomery HE, Sanders J, Dhamrait S, Luong L, Rumley A, Lowe GD, Humphries SE (2001) Interleukin-6 gene- 174g> c and- 572g> c promoter polymorphisms are strong predictors of plasma interleukin-6 levels after coronary artery bypass surgery. Arterioscler Thromb Vasc Biol 21:1458–1463

Burkhart CN, Burkhart CG (2003) Microbiology's principle of biofilms as a major factor in the pathogenesis of acne vulgaris. Int J Dermatol 42:925–927

Caillon F, O'Connell M, Eady EA, Jenkins GR, Cove JH, Layton AM, Mountford AP (2010) Interleukin-10 secretion from CD14+ peripheral blood mononuclear cells is downregulated in patients with acne vulgaris. Br J Dermatol 162:296–303

Chamaie-Nejad F, Saeidi S, Najafi F, Ebrahimi A, Rahimi Z, Shakiba E, Rahimi Z (2018) Association of the CYP17 MSP AI (T-34C) and CYP19 codon 39 (Trp/Arg) polymorphisms with susceptibility to acne vulgaris. Clin Exp Dermatol 43:183–186

Chang S-W, Su C-H, Chen H-H, Huang C-W, Tsao L-P, Tsao Y-P, Chen S-L (2012) DDB2 is a novel AR interacting protein and mediates AR ubiquitination/degradation. The International Journal of Biochemistry & Cell Biology 44:1952–1961

Chen W, Obermayer-Pietsch B, Hong JB, Melnik B, Yamasaki O, Dessinioti C, Ju Q, Liakou A, Al-Khuzaei S, Katsambas A (2011) Acne-associated syndromes: models for better understanding of acne pathogenesis. J Eur Acad Dermatol Venereol 25:637–646

Choi EH, Ahn SK, Lee SH (1997) The changes of stratum corneum interstices and calcium distribution of follicular epithelium of experimentally induced comedones (EIC) by oleic acid. Exp Dermatol 6:29–35

Chronnell CM, Ghali LR, Quinn AG, Bull JJ, McKay IA, Philpott MP, Müller-Röver S, Ali RS, Holland DB, Cunliffe WJ (2001) Human β defensin-1 and-2 expression in human pilosebaceous units: upregulation in acne vulgaris lesions. J Invest Dermatol 117:1120–1125

Cordain L, Lindeberg S, Hurtado M, Hill K, Eaton SB, Brand-Miller J (2002) Acne vulgaris: a disease of Western civilization. Arch Dermatol 138:1584–1590

Cugno M, Borghi A, Marzano AV (2017) PAPA, PASH and PAPASH syndromes: pathophysiology, presentation and treatment. Am J Clin Dermatol 18:555–562

Dessinioti C, Katsambas AD (2010) The role of Propionibacterium acnes in acne pathogenesis: facts and controversies. Clin Dermatol 28:2–7

Dominici R, Cattaneo M, Malferrari G, Archi D, Mariani C, Grimaldi LM, Biunno I (2002) Cloning and functional analysis of the allelic polymorphism in the transcription regulatory region of interleukin-1 alpha. Immunogenetics 54:82–86

Ehm MG, Aponte JL, Chiano MN, Yerges-Armstrong LM, Johnson T, Barker JN, Cook SF, Gupta A, Hinds DA, Li L (2017) Phenome-wide association study using research participants' self-reported data provides insight into the Th17 and IL-17 pathway. PloS One 12:e0186405.

El-Tahlawi SM, Abdel-Halim MR, Hamid MFA, Mohammad KS, Wafai H, El-Sayed AH (2014) Gene polymorphism and serum levels of insulin-like growth factor-I in Egyptian acne patients. J Egypt Women's Dermatol Soc 11:45–49

El-Taweel A, Mustafa A, Abdul Haleem W, El-Motaleb A (2021) Serum level of follistatin in patients with scarring and non scarring acne vulgaris. Benha J Appl Sci 5:1–4

Escobar-Morreale HF, Calvo RM, Sancho J, San Millán JL (2001) TNF-alpha and hyperandrogenism: a clinical, biochemical, and molecular genetic study. J Clin Endocrinol Metab 86:3761–3767

Evans DM, Kirk KM, Nyholt DR, Novac C, Martin NG (2005) Teenage acne is influenced by genetic factors. Br J Dermatol 152:579–581

Farag AGA, Badr EA, Eltorgoman AMA, Assar MF, Elshafey EN, Tayel NR, Aboutaleb HE (2019) Role of 11β HSD 1, rs12086634, and rs846910 single-nucleotide polymorphisms in metabolic-related skin diseases: a clinical, biochemical, and genetic study. Clin, Cosmet Invest Dermatol 12:91

Furue K, Ito T, Tsuji G, Ulzii D, Vu YH, Kido-Nakahara M, Nakahara T, Furue M (2019) The IL-13–OVOL 1–FLG axis in atopic dermatitis. Immunology 158:281–286

Ganceviciene R, Fimmel S, Glass E, Zouboulis CC (2006) Psoriasin and follicular hyperkeratinization in acne comedones. Dermatology 213:270

Giamarellos-Bourboulis EJ, Platzer M, Karagiannidis I, Kanni T, Nikolakis G, Ulrich J, Bellutti M, Gollnick H, Bauer M, Zouboulis CC (2016) High copy numbers of β-defensin cluster on 8p23. 1, confer genetic susceptibility, and modulate the physical course of hidradenitis suppurativa/acne inversa. J Invest Dermatol 136:1592–1598

Goulden V, McGeown CH, Cunliffe WJ (1999) The familial risk of adult acne: a comparison between first-degree relatives of affected and unaffected individuals. Br J Dermatol 141:297–300

Grech I, Giatrakos S, Damoraki G, Kaldrimidis P, Rigopoulos D, Giamarellos-Bourboulis EJ (2014) Impact of TNF haplotypes in the physical course of acne vulgaris. Dermatology 228:152–157

Ham S, Harrison C, de Kretser D, Wallace EM, Southwick G, Temple-Smith P (2020) Potential treatment of keloid pathogenesis with follistatin 288 by blocking the activin molecular pathway. Exp Dermatol.

Haneklaus M, O'Neill LA, Coll RC (2013) Modulatory mechanisms controlling the NLRP3 inflammasome in inflammation: recent developments. Curr Opin Immunol 25:40–45

Hans M, Madaan Hans V (2014) Epithelial antimicrobial peptides: guardian of the oral cavity. Int J Peptides.

Harder J, Gläser R, Schröder J-M (2007) Human antimicrobial proteins—Effectors of innate immunity. J Endotoxin Res 13:317–338

Harder J, Schröder J-M (2002) RNase 7, a novel innate immune defense antimicrobial protein of healthy human skin. J Biol Chem 277:46779–46784

Harder J, Tsuruta D, Murakami M, Kurokawa I (2013) What is the role of antimicrobial peptides (AMP) in acne vulgaris? Exp Dermatol 22:386–391

He L, Wu W-J, Yang J-K, Cheng H, Zuo X-B, Lai W, Gao T-W, Ma C-L, Luo N, Huang J-Q (2014) Two new susceptibility loci 1q24. 2 and 11p11. 2 confer risk to severe acne. Nat Commun 5:1–7

Heng AHS, Say Y-H, Sio YY, Ng YT, Chew FT (2021) Gene variants associated with acne vulgaris presentation and severity: a systematic review and meta-analysis. BMC Med Genomics 14:1–42

Herane MI, Ando I (2003) Acne in infancy and acne genetics. Dermatology 206:24–28

Hollox EJ, Huffmeier U, Zeeuwen PL, Palla R, Lascorz J, Rodijk-Olthuis D, Van De Kerkhof PC, Traupe H, De Jongh G, Den Heijer M (2008) Psoriasis is associated with increased β-defensin genomic copy number. Nat Genet 40:23–25

Hoogendoorn B, Coleman SL, Guy CA, Smith K, Bowen T, Buckland PR, O'Donovan MC (2003) Functional analysis of human promoter polymorphisms. Hum Mol Genet 12:2249–2254

Huang PY, Kandyba E, Jabouille A, Sjolund J, Kumar A, Halliwill K, McCreery M, DelRosario R, Kang HC, Wong CE (2017) Lgr6 is a stem cell marker in mouse skin squamous cell carcinoma. Nat Genet 49:1624

Hussain S, Faraz A, Iqbal T (2015a) The RETN gene rs1862513 polymorphism as a novel predisposing marker for familial Acne vulgaris in a Pakistani population. Iran J Basic Med Sci 18:526–528

Hussain S, Iqbal T, Sadiq I, Feroz S, Shafique Satti H (2015b) Polymorphism in the IL-8 Gene Promoter and the Risk of Acne Vulgaris in a Pakistani Population. Iran J Allergy Asthma Immunol 14:443–449

Ibrahimi OA, Eliseenkova AV, Plotnikov AN, Yu K, Ornitz DM, Mohammadi M (2001) Structural basis for fibroblast growth factor receptor 2 activation in Apert syndrome. Proc Natl Acad Sci 98:7182–7187

Ivetic A, Hoskins Green HL, Hart SJ (2019) L-selectin: a major regulator of leukocyte adhesion, migration and signaling. Front Immunol 10:1068

Jahns AC, Alexeyev OA (2014) Three dimensional distribution of P ropionibacterium acnes biofilms in human skin. Exp Dermatol 23:687–689

Jahns AC, Lundskog B, Ganceviciene R, Palmer RH, Golovleva I, Zouboulis C, McDowell A, Patrick S, Alexeyev OA (2012) An increased incidence of Propionibacterium acnes biofilms in acne vulgaris: a case–control study. Br J Dermatol 167:50–58

Johnston A, Arnadottir S, Gudjonsson JE, Aphale A, Sigmarsdottir AA, Gunnarsson SI, Steinsson JT, Elder JT, Valdimarsson H (2008) Obesity in psoriasis: leptin and resistin as mediators of cutaneous inflammation. Br J Dermatol 159:342–350

Jugeau S, Tenaud I, Knol A, Jarrousse V, Quereux G, Khammari A, Dreno B (2005) Induction of toll-like receptors by Propionibacterium acnes. Br J Dermatol 153:1105–1113

Kang S, Cho S, Chung JH, Hammerberg C, Fisher GJ, Voorhees JJ (2005) Inflammation and extracellular matrix degradation mediated by activated transcription factors nuclear factor-kappaB and activator protein-1 in inflammatory acne lesions in vivo. Am J Pathol 166:1691–1699

Kelhälä H-L, Palatsi R, Fyhrquist N, Lehtimäki S, Väyrynen JP, Kallioinen M, Kubin ME, Greco D, Tasanen K, Alenius H (2014) IL-17/Th17 pathway is activated in acne lesions. PloS One 9:e105238.

Kim J, Ochoa M-T, Krutzik SR, Takeuchi O, Uematsu S, Legaspi AJ, Brightbill HD, Holland D, Cunliffe WJ, Akira S (2002) Activation of toll-like receptor 2 in acne triggers inflammatory cytokine responses. J Immunol 169:1535–1541

Knaggs HE, Holland DB, Morris C, Wood EJ, Cunliffe WJ (1994) Quantification of cellular proliferation in acne using the monoclonal antibody Ki-67. J Invest Dermatol 102:89–92

Kobayashi Y, Yamamoto K, Saido T, Kawasaki H, Oppenheim JJ, Matsushima K (1990) Identification of calcium-activated neutral protease as a processing enzyme of human interleukin 1 alpha. Proc Natl Acad Sci 87:5548–5552

Kolczynska K, Loza-Valdes A, Hawro I, Sumara G (2020) Diacylglycerol-evoked activation of PKC and PKD isoforms in regulation of glucose and lipid metabolism: a review. Lipids Health Dis 19:1–15

Koster MI, Roop DR (2007) Mechanisms regulating epithelial stratification. Annu Rev Cell Dev Biol 23

Lai J-J, Chang P, Lai K-P, Chen L, Chang C (2012) The role of androgen and androgen receptor in skin-related disorders. Arch Dermatol Res 304:499–510

Layton A, Thiboutot D, Tan J (2021) Reviewing the global burden of acne: how could we improve care to reduce the burden? Br J Dermatol 184:219–225

Lee D-Y, Yamasaki K, Rudsil J, Zouboulis CC, Park GT, Yang J-M, Gallo RL (2008) Sebocytes express functional cathelicidin antimicrobial peptides and can act to kill propionibacterium acnes. J Invest Dermatol 128:1863

Lee SE, Kim J-M, Jeong SK, Jeon JE, Yoon H-J, Jeong M-K, Lee SH (2010) Protease-activated receptor-2 mediates the expression of inflammatory cytokines, antimicrobial peptides, and matrix metalloproteinases in keratinocytes in response to Propionibacterium acnes. Arch Dermatol Res 302:745–756

Lehrer RI (2004) Primate defensins. Nat Rev Microbiol 2:727–738

Leyden JJ, McGinley KJ, Mills OH, Kligman AM (1975) Propionibacterium levels in patients with and without acne vulgaris. J Invest Dermatol 65:382–384

Li ZJ, Choi DK, Sohn KC, Seo MS, Lee HE, Lee Y, Seo YJ, Lee YH, Shi G, Zouboulis CC (2014) Propionibacterium acnes activates the NLRP3 inflammasome in human sebocytes. J Invest Dermatol 134:2747–2756

Lichtenberger R, Simpson MA, Smith C, Barker J, Navarini AA (2017) Genetic architecture of acne vulgaris. J Eur Acad Dermatol Venereol 31:1978–1990

Liu H, Ippolito GC, Wall JK, Niu T, Probst L, Lee B-S, Pulford K, Banham AH, Stockwin L, Shaffer AL (2006) Functional studies of BCL11A: characterization of the conserved BCL11A-XL splice variant and its interaction with BCL6 in nuclear paraspeckles of germinal center B cells. Mol Cancer 5:1–16

Liu Y, Li Y, Li N, Teng W, Wang M, Zhang Y, Xiao Z (2016) TGF-β1 promotes scar fibroblasts proliferation and transdifferentiation via up-regulating MicroRNA-21. Scie Rep 6:1–9

Lo Celso C, Berta MA, Braun KM, Frye M, Lyle S, Zouboulis CC, Watt FM (2008) Characterization of bipotential epidermal progenitors derived from human sebaceous gland: contrasting roles of c-Myc and beta-catenin. Stem Cells 26:1241–1252

Lwin SM, Kimber I, McFadden JP (2014) Acne, quorum sensing and danger. Clin Exp Dermatol 39:162–167

Mälarstig A, Wallentin L, Siegbahn A (2007) Genetic variation in the interleukin-6 gene in relation to risk and outcomes in acute coronary syndrome. Thromb Res 119:467–473

McNairn AJ, Doucet Y, Demaude J, Brusadelli M, Gordon CB, Uribe-Rivera A, Lambert PF, Bouez C, Breton L, Guasch G (2013) TGFβ signaling regulates lipogenesis in human sebaceous glands cells. BMC Dermatol 13:1–12

Melnik B (2009) Role of FGFR2-signaling in the pathogenesis of acne. Dermato-Endocrinol 1:141–156

Melnik B (2010) Acne vulgaris. Role of diet. Hautarzt 61:115–125

Mill P, Mo R, Fu H, Grachtchouk M, Kim PC, Dlugosz AA, Hui C-c (2003) Sonic hedgehog-dependent activation of Gli2 is essential for embryonic hair follicle development. Genes Dev 17:282–294

Mina-Vargas A, Colodro-Conde L, Grasby K, Zhu G, Gordon S, Medland SE, Martin NG (2017) Heritability and GWAS analyses of acne in Australian adolescent twins. Twin Res Hum Gene 20:541–549

Mukherjee S, Hooper LV (2015) Antimicrobial defense of the intestine. Immunity 42:28–39

Müller F, Müller-Röver S, Korge B, Kapas S, Hinson J, Philpott M (2003) Adrenomedullin: expression and possible role in human skin and hair growth. Br J Dermatol 148:30–38

Nagy I, Pivarcsi A, Koreck A, Széll M, Urbán E, Kemény L (2005) Distinct strains of Propionibacterium acnes induce selective human β-defensin-2 and interleukin-8 expression in human keratinocytes through toll-like receptors. J Invest Dermatol 124:931–938

Nair M, Teng A, Bilanchone V, Agrawal A, Li B, Dai X (2006) Ovol1 regulates the growth arrest of embryonic epidermal progenitor cells and represses c-myc transcription. J Cell Biol 173:253–264

Najafi S, Mohammadzadeh M, Rajabi F, Zare Bidoki A, Yousefi H, Farhadi E, Rezaei N (2018) Interleukin-4 and interleukin-4 receptor alpha gene polymorphisms in recurrent aphthous stomatitis. Immunol Invest 47:680–688

Navarini AA, Simpson MA, Weale M, Knight J, Carlavan I, Reiniche P, Burden DA, Layton A, Bataille V, Allen M (2014) Genome-wide association study identifies three novel susceptibility loci for severe Acne vulgaris. Nat Commun 5:1–6

Ortega S, Ittmann M, Tsang SH, Ehrlich M, Basilico C (1998) Neuronal defects and delayed wound healing in mice lacking fibroblast growth factor 2. Proc Natl Acad Sci 95:5672–5677

Osawa H, Onuma H, Ochi M, Murakami A, Yamauchi J, Takasuka T, Tanabe F, Shimizu I, Kato K, Nishida W (2005) Resistin SNP-420 determines its monocyte mRNA and serum levels inducing type 2 diabetes. Biochem Biophys Res Commun 335:596–602

Ottaviani M, Mastrofrancesco A, Alestas T, Flori E, Zouboulis C, Picardo M (2005) Role of squalene peroxidation in the development of inflammation in acne vulgaris. J Invest Dermatol. Blackwell Publishing 9600 Garsington Rd, oxford ox4 2dq, Oxon, England, pp A37-A37.

Pang SS, Le YY (2006) Role of resistin in inflammation and inflammation-related diseases. Cell Mol Immunol 3:29–34

Pang Y, He CD, Liu Y, Wang KB, Xiao T, Wang YK, Zhu H, Wei B, Zhao N, Jiang Y, Wei HC, Chen HD (2008) Combination of short CAG and GGN repeats in the androgen receptor gene is associated with acne risk in North East China. J Eur Acad Dermatol Venereol 22:1445–1451

Petridis C, Navarini AA, Dand N, Saklatvala J, Baudry D, Duckworth M, Allen MH, Curtis CJ, Lee SH, Burden AD (2018) Genome-wide meta-analysis implicates mediators of hair follicle development and morphogenesis in risk for severe acne. Nature Communications 9:1–8

Phillips EH, Ryan S, Ferrari R, Green C (2003) Estratest and Estratest HS (esterified estrogens and methyltestosterone) therapy: a summary of safety surveillance data, January 1989 to August 2002. Clin Ther 25:3027–3043

Platsidaki E, Dessinioti C (2018) Recent advances in understanding Propionibacterium acnes (Cutibacterium acnes) in acne. F1000 Res 7

Plewig G, Fulton JE, Kligman AM (1971) Cellular dynamics of comedo formation in acne vulgaris. Archiv Für Dermatol Forsch 242:12–29

Plewig G, Melnik B, Chen W (2019) Acne pathogenesis. In: Plewig and Kligman's acne and Rosacea. Springer, pp 45–61

Presicce P, Giannelli S, Taddeo A, Villa ML, Della Bella S (2009) Human defensins activate monocyte-derived dendritic cells, promote the production of proinflammatory cytokines, and up-regulate the surface expression of CD91. J Leukoc Biol 86:941–948

Qin M, Pirouz A, Kim M-H, Krutzik SR, Garbán HJ, Kim J (2014) Propionibacterium acnes induces IL-1β secretion via the NLRP3 inflammasome in human monocytes. J Invest Dermatol 134:381–388

Ragab M, Hassan E, Elneily D, Fathallah N (2019) Association of interleukin-6 gene promoter polymorphism with acne vulgaris and its severity. Clin Exp Dermatol 44:637–642

Rahaman SMA, De D, Handa S, Pal A, Sachdeva N, Ghosh T, Kamboj P (2016) Association of insulin-like growth factor (IGF)-1 gene polymorphisms with plasma levels of IGF-1 and acne severity. J Am Acad Dermatol 75:768–773

Raina D, Kharbanda S, Kufe D (2004) The MUC1 oncoprotein activates the anti-apoptotic phosphoinositide 3-kinase/Akt and Bcl-xL pathways in rat 3Y1 fibroblasts. J Biol Chem 279:20607–20612

Raj PA, Dentino AR (2002) Current status of defensins and their role in innate and adaptive immunity. FEMS Microbiol Lett 206:9–18

Reinholz M, Ruzicka T, Schauber J (2012) Cathelicidin LL-37: an antimicrobial peptide with a role in inflammatory skin disease. Ann Dermatol 24:126

Rice DP (2008) Craniofacial sutures: development, disease and treatment. Karger Medical and Scientific Publishers

Romano R-A, Smalley K, Liu S, Sinha S (2010) Abnormal hair follicle development and altered cell fate of follicular keratinocytes in transgenic mice expressing ΔNp63α. Development 137:1431–1439

Saadi I, Alkuraya FS, Gisselbrecht SS, Goessling W, Cavallesco R, Turbe-Doan A, Petrin AL, Harris J, Siddiqui U, Grix AW Jr (2011) Deficiency of the cytoskeletal protein SPECC1L leads to oblique facial clefting. Am J Hum Genet 89:44–55

Saeidi S, Chamaie-Nejad F, Ebrahimi A, Najafi F, Rahimi Z, Vaisi-Raygani A, Shakiba E, Rahimi Z (2018) PPARγ Pro12Ala and C161T polymorphisms in patients with acne vulgaris: contribution to lipid and lipoprotein profile. Adv Med Sci 63:147–151

Sanjabi S, Oh SA, Li MO (2017) Regulation of the immune response by TGF-β: from conception to autoimmunity and infection. Cold Spring Harb Perspect Biol 9:a022236

Scott A, Weldon S, Buchanan PJ, Schock B, Ernst RK, McAuley DF, Tunney MM, Irwin CR, Elborn JS, Taggart CC (2011) Evaluation of the ability of LL-37 to neutralise LPS in vitro and ex vivo. PloS One 6: e26525

Serna-Tamayo C, Janniger CK, Micali G, Schwartz RA (2014) Neonatal and infantile acne vulgaris: an update. Cutis 94:13–16

Shen C, Wang Q, Shen Z, Yuan H, Yu W, Chen X, Xu H (2019) Genetic association between the NLRP3 gene and acne vulgaris in a Chinese population. Clin Exp Dermatol 44:184–189

Simonart T (2013) Immunotherapy for acne vulgaris: current status and future directions. Am J Clin Dermatol 14:429–435

Snodgrass RG, Huang S, Choi I-W, Rutledge JC, Hwang DH (2013) Inflammasome-mediated secretion of IL-1β in human monocytes through TLR2 activation; modulation by dietary fatty acids. J Immunol 191:4337–4347

Sobjanek M, Zablotna M, Glen J, Michajlowski I, Nedoszytko B, Roszkiewicz J (2013) Polymorphism in interleukin 1A but not in interleukin 8 gene predisposes to acne vulgaris in Polish population. J Eur Acad Dermatol Venereol 27:259–260

Sobjanek M, Zabłotna M, Nedoszytko B, Sokołowska-Wojdyło M, Włodarkiewicz A (2009) Lack of association between the promoter polymorphisms at positions -238 and -308 of the tumour necrosis factor alpha gene and acne vulgaris in Polish patients. J Eur Acad Dermatol Venereol 23:331–332

Stewart ME, Grahek MO, Cambier LS, Wertz PW, Downing DT (1986) Dilutional effect of increased sebaceous gland activity on the proportion of linoleic acid in sebaceous wax esters and in epidermal acylceramides. J Invest Dermatol 87:733–736

Stoyanova T, Roy N, Kopanja D, Bagchi S, Raychaudhuri P (2009) DDB2 decides cell fate following DNA damage. Proc Natl Acad Sci 106:10690–10695

Sun P, Vu R, Dragan M, Haensel D, Gutierrez G, Nguyen Q, Greenberg E, Chen Z, Wu J, Atwood S (2020) Ovol1 regulates psoriasis-like skin inflammation and epidermal hyperplasia. J Invest Dermatol

Swanson KV, Deng M, Ting JP-Y (2019) The NLRP3 inflammasome: molecular activation and regulation to therapeutics. Nat Rev Immunol 19:477–489

Szabó K, Kemény L (2011) Studying the genetic predisposing factors in the pathogenesis of acne vulgaris. Hum Immunol 72:766–773

Szabó K, Tax G, Kis K, Szegedi K, Teodorescu-Brinzeu D, Diószegi C, Koreck A, Széll M, Kemény L (2010) Interleukin-1A+ 4845 (G> T) polymorphism is a factor predisposing to acne vulgaris. Tissue Antigens 76:411–415

Szabó K, Tax G, Teodorescu-Brinzeu D, Koreck A, Kemény L (2011) TNFα gene polymorphisms in the pathogenesis of acne vulgaris. Arch Dermatol Res 303:19–27

Tan J, Kang S, Leyden J (2017) Prevalence and risk factors of acne scarring among patients consulting dermatologists in the USA. J Drugs Dermatol 16:97–102

Tanghetti EA (2013) The role of inflammation in the pathology of acne. J Clin Aesthet Dermatol 6:27–35

Tasli L, Turgut S, Kacar N, Ayada C, Coban M, Akcilar R, Ergin S (2013) Insulin-like growth factor-I gene polymorphism in acne vulgaris. J Eur Acad Dermatol Venereol 27:254–257

Tian L-M, Ke D (2021) Acne Vulgaris is associated with the human β-defensin 1-gene polymorphisms in Han Chinese ethnic group patients. Clin Cosmet Invest Dermatol 14:123

Tian L-M, Xie H-F, Yang T, Hu Y-H, Li J, Wang W-Z (2010) Association study of tumor necrosis factor receptor type 2 M196R and toll-like receptor 2 Arg753Gln polymorphisms with acne vulgaris in a Chinese Han ethnic group. Dermatology 221:276–284

Tripathi D, Kant S, Pandey S, Ehtesham NZ (2020) Resistin in metabolism, inflammation, and disease. FEBS J 287:3141–3149

Trivedi NR, Cong Z, Nelson AM, Albert AJ, Rosamilia LL, Sivarajah S, Gilliland KL, Liu W, Mauger DT, Gabbay RA (2006a) Peroxisome proliferator-activated receptors increase human sebum production. J Invest Dermatol 126:2002–2009

Trivedi NR, Gilliland KL, Zhao W, Liu W, Thiboutot DM (2006b) Gene array expression profiling in acne lesions reveals marked upregulation of genes involved in inflammation and matrix remodeling. J Invest Dermatol 126:1071–1079

Trivedi NR, Gilliland KL, Zhao W, Liu W, Thiboutot DM (2006c) Gene array expression profiling in acne lesions reveals marked upregulation of genes involved in inflammation and matrix remodeling. J Invest Dermatol 126:1071–1079

Tsuji G, Ito T, Chiba T, Mitoma C, Nakahara T, Uchi H, Furue M (2018) The role of the OVOL1–OVOL2 axis in normal and diseased human skin. J Dermatol Sci 90:227–231

Van Bokhoven H, Hamel BC, Bamshad M, Sangiorgi E, Gurrieri F, Duijf PH, Vanmolkot KR, van Beusekom E, van Beersum SE, Celli J (2001) p63 Gene mutations in EEC syndrome, limb-mammary syndrome, and isolated split hand–split foot malformation suggest a genotype-phenotype correlation. Am J Hum Gene 69:481–492

Walton S, Wyatt EH, Cunliffe WJ (1988) Genetic control of sebum excretion and acne–a twin study. Br J Dermatol 118:393–396

Wu L, Siddiqui A, Morris DE, Cox DA, Roth SI, Mustoe TA (1997) Transforming growth factor β3 (TGFβ3) accelerates wound healing without alteration of scar prominence: histologic and competitive reverse-transcription–polymerase chain reaction studies. Arch Surg 132:753–760

Xu M, Horrell J, Snitow M, Cui J, Gochnauer H, Syrett CM, Kallish S, Seykora JT, Liu F, Gaillard D (2017) WNT10A mutation causes ectodermal dysplasia by impairing progenitor cell proliferation and KLF4-mediated differentiation. Nat Commun 8:1–21

Xu SX, Wang HL, Fan X, Sun LD, Yang S, Wang PG, Xiao FL, Gao M, Cui Y, Ren YQ, Du WH, Quan C, Zhang XJ (2007) The familial risk of acne vulgaris in Chinese Hans—a case-control study. J Eur Acad Dermatol Venereol 21:602–605

Yamamoto T, Osaki T, Yoneda K, Ueta E (1994) Cytokine production by keratinocytes and mononuclear infiltrates in oral lichen planus. J Oral Pathol Med 23:309–315

Yang JH, Yoon JY, Moon J, Min S, Kwon HH, Suh DH (2018) Expression of inflammatory and fibrogenetic markers in acne hypertrophic scar formation: focusing on role of TGF-β and IGF-1R. Arch Dermatol Res 310:665–673

Yang JK, Wu WJ, Qi J, He L, Zhang YP (2014) TNF-308 G/A polymorphism and risk of acne vulgaris: a meta-analysis. PLoS One 9:e87806

Yang X-Y, Wu W-J, Yang C, Yang T, He J-D, Yang Z, He L (2013) Association of HSD17B3 and HSD3B1 polymorphisms with acne vulgaris in Southwestern Han Chinese. Dermatology 227:202–208

Yang Z, Yu H, Cheng B, Tang W, Dong Y, Xiao C, He L (2009) Relationship between the CAG repeat polymorphism in the androgen receptor gene and acne in the Han ethnic group. Dermatology 218:302–306

Younis S, Blumenberg M, Javed Q (2016) Resistin gene polymorphisms are associated with acne and serum lipid levels, providing a potential nexus between lipid metabolism and inflammation. Arch Dermatol Res 308:229–237

Younis S, Javed Q (2015) The interleukin-6 and interleukin-1A gene promoter polymorphism is associated with the pathogenesis of acne vulgaris. Arch Dermatol Res 307:365–370

Zaba R, Schwartz R, Jarmuda S, Czarnecka-Operacz M, Silny W (2011) Acne fulminans: explosive systemic form of acne. J Eur Acad Dermatol Venereol 25:501–507

Zhang A-Q, Zeng L, Gu W, Zhang L-Y, Zhou J, Jiang D-P, Du D-Y, Hu P, Yang C, Yan J (2011) Clinical relevance of single nucleotide polymorphisms within the entire NLRP3 gene in patients with major blunt trauma. Crit Care 15:1–10

Zhang M, Qureshi AA, Hunter DJ, Han J (2014) A genome-wide association study of severe teenage acne in European Americans. Hum Genet 133:259–264

The Immunogenetics of Morphea and Lichen Sclerosus

Pooya Khan Mohammad Beigi

Abstract

Morphea and lichen sclerosis et atrophicus (LSA) are two distinct immune-mediated diseases with a dominant presentation of dermal fibrosis and sclerosis. The two diseases have many similar clinical and histological features and tend to co-occur. Both diseases are thought to result from a derailment of the normal response to environmental triggers. Positive family history is more common in LSA than morphea but individuals with morphea have a higher frequency of concomitant and familial autoimmunity. These findings hint at the involvement of inheritance in susceptibility to LSA and morphea and thus provide a rationale for exploring the disease genetics. This chapter contains a comprehensive review of the pathogenesis of the two diseases and their known genetic associations including HLA class I and II genes.

Keywords

Immunogenetics · Morphea · Lichen sclerosus · Pathogenesis · Susceptibility genes

1 Introduction

Morphea, also known as localized scleroderma, and lichen sclerosus et atrophicus (LSA) are two distinct autoimmune diseases that manifest as single to multiple sclerotic plaques with dyschromia. Unlike LSA which is a skin-limited entity usually confined to small areas, morphea can involve virtually any part of the skin and extend to the underlying muscle, bone, and joint (Bevans et al. 2017; Fett 2013; Florez-Pollack et al. 2018). Several subtypes of morphea have been described with localized plaque-type and linear morphea being the most common forms. Based on the affected region, LSA lesions are also categorized as genital and extragenital.

The two diseases share similar histological features of increased collagen deposition and lymphocytic infiltration of the dermis. In LSA, there is a band-like infiltration in the papillary dermis, follicular plugging, and loss of elastin whereas morphea lesions have perivascular infiltration and involvement of the reticular dermis with the destruction of the adnexal structures (Nishioka 1997). Aside from the similarities in clinical and histological features, recent reports have shown that the two diseases tend to co-exist in a higher frequency than anticipated to occur by chance (Das et al. 2016; Kreuter et al. 2012; Lutz et al. 2012). Some have gone further to consider LSA is as a variant of morphea but this opinion is not very popular (Sehgal et al. 2002).

P. Khan Mohammad Beigi (✉)
Mismedicine Organization and Research Institute, Beverly Hills, CA, USA
e-mail: dr.pooyabeigi@marihc.com

N. Rezaei and F. Rajabi (eds.), *The Immunogenetics of Dermatologic Diseases*, Advances in Experimental Medicine and Biology 1367,
https://doi.org/10.1007/978-3-030-92616-8_7

Nevertheless, similar etiopathological factors may be involved in both diseases and perhaps they may even share similar susceptibility genes.

2 Epidemiology

2.1 Morphea

The incidence of morphea is 0.4–2.7 per 100,000 people (Fett 2013; Florez-Pollack et al. 2018). Morphea can affect patients of all ages but often has an onset during childhood and middle adulthood (Fett 2013). In a controlled study, researchers looked at 110 adult-onset and 77 juvenile-onset patients and determined the mean age of onset to be 45 and 10 years in respective groups (Dharamsi et al. 2013). Linear morphea is more common in children whereas the localized form is more common in adults. All races are affected but the occurrence of morphea is sporadic in populations of African origin. The prevalence of morphea is 2–3 times greater in women than men (Sehgal et al. 2002). Though there is a higher prevalence of autoimmune diseases in the family members of those affected, familial cases of morphea are rare (Leitenberger et al. 2009; Pham and Browning 2010; Wadud et al. 1989; Yurtsever et al. 2021).

2.2 Lichen Sclerosus

Lichen sclerosus can occur at any age and in either sex. The prevalence of the disease is bimodal, mainly affecting prepubertal and postmenopausal women with the latter as the predominant group meeting the diagnosis for lichen sclerosus. The disease affects women 6–10 times more than men and recent reports estimate the prevalence in women to be 1 in 60 (Pérez-López and Vieira-Baptista 2017). The disease occurs more in adults than children. Prevalence in children is estimated to be 1 in 900 (Nóbrega et al. 2016). According to Kirtschig et al., about 10% of patients have other family members with the same condition (Kirtschig 2016).

3 Clinical Features

3.1 Morphea

Based on the clinical presentation, three main subtypes (plaque-type, linear, and generalized) and several less common types of morphea (nodular, deep, guttate, and mixed variants) have been described.

The plaque-type morphea presents with few well-circumscribed reds to purple lesions with subtle induration on the truck of extremity that solely progresses to firm depressed patches with brown or white tint (Fig. 1a). These lesions are often asymptomatic with occasional itch and rarely pain. Once formed, the scar tissue rarely fades completely (Fett 2013).

Generalized morphea is the most severe form of this disease. At the onset, this form appears the same as circumscribed form but as the disease progresses, lesions will increase in number and size becoming confluent. This will result in indurated plaques with hyperpigmentation covering almost all the trunk except for the nipples (Werth et al. 1992).

Linear morphea is more commonly seen in children and appears as single unilateral linear bands along an extremity. As it extends deep to the tissue and runs over the joint, it can affect bone growth and cause severe deformities and limited limb mobility (Fig. 1b) (Chu et al. 2011). The clinical characteristics of morphea subtypes are summarized in Table 1.

Linear Morphea can also affect the face and scalp creating two distinct phenotypes called en-coup-de-saber and Parry-Romberg. En-coup-de-sabre presents as a linear streak along the forehead and since it extends into the brain it can cause seizures. Parry-Romberg presents with hemifacial atrophy (Fett 2013).

Pansclerotic morphea involves generalized full-thickness sclerosis of the trunk, extremities, face, and scalp. This represents a rare but the most disabling form of morphea. It generally affects children younger than age 14. Sclerosis extends beyond the dermis causing panniculitis, fasciitis, compromising the muscle, and

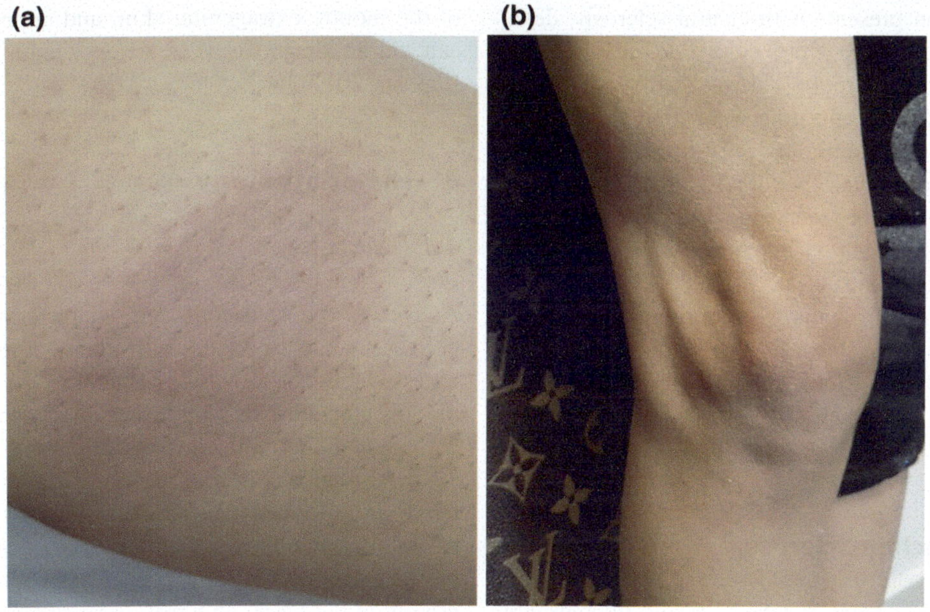

Fig. 1 Morphea. **a** Active plaque-type morphea presenting as a violaceous firm lesion on the trunk. **b** Deep linear morphea. Courtesy of Dr. Nasim Niknezhad

Table 1 Subtypes of circumscribed Morphea (Sehgal et al. 2002)

Morphea subtype	Clinical characteristics
Morphea en plaque	• Few affected areas • Erythematous halo progressing to sclerosis • Hyper or hypopigmented scarring
Guttate morphea	• Multiple small chalk-white patched • Chest, neck, shoulders, or upper back • Flat or slightly depressed mildly firm patches
Atrophoderma of Pasini and Pierini	• Asymptomatic • Hyperpigmented • Atrophic plaques • No sclerosis • "Cliff drop" borders with depressed center • Trunk
Keloid morphea	• Rare • Nodular lesions in association with typical morphea lesions

sometimes the bone (Florez-Pollack et al. 2018) The absence of the Raynaud phenomenon and internal organ involvement distinguished the subtype from systemic sclerosis (Fett 2013).

The diagnosis of morphea is generally made clinically and confirmed by skin biopsy. Additional to clinical assessment, evaluation of the history and evolution of the disease is needed to assess the activity. Active morphea may appear bruise-like and present with erythema and induration. Deep active inflammatory lesions are poorly circumscribed and may be easier to evaluate by palpation. Erythema around the borders of the lesion is another sign of disease activity (Florez-Pollack et al. 2018). In inactive erythema is replaced by hyperpigmentation and the lesion presents with central sclerosis, developing a yellow-white color. Sclerosis is then replaced by atrophy. Dermal atrophy presents with a shiny appearance of the skin, visible underlying vessels, and cliff-drop deformity. If lesions extend deeper than the dermis, telangiectasia can be seen. In these cases, loss of adnexa and hair is apparent at the site of the lesion (Dharamsi et al. 2013).

In some patients with morphea, especially those with the linear and generalized types high titers of anti nucleic acid antibodies (ANA), antihistone antibodies, and anti ssDNA antibodies could be found (Khatri et al. 2019).

3.2 Lichen Sclerosus

LSA presents as patches of scar-like atrophic tissue and erosions with a blue-white hue. A typical pattern of lichen sclerosus is when both the vulva and perianal area are involved in the 'figure of 8' or 'key-hole sign' (Pérez-López and Vieira-Baptista 2017). Other reported types of lesions include fissures, petechiae, purpura, ulcerations, edema, hyper- or hypopigmentation, and cigarette paper wrinkling. In the genitals, the most common area involved, scarring can significantly change the architecture of the genitals due to fibrosis and ulceration (Fistarol and Itin 2013). Extensive scarring could lead to burying of the clitoris or vaginal introitus (Kirtschig 2016). Unlike Morphea, LSA is often symptomatic. In women, symptoms vary in severity. Most report burning, itching, and soreness. Some report dysuria, dyspareunia, voiding dysfunction, and bleeding.

Men may develop sclerosis and narrowing of the foreskin, preventing erections. The disease may be limited to the glans of the penis and prepuce but could also affect the penile shaft and scrotum. Complications can include fibrosis of the meatus and urethra, leading to urethral stenosis (Kirtschig 2016).

15–20% of patients have extragenital manifestations either with or without primary anogenital lesions (Fig. 2) (Bevans et al. 2017). Therefore complementation clinical assessment of the mouth, extragenital skin, and appendages can aid in diagnosis (Pérez-López and Vieira-Baptista 2017).

4 Histopathology

4.1 Morphea

Active morphea lesions are characterized by perivascular and periadnexal inflammatory infiltrates which can sometimes extend to the septae of subcutaneous fat. Infiltrates are commonly composed of lymphocytes, plasma cells, histiocytes, and eosinophils in the lower dermis scattered amongst collagen bundles (Florez-Pollack et al. 2018; Sehgal et al. 2002). Plasma cells are also apparent in the infiltrates. If eosinophils are present in the fascia, this may indicate an overlap with eosinophilic fasciitis. Inactive lesions show thinning of the epidermis and loss of adnexal structure (Florez-Pollack et al. 2018). Collagen changes, such as eosinophilia, broadening of collagen bundles, and a reduction in inter bundle spaces can be seen in the lower part of the dermis and subcutaneous tissue (Sehgal et al. 2002).

4.2 Lichen Sclerosus

Classical histological features of lichen sclerosus include epidermal atrophy, follicular plugging, dermal edema with deposition of homogenized collagen, and lichenoid lymphocytic infiltrate (Dalal et al. 2017).

5 Pathogenesis

5.1 Morphea

The etiology of morphea is not well understood. It has been suggested that an interplay between genetic and environmental factors contributes to the development of the disease. However, a clear scenario of the involvement of each factor remains to be elucidated and most of the theories are extrapolated from studies on scleroderma.

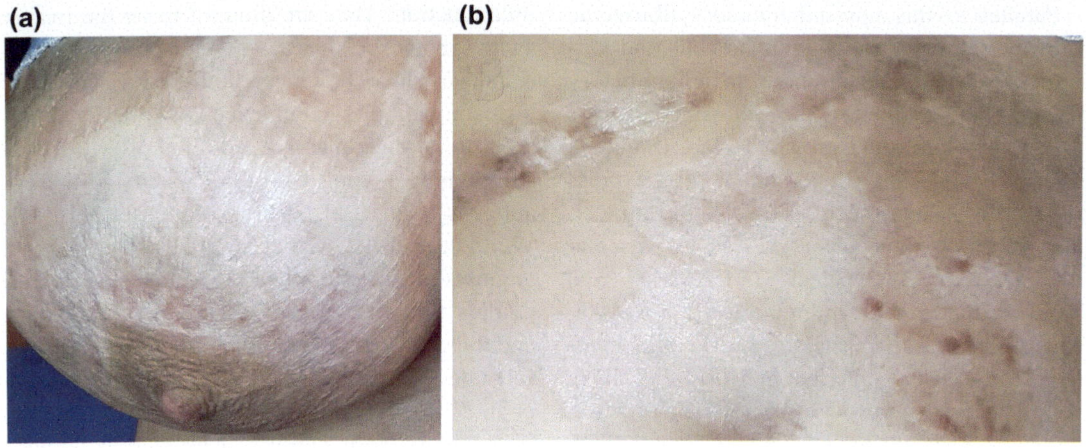

Fig. 2 Extragenital lichen sclerosus et atrophicus (LSA)

Perhaps the most widely agreed upon pathogenesis theory is the insult/dysregulated repair theory that applies to most of the diseases in the greater category of fibrotic disorders ranging from cirrhosis, cardiac, and pulmonary fibrosis to systemic sclerosis, morphea, and keloids (Stone et al. 2020). The distinct diseases in this vast category share many pathological pathways as apparent from cytokine profiling, genetic association, and transcriptome studies (Stone et al. 2020). This theory states that in susceptible individuals, site-specific injuries initiate an unbalanced inflammatory response that would persistently fuel fibrogenic pathways (Matucci-Cerinic et al. 2013). Though the endothelial lining of the small vessels is believed to be the initial site of injury in scleroderma and morphea recent studies have also highlighted the role of stressed keratinocytes (Abraham and Distler 2007; Kobayasi and Serup 1985; Nikitorowicz-Buniak et al. 2014; Saracino et al. 2017; Sartori-Valinotti and Tollefson 2013). Many environmental factors have been suggested to impose this stress including insect bites, trauma, vaccine and drug injections, radiation, and borrelial infection (Akay et al. 2010; Fett and Werth 2011; Goodlad et al. 2002; Grabell et al. 2014; Khaled et al. 2012; Peroni et al. 2008; Prinz et al. 2009). Endothelial injury can alter blood flow in small capillaries and induce tissue hypoxia. The reduced oxygen content in the cell cytoplasm decreases the proline hydroxylation of the hypoxia-inducible factor-α (HIFα) and thus rescues it from degradation by proteasomes. The HIFα would then enter the nucleus, form a heterodimer with HIFβ that is constitutively expressed in the nucleus, and initiate the transcription of genes with a hypoxia response element (HRE) at their promoters including genes encoding vascular endothelial growth factor (VEGF), transforming growth factor-β (TGFβ), and connective tissue growth factor (CTGF) (Kaelin and Ratcliffe 2008; Higgins et al. 2004; Kimura et al. 2000; Qian et al. 2015). TGFβ increases the production of collagen and proteoglycans and reduces the degradation of the extracellular matrix by inhibiting the matrix metalloproteinases (MMP) (Asano et al. 2006; Higley et al. 1994; Yamamoto 2006). While TGFβ is required for induction of fibrosis, the CTGF has a pivotal role in the maintenance of fibrosis (Mori et al. 1999). HIF also directly promotes collagen and extracellular matrix synthesis and is involved in the epithelial-to-mesenchymal transition of cells under hypoxic conditions which further assists fibrosis (Higgins et al. 2007; Xiong and Liu 2017). Multiple studies have been able to demonstrate the higher expression of HIFα, VEGF, CTGF, and TGFβ on sclerodermoid skin, and the role of TGFβ and CTGF in the pathogenesis of morphea is well documented (Igarashi et al. 1996; Ioannou et al. 2013; Leask et al. 2002).

Parallel to this non-inflammatory fibrogenic pathway, the insult on endothelial cells and keratinocytes could also promote an inflammatory cascade that facilitates the fibrosing process through cytokines and growth factors (Saracino et al. 2017). Damaged endothelial cells express adhesion molecules such as E-selectin, intracellular adhesion molecule-1 (ICAM-1), vascular cell adhesion molecule-1 (VCAM-1), and CXCL-8 that recruit immune cells (Wolska-Gawron et al. 2020). The stressed keratinocytes express S100A9, interleukin-1 (IL-1), IL-6, platelet-derived growth factor (PDGF) factor, tumor necrosis factor-α (TNFα), and CTGF (Russo et al. 2020; Saracino et al. 2017). The S100A9 protein activates toll-like receptor-4 (TLR4) and stimulates the production of type I interferon-dominant innate immune response (Magee et al. 2013; Nikitorowicz-Buniak et al. 2014). IL-1 and PDGF are known mediators of wound healing that promote fibroblast activation and collagen production. TLRs, in particular, TLR3 and 4 promote fibrosis through potentiating TGFβ and reducing the amount of anti-fibrosis micro-RNAs (miRNAs) (Bhattacharyya et al. 2012; Meyer et al. 2011; Nikitorowicz-Buniak et al. 2014).

Eventually, in the presence of intense TLR-stimulated type-I IFN response, dendritic cells (DC) can escape the tolerogenic signals and activate the adaptive immune response by presenting self-antigens to T-cells (Osmola-Mańkowska et al. 2015; Rajabi et al. 2018). Both plasmacytoid dendritic cells (PDCs) and myeloid dendritic cells (MDCs) are assumed to be involved (Osmola-Mańkowska et al. 2015). MDCs are the most common antigen-presenting cells residing in non-lymphoid tissue that constantly inspect their surrounding environment and upon encountering new antigens travel to lymph nodes to educate naïve T-cells. A subset of MDCs that express CD205, a scavenger receptor that uptakes self-antigens from apoptotic cells, are responsible for the induction of self-tolerance through promoting the differentiation of regulatory T-cells (T-reg) (Shrimpton et al. 2009; Tarbell et al. 2006). PDCs reside in lymphoid tissues and are recruited to the skin upon inflammation. They are thought to be the master switch between innate and adaptive immune responses since they carry both TLRs and major histocompatibility complexes (MHCs) enabling them to produce massive amounts of type I IFN (IFNα and β) along with the capacity to present antigens (Chu et al. 2011; Colonna et al. 2004; Werth et al. 1992; Wu et al. 2012). The massive amounts of TLR stimulated IFN release by PDCs renders the MDCs resistant to T-reg inhibition and thus by presenting autoantigens to T-cells the self-tolerance is breached (Osmola-Mańkowska et al. 2015). The role of DCs in the pathogenesis of the morphea is confirmed by studies demonstrating the infiltration of the PDCs and the strong type I IFN signature in morphea lesions plus the capability of type I IFNs (especially IFNβ) to induce morphea like lesions (Ghoreishi et al. 2012; Lee and Glassman 2016; Ozlu et al. 2019; Wollenberg et al. 2002).

In the primary inflammatory stages of morphea, the T helper-1 (Th1) response is dominant with its cytokines such as IL-2, IL-6, and TNFα (Torok et al. 2015). Humoral immunity is also involved from early on as apparent from the presence of autoantibodies (Badea et al. 2009; Khatri et al. 2019). IL-2 and IL-6 induce the production of Th17 cells marking the secondary fibrotic phase with the dominance of, IL-17, IL-22, and TGFβ (Kurzinski and Torok 2011). Subsequently, the increase in the number of Th2 mediated cytokines (IL-4 and IL-13) and B-cells mark the burnt-out atrophic phase of morphea (Torok et al. 2015). Many cytokines released throughout the disease can promote fibrosis. IL-1 and IL-6 promote fibroblast proliferation (Maas-Szabowski and Fusenig 1996), IL-17A, IL-17E, and IL-22 activate a profibrotic response in fibroblasts (Furuzawa-Carballeda et al. 2012), IL-4 and IL-13 induce collagen synthesis and reduce collagenase activity (Fedarko et al. 2000). Figure 3 summarizes the presumed pathogenic scenario of morphea.

In addition to the above-mentioned pathways, genome expression profiling has been able to demonstrate the involvement of chemokines and chemokine receptors such as CXCR3, CXCL9, CCL2, CCL18, and IFNγ inducible protein-10

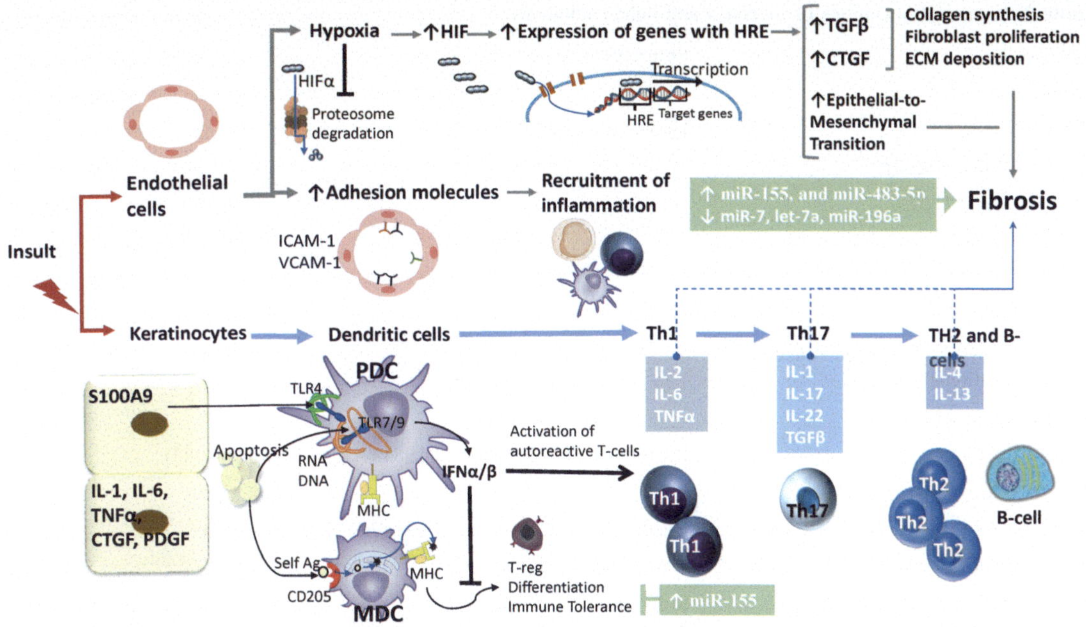

Fig. 3 The pathogenesis of morphea. HIF, hypoxia-inducible factor; TGFβ, transforming growth factor-beta; CTGF, connective tissue growth factor; ICAM-1, intercellular Adhesion Molecule-1; VCAM-1, vascular cell adhesion molecule-1; IL, interleukin; TNFα, tumor necrosis factor-alpha; PDGF, platelet-derived growth factor; PDC, plasmacytoid dendritic cell; MDC, myeloid dendritic cell; IFN, interferon; Th, T helper; TLR, toll-like receptor

(IP-10, also known as CXCL10) in the pathogenesis of morphea (Mertens et al. 2019; O'Brien et al. 2017; Saracino et al. 2017).

5.2 The Immunogenetics of Morphea

As mentioned earlier, the whole pathogenic process in morphea is a derailment from a regular healing process by a stimulus that results in tissue hypoxia. In normal circumstances, the inflammation would resolve to leave behind a somewhat normal amount of fibrous tissue. But in a susceptible individual defective tissue remodeling and/or a continuous inflammatory cycle would allow widespread fibrosis to ensue. This vicious cycle continues with extensive microangiopathy and progressive narrowing of the vessel lumens that intensifies hypoxia.

The susceptibility to morphea has been attributed to both genetic and epigenetic factors. Hypothetically, genes could affect the pathogenesis through two main paths, polymorphisms in genes involved in immunological, fibrotic, and anti-fibrotic pathways, and postzygotic mutations resulting in mosaicism.

Very few studies have investigated single nucleotide polymorphisms in individuals with morphea and thus only the association of morphea with human leucocyte antigen (HLA) subtypes have been confirmed (Table 2). The *HLA-DQA1*03:01*, *DRB1*04:04*, *DQA1*03:00*, *DRB1*03:01*, and *DQB1*02:01* from MHC class II and *HLA-B*37*, *C*08*, and *C*15* from MHC class I cluster confer susceptibility to morphea (Jacobe et al. 2014). Within these alleles, the HLA-DRB1*04:04 and HLAB*37 have the highest association with morphea, and HLA-DRB1*15:01 confers susceptibility to the generalized subtype of morphea (Jacobe et al. 2014).

Some of these alleles also confer susceptibility to other autoimmune diseases such as

Table 2 Genetic associations of morphea and lichen sclerosus

Disease		References
Morphea		
HLA-	*DRB1*04*	Jacobe et al. (2014)
	*DRB1*03:01*	
	*DQB1*02:01*	
	*B*37*	
	*C*08*	
	*C*15*	
	*DRB1*15:01* (generalized subtype)	
Lichen sclerosus		
HLA-	*B40*	Harrington and Gelsthorpe (1981), Pa and Darke (1983)
	Aw31	
	B44	Friedrich and MacLaren (1984), Purcell et al. (1990)
	BRW6	
	B21	Sideri et al. (1988)
	DR5	
	DR7	
	A29	Purcell et al. (1990)
	B8	
	DR3	
	DQ7	Azurdia et al. (1999), Farrell et al. (2000), Marren et al. (1995), Powell et al. (2000)
	DQ8	
	DQ9	
	DR11	Azurdia et al. (1999)
	DR12	
	*B*08*	Şentürk et al. (2004)
	*B*18*	
	*DRB1*12*	Gao et al. (2005)
	*B*15*	Aslanian et al. (2006)
	*B*57*	
	*CW*03*	
	*CW*07*	
	*CW*18*	
	*DRB1*04*	
	*BRB1*07*	
	DRB4	
	*A*11*	Liu et al. (2015)
	*B*13*	
	*B*15*	
Interleukin 1 receptor antagonist		Clay et al. (1994)

*DRB1*04:04* for rheumatoid arthritis (RA), *DRB1*15:01* for multiple sclerosis (MS) *DRB1*03:01* for diabetes mellitus type I, and *DQB1*02:01*, *DRB1*03:01*, and *DRB1*04* for autoimmune thyroid disease (Leitenberger et al. 2009; Oksenberg et al. 2001; Simmonds and Gough 2004; Weyand et al. 1992). The co-occurrence of morphea and RA, autoimmune thyroid disease, and MS has also been confirmed in population-based studies (Leitenberger et al. 2009). Up to 46% of patients diagnosed with morphea, especially those with the generalized or linear subtype, have a personal or family history of autoimmune disease (Christen-Zaech et al. 2008; Pequet et al. 2014; Zulian et al. 2006) and nearly half of them have elevated levels of anti-nuclear antibodies (ANA), anti-histone antibodies (AHA), and/or anti-ssDNA (Khatri et al. 2019).

It has been hypothesized that genetic mosaicism may explain the regional genetic vulnerability in linear morphea. Genetic mosaicism could perhaps alter the keratinocyte- fibroblast communication or it could trigger an immune response by expressing antigenic diversity (Attili and Attili 2013; Paller 2007; Saracino et al. 2017). However, there is no actual evidence of the presence of genetic mosaicism in linear morphea besides the blaschkoid pattern of the lesions (Jue et al. 2011; Molho-Pessach and Schaffer 2011).

Epigenetic mechanisms including DNA methylation, histone acetylation, and non-coding RNA regulations are involved in the pathogenesis of autoimmune diseases by altering gene expression. The genetic regulation by non-coding micro-RNAs (miRNA) is the most extensively studied epigenetic mechanism in morphea and scleroderma. These small nucleotide chains bind to messenger-RNA (mRNA) molecules and based on their complementarity either repress their translation or initiate their degradation. The miRNAs can affect fibrotic and anti-fibrotic pathways by targeting TFGβ, CTGF, epithelial-to-mesenchymal transition, and myofibroblast proliferation. Alteration in the pattern of miRNA expression has been documented in morpheic lesions with lower levels of miR-7, miRNA let-7a, and miR-196a along with higher levels of miR-155, and miR-483-5p. The first three sets of miRNAs (miR-7, miRNA let-7a, and miR-196a) possess anti-fibrotic properties by lowering the production of type I collagen (Wolska-Gawron et al. 2020). The miR-155 up-regulates the epithelial-to-mesenchymal transition and is thus considered pro-fibrotic (Paul et al. 2018). The miR-483-5p promotes myofibroblast differentiation it also negatively regulates an extracellular matrix inhibitor known as friend leukemia virus integration-1 (Fli-1) (Chouri et al. 2018). Elevated levels of miR-155 can also reduce the activity of T-reg cells (Corthay 2009).

5.3 Lichen Sclerosus

Much like morphea, the pathogenesis of lichen sclerosus is not very well understood. There is a lot of evidence that points to the involvement of autoimmunity in the pathogenesis of lichen sclerosus including the highly common co-occurrence of autoimmune diseases such as thyroiditis, alopecia areata, vitiligo, and pernicious anemia (Cooper et al. 2008; Kreuter et al. 2013), the lymphocytic infiltration beneath the hyalinized collagen in early stages (Niamh et al. 2009), the presence of autoantibodies in up 74% of female cases of lichen sclerosus (Oyama et al. 2003), and the autoimmune signature of the gene expression profile (Edmonds et al. 2011; Terlou et al. 2012). The gene expression and immunohistochemical studies also demonstrate an integral role in fibrogenic pathways (Carli et al. 1997; Edmonds et al. 2011; Gambichler et al. 2012). It has been suggested that an interplay between genetic and environmental factors simultaneously activates these two main pathways (Fergus et al. 2020; Tran et al. 2019).

The most important environmental trigger of lichen sclerosus is the occluded contact with urine in situations that are associated with post-micturition micro-incontinence or ineffective cleaning of the skin such as lack of circumcision, presence of exaggerated skin folding in female obese patients, pseudo-foreskin in obese male patients, and areas near urostomies (Al-Niaimi and Lyon 2013; Doiron and Bunker 2017; Erickson et al. 2016b; Gupta et al. 2010; Shim et al. 2012). Contact with urine explains the predilection of the lesions to the genital area and the substantially higher rate of lichen sclerosus in uncircumscribed men.

Other environmental triggering factors include skin irritation associated with urethritis, balanitis, catheterization, surgeries, sunburn, radiation, and frequent friction due to higher body mass index and genital jewelry (Bjekić et al. 2011; Bunker 2013; Erickson et al. 2016a; Hofer et al. 2014; Milligan et al. 1988; Yates et al. 1985). Lastly, some studies have drawn an association between different infectious agents and lichen sclerosus including Borrelia burgdorferi, Epstein Barr virus (EBV), and human papillomavirus (HPV) (Eisendle et al. 2008; Fergus et al. 2020; Zhang et al. 2016).

The precise scenario in which the triggering factors could provoke autoimmunity and fibrogenesis is not well elucidated. It has been postulated that they could promote sustained inflammation and fibrogenesis through the formation of reactive oxygen species (ROS) (Sander et al. 2004).

High levels of superoxide anions can epigenetically silence the expression of antioxidant enzymes such as superoxide dismutase (SOD) which creates a positive feedback loop that further increases ROS (Cyr et al. 2013). The ROS promotes fibrosis through multiple pathways with positive feedforward and feedback loops (Richter and Kietzmann 2016). The ROS-forming reactions can alter the functions of DNA/histone demethylase enzymes by consuming their cofactors. Thus the epigenetic landscape is reformed in a way that could promote fibrosis. These epigenetic changes could also explain the neoplastic transformation in fibrotic disorders (Cyr et al. 2013; Richter and Kietzmann 2016). ROS can promote fibrosis by directly facilitating the release of active TGFβ from the latent TGFβ complex (Jobling et al. 2006). TGFβ, in turn, increases the amount of ROS by inducing the expression of ROS-producing enzymes such as NOX4 (NAD (P) H oxidase) and decreasing the expression of antioxidant enzymes such as glutathione (GSH) (Arsalane et al. 1997; Sturrock et al. 2006; Tiitto et al. 2004). NOX4 also contributes to fibrosis by activating the myofibroblasts (Hecker et al. 2009).

ROS damages proteins, lipids, and nucleic acids through different chemical reactions (Sander et al. 2004). Oxidative stress causes DNA fragmentation, telomere erosion, and alters the nucleic acid translation and transcription processes (Guachalla and Rudolph 2010). The accumulation of DNA damage could result in cell-cycle arrest and apoptosis through the production of tumor suppressor proteins such as $p16^{INK4}$, and $p27^{Kip1}$ (Zannoni et al. 2006). The increased rate of apoptosis could provoke autoimmunity by allowing the immune system to encounter sequestered intracellular antigens. The inflammatory response caused by the autoimmune attack, on the other hand, boosts the development of ROS and thus creates a positive feedback loop (Chen et al. 2016). DNA damage could also result in genetic mutation of tumor suppressor genes such as P53 and thus explain the malignant transformation in lichen sclerosus (Gambichler et al. 2011; Hantschmann et al. 2005; Rolfe et al. 2003).

The peroxidation of intra- and extracellular lipids produces 4-hydroxynonenal (4-HNE) and malondialdehyde (MDA). These unsaturated aldehydes can provoke autoimmunity by attaching to proteins and forming neo-antigens (Amara et al. 1995; Vay et al. 2001). These protein adducts can also promote mutagenesis (Marnett 1999).

Oxidation can directly alter the three-dimensional structure of proteins. This post-transcriptional modification creates neo-epitopes that can engage with the pattern recognition receptors (PRR) of the innate immune system (Ryan et al. 2014).

Along with the ROS-mediated activation of the innate immune responses, the environmental triggers could also directly stimulate innate immunity. Two antimicrobial peptides (AMP) related to the innate response, human beta-defensin-2 (HBD-2) and psoriasin are highly expressed in lichen sclerosus lesions (Gambichler et al. 2009). These peptides are increased in response to colonization of *Escherichia coli*, *Pseudomonas aeruginosa*, and *Candida albicans* in macerated areas (Schittek et al. 2008). Psoriasin and HBD-2 can induce the expression of various inflammatory cytokines and chemoattractants that recruit neutrophils and T-cells (Niyonsaba et al. 2007; Zheng et al. 2008). Studies on lichen sclerosus lesions have also documented an increased infiltration of plasmacytoid dendritic cells and elevated levels of innate immunity cytokines such as type I IFN, CXCR3, and IP-10 (Wenzel 2007). The sustained stimulation of the innate immune system and the aberrant expression of AMPs could contribute to the progression to autoimmunity by promoting the adaptive immune responses (Liang and Diana 2020; Zhang and Yang 2020).

Lichen sclerosus is a Th1 dominant disease with high expression levels of IL-1, IL-2, IL-5, IL-7, IL-10, IL-12, IL-15, TNFα, and IFNγ, increased levels of perforin and granzyme-B, and clonal expansion of T-cell against the NC16A domain of bullous pemphigoid antigen 180 kDa (BP180) (Baldo et al. 2010; Gross et al. 2001; Terlou et al. 2012).

The B-cell mediated humoral immunity is also involved in the pathogenesis of lichen sclerosus. Circulating antibodies against the extracellular matrix 1 (ECM1) and BP180 are present in the sera of patients with lichen sclerosus (Oyama et al. 2003). However, the passive transfer of anti-ECM1 antibodies is only able to induce some of the pathological features of lichen sclerosus such as edema, dilated blood vessels, and inflammation without the prominent hyalinosis and scarring (Oyama et al. 2004). It has been postulated that the autoantibodies contribute to the progression of the already established disease by interfering with the functions of ECM1. The ECM1 is a soluble glycoprotein that is ubiquitously expressed throughout all layers of the skin. The ECM1 is connected to multiple molecules such as collagen-4, plectin, TGFβ, fibronectin, fibulin-3, laminin 332, MMP-9, cartilage oligomeric matrix protein (COMP), chondroitin sulfate, and hyaluronic acid (Oyama and Merregaert 2017) and is thus involved in numerous functions such as dermo-epidermal communication, keratinocyte differentiation, angiogenesis, tumor progression, and T-cell mediated immune responses (Oyama and Merregaert 2017). An analysis of the sera of patients with lichen sclerosus demonstrated heterogenous IgG reactivity toward different parts of the ECM1 molecule but the distal COOH-terminus (amino acids 359 to 559) was the most common epitope (Oyama et al. 2004). Though only COMP, perlecan, heparin, chondroitin sulfate, and hyaluronic acid directly bind to the C-terminal of the ECM1 protein, its interaction with other molecules is also tampered because of the structural changes instilled upon ECM1 through antibody binding (Oyama and Merregaert 2017). Hypothetically, anti-ECM1 antibodies could disturb its connections to MMP9, allowing unleashed activity of the enzyme dissolving the extracellular matrix and releasing growth factors such as TGFβ, tumstatin, and perlecan. TFGβ increases collagen production and a perlecan-derived molecule with antiangiogenetic capacities known as endorepellin promote the vascular changes of lichen sclerosus (Fujimoto et al. 2006). The lesion of lichen sclerosus also demonstrates decreased levels of angiogenic vascular endothelial growth factor (VEGF) which could further explain the disorganization of the capillary architectural (Li et al. 2009). The vascular changes are associated with reduced blood supply to the skin and hypoxia. The hypoxia results in ultrastructural changes in oxygen-dependent organelles such as mitochondria and endoplasmic reticulum and increased expression of glucose transporter-1 (Glut-1) which is a marker of metabolic adaptation to hypoxia and anaerobic glycolysis (Li et al. 2009). Hypoxia-related stress could also explain the increased expression of P53 in lesions of lichen sclerosus (Liegl and Regauer 2006). P53 induces the expression of a glycan-binding protein known as Galectin-7 (Chen et al. 2004). Galectin-7 is expressed throughout the epidermis (both in the nucleus and in the cytoplasm) and is involved in apoptosis and epidermal hemostasis after injury (Bernerd et al. 1999; Gendronneau et al. 2008; Zhao et al. 2018). In lichen sclerosus, galectin-7 contributes to the progression of fibrosis (Zhao et al. 2018). It increased the expression of type I and III collagen and reduces the viability of fibroblasts (Zhao et al. 2018). Galectin-7 also possesses proinflammatory properties. It enhances the proliferation of activated CD4+ T-cells and promotes a Th1 polarization through increasing the production of IFNγ and TNFα and decreasing the production of IL-10 (Luo et al. 2018). On the molecular level the proinflammatory functions of the Galectin-7 are attributed to the blockade of TGF-Smad3 pathway (Luo et al. 2018).

5.4 The Immunogenetics of Lichen Sclerosus

As mentioned earlier, genetic susceptibility plays an integral role in the pathogenesis of lichen sclerosus. Over 10% of patients with lichen sclerosus report relatives with the same disease (Sherman et al. 2010). An association with HLA genes has also been documented in multiple studies (Table 2) (Fergus et al. 2020). Two class II HLAs, *HLA-DQ7* and *HLA-DRB1*0201*, occur more frequently in patients with lichen sclerosus (Marren et al. 1995; Setterfield et al. 2006). *HLA-DQ8* and *DQ9* have been found more frequently in female patients and *HLA-DR11* and *DR12* were more common in males. Other genetic associations that have been reported include *HLA-B*08–B*18*, *-B*15*, *-B*57*, *-CW*03*, *-CW*07*, *-CW*18*, *-DRB1*04*, *-DRB4**, *-DRB1*07*, *-DRB1*12*, and the haplotype *DRB1*12/DQB1*0301/04/09/010* (Fistarol and Itin 2013; Gao et al. 2005; Marren et al. 1995). Individuals with *HLA-DR17* have a lower risk for developing lichen sclerosus and those with *HLA-DRB1*13* are less likely to have an accompanying autoimmune disease (Gao et al. 2005). Variable tandem repeat polymorphisms within the gene encoding interleukin-1 receptor antagonist (IL1RN) are also associated with susceptibility to lichen sclerosus (Clay et al. 1994).

Epigenetic inheritance such micro-RNAs also contribute to the pathogenesis of lichen sclerosus. High levels of miR-155 have been detected in lesions of lichen sclerosus (Terlou et al. 2012). The mi-155, as mentioned previously in the pathogenesis of morphea, possesses multiple regulatory functions. The overexpression of miR-155 promotes autoimmunity by disrupting the production of IL-10 by T-regs, decreasing the susceptibility of CD4+ T-cells toward T-regs, and skewing the immune response toward Th1 (Corthay 2009; Terlou et al. 2012). Though the number of T-regs does not significantly differ between lichen sclerosus lesions and normal skin, their functions and the production of immune regulatory cytokines such as IL-10 are lower in lichen sclerosus (Terlou et al. 2012). The miR-155 is also involved in the progression of sclerosis (Ren et al. 2018). The increased production of collagen and the accelerated proliferation of fibroblasts are attributed to the down-regulation of two tumor suppressors, *FOXO3* and *CDKN1B*, by miR-155 (Ren et al. 2018).

6 Conclusion

Due to the substantial shortage of genetic studies on morphea and LSA, our knowledge about the contribution of genes to disease susceptibility is limited. Thus far only specific HLAs have been linked to morphea and LSA which do not provide meaningful insight into the pathogenic mechanisms. This might reflect the fact that both diseases are relatively rare and have little familial clustering that might underestimate the involvement of inheritance. Future investigations should focus on screening for polymorphisms in other genes besides the HLAs using modalities such as genome association studies.

References

Abraham D, Distler O (2007) How does endothelial cell injury start? The role of endothelin in systemic sclerosis. Arthritis Res Ther 9:1–8

Akay B, Sanli H, Heper A (2010) Postirradiation linear morphoea. Clin Exp Dermatol Clin Dermatol 35: e106–e108

Al-Niaimi F, Lyon C (2013) Peristomal lichen sclerosus: the role of occlusion and urine exposure? Br J Dermatol 168:643–646

Amara A, Constans J, Chaugier C, Sebban A, Dubourg L, Peuchant E, Pellegrin JL, Leng B, Conri C, Geffard M (1995) Autoantibodies to malondialdehyde-modified epitope in connective tissue diseases and vasculitides. Clin Exp Immunol 101:233–238

Arsalane K, Dubois CM, Muanza T, Bégin R, Boudreau F, Asselin C, Cantin AM (1997) Transforming growth factor-β1 is a potent inhibitor of glutathione synthesis in the lung epithelial cell line A549: transcriptional effect on the GSH rate-limiting enzyme γ-glutamylcysteine synthetase. Am J Respir Cell Mol Biol 17:599–607

Asano Y, Ihn H, Jinnin M, Mimura Y, Tamaki K (2006) Involvement of αvβ5 integrin in the establishment of autocrine TGF-β signaling in dermal fibroblasts derived from localized scleroderma. J Investig Dermatol 126:1761–1769

Aslanian FM, Marques MTQ, Matos HJ, Pontes LF, Porto LCS, Azevedo LM, Filgueira AL (2006) HLA markers in familial lichen sclerosus. JDDG Journal der Deutschen Dermatologischen Gesellschaft 4:842–847

Attili VR, Attili SK (2013) Segmental and generalized vitiligo: both forms demonstrate inflammatory histopathological features and clinical mosaicism. Indian J Dermatol 58:433

Azurdia R, Luzzi G, Byren I, Welsh K, Wojnarowska F, Marren P, Edwards A (1999) Lichen sclerosus in adult men: a study of HLA associations and susceptibility to autoimmune disease. Br J Dermatol 140:79–83

Badea I, Taylor M, Rosenberg A, Foldvari M (2009) Pathogenesis and therapeutic approaches for improved topical treatment in localized scleroderma and systemic sclerosis. Rheumatology 48:213–221

Baldo M, Bailey A, Bhogal B, Groves R, Ogg G, Wojnarowska F (2010) T cells reactive with the NC16A domain of BP180 are present in vulval lichen sclerosus and lichen planus. J Eur Acad Dermatol Venereol 24:186–190

Bernerd F, Sarasin A, Magnaldo T (1999) Galectin-7 overexpression is associated with the apoptotic process in UVB-induced sunburn keratinocytes. Proc Natl Acad Sci 96:11329–11334

Bevans SL, Keeley JM, Sami N (2017) Oral lichen sclerosus—a review of clinical presentation, treatment, and clinical outcomes. Oral Surg Oral Med Oral Pathol Oral Radiol 124:e243–e248

Bhattacharyya S, Wei J, Varga J (2012) Understanding fibrosis in systemic sclerosis: shifting paradigms, emerging opportunities. Nat Rev Rheumatol 8:42

Bjekić M, Šipetić S, Marinković J (2011) Risk factors for genital lichen sclerosus in men. Br J Dermatol 164:325–329

Bunker C (2013) Atopy, the barrier, urine and genital lichen sclerosus. Br J Dermatol 1951:169

Carli P, Moretti S, Spallanzani A, Berti E, Cattaneo A (1997) Fibrogenic cytokines in vulvar lichen sclerosus. An immunohistochemical study. J Reprod Med 42:161–165

Chen J, He QY, Yuen APW, Chiu JF (2004) Proteomics of buccal squamous cell carcinoma: the involvement of multiple pathways in tumorigenesis. Proteomics 4:2465–2475

Chen X, Song M, Zhang B, Zhang Y (2016) Reactive oxygen species regulate T cell immune response in the tumor microenvironment. Oxidative Med Cell Longev

Chouri E, Servaas NH, Bekker CP, Affandi AJ, Cossu M, Hillen MR, Angiolilli C, Mertens JS, van den Hoogen LL, Silva-Cardoso S (2018) Serum microRNA screening and functional studies reveal miR-483-5p as a potential driver of fibrosis in systemic sclerosis. J Autoimmun 89:162–170

Christen-Zaech S, Hakim MD, Afsar FS, Paller AS (2008) Pediatric morphea (localized scleroderma): review of 136 patients. J Am Acad Dermatol 59:385–396

Chu S-Y, Chen Y-J, Tseng W-C, Lin M-W, Chen T-J, Hwang C-Y, Chen C-C, Lee D-D, Chang Y-T, Wang W-J (2011) Comorbidity profiles among patients with alopecia areata: the importance of onset age, a nationwide population-based study. J Am Acad Dermatol 65:949–956

Clay FE, Cork MJ, Tarlow JK, Blakemore AI, Harrington CI, Lewis F, Duff GW (1994) Interleukin 1 receptor antagonist gene polymorphism association with lichen sclerosus. Hum Genet 94:407–410

Colonna M, Trinchieri G, Liu Y-J (2004) Plasmacytoid dendritic cells in immunity. Nat Immunol 5:1219–1226

Cooper SM, Ali I, Baldo M, Wojnarowska F (2008) The association of lichen sclerosus and erosive lichen planus of the vulva with autoimmune disease: a case-control study. Arch Dermatol 144:1432–1435

Corthay A (2009) How do regulatory T cells work? Scand J Immunol 70:326–336

Cyr AR, Hitchler MJ, Domann FE (2013) Regulation of SOD2 in cancer by histone modifications and CpG methylation: closing the loop between redox biology and epigenetics. Antioxid Redox Signal 18:1946–1955

Dalal V, Kaur M, Rai CB, Singh A, Ramesh V (2017) Histopathological spectrum of lichen sclerosus Et atrophicus. Indian J Dermatopathol Diagnos Dermatol 4:8

Das A, Gupta S, Singh S, Pant L (2016) Coexisting morphea with lichen sclerosus et atrophicus in a single lesion-a rare case report. Bangladesh J Med Sci 15:145–147

Dharamsi JW, Victor S, Aguwa N, Ahn C, Arnett F, Mayes MD, Jacobe H (2013) Morphea in adults and children cohort III: nested case-control study—the clinical significance of autoantibodies in morphea. JAMA Dermatol 149:1159–1165

Doiron P, Bunker C (2017) Obesity-related male genital lichen sclerosus. J Eur Acad Dermatol Venereol 31:876–879

Edmonds E, Barton G, Buisson S, Francis N, Gotch F, Game L, Haddad M, Dinneen M, Bunker C (2011)

Gene expression profiling in male genital lichen sclerosus. Int J Exp Pathol 92:320–325

Eisendle K, Grabner T, Kutzner H, Zelger B (2008) Possible role of borreliaburgdorferi sensu lato infection in lichen sclerosus. Arch Dermatol 144:591–598

Erickson B, Elliott S, Myers J, Voelzke B, Smith T 3rd, McClung C, Alsikafi N, Vanni A, Brant W, Broghammer J (2016a) Trauma and urologic reconstructive network of surgeons. Understanding the relationship between chronic systemic disease and lichen sclerosus urethral strictures. J Urol 195:363–368

Erickson BA, Elliott SP, Myers JB, Voelzke BB, Smith TG, McClung CD, Alsikafi NF, Vanni AJ, Brant WO, Broghammer JA (2016b) Understanding the relationship between chronic systemic disease and lichen sclerosus urethral strictures. J Urol 195:363–368

Farrell A, Marren P, Wojnarowska F (2000) Genital lichen sclerosus associated with morphoea or systemic sclerosis: clinical and HLA characteristics. Br J Dermatol 143:598–603

Fedarko NS, Pacocha SE, Huang S-K, Lichtenstein LM, Essayan DM (2000) Interleukin-13 modulates collagen homeostasis in human skin and keloid fibroblasts. J Pharmacol Exp Ther 292:988–994

Fergus KB, Lee AW, Baradaran N, Cohen AJ, Stohr BA, Erickson BA, Mmonu NA, Breyer BN (2020) Pathophysiology, clinical manifestations, and treatment of lichen sclerosus: a systematic review. Urology 135:11–19

Fett NM (2013) Morphea (localized scleroderma). JAMA Dermatol 149:1124–1124

Fett N, Werth VP (2011) Update on morphea: part I. Epidemiology, clinical presentation, and pathogenesis. J Am Acad Dermatol 64:217–228

Fistarol SK, Itin PH (2013) Diagnosis and treatment of lichen sclerosus. Am J Clin Dermatol 14:27–47

Florez-Pollack S, Kunzler E, Jacobe HT (2018) Morphea: current concepts. Clin Dermatol 36:475–486

Friedrich EG Jr, MacLaren NK (1984) Genetic aspects of vulvar lichen sclerosus. Am J Obstet Gynecol 150:161–166

Fujimoto N, Terlizzi J, Aho S, Brittingham R, Fertala A, Oyama N, McGrath JA, Uitto J (2006) Extracellular matrix protein 1 inhibits the activity of matrix metalloproteinase 9 through high-affinity protein/protein interactions. Exp Dermatol 15:300–307

Furuzawa-Carballeda J, Ortíz-Ávalos M, Lima G, Jurado-Santa Cruz F, Llorente L (2012) Subcutaneous administration of polymerized type I collagen downregulates interleukin (IL)-17A, IL-22 and transforming growth factor-β1 expression, and increases Foxp3-expressing cells in localized scleroderma. Clin Exp Dermatol Clin Dermatol 37:599–609

Gambichler T, Skrygan M, Tigges C, Kobus S, Gläser R, Kreuter A (2009) Significant upregulation of antimicrobial peptides and proteins in lichen sclerosus. Br J Dermatol 161:1136–1142

Gambichler T, Kammann S, Tigges C, Kobus S, Skrygan M, Meier JJ, Köhler CU, Scola N, Stücker M, Bechara FG (2011) Cell cycle regulation and proliferation in lichen sclerosus. Regul Pept 167:209–214

Gambichler T, Skrygan M, Czempiel V, Tigges C, Kobus S, Meier J, Köhler C, Scola N, Stücker M, Altmeyer P (2012) Differential expression of connective tissue growth factor and extracellular matrix proteins in lichen sclerosus. J Eur Acad Dermatol Venereol 26:207–212

Gao X-H, Barnardo MC, Winsey S, Ahmad T, Cook J, Agudelo JD, Zhai N, Powell JJ, Fuggle SV, Wojnarowska F (2005) The association between HLA DR, DQ antigens, and vulval lichen sclerosus in the UK: HLA DRB1* 12 and its associated DRB1* 12/DQB1* 0301/04/09/010 haplotype confers susceptibility to vulval lichen sclerosus, and HLA DRB1* 0301/04 and its associated DRB1* 0301/04/DQB1* 0201/02/03 haplotype protects from vulval lichen sclerosus. J Investig Dermatol 125:895–899

Gendronneau G, Sidhu SS, Delacour D, Dang T, Calonne C, Houzelstein D, Magnaldo T, Poirier F (2008) Galectin-7 in the control of epidermal homeostasis after injury. Mol Biol Cell 19:5541–5549

Ghoreishi M, Vera Kellet C, Dutz JP (2012) Type 1 IFN-induced protein MxA and plasmacytoid dendritic cells in lesions of morphea. Exp Dermatol 21:417–419

Goodlad J, Davidson M, Gordon P, Billington R, Ho-Yen D (2002) Morphoea and Borrelia burgdorferi: results from the Scottish Highlands in the context of the world literature. Mol Pathol 55:374

Grabell D, Hsieh C, Andrew R, Martires K, Kim A, Vasquez R, Jacobe H (2014) The role of skin trauma in the distribution of morphea lesions: a cross-sectional survey of the Morphea in Adults and Children cohort IV. J Am Acad Dermatol 71:493–498

Gross T, Wagner A, Ugurel S, Tilgen W, Reinhold U (2001) Identification of TIA-1+ and granzyme B+ cytotoxic T cells in lichen sclerosus et atrophicus. Dermatology 202:198–202

Guachalla LM, Rudolph KL (2010) ROS induced DNA damage and checkpoint responses: influences on aging? Cell Cycle 9:4058–4060

Gupta S, Malhotra AK, Ajith C (2010) Lichen sclerosus: role of occlusion of the genital skin in the pathogenesis. Indian J Dermatol Venereol Leprol 76:56

Hantschmann P, Sterzer S, Jeschke U, Friese K (2005) P53 expression in vulvar carcinoma, vulvar intraepithelial neoplasia, squamous cell hyperplasia and lichen sclerosus. Anticancer Res 25:1739–1745

Harrington CI, Gelsthorpe K (1981) The association between lichen sclerosus et atrophicus and HLA-B40. Br J Dermatol 104:561–562

Hecker L, Vittal R, Jones T, Jagirdar R, Luckhardt TR, Horowitz JC, Pennathur S, Martinez FJ, Thannickal VJ (2009) NADPH oxidase-4 mediates myofibroblast activation and fibrogenic responses to lung injury. Nat Med 15:1077–1081

Higgins DF, Biju MP, Akai Y, Wutz A, Johnson RS, Haase VH (2004) Hypoxic induction of Ctgf is directly mediated by Hif-1. Am J Physiol Renal Physiol 287:F1223–F1232

Higgins DF, Kimura K, Bernhardt WM, Shrimanker N, Akai Y, Hohenstein B, Saito Y, Johnson RS, Kretzler M, Cohen CD (2007) Hypoxia promotes fibrogenesis in vivo via HIF-1 stimulation of epithelial-to-mesenchymal transition. J Clin Investig 117:3810–3820

Higley H, Persichitte K, Chu S, Waegell W, Vancheeswaran R, Black C (1994) Immunocytochemical localization and serologic detection of transforming growth factor β1. Arthritis Rheum Off J Am Coll Rheumatol 37:278–288

Hofer MD, Meeks JJ, Mehdiratta N, Granieri MA, Cashy J, Gonzalez CM (2014) Lichen sclerosus in men is associated with elevated body mass index, diabetes mellitus, coronary artery disease and smoking. World J Urol 32:105–108

Igarashi A, Nashiro K, Kikuchi K, Sato S, Ihn H, Fujimoto M, Grotendorst GR, Takehara K (1996) Connective tissue growth factor gene expression in tissue sections from localized scleroderma, keloid, and other fibrotic skin disorders. J Investig Dermatol 106:729–733

Ioannou M, Pyrpasopoulou A, Simos G, Paraskeva E, Nikolaidou C, Venizelos I, Koukoulis G, Aslanidis S, Douma S (2013) Upregulation of VEGF expression is associated with accumulation of HIF-1α in the skin of naive scleroderma patients. Mod Rheumatol 23:1245–1248

Jacobe H, Ahn C, Arnett FC, Reveille JD (2014) Major histocompatibility complex class I and class II alleles may confer susceptibility to or protection against morphea: findings from the Morphea in Adults and Children cohort. Arthritis Rheumatol 66:3170–3177

Jobling MF, Mott JD, Finnegan MT, Jurukovski V, Erickson AC, Walian PJ, Taylor SE, Ledbetter S, Lawrence CM, Rifkin DB (2006) Isoform-specific activation of latent transforming growth factor β (LTGF-β) by reactive oxygen species. Radiat Res 166:839–848

Jue MS, Kim MH, Ko JY, Lee CW (2011) Digital image processing for the acquisition of graphic similarity of the distributional patterns between cutaneous lesions of linear scleroderma and Blaschko's lines. J Dermatol 38:778–783

Kaelin WG Jr, Ratcliffe PJ (2008) Oxygen sensing by metazoans: the central role of the HIF hydroxylase pathway. Mol Cell 30:393–402

Khaled A, Kharfi M, Zaouek A, Rameh S, Zermani R, Fazaa B, Kamoun MR (2012) Postvaccination morphea profunda in a child. Pediatr Dermatol 29:525–527

Khatri S, Torok KS, Mirizio E, Liu C, Astakhova K (2019) Autoantibodies in morphea: an update. Front Immunol 10:1487

Kimura H, Weisz A, Kurashima Y, Hashimoto K, Ogura T, D'Acquisto F, Addeo R, Makuuchi M, Esumi H (2000) Hypoxia response element of the human vascular endothelial growth factor gene mediates transcriptional regulation by nitric oxide: control of hypoxia-inducible factor-1 activity by nitric oxide. Blood J Am Soc Hematol 95:189–197

Kirtschig G (2016) Lichen sclerosus–Beratungsanlass, Diagnose und therapeutisches Procedere. Deutsches Ärzteblatt 113:337–343

Kobayasi T, Serup J (1985) Vascular changes in morphea. Acta Derm-Venereol 65:116–120

Kreuter A, Wischnewski J, Terras S, Altmeyer P, Stücker M, Gambichler T (2012) Coexistence of lichen sclerosus and morphea: a retrospective analysis of 472 patients with localized scleroderma from a German tertiary referral center. J Am Acad Dermatol 67:1157–1162

Kreuter A, Kryvosheyeva Y, Terras S, Moritz R, MöLLENHOff K, Altmeyer P, Scola N, Gambichler T (2013) Association of autoimmune diseases with lichen sclerosus in 532 male and female patients. Acta Derm Venereol 93:238–241

Kurzinski K, Torok KS (2011) Cytokine profiles in localized scleroderma and relationship to clinical features. Cytokine 55:157–164

Leask A, Holmes A, Abraham DJ (2002) Connective tissue growth factor: a new and important player in the pathogenesis of fibrosis. Curr Rheumatol Rep 4:136–142

Lee EY, Glassman SJ (2016) Deep morphea induced by interferon-β1b injection. JAAD Case Reports 2:236–238

Leitenberger JJ, Cayce RL, Haley RW, Adams-Huet B, Bergstresser PR, Jacobe HT (2009) Distinct autoimmune syndromes in morphea: a review of 245 adult and pediatric cases. Arch Dermatol 145:545–550

Li YZ, Wu Y, Zhang QH, Wang Y, Zhen JH, Li SL (2009) Hypoxia–ischaemia is involved in the pathogenesis of vulvar lichen sclerosus. Clin Exp Dermatol 34:e531–e536

Liang W, Diana J (2020) The dual role of antimicrobial peptides in autoimmunity. Front Immunol 11:2077

Liegl B, Regauer S (2006) p53 immunostaining in lichen sclerosus is related to ischaemic stress and is not a marker of differentiated vulvar intraepithelial neoplasia (d-VIN). Histopathology 48:268–274

Liu G, Cao F, Zhao M, Shi J, Liu S (2015) Associations between HLA-A\B\DRB1 polymorphisms and risks of vulvar lichen sclerosus or squamous cell hyperplasia of the vulva. Genet Mol Res 14:15962–15971

Luo Z, Ji Y, Tian D, Zhang Y, Chang S, Yang C, Zhou H, Chen ZK (2018) Galectin-7 promotes proliferation and Th1/2 cells polarization toward Th1 in activated CD4+ T cells by inhibiting The TGFβ/Smad3 pathway. Mol Immunol 101:80–85

Lutz V, Bessis D, Cosnes A, Kluger N, Godet J, Sauleau E, Lipsker D (2012) High frequency of genital lichen sclerosus in a prospective series of 76 patients with morphea: toward a better understanding of the spectrum of morphea. Arch Dermatol 148:24–28

Maas-Szabowski N, Fusenig NE (1996) Interleukin-1-induced growth factor expression in postmitotic and resting fibroblasts. J Investig Dermatol 107:849–855

Magee KE, Kelsey CE, Kurzinski KL, Ho J, Mlakar LR, Feghali-Bostwick CA, Torok KS (2013) Interferon-gamma inducible protein-10 as a potential biomarker in localized scleroderma. Arthritis Res Ther 15:1–8

Marnett L (1999) Chemistry and biology of DNA damage by malondialdehyde. IARC Scientific Publications, pp 17–27

Marren P, Jell J, Charnock F, Bunce M, Welsh K, Wojnarowska F (1995) The association between lichen sclerosus and antigens of the HLA system. Br J Dermatol 132:197–203

Matucci-Cerinic M, Kahaleh B, Wigley FM (2013) Evidence that systemic sclerosis is a vascular disease. Arthritis Rheum 65:1953–1962

Mertens J, de Jong E, van den Hoogen L, Wienke J, Thurlings R, Seyger M, Hoppenreijs E, Wijngaarde C, van Vlijmen-Willems I, van den Bogaard E (2019) The identification of CCL18 as biomarker of disease activity in localized scleroderma. J Autoimmun 101:86–93

Meyer M, Müller A-K, Yang J, Šulcová J, Werner S (2011) The role of chronic inflammation in cutaneous fibrosis: fibroblast growth factor receptor deficiency in keratinocytes as an example. In: Journal of Investigative Dermatology symposium proceedings. Elsevier, pp 48–52

Milligan A, Graham-Brown R, Burns D (1988) Lichen sclerosus et atrophicus following sunburn. Clin Exp Dermatol (print) 13:36–37

Molho-Pessach V, Schaffer JV (2011) Blaschko lines and other patterns of cutaneous mosaicism. Clin Dermatol 29:205–225

Mori T, Kawara S, Shinozaki M, Hayashi N, Kakinuma T, Igarashi A, Takigawa M, Nakanishi T, Takehara K (1999) Role and interaction of connective tissue growth factor with transforming growth factor-β in persistent fibrosis: a mouse fibrosis model. J Cell Physiol 181:153–159

Niamh L, Naveen S, Hazel B (2009) Diagnosis of vulval inflammatory dermatoses: a pathological study with clinical correlation. Int J Gynecol Pathol 28:554–558

Nikitorowicz-Buniak J, Shiwen X, Denton CP, Abraham D, Stratton R (2014) Abnormally differentiating keratinocytes in the epidermis of systemic sclerosis patients show enhanced secretion of CCN2 and S100A9. J Investig Dermatol 134:2693–2702

Nishioka S (1997) Histological comparison of morphea and lichen sclerosus et atrophicus. Kurume Med J 44:83–90

Niyonsaba F, Ushio H, Nakano N, Ng W, Sayama K, Hashimoto K, Nagaoka I, Okumura K, Ogawa H (2007) Antimicrobial peptides human β-defensins stimulate epidermal keratinocyte migration, proliferation and production of proinflammatory cytokines and chemokines. J Investig Dermatol 127:594–604

Nóbrega MM, Cabral F, Corrêa MC, Barcaui CB, Bressan AL, Gripp AC (2016) Lichen sclerosus associated with localized scleroderma: dermoscopy contribution. Anais Brasileiros de Dermatologia 91:534–536

O'Brien JC, Rainwater YB, Malviya N, Cyrus N, Auer-Hackenberg L, Hynan LS, Hosler GA, Jacobe HT (2017) Transcriptional and cytokine profiles identify CXCL9 as a biomarker of disease activity in morphea. J Investig Dermatol 137:1663–1670

Oksenberg JR, Baranzini SE, Barcellos LF, Hauser SL (2001) Multiple sclerosis: genomic rewards. J Neuroimmunol 113:171–184

Osmola-Mańkowska A, Teresiak-Mikołajczak E, Dańczak-Pazdrowska A, Kowalczyk M, Żaba R, Adamski Z (2015) The role of dendritic cells and regulatory T cells in the pathogenesis of morphea. Central Eur J Immunol 40:103

Oyama N, Chan I, Neill SM, Hamada T, South AP, Wessagowit V, Wojnarowska F, D'Cruz D, Hughes GJ, Black MM (2003) Autoantibodies to extracellular matrix protein 1 in lichen sclerosus. Lancet 362:118–123

Oyama N, Chan I, Neill SM, South AP, Wojnarowska F, Kawakami Y, D'Cruz D, Mepani K, Hughes GJ, Bhogal BS (2004) Development of antigen-specific ELISA for circulating autoantibodies to extracellular matrix protein 1 in lichen sclerosus. J Clin Investig 113:1550–1559

Oyama N, Merregaert J (2017) The extracellular matrix protein 1 (ECM1) in molecular-based skin biology. Textbook of aging skin. Springer, Berlin, Heidelberg, pp 91–110

Ozlu E, Karadag AS, Akdeniz N, Uzuncakmak TK, Zemheri E, Ozkanli S (2019) Morphea secondary to interferon beta1b injection: a case and review of the literature. Dermatology (online journal) 25

Pa HOLT, Darke C (1983) HLA antigens and Bf allotypes in lichen sclerosus et atrophicus. Tissue Antigens 22:89–91

Paller AS (2007) Wnt signaling in focal dermal hypoplasia. Nat Genet 39:820–821

Paul P, Chakraborty A, Sarkar D, Langthasa M, Rahman M, Bari M, Singha RS, Malakar AK, Chakraborty S (2018) Interplay between miRNAs and human diseases. J Cell Physiol 233:2007–2018

Pequet M, Holland K, Zhao S, Drolet B, Galbraith S, Siegel D, Chiu Y (2014) Risk factors for morphoea disease severity: a retrospective review of 114 paediatric patients. Br J Dermatol 170:895–900

Pérez-López F, Vieira-Baptista P (2017) Lichen sclerosus in women: a review. Climacteric 20:339–347

Peroni A, Zini A, Braga V, Colato C, Adami S, Girolomoni G (2008) Drug-induced morphea: report of a case induced by balicatib and review of the literature. J Am Acad Dermatol 59:125–129

Pham CM, Browning JC (2010) Morphea affecting a father and son. Pediatr Dermatol 27:536–537

Powell J, Wojnarowska F, Winsey S, Marren P, Welsh K (2000) Lichen sclerosus premenarche: autoimmunity and immunogenetics. Br J Dermatol 142:481–484

Prinz JC, Kutasi Z, Weisenseel P, Pótó L, Battyáni Z, Ruzicka T (2009) "Borrelia-associated early-onset morphea": a particular type of scleroderma in childhood and adolescence with high titer antinuclear antibodies? Results of a cohort analysis and presentation of three cases. J Am Acad Dermatol 60:248–255

Purcell KG, Spencer LV, Simpson PM, Helman SW, Oldfather JW, Fowler JF (1990) HLA antigens in lichen sclerosus et atrophicus. Arch Dermatol 126:1043–1045

Qian F, He M, Duan W, Mao L, Li Q, Yu Z, Zhou Z, Zhang Y (2015) Cross regulation between hypoxia-inducible transcription factor-1α (HIF-1α) and transforming growth factor (TGF)-ß1 mediates nickel oxide nanoparticles (NiONPs)-induced pulmonary fibrosis. Am J Transl Res 7:2364

Rajabi F, Drake L, Senna M, Rezaei N (2018) Alopecia areata: a review of disease pathogenesis. Br J Dermatol 179:1033–1048

Ren L, Zhao Y, Huo X, Wu X (2018) MiR-155-5p promotes fibroblast cell proliferation and inhibits FOXO signaling pathway in vulvar lichen sclerosis by targeting FOXO3 and CDKN1B. Gene 653:43–50

Richter K, Kietzmann T (2016) Reactive oxygen species and fibrosis: further evidence of a significant liaison. Cell Tissue Res 365:591–605

Rolfe K, MacLean A, Crow J, Benjamin E, Reid W, Perrett C (2003) TP53 mutations in vulval lichen sclerosus adjacent to squamous cell carcinoma of the vulva. Br J Cancer 89:2249–2253

Russo B, Brembilla NC, Chizzolini C (2020) Interplay between keratinocytes and fibroblasts: a systematic review providing a new angle for understanding skin fibrotic disorders. Front Immunol 11

Ryan BJ, Nissim A, Winyard PG (2014) Oxidative post-translational modifications and their involvement in the pathogenesis of autoimmune diseases. Redox Biol 2:715–724

Sander C, Ali I, Dean D, Thiele J, Wojnarowska F (2004) Oxidative stress is implicated in the pathogenesis of lichen sclerosus. Br J Dermatol 151:627–635

Saracino A, Denton C, Orteu C (2017) The molecular pathogenesis of morphoea: from genetics to future treatment targets. Br J Dermatol 177:34–46

Sartori-Valinotti JC, Tollefson MM, Reed AM (2013) Updates on morphea: role of vascular injury and advances in treatment. Autoimmune Dis

Schittek B, Paulmann M, Senyurek I, Steffen H (2008) The role of antimicrobial peptides in human skin and in skin infectious diseases. Infect Disord Drug Targets (Formerly Current Drug Targets-Infectious Disorders) 8:135–143

Sehgal VN, Srivastava G, Aggarwal AK, Behl PN, Choudhary M, Bajaj P (2002) Localized scleroderma/morphea. Int J Dermatol 41:467–475

Şentürk N, Aydın F, Birinci A, Yildiz L, Cantürk T, Durupınar B, Turanlı AY (2004) Coexistence of HLA-B* 08 and HLA-B* 18 in four siblings with lichen sclerosus. Dermatology 208:64–66

Setterfield JF, Neill S, Shirlaw PJ, Theron J, Vaughan R, Escudier M, Challacombe SJ, Black MM (2006) The vulvovaginal gingival syndrome: a severe subgroup of lichen planus with characteristic clinical features and a novel association with the class II HLA DQB1∗ 0201 allele. J Am Acad Dermatol 55:98–113

Sherman V, McPherson T, Baldo M, Salim A, Gao X, Wojnarowska F (2010) The high rate of familial lichen sclerosus suggests a genetic contribution: an observational cohort study. J Eur Acad Dermatol Venereol 24:1031–1034

Shim T, Patel N, Bunker C (2012) Urinary voiding symptomatology (microincontinence) in male genital lichen sclerosus: P54. Br J Dermatol 167:45–46

Shrimpton RE, Butler M, Morel A-S, Eren E, Hue SS, Ritter MA (2009) CD205 (DEC-205): a recognition receptor for apoptotic and necrotic self. Mol Immunol 46:1229–1239

Sideri M, Rognoni M, Rizzolo L, Micheletti L, Barbero M, Origoni M, Garsia S (1988) Antigens of the HLA system in women with vulvar lichen sclerosus. Association with HLA-B21. J Reprod Med 33:551–554

Simmonds M, Gough S (2004) Unravelling the genetic complexity of autoimmune thyroid disease: HLA, CTLA-4 and beyond. Clin Exp Immunol 136:1–10

Stone RC, Chen V, Burgess J, Pannu S, Tomic-Canic M (2020) Genomics of human fibrotic diseases: disordered wound healing response. Int J Mol Sci 21:8590

Sturrock A, Cahill B, Norman K, Huecksteadt TP, Hill K, Sanders K, Karwande S, Stringham JC, Bull DA, Gleich M (2006) Transforming growth factor-β1 induces Nox4 NAD (P) H oxidase and reactive oxygen species-dependent proliferation in human pulmonary artery smooth muscle cells. Am J Physiol Lung Cell Mol Physiol 290:L661–L673

Tarbell KV, Yamazaki S, Steinman RM (2006) The interactions of dendritic cells with antigen-specific, regulatory T cells that suppress autoimmunity. In: Seminars in immunology. Elsevier, pp 93–102

Terlou A, Santegoets LA, Van Der Meijden WI, Heijmans-Antonissen C, Swagemakers SM, Van Der Spek PJ, Ewing PC, Van Beurden M, Helmerhorst TJ, Blok LJ (2012) An autoimmune phenotype in vulvar lichen sclerosus and lichen planus: a Th1 response and high levels of microRNA-155. J Investig Dermatol 132:658–666

Tiitto LH, Peltoniemi MJ, Kaarteenaho-Wiik RL, Soini YM, Pääkkö PK, Sormunen RT, Kinnula VL (2004) Cell-specific regulation of gamma-glutamylcysteine synthetase in human interstitial lung diseases. Hum Pathol 35:832–839

Torok KS, Kurzinski K, Kelsey C, Yabes J, Magee K, Vallejo AN, Medsger Jr T, Feghali-Bostwick CA (2015) Peripheral blood cytokine and chemokine profiles in juvenile localized scleroderma: T-helper cell-associated cytokine profiles. In: Seminars in arthritis and rheumatism. Elsevier, pp 284–293

Tran DA, Tan X, Macri CJ, Goldstein AT, Fu SW (2019) Lichen Sclerosus: an autoimmunopathogenic and genomic enigma with emerging genetic and immune targets. Int J Biol Sci 15:1429

Vay D, Parodi M, Rolla R, Mottaran E, Vidali M, Bellomo G, Albano E (2001) Circulating antibodies recognizing malondialdehyde-modified proteins in healthy subjects. Free Radical Biol Med 30:277–286

Wadud M, Bose B, Al Nasir T (1989) Familial localised scleroderma from Bangladesh: two case reports. Bangladesh Med Res Counc Bull 15:15–19

Wenzel J, Wiechert A, Merkel C, Bieber T, Tüting T (2007) IP10/CXCL10–CXCR3 interaction: a potential self-recruiting mechanism for cytotoxic lymphocytes in lichen sclerosus et atrophicus. Acta Derm Venereol 87:112–117

Werth VP, White WL, Sanchez MR, Franks AG (1992) Incidence of alopecia areata in lupus erythematosus. Arch Dermatol 128:368–371

Weyand CM, Hicok KC, Conn DL, Goronzy JJ (1992) The influence of HLA-DRB1 genes on disease severity in rheumatoid arthritis. Ann Intern Med 117:801–806

Wollenberg A, Günther S, Moderer M, Wetzel S, Wagner M, Towarowski A, Tuma E, Rothenfusser S, Endres S, Hartmann G (2002) Plasmacytoid dendritic cells: a new cutaneous dendritic cell subset with distinct role in inflammatory skin diseases. J Investig Dermatol 119:1096–1102

Wolska-Gawron K, Bartosińska J, Krasowska D (2020) MicroRNA in localized scleroderma: a review of literature. Arch Dermatol Res 312:317–324

Wu JJ, Nguyen TU, Poon K-YT, Herrinton LJ (2012) The association of psoriasis with autoimmune diseases. J Am Acad Dermatol 67:924–930

Xiong A, Liu Y (2017) Targeting hypoxia inducible factors-1α as a novel therapy in fibrosis. Front Pharmacol 8:326

Yamamoto T (2006) Chemokines and chemokine receptors in scleroderma. Int Arch Allergy Immunol 140:345–356

Yates VM, King CM, Dave VK (1985) Lichen sclerosus et atrophicus following radiation therapy. Arch Dermatol 121:1044–1047

Yurtsever I, Łukomska M, Sobolewski P, Szymańska E, Owczarek W, Walecka I (2021) Familial localized scleroderma with paediatric onset: a review. Adv Dermatol Allergol/Postepy Dermatologii i Alergologii 38

Zannoni GF, Faraglia B, Tarquini E, Camerini A, Vrijens K, Migaldi M, Cittadini A, Sgambato A (2006) Expression of the CDK inhibitor p27 kip1 and oxidative DNA damage in non-neoplastic and neoplastic vulvar epithelial lesions. Mod Pathol 19:504–513

Zhang C, Yang M (2020) The role and potential application of antimicrobial peptides in autoimmune diseases. Front Immunol 11:859

Zhang Y, Fu Q, Zhang X (2016) The presence of human papillomavirus and Epstein-Barr virus in male Chinese lichen sclerosus patients: a single center study. Asian J Androl 18:650

Zhao Y, Zhao S, Li H, Qin X, Wu X (2018) Expression of galectin-7 in vulvar lichen sclerosus and its effect on dermal fibroblasts. Oncol Lett 16:2559–2564

Zheng Y, Niyonsaba F, Ushio H, Ikeda S, Nagaoka I, Okumura K, Ogawa H (2008) Microbicidal protein psoriasin is a multifunctional modulator of neutrophil activation. Immunology 124:357–367

Zulian F, Athreya B, Laxer R, Nelson A, Feitosa de Oliveira S, Punaro M, Cuttica R, Higgins G, Van Suijlekom-Smit L, Moore T (2006) Juvenile localized scleroderma: clinical and epidemiological features in 750 children. An international study. Rheumatology 45:614–620

The Immunogenetics of Autoimmune Blistering Diseases

Diana Kneiber, Eric H. Kowalski, and Kyle T. Amber

Abstract

Dermatological conditions constituting the group of autoimmune blistering diseases (AIBD) are characterized by loss of immunotolerance and humoral, as well as cellular, autoimmune responses that result in the development of bullae and erosions on the skin and mucous membranes. AIBDs are broadly categorized into pemphigus and pemphigoid classes with several distinct subtypes amongst them. Advances in genetics have allowed for the study and identification of alleles, and even single nucleotide polymorphisms, that harbor increased susceptibility or confer protection for the development of these conditions. The focus of this chapter pertains to a comprehensive review of the known genetic associations with AIBDs, including HLA class I-III, as well as non-HLA genes and non-coding sequences that influence cellular processes and signaling pathways.

D. Kneiber · E. H. Kowalski
Department of Dermatology, University of Illinois at Chicago, Chicago, USA

K. T. Amber (✉)
Division of Dermatology, Rush University Medical Center, Chicago, USA
e-mail: kyle_amber@rush.edu

Department of Internal Medicine, Rush University Medical Center, Chicago, USA

Keywords

Pemphigus vulgaris · Pemphigus foliaceus · Paraneoplastic autoimmune multiorgan syndrome · Bullous pemphigoid · Epidermolysis bullosa acquisita

1 Introduction

Autoimmune blistering diseases (AIBD) are skin conditions distinguished by autoantibody-mediated development of bullae and erosions on the skin and mucous membranes. They can be subdivided into two groups, the epidermal class, pemphigus, or the peridermal pemphigoids. Diagnosis is established by the clinical presentation, immunofluorescence, and serology. These conditions lead to significant morbidity and mortality in these patients with 21% and 23.5% of patients with pemphigus and bullous pemphigoid, respectively, passing away within 1 year of diagnosis (Kridin et al. 2017, 2019). Management has traditionally been centered around the use of systemic corticosteroids, however, advancements in our understanding of the pathogenesis of these conditions have led to novel treatments that are efficacious and have better safety profiles (Ahmed and Kaveri 2018; Amber et al. 2018a; Caillot et al. 2018; Colliou et al. 2013; Hertl et al. 2015; Joly et al. 2007; Kridin 2018a; Nagel et al. 2009; Yamagami 2018). As our comprehension of the relationship

N. Rezaei and F. Rajabi (eds.), *The Immunogenetics of Dermatologic Diseases*, Advances in Experimental Medicine and Biology 1367,
https://doi.org/10.1007/978-3-030-92616-8_8

between the human genome and the immune system has evolved, it has become clear that genetic susceptibility plays a key role in the development of AIBDs. Multiple human leukocyte antigen (HLA) genes have been associated with predisposition to disease development, confirming the key role of Th2 cells in the induction of these conditions. Likewise, several HLA genes have also been associated with protection. Non-coding sequences and non-HLA gene polymorphisms have also been identified, strengthening the importance of signaling pathway alterations in combination with pathways involved in autoantibody production. We hereby review the known genetic associations in patients with AIBDs.

2 Pemphigus

Pemphigus is a rare group of autoimmune blistering disorders characterized by the formation of autoantibodies against proteins involved in epidermal cell adhesion. The two most common forms are pemphigus vulgaris (PV) and pemphigus foliaceous (PF). Paraneoplastic autoimmune multiorgan syndrome (PAMS) occurs in the setting of an underlying malignancy or lymphoproliferative disorder (Kaplan et al. 2004). In all, epidermal acantholysis ensues with flaccid bullae and erosion development.

In pemphigus vulgaris, autoantibody formation to desmogleins 1 and 3 and other keratinocyte proteins leads to painful erosions and bullae formation on the skin and mucous membranes (Amagai et al. 1991; Amber et al. 2018c; Calvanico et al. 1991; Chernyavsky et al. 2019; Korman et al. 1989). In pemphigus foliaceous, patients develop autoantibodies primarily against desmoglein 1 and have sparing of the mucosal membranes (Koulu et al. 1984; Stanley et al. 1986). In PAMS, autoantibodies form against desmoplakins and a wide array of proteins with severe mucocutaneous eruption ensuing (Amber et al. 2018d; Joly et al. 2000). Histologically pemphigus is characterized by apoptolysis, a unique combination of acantholysis and apoptosis (Grando et al. 2009; Joly et al. 2000). In pemphigus vulgaris, separation occurs between the basal and suprabasal epidermal cell layers while in pemphigus foliaceous the split occurs higher, between the suprabasal and granular cell layers (Arundhathi et al. 2013). In PAMS, separation can occur at various levels and interface dermatitis can be present (Amber et al. 2018d). The direct pathogenesis of anti-desmoglein antibodies is portrayed by passive transfer mouse models demonstrating blister formation and epidermal IgG deposits following injection of patient sera (Anhalt et al. 1982; Ishii et al. 2008; Payne et al. 2005; Rock et al. 1990). The diagnosis of pemphigus is made with direct immunofluorescence (DIF) showing the presence of autoantibodies bound to lesional tissue, indirect immunofluorescence (IIF) using monkey and guinea pig esophagus, or ELISA confirming the presence of circulating autoantibodies (Hofmann et al. 2018).

Pemphigus is a multifactorial disease with genetic and environmental factors playing a significant role in the development of pemphigus. Pemphigus occurs at a rate of 2–10 cases per million and is more frequently seen in people of Ashkenazi Jewish, Serbian, Tunisian, Mediterranean, and Macedonian descent (Alpsoy et al. 2015; Kridin et al. 2016; Langan et al. 2008; Mimouni et al. 2008; Uzun et al. 2006; V'lckova-Laskoska et al. 2007). Although rare, familial cases of pemphigus have been reported (Feinstein et al. 1991; Katzenelson et al. 1990; Laskaris et al. 1989; Stavropoulos et al. 2001). In addition, there is an increased rate of autoimmune conditions in patients with pemphigus and their family members (Chiu et al. 2017; Firooz et al. 1994; Heelan et al. 2015; Parameswaran et al. 2015). As such, the role of underlying genetic predispositions plays an important part in its pathogenesis.

2.1 Pemphigus Vulgaris

Pemphigus vulgaris is a characteristic autoimmune disease generated by the formation of autoantibodies against epidermal adhesion molecules. Anti-desmoglein IgG autoantibodies predominate, although autoantibodies to mitochondrial proteins, thyroid peroxidase, and muscarinic acetylcholine receptors also play a role (Kalantari-Dehaghi et al. 2013; Marchenko et al. 2010; Sajda et al. 2016). Desmoglein 1 and 3 are transmembrane cadherin adhesion molecules (Getsios et al. 2004). Each desmoglein is comprised of 5 extracellular (EC) subdomains, EC1-EC5. In PV and PF, the N-terminal EC1 and EC2 subdomains form the critical epitopes for anti-desmoglein antibodies (Chan et al. 2010; Futei et al. 2000; Sekiguchi et al. 2001). Together, EC1 and EC2 mediate trans interactions between molecules on opposing cell membranes and cis interactions between proteins on the same cell surface (Boggon et al. 2002; Nagar et al. 1996; Nose et al. 1990). The cytoplasmic regions mediate cytoskeletal alterations through catenins (Kemler 1993; Nagar et al. 1996). Disruption of cis and trans interactions between desmoglein 3 molecules, triggers an intracellular signaling cascade that initiates cytoskeleton remodeling, resulting in keratinocyte shrinkage, detachment from neighboring cells, and apoptolysis (Zenzo et al. 2012; Heupel et al. 2008; Orlov et al. 2006; Sharma et al. 2007). Autoantigen presentation on HLA Class II molecules activates CD4+ T-cells, with a predominance of Th2 cells in the early disease course (Veldman et al. 2003). CD40–CD40 ligand interactions result in B-cell anti-desmoglein autoantibody formation (Eming et al. 2014).

2.1.1 MHC Class II, DR

Within HLA Class II alleles, DRB1*04, DRB1*08, and DRB1*14 confer strong susceptibility to PV (Table 1) (Yan et al. 2012). HLA-DRB1*04 and DRB1*14 phenotypes are found in higher frequency across multiple ethnicities and geographic locations (Haase et al. 2015; Harfouch and Daoud 2014; Párnická et al. 2013; Yan et al. 2012; Zhang et al. 2018b). Amongst, HLA-DRB*04 alleles, 04:02 is the predominant genotype associated with PV in Jewish and non-Jewish patients from all around the world (Brochado et al. 2016; Gil et al. 2017; Haase et al. 2015; Harfouch and Daoud 2014; Lee et al. 2006; Párnická et al. 2013; Sáenz-Cantele et al. 2007; Saha et al. 2010; Shams et al. 2009; Weber et al. 2011; Zivanovic et al. 2016). In patients with mucocutaneous type PV, it is the predominant allele (Svecova et al. 2015). DRB1*04 has two negatively charged amino acid residues, aspartate, and glutamate, at positions 70 and 71, which allow it to bind to positively charged residues (190–204) on desmoglein 3 (Wucherpfennig et al. 1995). In contrast, DRB1*04:01 and 04:03, are protective, in Germans and Syrians respectively, due to the lack of these two negatively charged residues (Haase et al. 2015; Harfouch and Daoud 2014).

Based on the reactivity of HLA DRB1*04:02 on desmoglein 3, it becomes apparent how HLA molecules may predispose to reactivity with pathogenic peptide sequences in these autoantigens (Fig. 1).

HLA DRB1*14:01, 14:04, 14:05, 14:54 increase the likelihood of developing PV (Párnická et al. 2013; Xiao et al. 2009; Zhang et al. 2018b). DRB1*08 is found to predispose patients of multiple ethnicities with 08:04 playing a major role in patients of mixed Brazilian and Egyptian descent (Brochado et al. 2016; Gil et al. 2017; Haase et al. 2015; Weber et al. 2011; Yan et al. 2012; Zhang et al. 2018b). Other classes of HLA alleles are found to predispose patients from distinct ethnicities to PV. In Han Chinese patients, DRB1*12 is higher in patients with PV (Geng et al. 2005).

HLA-DRB1*03, DRB1*07, and DRB1*15 are protective across ethnicities (Sáenz-Cantele et al. 2007; Yan et al. 2012). In particular, 03:01 is found to be more common in healthy patients without PV (Saha et al. 2010; Shams et al. 2009). In Caucasian patients and those of mixed ethnicities, DRB1*07 confers protection (Yan et al. 2012). In Chinese patients, DRB1*09:01 reduces the risk of disease (Zhang et al. 2018b). In patients from Pakistan, DRB1*10 prevents disease, while DRB1*11 protects patients of Serbian, Turkish, Syrian, and Iranian descent (Birol et al. 2002; Harfouch and Daoud 2014; Khan et al. 2015; Lee et al. 2006; Shams et al. 2009; Zivanovic et al. 2016). Likewise, DRB1*13 confers reduced risk in Brazilian, German, Syrian, and Slovakian patients (Gil et al. 2017;

Table 1 HLA MHC Class II DRB1 allele associations in patients with pemphigus vulgaris

Pemphigus vulgaris						
HLA-DRB1 Allele	References	Study type	Ethnicity	Effect	*N*	*P*-value
*01	Yan et al. (2012)	Meta-analysis	–	P	730	NS
*03	Yan et al. (2012)	Meta-analysis	–	P	988	Allele **** Phenotype ***
*03:01	Shams et al. (2009)	Case–control	Iranian Non-Jewish	P	52	*
	Lee et al. (2006)	Case–control	North American Caucasian, Ashkenazi Jewish, and Non-Jewish	P	Non-AJ 26, AJ 32	NAJ NS AJ***
	Saha et al. (2010)	Case–control	White European or Indo-Asians	P	96	WE***
*04	Yan et al. (2012)	Meta-analysis	–	S	1150	Allele * Phenotype *
	Haase et al. (2015)	Case–control	Egyptians and Germans	S	73 E, 46 G	E **** G ***
	Zivanovic et al. (2016)	Case–control	Serbian	S	72	****
	Harfouch and Daoud (2014)	Case–control	Syrian	S	91	****
	Párnická et al. (2013)	Case–control	Slovakian	S	43	***
*04:01	Haase et al. (2015)	Case–control	Egyptians and Germans	P	73 E, 46 G	E NS G *
*04:02	Brochado et al. (2016)	Case–control	Brazilian	S	83	****
	Zivanovic et al. (2016)	Case–control	Serbian	S	72	****
	Haase et al. (2015)	Case–control	Egyptians and Germans	S	73 E, 46 G	E **** G ****
	Harfouch et al. (2014)	Case–control	Syrian	S	91	**
	Párnická et al. (2013)	Case–control	Slovakian	S	43	****
	Weber et al. (2011)	Case–control	Brazilian	S	36	*
	Saha et al. (2010)	Case–control	White European or Indo-Asians	S	96 WE, 57 IA	WE **** IA ***
	Shams et al. (2009)	Case–control	Iranian non-Jewish	S	52	****
	Sáenz-Cantele et al. (2007)	Case–control	Venezuelan	S	49	****
	Lee et al. (2006)	Case–control	North American Caucasian, Ashkenazi Jewish, and Non-Jewish	S	Non-AJ 26, AJ 32	NAJ **** AJ ****
*04:03	Harfouch et al. (Harfouch and Daoud 2014)	Case–control	Syrian	P	91	****

(continued)

Table 1 (continued)

Pemphigus vulgaris

HLA-DRB1 Allele	References	Study type	Ethnicity	Effect	*N*	*P*-value
*04:04	Párnická et al. (2013)	Case–control	Slovakian	S	43	***
	Zhang et al. (2018b)	Case–control	Chinese	S	365	***
*07	Yan et al. (2012)	Meta-analysis	–	P	962	Allele***
*08	Yan et al. (2012)	Meta-analysis	–	S	630	Allele* Phenotype***
	Zhang et al. (2018b)	Case–control	Chinese	P	365	***
	Gil et al. (2017)	Case–control	Brazilian	S	102	**
	Haase et al. (2015)	Case–control	Egyptians and Germans	S	73 E, 46 G	E ** G NS
*08:04	Weber et al. (2011)	Case–control	Brazilian	S	36	*
	Brachado et al. (2016)	Case–control	Brazilian	S	83	****
*09:01	Zhang et al. (2018b)	Case–control	Chinese	P	365	****
*10	Yan et al. (2012)	Meta-analysis	–	–	538	NS
	Khan et al. (2015)	Case–control	Pakistani	P	28	*
*11	Yan et al. (2012)	Meta-analysis	–	P	604	Allele ****
	Zivanovic et al. (2016)	Case–control	Serbian	P	72	**
	Harfouch and Daoud (2014)	Case–control	Syrian	P	91	****
*11:04	Lee et al. (2006)	Case–control	North American Caucasian, Ashkenazi Jewish, and Non-Jewish	P	Non-AJ 26, AJ 32	NAJ NS AJ ***
*12	Yan et al. (2012)	Meta-analysis	–	–	538	NS
	Geng et al. (2005)	Requested	Chinese	S	27	**
*13	Yan et al. (2012)	Meta-analysis			566	NS
	Gil et al. (2017)	Case–control	Brazilian	P	102	*
	Haase et al. (2015)	Case–control	Egyptians and Germans	P	73 E, 46 G	Egyptian NS German *
	Harfouch and Daoud (2014)	Case–control	Syrian	P	91	*
	Párnická et al. (2013)	Case–control	Slovakian	P	43	*

(continued)

Table 1 (continued)

Pemphigus vulgaris						
HLA-DRB1 Allele	References	Study type	Ethnicity	Effect	*N*	*P*-value
*14	Yan et al. (2012)	Meta-analysis		S	1048	Allele **** Phenotype ****
	Haase et al. (2015)	Case–control	Egyptians and Germans	S	73 E, 46 G	Egyptian** German****
	Harfouch and Daoud (2014)	Case–control	Syrian	S	91	****
	Párnická et al. (2013)	Case–control	Slovakian	S	43	****
	Zhang et al. (2018b)	Case–control	Chinese	S	365	****
*14:01	Shams et al. (2009)	Case–control	Iranian non-Jewish	S	52	***
	Lee et al. (2006)	Case–control	North American Caucasian Non-Ashkenazi Jewish and Ashkenazi Jewish	S	Non-AJ 26, AJ 32	NAJ **** AJ NS
*14:04	Saha et al. (2010)	Case–control	White European or Indo-Asians	S	96 WE, 57 IA	WE *** IA ****
	Zivanovic et al. (2016)	Case–control	Serbian	S	72	****
	Párnická et al. (2013)	Case–control	Slovakian	S	43	**
	Lee et al. (2006)	Case–control	North American Caucasian Non-Ashkenazi Jewish and Ashkenazi Jewish	S	Non-AJ 26, AJ 32	NAJ **** AJ NS
	Zhang et al. (2018b)	Case–control	Chinese	S	365	****
*14:05	Párnická et al. (2013)	Case–control	Slovakian	S	43	*
	Zhang et al. (2018b)	Case–control	Chinese	S	365	****
*14:54	Saha et al. (2010)	Case–control	White European or Indo-Asians	S	96 WE, 57 IA	WE **** IA NS
	Párnická et al. (2013)	Case–control	Slovakian	S	43	***
*15	Yan et al. (2012)	Meta-analysis	–	P	736	Allele **
	Zhang et al. (2018b)	Case–control	Chinese	P	365	****
	Geng et al. (2005)	Requested	Chinese	P	27	*
*15:01	Zhang et al. (2018b)	Case–control	Chinese	P	365	****
*16	Zhang et al. (2018b)	Case–control	Chinese	P	365	****
*16:02	Zhang et al. (2018b)	Case–control	Chinese	P	365	****

* = $p < 0.05$, ** = $p < 0.01$, *** = $p < 0.001$, **** = $p < 0.0001$. *P* = protective, *S* = increased susceptibility, *NS* = no significant difference, *AJ* = Ashkenazi Jewish, *E* = Egyptian, *G* = German, *WE* = white European, *IA* = Indo-Asian

```
  1 mmglfprttg alaifvvvil vhgelrietk gqydeeemtm qqakrrqkre wvkfakpcre
 61 gednskrnpi akitsdydat qkityrisgv gidqppfgif vvdkntgdin itaivdreet
121 psflitcral naqgldvekp liltvkildi ndnppvfsqq ifmgeieens asnslvmiln
181 atdadepnhl nskiafkivs qepagtpmfl lsrntgevrt ltnsldreqa ssyrlvvsga
241 dkdgeglstq cecnikvkdv ndnfpmfrds qysarieeni lssellrfqv tdldeeytdn
301 wlavyfftsg negnwfeiqt dprtnegilk vvkaldyeql qsvklsiavk nkaefhqsvi
361 sryrvqstpv tiqvinvreg iafrpasktf tvqkgisskk lvdyilgtyq aidedtnkaa
421 snvkyvmgrn dggylmidsk taeikfvknm nrdstfivnk titaevlaid eytgktstgt
481 vyvrvpdfnd ncptavlekd avcssspsvv vsartlnnry tgpytfaled qpvklpavws
541 ittlnatsal lraqeqippg vyhislvltd sqnnrcempr sltlevcqcd nrgicgtsyp
601 ttspgtrygr phsgrlgpaa iglllglll lllaplllt cdcgagstgg vtggfipvpd
661 gsegtihqwg iegahpedke itnicvppvt angadfmess evctntyarg tavegtsgme
721 mttklgaate sggaagfatg tvsgaasgfg aatgvgicss gqsgtmrtrh stggtnkdya
781 dgaismnfld syfsqkafac aeeddgqean dclliydneg adatgspvgs vgccsfiadd
841 lddsfldslg pkfkklaeis lgvdgegkev qppskdsgyg iescghpiev qqtgfvkcqt
901 lsgsqgasal stsgsvqpav sipdplqhgn ylvtetysas gslvqpstag fdplltqnvi
961 vtervicpis svpgnlagpt qlrgshtmlc tedpcsrli
```

Matrix: HLA_DR4oDRB1s0402c.p.mtx
Consensus: ICFWHNHNM
Optimal Score: 44.604
Binding Threshold: 11.44

RANK	POS.	N	SEQUENCE	C	MW (Da)	SCORE	% OPT.
1	606	SPG	TRYGRPHSG	RLG	1012.1	17.99	40.33 %
2	766	SGT	MRTRHSTGG	TNK	984.09	17.387	38.98 %
3	194	NSK	IAFKIVSQE	PAG	1016.21	15.149	33.96 %
4	444	TAE	IKFVKNMNR	DST	1131.39	15.046	33.73 %
5	423	ASN	VKYVMGRND	GGY	1063.23	14.554	32.63 %
6	83	TQK	ITYRISGVG	IDQ	947.1	13.746	30.82 %
7	813	NDC	LLIYDNEGA	DAT	989.1	12.572	28.19 %
8	70	RNP	IAKITSDYQ	ATQ	1020.15	12.438	27.89 %
9	360	QSV	ISRYRVQST	PVT	1091.24	11.643	26.10 %
10	304	WLA	VYFFTSGNE	GNW	1045.12	11.59	25.98 %
11	218	TGE	VRTLTNSLD	REQ	1000.11	11.507	25.80 %

1. Major immunogenic domain in PV responsible for calcium dependent cell-cell adhesion
2. Pathogenic epitope in patients with pemphigus vulgaris
3. Non-calcium dependent binding site, pathogenic in PV

Fig. 1 The RankPep server identifies HLA-DRB:04*02 avidity for key pathogenic binding on Dsg3 known to have a significant role in PV. The RankPep server (http://imed.med.ucm.es/tools/rankpep.html) was used to evaluate the predicted binding of HLA-DRB:04*02 with Dsg3 using the protein sequence from UniProtKB (P32926, DSG3_human). Known physiologically relevant immunogenic sites (Futei et al. 2003; Sekiguchi et al. 2001; Tsunoda et al. 2003) including the calcium-dependent domain (1–161), the non-calcium domain (403–565), and the sequences (25–88) and (78–94) were confirmed by modeling software

Haase et al. 2015; Harfouch and Daoud 2014; Párnická et al. 2013). In Chinese patients, DRB1*16, and specifically, 16:02, provide protection (Zhang et al. 2018b).

Patients of Ashkenazi Jews are particularly susceptible to PV and are treated as their ethnic population (Kridin et al. 2016). Examining them separately, we find that the HLA-DRB1*04:02 allele confers susceptibility while DRB1*03:01, DRB1*07, and DRB1*11:04 alleles are protective, similar to other patient populations (Lee et al. 2006; Yan et al. 2012).

2.1.2 MHC Class II, DQ

HLA-DQA1*01:04, 03:01, and 05:05 predispose to PV (Brochado et al. 2016; Lee et al. 2006; Shams et al. 2009). while DQA1*01:01, 01:02, 01:03, 02, 05, 05:01 are protective (see Table 2) (Lee et al. 2006; Shams et al. 2009; Zhang et al. 2018b). In the DQB1 region, DQB1*02 protects against PV, especially the 02:01 and 02:02 alleles (Gil et al. 2017; Lee et al. 2006; Li et al. 2018; Loiseau et al. 2000; Saha et al. 2010; Shams et al. 2009). DQB1*03 increases the risk of developing PV with the majority of cases attributable to the 03:02 allele (Li et al. 2018). 03:02 is also associated with increased disease severity (Loiseau et al. 2000; Svecova et al. 2015). In contrast, the 03:03 allele is protective and is found more commonly in healthy individuals (Li et al. 2018; Zhang et al. 2018b). DQB1*05:03 confers increased risk for disease and is found globally in patients with PV (Brochado et al. 2016; Geng et al. 2005; Gil et al. 2017; Lee et al. 2006; Li et al. 2018; Loiseau et al. 2000; Párnická et al. 2013; Saha et al. 2010; Sun et al. 2019; Zhang et al. 2018b; Zivanovic et al. 2016). 05:03 has similar binding motifs on desmoglein 3 as DRB1*04:02 suggesting that overlapping epitopes may be responsible in patients with either allele (Tong et al. 2006). In contrast, 05:01 and 06:01 confer protection (Li et al. 2018). DQB1*0601 is preventative across different ethnicities while 06:02 reduces the risk of PV in patients of Brazilian and non-Jewish Iranian descent (Brochado et al. 2016; Li et al. 2018; Shams et al. 2009).

In the DQ region of patients of Ashkenazi Jewish descent, DQA1*03 and 05:05 increase the risk, and DQA1*01:01, 01:02, 02:01, and 05:01 decrease the risk of developing PV (Lee et al. 2006). In the DQB1 region, 02:01 and 02:02 confer protection (Lee et al. 2006). Interestingly, DQD1*03:02 has also been found at a higher frequency in patients with PV and Ashkenazi Jewish descent, although this does not

Table 2 HLA MHC Class II DQA1 and DQB1 allele associations in patients with pemphigus vulgaris

Pemphigus vulgaris						
HLA-DQA1 Allele	References	Study type	Ethnicity	Effect	N	P-value
*01:01	Shams et al. (2009)	Case–control	Iranian Non-Jewish	P	52	***
	Lee et al. (2006)	Case–control	North American Caucasian Non-Ashkenazi Jewish and Ashkenazi Jewish	P	Non-AJ 26, AJ 32	NAJ NS AJ ****
	Zhang et al. (2018b)	Case–control	Chinese	S	365	****
*01:02	Lee et al. (2006)	Case–control	North American Caucasian Non-Ashkenazi Jewish and Ashkenazi Jewish	P	Non-AJ 26, AJ 32	NAJ NS AJ ***
	Zhang et al. (2018b)	Case–control	Chinese	P	365	****
*01:03	Shams et al. (2009)	Case–control	Iranian Non-Jewish	P	52	*
*01:04	Shams et al. (2009)	Case–control	Iranian Non-Jewish	S	52	****
	Lee et al. (2006)	Case–control	North American Caucasian Non-Ashkenazi Jewish and Ashkenazi Jewish	S	Non-AJ 26, AJ 32	NAJ **** AJ NS
*02:01	Shams et al. (2009)	Case–control	Iranian Non-Jewish	P	52	**
	Lee et al. (2006)	Case–control	North American Caucasian Non-Ashkenazi Jewish and Ashkenazi Jewish	P	Non-AJ 26, AJ 32	NAJ NS AJ ***
*03	Lee et al. (2006)	Case–control	North American Caucasian Non-Ashkenazi Jewish and Ashkenazi Jewish	S	Non-AJ 26, AJ 32	NAJ NS AJ ****
*03:01	Shams et al. (2009)	Case–control	Iranian Non-Jewish	S	52	**
	Lee et al. (2006)	Case–control	North American Caucasian Non-Ashkenazi Jewish and Ashkenazi Jewish	S	Non-AJ 26, AJ 32	NAJ **** AJ NS
	Brochado et al. (2016)	Case–control	Brazilian	S	83	***
*05	Shams et al. (2009)	Case–control	Iranian Non-Jewish	P	52	***
	Zhang et al. (2018b)	Case–control	Chinese	P	365	****

(continued)

Table 2 (continued)

Pemphigus vulgaris						
HLA-DQA1 Allele	References	Study type	Ethnicity	Effect	N	P-value
*0501	Lee et al. (2006)	Case–control	North American Caucasian Non-Ashkenazi Jewish and Ashkenazi Jewish	P	Non-AJ 26, AJ 32	NAJ **** AJ ****
	Zhang et al. (2018b)	Case–control	Chinese	P	365	****
*05:05	Lee et al. (2006)	Case–control	North American Caucasian Non-Ashkenazi Jewish and Ashkenazi Jewish	S	Non-AJ 26, AJ 32	NAJ **** AJ ****
HLA-DQB1 Allele						
*02	Li et al. (2018)	Meta-analysis	–	P	–	Allele ** Phenotype **
*02:01	Shams et al. (2009)	Case–control	Iranian Non-Jewish	P	52	****
*02:01/02:02	Lee et al. (2006)	Case–control	North American Caucasian	S	58, Non-AJ 26, AJ 32	NAJ NS AJ ****
*03	Li et al. (2018)	Meta-analysis	–	S	–	Allele *** Phenotype NS
*03:01	Li et al. (2018)	Meta-analysis	–	P	–	Allele ****
*03:02	Li et al. (2018)	Meta-analysis	–	S	–	Allele ****
*03:03	Li et al. (2018)	Meta-analysis	–	P	–	Allele *
	Zhang et al. (2018b)	Case–control	Chinese	P	365	****
*03:05	Shams et al. (2009)	Case–control	Iranian Non-Jewish	S	52	*
*05	Li et al. (2018)	Meta-analysis	–	S	–	Allele *** Phenotype *
	Zhang et al. (2018b)	Case–control	Chinese	S	365	****
*05:01	Li et al. (2018)	Meta-analysis	–	P	–	Alelle ****
*05:02	Shams et al. (2009)	Case–control	Iranian Non-Jewish	S	52	****

(continued)

Table 2 (continued)

Pemphigus vulgaris						
HLA-DQA1 Allele	References	Study type	Ethnicity	Effect	N	P-value
*05:03	Li et al. (2018)	Meta-analysis	–	S	–	****
	Zhang et al. (2018b)	Case–control	Chinese	S	365	****
	Sun et al. (2019)	Case–control	Chinese	S	210	****
*06	Zhang et al. (2018b)	Case–control	Chinese	S	365	****
	Li et al. (2018)	Meta-analysis	–	P	–	Allele *** Phenotype NS
*06:01	Li et al. (2018)	Meta-analysis	–	P	–	Allele **
*06:02	Saha et al. (2010)	Case–control	White European or Indo-Asians	P	153, 96 WE, 57 IA	WE ** IA NS
	Li et al. (2018)	Meta-analysis	–	P	–	Allele *
	Shams et al. (2009)	Case–control	Iranian Non-Jewish	P	52	**
	Brochado et al. (2016)	Case–control	Brazilian	P	83	**
*06:03	Shams et al. (2009)	Case–control	Iranian Non-Jewish	S	52	**

* = $p < 0.05$, ** = $p < 0.01$, *** = $p < 0.001$, **** = $p < 0.0001$. *P* = protective, *S* = increased susceptibility, *NS* = no significant difference, *AJ* = Ashkenazi Jewish, *WE* = white European, *IA* = Indo-Asian

appear to play a major role in other ethnicities (Lee et al. 2006).

2.1.3 MHC Class II, Haplotypes

Specific haplotypes increase the risk of having PV (see Table 3). The HLA DRB1*04:02/DQB1*03:02 and DRB1*14:54/DQB1*05:03 are found in greater than 90% of patients with PV (Párnická et al. 2013). DRB1*04:02/DQB1*03:02 is associated with a significantly higher risk of PV and increased disease severity (Gil et al. 2017; Lee et al. 2006; Párnická et al. 2013; Shams et al. 2009; Svecova et al. 2015; Tunca et al. 2010; Zivanovic et al. 2016). Patients with DRB1*04:02/DQB1*03:02 have up to an 18 × greater risk of having PV, whereas, patients with DRB1*04:02 and not DQB1*03:02 have up to a 40 × greater risk (Sáenz-Cantele et al. 2007). When separating the risk provided by each allele, the association with 03:02 disappears (Lee et al. 2006). Linkage disequilibrium is the cause of increased DQB1*03:02, and not its inherent ability to predispose to PV (Lee et al. 2006). Thus HLA-DRB1*04:02 is the disease conferring allele in this haplotype (Lee et al. 2006). In patients of

Table 3 HLA haplotype associations in patients with pemphigus vulgaris

Pemphigus vulgaris-haplotypes						
Haplotype	Authors	Study type	Ethnicity	Effect	N	P-value
DRB1*01/DQB1*05	Zivanovic et al. (2016)	Case–control	Serbian	P	72	*
DRB1*03/DQB1*02	Zivanovic et al. (2016)	Case–control	Serbian	P	72	*
DRB1*03:01/DQA1*05:011/DQB1*02:01	Shams et al. (2009)	Case–control	Iranian Non-Jewish	P	52	*
DRB1*04/DQB1*03	Zivanovic et al. (2016)	Case–control	Serbian	S	72	****
	Tunca et al. (2010)	Case–control	Turkish	S	25	***
DRB1*04/DQB1*03:02	Párnická et al. (2013)	Case–control	Slovakian	S	43	****
DRB1*04:02/DQA1*03:01	Lee et al. (2006)	Case–control	North American Caucasian	S	26	****
DRB1*04/DQA1*03:01/DQB1*03:02	Gil et al. (2017)	Case–control	Brazilian	S	102	****
	Shams et al. (2009)	Case–control	Iranian Non-Jewish	P	52	****
DRB1*04:02/DQB1*03:02	Párnická et al. (2013)	Case–control	Slovakian	S	43	****
	Zivanovic et al. (2016)	Case–control	Serbian	S	72	****
	Lee et al. (2006)	Case–control	North American Caucasian	S	26	****
	Sáenz-Cantele et al. (2007)	Case–control	Venezuelan	S	49	****
DRB1*04:04/DQB1*03:02	Párnická et al. (2013)	Case–control	Slovakian	S	43	**
DRB1*07/DQA1*02:01/DQB1*02:01	Shams et al. (2009)	Case–control	Iranian Non-Jewish	P	52	*
DRB1*11/DQB1*03	Zivanovic et al. (2016)	Case–control	Serbian	P	72	*
DRB1*14/DQB1*05	Zivanovic et al. (2016)	Case–control	Serbian	S	72	****
	Tunca et al. (2010)	Case–control	Turkish	S	25	**
DRB1*14/DQB1*05:03	Párnická et al. (2013)	Case–control	Slovakian	S	43	****
DRB1*14/DQA1*01:01/DQB1*05:03	Gil et al. (2017)	Case–control	Brazilian	S	102	***

(continued)

Table 3 (continued)

Pemphigus vulgaris-haplotypes						
Haplotype	Authors	Study type	Ethnicity	Effect	N	P-value
DRB1*14:01/DQB1*05:03	Lee et al. (2006)	Case–control	North American Caucasian	S	26	****
	Sáenz-Cantele et al. (2007)	Case–control	Venezuelan	S	49	****
DRB1*14:01/DQA1*01:04/DQB1*05:02	Shams et al. (2009)	Case–control	Iranian Non-Jewish	S	52	****
DRB1*14:04/DQB1*05:03	Párnická et al. (2013)	Case–control	Slovakian	S	43	**
	Zivanovic et al. (2016)	Case–control	Serbian	S	72	****
DRB1*14:54/DQB1*05:03	Párnická et al. (2013)	Case–control	Slovakian	S	43	***
DQB1*05:03/DQA1*01:04	Lee et al. (2006)	Case–control	North American Caucasian	S	58, Non-AJ 26, AJ 32	****
DRB1*15/DQA1*03:01/DQB1*06:011	Shams et al. (2009)	Case–control	Iranian Non-Jewish	P	52	*

* = $p < 0.05$, ** = $p < 0.01$, *** = $p < 0.001$, **** = $p < 0.0001$. *P* = protective, *S* = increased susceptibility, *NS* = no significant difference

Ashkenazi Jewish descent, DRB1*04:02/DQB1*03:02 similarly confers a higher risk of PV, however, due to extreme linkage disequilibrium, it cannot be determined if this association is due to the synergistic effect of the two alleles or due to a single allele providing susceptibility (Lee et al. 2006).

The DRB1*14/DQB1*05:03 haplotype is also more commonly found in patients with PV (Gil et al. 2017; Miyagawa et al. 2002; Párnická et al. 2013; Sáenz-Cantele et al. 2007; Shams et al. 2009; Tunca et al. 2010; Zivanovic et al. 2016). Similar to the above relation, when determining disease susceptibility for each allele individually, the association with PV ceases to exist for DRB1*14:01. Thus DQB1*05:03 is the predominant disease-promoting allele in these patients (Lee et al. 2006). Other haplotypes that are associated with protection against PV include: HLA-DRB1*11/DQB1*03, DRB1*01/DQB1*05, DRB1*03/DQB1*02, DRB1*15/DQA1*03:01/DQB1*06:011, DRB1*07/DQA1*02:01/DQB1*02:01 (Shams et al. 2009; Zivanovic et al. 2016). In rare instances, patients who had a prior diagnosis of pemphigoid develop pemphigus or vice versa. In these patients a mix of HLA-DRB1*04:02, DQB1*03:01, DQB1*03:02, DQB1*05:03, DQB1*06:02 and DQB1*06:03 can be found. Epitope spreading can begin to explain this phenomenon as Desmoglein 3, BP180, BP230, alpha 6 integrin, and beta 4 integrin have binding epitopes on both DRB1*04:02 and DQB1*03:01 (Zakka et al. 2010).

2.1.4 MHC Class I

MHC Class I genes have been hypothesized to play a role in the pathogenesis of pemphigus. HLA-A*3 has been associated with higher rates of PV in patients of Han Chinese and Brazilian descent (Brochado et al. 2016; Geng et al. 2005). Likewise, HLA-A*10 is seen to be more frequent in patients with PV of Japanese descent and HLA-A*26 in patients of Han Chinese descent in comparison to unaffected patients (Hashimoto et al. 1977). In the HLA-B subdomain, HLA B*15 is preventative in Brazilian patients (Brochado et al. 2016; Gil et al. 2017). In Japanese patients, B*15, and specifically, B*15:07, confer risk (Miyagawa et al. 2002). B*35 and 44 also predispose patients of Turkish descent as do B*38, B*42, and B*57 in patients of Brazilian descent (Birol et al. 2002; Brochado et al. 2016; Gil et al. 2017). B*38 is also increased in PV patients of Spanish descent (González-Escribano et al. 1998). In Han Chinese patients, B*60 increases the risk of developing PV (Geng et al. 2005).

In the HLA-C subdomain, C*w4 is associated with increased PV risk in Turkish patients (Birol et al. 2002). C*04:01, 15:02, 16:01 pose susceptibility in Iranian patients while 06:02 and 18:01 are protective (Mortazavi et al. 2013). C*15:02 allele is also found more commonly in Japanese PV patients (Miyagawa et al. 2002). In Brazilian patients, C*12 and C*15 occur more frequently in patients with PV (Brochado et al. 2016; Gil et al. 2017).

The HLA-E*0103X allele is associated with PV in North American patients of Caucasian and Ashkenazi Jewish descent, while the 01:01 allele is protective (Bhanusali et al. 2013). In these patients, the genotypes E*01:01/01:01, *01:01/*01:032 confer protection (Bhanusali et al. 2013). Whereas *01:03X genotypes, including *01:031/01:031, *01:031/01:032, *01:032/01:032, predispose to PV (Bhanusali et al. 2013). In patients of Turkish descent, E*01:03X/01:03X is protective in male patients while E*01:01/01:03X genotype increases the risk of PV, and in particular, mucocutaneous PV (Altun et al. 2017). Mucosal type is associated with HLA-E*01:01/01:01 (Altun et al. 2017) In the HLA-G region, a 14 base pair deletion in exon 8 also appears to confer an increased risk of PV by increasing HLA-G gene transcription in Non-Ashkenazi Jewish patients (Gazit et al. 2004; Hviid et al. 2003). In lesional PV skin, HLA-G is expressed by keratinocytes, a finding not seen in healthy controls (Yari et al. 2008). In Ashkenazi Jewish patients, HLA-A*26 and B*38 appear to play the greatest role amongst the MHC Class I alleles in the development of PV (Ahmed et al. 1990). HLA-E*01:03X has also been associated with PV in Ashkenazi Jewish patients (Bhanusali et al. 2013).

2.2 Pemphigus Foliaceous

Pemphigus foliaceous (PF) is identified by widespread fragile bullae which rupture leaving erosions, crusting, and scaling. In contrast to pemphigus vulgaris, bullae develop on the skin and spare the mucous membranes. As in PV, a Th2 type response drives IgG4 autoantibody formation, with desmoglein 1 as the major autoantigen (Zenzo et al. 2016; Funakoshi et al. 2012). Thus, a patient's HLA class II molecules play a role in predisposition to PF.

2.2.1 MHC Class II, DR

In the HLA DR region, DRB1*01:01 and 01:02 confer risk for the development of sporadic PF in patients living in Brazil and France (Brochado et al. 2016; Loiseau et al. 2000). DRB1*04, and in particular the 04:01, 04:04, and 04:06 alleles, predispose patients of White British, French, Dutch, Indian, and Asian descent (de Sena Nogueira Maehara et al. 2018; Loiseau et al. 2000; Saha et al. 2018; Sun et al. 2019; Zhang et al. 2018b). Likewise, DRB*14, and in particular, 14:01, 14:05, and 14:04 increase PF risk in patients of Italian, Indian and Asian descent, but not of white British descent (Lombardi et al. 1999; Saha et al. 2018; Zhang et al. 2018b). In contrast, DRB1*08:01, 11:01, and 13:01 protect against PF (Brochado et al. 2016; Saha et al. 2018).

2.2.2 MHC Class II, DQ

In the DQ region, DQA1*01:02 increases the risk of PF in patients of Brazilian descent while DQA1*02:01 decreases the risk (Brochado et al. 2016; Zhang et al. 2018b). HLA-DQB1*03:02, 05:01, 05:02, and 05:03 likewise increase the risk of PF while 03:01 and 06:03 reduce the risk (Brochado et al. 2016; Loiseau et al. 2000; Saha et al. 2018; Sun et al. 2019; Zhang et al. 2018b). Particular haplotypes also play a role in the pathogenesis of sporadic PF as seen in PV. In patients of Indian and Asian ethnicities, DRB1*14:04/DQB1*05:03 is found in higher frequency in patients of PF, while in white British patients, DRB1*04:01/DQB1*03:02 and DRB1*04:04/DQB1*03:02 confer risk for PF disease development (Saha et al. 2018).

2.2.3 MHC Class I

MHC Class I HLA-A and HLA-B alleles have also been associated with sporadic PF. HLA-A2 is preventative while HLA-A11, A33, and B14 confer risk to patients of Brazilian descent (Brochado et al. 2016). Additionally, HLA-Bw4 epitope 80 T reduces the risk of disease while Bw6 confers risk in Euro-Brazilian patients living in urban regions (Augusto et al. 2012). In Japanese patients, HLA-A10 and C04 increase the risk of PF (Hashimoto et al. 1977; Miyagawa et al. 2002).

2.3 Endemic Pemphigus Foliaceous

Endemic pemphigus foliaceous (Fogo selvagem, FS) is a variant of pemphigus foliaceous which is thought to have an environmental trigger. In contrast to sporadic pemphigus foliaceous, which occurs worldwide, endemic pemphigus foliaceous is seen most commonly in Brazil and Tunisia. Antigenic mimicry against local insects results in autoantibody formation against desmoglein 1 (Aoki et al. 2015). In healthy patients, non-pathogenic IgG1 autoantibodies are produced against the EC5 subunit of desmoglein 1 (Zenzo et al. 2016; Li et al. 2003; Warren et al. 2003). However, in patients with particular HLA susceptibility genes, epitope spreading leads to the assembly of pathogenic IgG4 autoantibodies against the EC1 and EC2 subunits resulting in disease onset (Zenzo et al. 2016; Li et al. 2003; Warren et al. 2003).

In Brazil, FS is diagnosed more commonly in rural areas near streams and creeks in the Southern and Midwest states (Aoki et al. 2015). HLA-DR1*01:01, 01:02, 04:04, 04:06, and 16 predispose patients to disease (see Table 4) (de Sena Nogueira Maehara et al. 2018; Piovezan and Petzl-Erler 2013). Whereas, 03:01, 07:01, 11:01, 11:04, 13:01, 13:03 prevent FS (de Sena Nogueira Maehara et al. 2018; Piovezan and Petzl-Erler 2013) In the DQ region, DQB1*05 confers susceptibility to FS while DQB1*02 is protective (de Sena Nogueira Maehara et al. 2018). In Tunisia, sporadic and endemic PF occurs with the endemic type found more frequently in the southern-most regions of the country. HLA-DRB1*03 confers risk for Tunisian FS development while DRB1*11 and 15 alleles are protective (Abida et al. 2009). In the DQ region, DQB1*03:02 predisposes patients while 03:01 and 06 are negatively associated with disease (Abida et al. 2009).

2.4 Paraneoplastic Autoimmune Multiorgan Syndrome

The paraneoplastic autoimmune multiorgan syndrome is an uncommon subtype of pemphigus distinguished by multi-organopathy and autoantibody formation to plakins. Lymphoproliferative disorders/malignancies, including non-Hodgkin lymphoma, chronic lymphocytic leukemia, and Castleman's disease are most commonly associated, while non-hematologic neoplasms can be seen in up to 16% of patients (Kaplan et al. 2004). Diffuse inflammation of the oral mucosa with extension to the digestive tract or the airways develops with erythema, erosions, and crusting (Joly et al. 2000). Polymorphous cutaneous eruptions occur and can mimic erythema multiforme, lichen planus, or graft-vs-host disease (Joly et al. 2000). Complications include corneal ulceration and perforation, bronchiolitis obliterans, and respiratory failure with a mortality rate of 90% (Anan et al. 2011; Lee et al. 2015; Nousari et al. 1999; Piscopo et al. 2018).

Autoantibodies are most commonly found in members of the plakin family including desmoplakin I and II, envoplakin, periplakin, plectin, and BP 230 although antibodies to desmoglein 1

Table 4 HLA MHC Class II DRB1 and DQB1 allele associations in patients with endemic pemphigus foliaceous

Pemphigus foliaceous-endemic						
HLA-DRB1 Allele	References	Study type	Ethnicity	Effect	*N*	*P*-value
*01	Piovezan and Petzl-Erler (2013)	Case–control	Brazilians	S	206	****
*01:01	Piovezan and Petzl-Erler (2013)	Case–control	Brazilians	S	206	*
*01:02	Piovezan and Petzl-Erler (2013)	Case–control	Brazilians	S	206	****
*03	Abida et al. (2009)	Case–control	Tunisian	S	50	***
*03:01	Piovezan and Petzl-Erler (2013)	Case–control	Brazilians	P	206	*
*04	Piovezan and Petzl-Erler (2013)	Case–control	Brazilians	S	206	**
	de Sena Nogueira Maehara et al. (2018)	Case–control	Brazilian	S	42	****
	Abida et al. (2009)	Case–control	Tunisian	S	50	***
*04:04	Piovezan and Petzl-Erler (2013)	Case–control	Brazilians	S	206	*
*04:06	Piovezan and Petzl-Erler (2013)	Case–control	Brazilians	S	206	*
*07	Piovezan and Petzl-Erler (2013)	Case–control	Brazilians	P	206	****
	de Sena Nogueira Maehara et al. (2018)	Case–control	Brazilian	P	42	*
*07:01	Piovezan and Petzl-Erler (2013)	Case–control	Brazilians	P	206	****
*11	Piovezan and Petzl-Erler (2013)	Case–control	Brazilians	P	206	****
	Abida et al. (2009)	Case–control	Tunisian	P	50	*
*11:01	Piovezan and Petzl-Erler (2013)	Case–control	Brazilians	P	206	****
*11:04	Piovezan and Petzl-Erler (2013)	Case–control	Brazilians	P	206	**
*13	Piovezan and Petzl-Erler (2013)	Case–control	Brazilians	P	206	**
*13:01	Piovezan and Petzl-Erler (2013)	Case–control	Brazilians	P	206	**
*13:03	Piovezan and Petzl-Erler (2013)	Case–control	Brazilians	P	206	*
*15	Abida et al. (2009)	Case–control	Tunisian	P	50	*
*16	Piovezan and Petzl-Erler (2013)	Case–control	Brazilians	S	206	*
	de Sena Nogueira Maehara et al. (2018)	Case–control	Brazilian	S	42	*
HLA-DQB1 Allele						
*02	de Sena Nogueira Maehara et al. (2018)	Case–control	Brazilian	P	42	**
*03:01	Abida et al. (2009)	Case–control	Tunisian	S	50	**
*06	Abida et al. (2009)	Case–control	Tunisian	P	50	*

* = $p < 0.05$, ** = $p < 0.01$, *** = $p < 0.001$, *** * = $p < 0.0001$. P = protective, S = increased susceptibility. NS = no significant difference

and 3, desmocollin 1/2/3, BP180, and alpha-2 microglobulin-like 1 can also be detected (Amber et al. 2018d). Despite sharing similar antigens to PV and PF patients, patients with PAMS recognize a distinct pattern of epitopes. EC4 and EC5 act as the major auto-antigens in while IgG1, IgG2, and IgG3 are the predominant autoantibody isotypes formed (Brandt et al. 2012). Damage occurs through a cell-mediated process demonstrated by the predominance of CD8+ T-cells, natural killer cells, and macrophages on histology (Nguyen et al. 2001). Little data exists to confirm an association between HLA genes and PAMS. HLA-DRB1*03 predisposes Caucasian patients from North France to PAMS. HLA-Cw*14, specifically Cw*14:02, confers risk for PAMS in Chinese patients (Liu et al. 2008).

2.5 Non-HLA Genes and Polymorphisms Involved in Pemphigus Vulgaris

The investigation of non-HLA genes in pemphigus has yielded mixed results, and for the majority of these associations, has proven to be ethnicity dependent with conflicting data between different populations. As increased production of various cytokines is seen in patients with pemphigus, and as single nucleotide polymorphisms (SNP) can potentiate or diminish the expression of genes, the finding of SNP differences in patients with pemphigus directs us to a possible mechanism of action leading to these cytokine alterations.

2.5.1 TNF-A, IL-6, and IL-10

The most studied gene polymorphism of tumor necrosis factor-alpha (TNF-α) is the (−308) promoter region. A guanine at this position leads to decreased TNF-alpha production while an adenine leads to increased gene expression. In PV patients of Slovak origin, the *TNFα* (−308 G/−238 G) haplotype is increased, however, no significant variation is seen in patients of Polish, Egyptian or Argentinian descent (Javor et al. 2010; Mosaad et al. 2012; Torzecka et al. 2003). The (−308 A/G) gene polymorphism is in high linkage disequilibrium with the HLA-DRB1*0301 allele in specific populations, which is reduced in patients. It is unclear at this time if the higher frequency of the (−308 G) allele and lower frequency of the (−308 A) are due to their disequilibrium or their direct role in PV (Kumar et al. 2007).

Interleukin (IL)-6 functions as a pro-inflammatory Th2 cytokine and is increased in several autoimmune conditions (Camporeale and Poli 2012). In the Egyptian population, the *IL-6* (−174 C) SNP predisposes patients to PV (Mosaad et al. 2012).

IL-10 is an immunomodulatory cytokine that functions to limit the inflammatory response. In Argentinian patients with PV, the *IL-10* (−819 T) polymorphism is increased along with the −1082/−819A/T haplotype (Eberhard et al. 2005). Reduced IL-10 contributes to disinhibition of the inflammatory response while in unaffected patients the lack of these alleles is protective (Cho et al. 2015).

2.5.2 Suppression of Tumorgenicity 18 (ST18) and VH3

Suppression of tumorgenicity 18 (ST18) is a transcription factor that is overexpressed in the non-lesional skin of patients (Vodo et al. 2016). ST18 functions as a regulator of apoptosis and inflammation. In the presence of PV IgG, ST18 promotes the secretion of TNFα, IL-1α, and IL-6 and keratinocyte disadhesion (Vodo et al. 2016; Yang et al. 2008). Polymorphisms in the region near the *ST18* gene predispose patients of Jewish descent to PV (*rs4074067, rs10504140, rs2304365*) (Sarig et al. 2012). *rs2304365*, in particular, is also associated with disease in the Egyptian and Iranian population but not in German or Chinese patients (Etesami et al. 2018; Sarig et al. 2012; Yue et al. 2014). Additionally, the *ST18 rs2304365* A allele is associated with greater disease severity and higher age of disease onset (Etesami et al. 2018).

Another gene, *VH3*, codes for the variable region of antibody heavy chains. The *VH3f-R4* SNP predisposes patients to PV (Gibson et al. 1994). In contrast to date, no polymorphisms have been found in the constant light chain or heavy chain regions (Zitouni et al. 2002).

2.5.3 IgG3

Genetic differences in immunoglobulins confer differential risk for disease development. IgG3, encoded by *IGHG3*, is a potent complement activator and promoter of the innate immune response. Due to its decreased affinity to FcRn, a molecule that rescues IgG from lysosomal degradation, IgG3 has a reduced half-life compared to the other IgG subclasses (Stapleton et al.

2011). An amino acid substitution at position 435 results in increased FcRn affinity and bioavailability (Stapleton et al. 2011). In patients of German descent, histidine to arginine substitution at position 435 results in an increased risk for PV and not BP (Recke et al. 2018).

2.5.4 FCγR

Additionally, polymorphisms in the FCγR have also been attributed to disease development (Recke et al. 2015). Increased disease risk occurs in patients with *FCGRB.ORF/STOP* while decreased risk occurs in those with the *FCGRB.G (-385* C) allele, a polymorphism that enhances expression of FCγRIIb (Recke et al. 2015). FCγRIIb functions in B-cell tolerance through inhibition of immunoglobulin G production and its function in PV has not yet been determined.

2.5.5 Other Immunomodulatory SNPs

As pemphigus diseases develop due to loss of self-tolerance, several gene polymorphisms associated with immune modulation have been discovered in patients with PV. *TAP2*, a gene located within the major histocompatibility complex (MHC) class II region, codes for an ATP binding cassette transporter which functions in the transport of molecules across cell membranes, in antigen presentation, and the expression of MHC class I molecules. The *TAP2* (−655 A) gene variant is more prevalent in Jewish patients with PV (Slomov et al. 2005). Specific *BTNL2, MICB, and NOTCH4* gene polymorphisms are also found in Jewish PV patients within the MHC locus (Sarig et al. 2012). *BTNL2* codes for an immunoglobulin-like variable domain and an immunoglobulin-like constant region which function in T-cell activation and inhibition through a similar mechanism as CD80 and CD86 molecules (Simmonds et al. 2006). Likewise, *MICB* products function in T-cell silencing while *NOTCH4* products modulate keratinocyte differentiation (Groh et al. 2002; Okuyama et al. 2008). Together these genes are thought to play a role in the T-cell response seen in pemphigus. *CD86* is a gene that codes for a protein expressed on antigen-presenting cells, which functions to activate naïve T-cells and promotes B-cells IgG4 production (Jeannin et al. 1997). The *CD86 rs1129055* A allele predisposes Serbian patients while the GG genotype is protective (Tanasilovic et al. 2017). Given that IgG4 is the main pathogenic antibody isoform produced, these Serbian patients may have an increased risk for alterations in this pathway.

2.5.6 Desmoglein 3

Polymorphisms in DSG3 itself may play a role in susceptibility to PV. In British patients, the DSG3*TCCTC haplotype predisposes to PV while in Indian patients the DSG3*TCCCC haplotype confers risk of PV (Capon et al. 2006).

2.6 Non-HLA Genes in Pemphigus Foliaceous

Several polymorphisms have also been associated with the development of pemphigus foliaceous.

2.6.1 Ras-Related Nuclear Protein

RAN encodes Ras-related nuclear protein, a protein that functions in microtubule polymerization and GTP hydrolysis. In sporadic PF patients of Chinese descent, RAN is upregulated in affected lesions (Sun et al. 2019). The rs2178077 SNP on 12q24.33 is also found more commonly in these patients, and as this SNP holds the RAN gene, it supports its role in PF (Sun et al. 2019).

2.6.2 TNF-A, IL-4, and IL-6

As in patients with PV, specific polymorphisms in the TNFα and IL-6 genes are associated with sporadic PF susceptibility. The TNFα (-308) A allele is found more frequently in patients while the G allele appears to be protective in patients of Polish descent (Torzecka et al. 2003). Likewise, the IL-6 (-174) C allele increases the risk of PF while the G allele is protective (Mosaad et al. 2012). Polymorphisms in IL-4 also modify the risk of PF in Tunisian patients. The IL-4 rs2243250 (−590) T allele and the TT genotype confer increased disease risk while the C variant and CC genotype have protective effects

(Toumi et al. 2013). In contrast, there is no association with the IL-4 receptor, IL-13, or the IL-13 receptor (Toumi et al. 2013).

2.6.3 FoxP3

Forkhead protein 3 (FOXP3) is a transcription factor that plays a role in the development and function of T regulatory cells. FOXP3 is located on chromosome Xp11.23 and is linked to several autoimmune conditions, especially those with a female predominance (Bassuny et al. 2003; Gao et al. 2010; Park et al. 2005). In Tunisian patients with endemic PF, FOXP3 rs3761549C > T, rs3761548A > C, and rs2294021C > T predispose to disease while in patients with sporadic PF, rs3761549C > T and the GG genotype of rs3761547 are predisposed to disease (Ben Jmaa et al. 2017). Furthermore, the rs3761548 > AA and rs3761548 > AC genotypes are correlated with positive Nikolsky's sign while rs2294021 > CC is associated with generalized pemphigus. In contrast, rs2294021 > TT is protective and is found more commonly in patients with pemphigus herpetiformis (Ben Jmaa et al. 2017).

2.6.4 B-cell Stimulation

CD40 (Tumor necrosis factor 5, TNFR-5) is a co-stimulatory molecule found on B-cells, follicular dendritic cells, monocytes, and non-hematopoietic cells including thymic epithelial cells, vascular endothelial cells, and keratinocytes (Denfeld et al. 1996; Vogel and Noelle 1998). CD40 is necessary for B-cell activation, proliferation, survival, germinal center formation, memory cell generation, and isotype switching (Vogel and Noelle 1998). CD40 binds to its ligand (CD40L, CD154) which is expressed on activated T-cells (Roy et al. 1993; Vogel and Noelle 1998). Inhibition of CD40-CD40L binding prevents the development of anti-desmoglein 3 autoantibodies in animal models (Aoki-Ota et al. 2006). In Euro- and Afro-Brazilian patients the CD40L -726 T allele predisposes patients to endemic PF while the C allele is protective (Malheiros and Petzl-Erler 2009). The CD40 -1C allele also confers susceptibility while the T allele is protective in Euro-Brazilian patients (Malheiros and Petzl-Erler 2009). This correlates with the finding that patients with the CD40 T allele have decreased CD40 translation so that having the C allele allows patients to have sufficient amounts of CD40 to promote the development of pemphigus (Jacobson et al. 2005).

B-lymphocyte stimulator (BLYS, BAFF, TALL-1, zTNF4) is a tumor necrosis family member and is expressed on numerous cell types including T-cells and dendritic cells (Moore et al. 1999; Schneider et al. 1999). BLYS receptors are found on B-cells, and upon binding, promote B-cell proliferation, autoantibody production, and differentiation (Moore et al. 1999; Schneider et al. 1999). Upregulation of BLYS has been associated with several autoimmune diseases (Cheema et al. 2001; Groom et al. 2002). In Brazilian patients, the BLYS -871 T allele reduces susceptibility to endemic PF (Malheiros and Petzl-Erler 2009). Interestingly, the BLYS-871 T allele is associated with higher BLYS mRNA levels in monocytes, how this relates to pemphigus pathogenesis is unclear at this time (Kawasaki et al. 2002). Looking at the genes simultaneously, having the CD40-1 T allele or the CD40L-762C allele and the BLYS-871 T allele is protective against disease while having either of the two alleles without BLYS-871 T does not reduce disease susceptibility. Additionally, having the CD40L-762C and BLYS-871 T alleles provides a compound effect.

2.6.5 Killer Cell Lectin-Like Subfamily G Member 1

Killer cell lectin-like subfamily G member 1 (KLRG1) is a protein that functions as an inhibitory receptor on NK cells preventing their autoreactivity (Li et al. 2009). In patients with pemphigus, the KLRG1 gene expression is upregulated (Cipolla et al. 2016). The KLRG1 rs1805672 A/G allele is associated with susceptibility to PF in Brazilian patients. This SNP alters the mi-R584-5p binding site, thus preventing miR-584-5p from downregulating KLRG1 mRNA translation (Cipolla et al. 2016). Killer-cell immunoglobulin-like receptors (KIR) bind to HLA class I ligands and regulate natural killer (NK) cell function. KIR3DL1, an inhibitory receptor that binds to Bw4, is associated with disease in Euro-Brazilians but not in Afro-Brazilians living in urban regions (Augusto et al. 2012). In contrast, KIR2DS1 (activating), KIR2DS3 (activating), KIR3DS1 (activating) and KIR2DL5 (inhibitory) are protective (Augusto et al. 2012). Additionally, having 3 or more activating KIR genes is protective (Augusto et al. 2012). Separating into haplogroups, the AA genotype of the KIR A haplogroup (having only KIR2DS4 as the activating gene) confers susceptibility, while the presence of the B haplogroup is protective (Augusto et al. 2012). The combination of KIR3DL1 or KIR3DS1 and HLA-Bw4 awards greater protection than either alone (Augusto et al. 2012). The direct role of these NK cell receptors in pemphigus has yet to be determined.

2.6.6 Leukocyte Receptor Complex

Leukocyte receptor complex polymorphisms have also been found (Farias et al. 2019). In endemic PF patients of Brazilian descent, the intergenic rs465169 A allele and leukocyte receptor cluster member 8 (LENG8) rs35336528 increase susceptibility to PF (Farias et al. 2019). The intergenic rs465169 A allele, based on its location, is thought to modulate the avian musculoaponeurotic fibrosarcoma oncogene homolog (MAF). MAF plays a key role in epidermal differentiation, T-cell apoptosis, IL-4 expression on TH2 cells, in addition to, regulating several other LRC genes including LILRB2 and LAIR1 which are increased in PF (Camargo et al. 2016; Köck et al. 2014; Lopez-Pajares et al. 2015; Malheiros et al. 2014). In contrast, the Fc fragment of IgA receptor (FCAR/CD89) rs1865097 A allele is protective in endemic PF in patients of Brazilian descent (Farias et al. 2019). CIITA (major histocompatibility complex class II transactivator, MHC2TA) is a transcriptional coactivator necessary for the expression of the genes encoding the MHC class II α and β chains. The CIITA gene SNP, rs3087456 (−168A > G) G allele, results in reduced CITTA and MHC Class II mRNA (Swanberg et al. 2005) The G allele has been associated with rheumatoid arthritis and myocardial infarctions, and in Euro-Brazilian patients, leads to increased susceptibility to endemic PF (Piovezan and Petzl-Erler 2013; Swanberg et al. 2005).

2.6.7 Complement Pathway

Complement pathway gene variants have also been found in patients with endemic PF (Bumiller-Bini et al. 2018). Having two intronic C3 rs4807895*T alleles increases susceptibility in Brazilian patients possibly through upregulation of C3 gene expression (Bumiller-Bini et al. 2018). Likewise, polymorphisms in the alternative and lectin pathways have been found. Homozygosity for intronic complement factor H (CFH) rs34388368*T, a regulator of the alternative pathway, results in higher CFH mRNA levels and an increased risk of disease development (Bumiller-Bini et al. 2018). MASP1 is a gene whose products (MASP-1 and MASP-3) are important activators and inhibitors of the lectin and alternative pathways, coagulation, intracellular signaling, and bradykinin systems. Specifically, MASP-1 launches the lectin pathway through autoactivation while MASP-3 activates the alternative pathway and the p38 mitogen-associated protein kinase (MAPK) pathway. Patients with the MASP1 rs13094773*G and rs850309*G polymorphisms have a lower risk of PF while those with the rs3864098*C and rs698104*T alleles have increased disease susceptibility (Bumiller-Bini et al. 2018). Additionally, a missense mutation at rs72549154*T leads to increased MASP-3 and decreased MASP-1 levels, resulting in protection against PF (Bumiller-Bini et al. 2018).

Polymorphisms of the membrane attack complex (MAC) have also been associated with endemic PF (Bumiller-Bini et al. 2018). Increased disease prevalence occurs in Brazilian patients with the C8A rs11206934*C or C9 rs187875*T alleles (Bumiller-Bini et al. 2018). Whereas protection occurs in those with the C9 rs700218*A allele variant (Bumiller-Bini et al. 2018). The 5'UTR C5AR1 rs10404456*C allele, which decreases expression of the C5a receptor, increases susceptibility to disease (Bumiller-Bini et al. 2018). Reduced CD59 levels also predispose patients to PF by way of the rs1047581*G allele in the 3'UTR of the CD59 gene (Bumiller-

Bini et al. 2018). Opsonin-binding complement receptors have also been associated with endemic PF in Brazilian patients (Bumiller-Bini et al. 2018). The CR1 rs6656401*G allele confers increased risk while the CR2 rs2182911*C, ITGAM (CR3) rs1298810*A, and ITGAX (CR4) rs11574637*C allele are protective (Bumiller-Bini et al. 2018).

CD59 is a powerful inhibitor of MAC and functions in T-cell activation and signal transduction, neutrophil activation, and induction of cell death (Das et al. 2013; Davies and Lachmann 1993; Deckert et al. 1992; Farkas et al. 2002; Gorter and Meri 1999; Monleón et al. 2000; Sivasankar et al. 2007; Berg et al. 1995; Zhang et al. 2018a). Altered expression of CD59 is associated with susceptibility to rheumatoid arthritis, systemic lupus erythematosus, and several other autoimmune diseases (Das et al. 2013; Konttinen et al. 1996; Song 2006). Deficiency in CD59 leads to paroxysmal nocturnal hematuria (Song 2006). Carriers of the CD59 rs861256*G allele have increased CD59 mRNA expression and a higher risk of developing endemic PF in Afro-Brazilian and Euro Brazilian patients (Salviano-Silva et al. 2017). Euro-Brazilian females also have an increased risk with the rs831625*G allele, which is in high linkage disequilibrium with the CD59 rs861256*G allele (Salviano-Silva et al. 2017). In Afro-Brazilian patients only, there is also an association with the rs704701*C allele regardless of age and sex, while the rs704697*A allele confers increased risk in Euro-Brazilian females only (Salviano-Silva et al. 2017).

2.7 Non-Coding Sequences in Pemphigus

The microRNAs (miRNA) are non-coding mRNA sequences that regulate cell differentiation, maturation, apoptosis, growth, and signal transduction. The miRNA bind to miRNA-induced silencing complexes (miRISC) and together, they bind complementary mRNA sequences and inhibit translation (Simpson and Ansel 2015). In patients with pemphigus, there is a >1,500 fold increase in peripheral blood monocular cell miR-424-5p with targets including the MAPK signaling pathway, T-cell receptor signaling, intracellular signaling cascades, phosphate metabolism, and kinase activity (Wang et al. 2017).

Long non-coding RNA genes (lncRNA) encode RNA sequences which when transcribed, participate in the regulation of many cellular functions including chromatin remodeling, gene expression, nuclear and cytoplasmic trafficking, and as competitor endogenous RNAs (ceRNAs) (Rinn and Chang 2012; Salviano-Silva et al. 2018b). The lncRNA *AL110292.1 rs7144332*T,* located on chromosome 14, has a strong association with endemic PF in patients of Brazilian descent (Lobo-Alves et al. 2019). Likewise, *rs6095016*A in lnc-PREXI-7:1*, *rs7195536*G in AC009121.1*, *rs1542604*T in AC133785.1*, *rs6942557*C in linc01176*, and *rs17774133*T* in *linc01119* are associated with increased susceptibility to disease (Lobo-Alves et al. 2019). These polymorphisms are within alternative splicing regions and thus can either be present or absent in mature lncRNA isoforms (Lobo-Alves et al. 2019). Although the function of these lncRNA sequences has not yet been established, they appear to predispose patients to disease development. Similarly, *rs2655420* in *CASC15, rs12192707*A* in *LY86-AS1, and rs674485*G* in *NEAT1* increase the risk of endemic PF development (Salviano-Silva et al. 2018a). In contrast, *rs102280404*A* in *LINC-PINT* and *rs1884537*T* in *MEG3* confer protection against disease (Salviano-Silva et al. 2018a).

3 Pemphigoids

The pemphigoid group of AIBDs bears considerable similarities in their clinical presentations and immunopathogenesis (Schmidt and Zillikens 2013). Pemphigoids are characterized by an autoimmune response targeting distinct components of the basement membrane zone. Because of variance in clinical presentation diagnosis may be challenging and benefits from immunofluorescence and immunoserology studies (Amber et al.

2018b). Here we discuss the genetic influence on disease development in each subtype.

3.1 Bullous Pemphigoid

Bullous pemphigoid (BP) is the most common subepithelial autoimmune blistering disease. Although it presents across all age groups, there is a predilection for the elderly population (Kridin and Ludwig 2018; Patsatsi et al. 2018). Characteristically BP presents with intense pruritus and large, tense bullae on the skin, although it can have a polymorphic presentation (Amber et al. 2017; Baum et al. 2014; Schmidt et al. 2014). BP is driven by the development of autoantibodies targeting components of the hemidesmosome complex at the dermal–epidermal junction leading to loss of adhesion between the basal keratinocytes and the underlying basement membrane (Amber et al. 2018b).

Specifically, two antibodies targeting antigens BP180 and BP230 lead to this loss of structural integrity at the basement membrane zone and blister formation. BP180 targets the ectodomain of collagen XVII (COLXVII) near the cell membrane, a transmembrane protein that links intracellular proteins to the extracellular matrix (Amber et al. 2018b). BP230 is a member of the desmoplakin family and is an intracellular protein that links intermediate filaments to the hemidesmosome complex. The non-collagenous domain 16 within BP180 is the immunodominant region recognized by autoreactive T and B-cells and is currently thought to be the main antigenic stimulus in BP pathogenesis (Thoma-Uszynski et al. 2006).

3.1.1 MHC Class II Alleles

The most significant association has been found in patients harboring the HLA-DQB1*03:01 across a variety of ethnic groups including Caucasians, Iranians, Brazilians, and Chinese (Table 5) (Büdinger et al. 1998; Chagury et al. 2018; Delgado et al. 1996; Esmaili et al. 2013; Fang et al. 2018; Vaira et al. 2013). There are however important differences in HLA alleles that lend susceptibility to disease development across different ethnic groups. Notably, the northern Chinese and general Japanese populace

Table 5 MHC Class II HLA allele associations in patients with bullous pemphigoid

Bullous pemphigoid						
HLA Allele D	Authors	Study type	Ethnicity	Effect	N	*P*-value
D	Venning et al. (1992)	Population	British	–	13	NS
	Ahmed et al. (1984)	Population	American	–	42	NS
DQ7	Banfield et al. (1998)	Population	British Caucasian men	S	34	**
HLA-DQA1						
*01:02	Fang et al. (2018)	Population	Northern Chinese	P	105	***
*01:03	Fang et al. (2018)	Population	Northern Chinese	P	105	*
	Ujie et al. (2018)	Cohort	Japanese DPP-4i	p	21	****
	Chagury et al. (2018)	Population	Brazilian	S	17	**
*01:05	Fang et al. (2018)	Population	Northern Chinese	S	105	****
*05:01	Esmali et al. (2013)	Population	Iranian	S	50	*
*05:05	Chagury et al. (2018)	Population	Brazilian	S	17	***
	Ujie et al. (2018)	Cohort	Japanese DPP-4i	S	21	****
	Fang et al. (2018)	Population	Northern Chinese	S	105	***

(continued)

Table 5 (continued)

Bullous pemphigoid						
HLA Allele D	Authors	Study type	Ethnicity	Effect	N	*P*-value
*05:08	Fang et al. (2018)	Population	Northern Chinese	S	105	*
HLA-DQB1						
*02:01	Vaira et al. (2013)	Case	Italian	–	1	Qualitative
	Setterfield et al. (1997)	Case	British	–	1	Qualitative
*03:01	Minagawa et al. (2015)	Familial	Japanese	–	2	Qualitative
	Vaira et al. (2013)	Case	Italian	–	1	Qualitative
	Esmali et al. (2013)	Population	Iranian	S	50	*
	Zakka et al. (2010)	Cohort	American	–	7	Qualitative
	Büdinger et al. (1998)	Cohort	–	–	16	Qualitative
	Delgado et al. (1996)	Population	American	S	21	**
	Ujie et al. (2018)	Cohort	Japanese DPP-4i	S	21	****
	Fang et al. (2018)	Population	Northern Chinese	S	105	*
	Chagury et al. (2018)	Population	Brazilian	S	17	***
	Sun et al. (2018)	Population	Han Chinese	S	572	****
*03:02	Zakka et al. (2010)	Cohort	American	–	7	Qualitative
	Okazaki et al. (2000)	Cohort	Japanese	S	23	*
*03:03	Sun et al. (2018)	Population	Han Chinese	P	572	****
*04:01	Esmali et al. (2013)	Population	Iranian	S	50	*
*05:01	Fang et al. (2018)	Population	Northern Chinese	S	105	****
*05:03	Zakka et al. (2010)	Cohort	American	–	7	Qualitative
*06:01	Ujie et al. (2018)	Cohort	Japanese DPP-4i	P	21	****
	Sun et al. (2018)	Population	Han Chinese	P	572	****
*06:02	Zakka et al. (2010)	Cohort	American	–	7	Qualitative
HLA-DRB1						
DR	Venning et al. (1989)	Population	British	–	32	NS
	Schaller et al. (1991)	Population	German	–	57	NS
*04	Minagawa et al. (2015)	Familial	Japanese	–	2	Qualitative
	Okazaki et al. (2000)	Cohort	Japanese	–	23	Qualitative
*07:01	Fang et al. (2018)	Population	Northern Chinese	P	105	**
*08	Gao et al. (2002)	Population	Northern Chinese	P	25	*
*10:01	Fang et al. (2018)	Population	Northern Chinese	S	105	****
*11:01	Ujie et al. (2018)	Cohort	Japanese DPP-4i	S	21	****
	Okazaki et al. (2000)	Cohort	Japanese	S	23	*
*12:01	Ujie et al. (2018)	Cohort	Japanese DPP-4i	S	21	****

* = $p < 0.05$, ** = $p < 0.01$, *** = $p < 0.001$, **** = $p < 0.0001$. *P* = protective, *S* = increased susceptibility, *NS* = no significant difference

do not have an association with DQB1*03:01 and BP (Gao et al. 2002; Okazaki et al. 2000). Although there are limited studies on these particular populations, the susceptibility to BP in the Japanese population is associated with alleles DRB1*1101 and DQB1*0302 as well as haplotypes DRB1*04/DQA1*0301/DQB1*0302 and DRB1*1101/DQA1*0505/DQB1*0302. Brazilian patients, similarly to western counterparts, showed an association with DQB1*03:01, and DQA1*05:05 which was also elevated in the Han Chinese. Additionally, one novel allele, DQA1*01:03, has so far only been found to be associated with BP in Brazilian patients (Chagury et al. 2018).

In a subgroup of Japanese patients who developed BP while receiving treatment for type II diabetes mellitus with dipeptidyl peptidase 4 inhibitors (DDP-4i), there was a higher prevalence of the DQB1*03:01 allele (Ujiie et al. 2018). Additionally, this subgroup had significant associations with DQA1*0505, DRB1*11:01, and DRB1*12:01. Two alleles were shown to be protective against DPP-4i induced BP; DQA1*01:03, DQB1*06:01.

The diversity of Chinese genetics is also vital to consider when interpreting potential genetic contributions to BP. The northern Chinese population, as mentioned, does not have a link between the DQB1*03:01 allele and BP. Rather, only one protective allele DRB1*08, and its haplotype DRB1*08/DQB1*06 have been identified (Gao et al. 2002). Investigations into the Han Chinese populace, however, identified numerous alleles including DQB1*03:01, DQA1*01:05, DQA1*05:05, DQA1*05:08, DQB1*03, DQB1*05:01, and DRB1*10:01 as genetic risk factors for BP (Fang et al. 2018; Sun et al. 2018). In contrast, these alleles were found to be protective against BP; DQA1*01:02, DQA1*01:03, DQB1*02:02, DRB1*07:01, DQB1*03:03, and DQB1*06:01 (Fang et al. 2018; Sun et al. 2018).

In an isolated study on Iranian patients, in addition to HLA-DQB1*03:01, DQA1*05:01 and DQB1*04:01 were shown to predispose to BP (Esmaili et al. 2013).

3.1.2 Collagen XVII

Genetic variation in the gene encoding COLXVII, *COL17A1*, which contains the major autoantigen associated with BP, could have substantial effects on the expression and immunological recognition of this protein and thus the development of BP. Numerous SNPs have been identified in coding and non-coding regions of *COL17A1* in a population of Northern European Caucasians however, none correlate with susceptibility or protection against BP (Winsey et al. 2004).

3.1.3 IgG

IgG3 is a potent activator of complement and immune effector cells (Recke et al. 2010). Certain polymorphisms produce amino acid conversions at position 435 from arginine to histidine resulting in greater half-life and increased FcRn affinity (Stapleton et al. 2011). BP is not associated with the SNP rs4042056 or the particular allotype G3m15 that confer risk in other autoimmune blistering diseases (Recke et al. 2018).

Kappa light chain Ig allotypes $Km^{1,2}$ and the genotype $Km^3/Km^{1,2}$ are risk factors for BP in French Caucasians (Jefferis and Lefranc 2009; Raux et al. 2000).

3.1.4 FcγR

The affinity of FcγRIIIa, expressed on macrophages and natural killer cells is mediated through an SNP at position 559. Results regarding the association of a low-affinity FcγRIIIa (F/F) allotype in European Caucasians and BP are conflicting (Guilabert et al. 2011; Recke et al. 2015; Weisenseel et al. 2007). There is, however, a negative association between high

FcγRIIIb and low FcγRIIc copy numbers in Germans (Recke et al. 2015). Paradoxically, high copy numbers of FcγRIIIb, which is expressed exclusively on neutrophils and is associated with increased reactive oxygen species (ROS) release, a crucial step in the pathogenesis of BP, exhibit this protective role (Recke et al. 2015).

3.1.5 IL-1β and TNF-A

IL-1β is a pleiotropic cytokine with a serum to blister gradient in BP (Ameglio et al. 1998; Fang et al. 2016; Schmidt et al. 1996; Sun et al. 2000). There is an increased frequency of two SNPs in the IL-1β gene at positions (-511 T) and (-31C) in the female Chinese BP population (Chang et al. 2006). The TNF-α-308G/A polymorphism does not appear to predispose to BP (Moravvej et al. 2018).

3.1.6 ATP-Binding Cassette Subfamily B Member 1

The ATP-binding cassette (ABC) superfamily includes the P-glycoprotein (P-gp), coded for by *ATP-binding cassette subfamily B member 1 (ABCB1)* gene, and are involved in extracellular transport of xenobiotics and endogenous substances such as cytokines (IL-2 and IFN-γ) (Park et al. 2003; Rychlik-Sych et al. 2017, 2018). Genetic alterations in *ABCB1* affect therapeutic efficacy and potentially contribute to disease development (Barańska et al. 2017; Kopp et al. 2015; Rychlik-Sych et al. 2017; Zhong et al. 2016). The 2677T allele and genotypes including it, 2677TT and 2677TA, confer susceptibility for BP in the Poles. These polymorphisms 2677T/A result in the amino acid conversion of alanine to serine or threonine at position 893 of P-gp. The 2677G allele and 2677GG genotype offer protection in the same population (Rychlik-Sych et al. 2017). Additionally, the 1236T-2677G-3435T haplotype confers protection in Poles (Rychlik-Sych et al. 2018). There was no association with either 3435C or 34345T alleles (Rychlik-Sych et al. 2017).

3.1.7 Cytochrome P450 Enzymes

In a similar vein, genetic variance in the cytochrome P450 family of enzymes can alter the metabolism of xenobiotics and endogenous compounds and are known to increase susceptibility to a host of diseases (Gao and Zhang 1999; Gołab-Janowska et al. 2007; Lee and Bae 2017; Mota et al. 2015; Rychlik-Sych et al. 2013; Skrętkowicz et al. 2011). Keratinocytes express these transmembrane transporters and metabolic enzymes (Merk 2009). The CYP2D6*3 alleles, and the CYP2D6*3/CYP2D6*4 genotypes confer risk for BP in Poles (Rychlik-Sych et al. 2015).

3.1.8 Mitochondrial ATP8

ROS contribute to blister formation and BP pathogenesis (Graauw et al. 2017; Schmidt and Zillikens 2013). Mutations in the mitochondrially encoded ATP8 synthase gene, *MT-ATP8*, result in increased levels of ROS production and are linked to greater disease severity in several autoimmune diseases (Hirose et al. 2015; Yu et al. 2009). Three potentially protective SNPs against BP in positions (−8388C), (−8473C), (−8557A) in *MT-ATP8* were more prevalent in the German control arm. Conversely, the SNP in position (−8519A), which causes a glutamic acid to lysine substitution, is more frequent among BP patients (Hirose et al. 2015).

3.2 Pemphigoid Gestationis

Pemphigoid gestationis (PG) is a rare autoimmune skin disease most often occurring during pregnancy or the puerperium. Clinically PG is grouped under the pemphigoid diseases, generating characteristic autoantibodies against COLXVII (Sadik et al. 2016). PG is unique in that the break-in immunotolerance occurs at a time when there is a sensitive uteroplacental immunological balance that is necessary to maintain the viability of the fetus. Characteristically, the outer trophoblast layers of the villous placenta and extraplacental chorionic membrane serve to protect the fetus from immunological recognition by the mother's adaptive immune system (Intong and Murrell 2011). The break in the tolerance that occurs in PG is believed to stem from the anomalous expression of MHC II molecules in the placenta (Borthwick et al. 1984; Kelly et al. 1989). This abnormal expression pattern plays a pivotal role in the presentation of BP180, which is expressed in the placenta and umbilical cord, to maternal MHC II molecules in the presence of paternal MHC II. The display of self-antigen, in this case, BP180, in the setting of paternal MHC is the likely culprit in generating an allogeneic response (Kelly et al. 1989).

Initially, notable relations between HLA-DR3 and DR4 maternal expression were shown through serological and immunofluorescence methods (Shornick et al. 1984, 1981). In an effort to determine whether specific anti-HLA antibodies play an important role in PG, paternal HLA expression was also investigated (Borthwick et al. 1984; Hines 1978; Shornick et al. 1983). Interestingly, over a quarter of normal, multiparous women have detectable anti-HLA antibodies (Shornick et al. 1983). There is contrasting evidence regarding an association between paternal HLA-DR2 and partners with PG (Hines 1978; Shornick et al. 1983). Furthermore, the majority of the maternal partners were positive for HLA-DR3 and DR4 expression which previously exhibited a strong association with PG (Shornick et al. 1984, 1981). Although most patients had detectable levels of anti-HLA class I and class II antibodies, the influence these have on disease development is unclear as anti-HLA antibodies were not shown to fix complement at the basement membrane zone (BMZ) (Shornick et al. 1983).

With the emergence of genetic sequencing techniques, specific polymorphisms in HLA class II alleles were able to be teased out. Alleles, DRB1*0301 and DRB1*0401/040X were found to individually have strong associations with PG, however, the haplotype containing both was found in about a quarter of patients (Shornick et al. 1995). Two alleles at the DQ locus, DQA1*2 and DQB1*0201, were found in higher frequencies in PG patients however, this is attributed to linkage disequilibrium with DRB1*0301 (Shornick et al. 1995).

Preliminary, small studies on various ethnic groups, including those of Mexican and Arab ancestry offer a window into the importance of genetic lineage when considering which alleles confer susceptibility for PG. Patients of Mexican lineage with PG were also found to have a preponderance of the HLA-DR3/DR4 haplotypes. Specifically, the HLA-DR3 haplotypes were all HLA-DRB1*0301, DQA1*0501, and DQB1*0201. Whereas the HLA-DR4 haplotypes were split between the DRB1*0401 subtype and DRB1*0407 with all being DQA1*03, DQB1*0302. Although the DRB1*0407 allele is the most frequent among Mexican patients, the association of a specific haplotype including this allele still lends weight to a relationship between this polymorphism and PG in this specific subset of patients (García-González et al. 1999). Kuwaiti patients displayed a strong association with HLA-DR3, but in contrast to previous findings had no connection with HLA-DR4 and exhibited a novel tie to HLA-DQ2 (Nanda et al. 2003).

Lastly, PG bears a significant relationship with an HLA class III C4 allele, C4*QO, but was not found to have an association with any C3 or factor B alleles (Shornick et al. 1993).

3.3 Mucous Membrane Pemphigoid

Mucous membrane pemphigoid (MMP) incorporates several autoimmune blistering diseases that all present with predominant mucosal involvement, and less common skin, secondary to autoantibodies targeting components of the BMZ. By international consensus, MMP encompasses a clinical phenotype identified by subepithelial blisters, erosions, and scarring of mucosal surfaces, and the skin (Murrell et al. 2015). Any mucosa such as the pharynx, larynx, nasal cavity, conjunctiva, and anogenital region may be involved. A multitude of autoantigens is targeted in MMP with patients often having autoantibodies targeting several BMZ proteins including BP180 and BP230. There is considerable overlap in the antigenic stimulus in BP and MMP. In addition to antibodies toward BP180, MMP patients also exhibit antibodies toward the ectodomain shedding products of BP180, such as the 120-kDa LAD-1, and 97-kDa LABD-97

(Oyama et al. 2006). In a subset of MMP patients, the disease is confined to the conjunctiva (Thorne et al. 2004). These individuals have autoantibodies targeting integrin β-4 and α-6 subunits (Rashid et al. 2006).

Although there is overlap in the autoantibodies present in the pemphigoid clinical variants, BP-associated autoantibodies target distinct epitopes (Oyama et al. 2006; Rashid et al. 2006). From a genetics perspective, however, many studies have shown significant associations between HLA-DQB1*0301 and all the clinical variants of pemphigoid. Computer models have verified experimental findings and provided specific recognition sites for HLA-DQB1*0301 on each of these unique antigens (Delgado et al. 1996; Zakka et al. 2011). This particular HLA allele confers increased susceptibility to the development of all the clinical pemphigoid variants.

3.3.1 Ocular Cicatricial Pemphigoid

The most significant and widely studied association in ocular cicatricial pemphigoid (OCP) patients is between HLA II allele DQB1*0301 (Ahmed et al. 1991; Chan et al. 1997, 1994; Haider et al. 1992; Minagawa et al. 2015; Yunis et al. 1994; Zaltas et al. 1989). Despite its significance in other pemphigoids, sequencing of the second and third exons, where the most polymorphisms are present, showed no significant differences between controls and OCP patients (Haider et al. 1992). Notably, a single study on British Caucasian patients failed to show evidence of increased DQB1*0301 frequency in patients with localized ocular involvement (Hübner et al. 2018). Additional associations were, however, found between HLA II alleles; DRB1*04, DQA1*03, DR4, and DR5 in OCP (Yunis et al. 1994; Zaltas et al. 1989).

Position 57 in the DQB1 polypeptide contains a peptide-binding groove and functions in peptide recognition (Kwok et al. 1996). OCP and oral pemphigoid (OP) patients harbor an aspartate residue in this position is significantly higher proportions (Yunis et al. 1994). Furthermore, several DQ alleles in these patient subsets, including DQB1*0301, share common amino acid residues at positions 71–77 with a yet unidentified role in MMP pathogenesis (Yunis et al. 1994).

Several HLA class I and III alleles have also been investigated. Initially, HLA-B12 was found to be associated with OCP however, later studies failed to support this information (Mondino et al. 1978, 1979; Venning et al. 1989; Zaltas et al. 1989). HLA-A2, B8, B35, and B49 were found to be associated in addition to several complements, HLA III, genes SC01, SC30, SC32, SC41, and SC42 (Ahmed et al. 1991).

3.3.2 Mucous Membrane Pemphigoid

The disease spectrum encompassing MMP, aside from predominant ocular involvement which was discussed in the preceding section, varies widely from minimal gingival inflammation to more severe cases involving the oropharynx and esophagus. The tendency for healing with scarring in MMP can result in disastrous consequences for those with lesions in these areas and potentially result in troubles with eating and breathing.

MHC Class II Alleles

The association between MMP and DQB1*0301 has been validated primarily in Caucasian populations including Americans, French, British, and Italians. (Carrozzo et al. 2001; Drouet et al. 1998; Hübner et al. 2018; Rabelo et al. 2014; Setterfield et al. 2001; Yunis et al. 1994). High-resolution sequencing of the DQB1*0301 allele was performed in an Egyptian family in which the only known case of pemphigoid was in a male child presenting with OP. Several other family members were found to harbor the DQB1*0301 allele without disease development. Carriers may be rendered more susceptible to pemphigoid, but disease development likely requires certain environmental triggers in the setting of this genetic predisposition (Mostafa et al. 2010, 2011).

Investigations into the DQB1*0301 allele frequency and correlations with site involvement have yielded slightly discordant results. The strength of the association between this allele and clinical phenotype varies amongst different patient populations. These differences highlight environmental triggers that may push a set of patients toward a certain pattern of disease on the MMP spectrum. French Caucasian patients also failed to show an association between DQB1*0301 and involved mucosa (Drouet et al. 1998). In the British Caucasian population, DQB1*0301 frequency was increased in all subsets and areas of clinical involvement except for the esophagus, larynx, and perianal region. These clinical sites of involvement, however, lacked power (Setterfield et al. 2001). In contrast, Italian patients with primarily oral lesions were more likely to be homozygous for the DQB1*0301 allele compared to healthy controls (Carrozzo et al. 2001).

Several HLA alleles found less frequently in MMP patients are thought to be protective. Across various populations, these include the generic DQB1*02 alleles in French and British Caucasians (Drouet et al. 1998; Hübner et al. 2018; Setterfield et al. 2001). DRB1*11 is also associated with MMP susceptibility in the British Caucasian population (Hübner et al. 2018; Setterfield et al. 2001), while DQB1*0302, DRB1*0301 appear protective (Hübner et al. 2018; Setterfield et al. 2001).

MHC Class I Alleles

Only a few studies regarding the significance of HLA class I alleles and their association with MMP have been conducted to date. These studies were performed before advancements in sequencing techniques. To this respect, no association between MMP and HLA class I A, B, or Cw was identified in British or American patients (Setterfield et al. 2001; Venning et al. 1989).

MHC Haplotypes

Several haplotypes are more prevalent in MMP patients. All haplotypes include the DQB1*0301 allele. Associations between MMP and certain individual alleles have not been established, and some are in linkage disequilibrium with DQB1*0301. Significant haplotypes identified in MMP include DRB1*04/DRB4*0101/DQA1*03/DQB1*0301 in Americans, DRB1*1101/DQB1*0301 in the French and British, and DRB1*04/DQB1*0301 only in the British (Drouet et al. 1998; Setterfield et al. 2001; Yunis et al. 1994). A single haplotype, DRB1*0701/DQB1*0202, including an aforementioned potentially protective allele, DQB1*02 was identified in French patients (Drouet et al. 1998).

SNPs

There is a dearth of studies regarding gene polymorphisms in MMP. Two studies centering on specific populations, Northern Italian and Germans, respectively, have been conducted. Polymorphisms of numerous pro-and anti-inflammatory cytokines were investigated in Northern Italian patients with predominantly oral MMP. A plethora of allele and genotype frequencies identified include: IL-1α (–889T/C), IL-1β (–511 C/T, +3962T/C), IL-12 (–1188 C/A), IFN-gamma (UTR 5644 A/T), TGF-β (codon 10 C/T, codon 25 G/C), TNF-α (–308 G/A, –238 G/A), IL-2 (–330 T/G, + 166 G/T), IL-4 (–1098 T/G, –590 T/C, –33T/C), IL-6 (–174 G/C, nt565 G/A), IL-10 (–1082 G/A, –819 C/T, –592 C/A), IL-1R (C/T pst1 1970), IL-1RA (T/C mspa1 11,100), IL-4RA (–1902 G/A) (23,557,074 (Carrozzo et al. 2014)). No significant differences in allele or genotype frequencies were found with the inclusion of the entire MMP cohort. An SNP in the IL-4RA gene at position 1902 was more frequent in patients with limited oral cavity involvement compared to healthy controls (Carrozzo et al. 2014; Hershey et al. 1997).

Genome-wide association studies on British and German cohorts identified two novel SNPs with unidentified relevance in MMP pathogenesis. Notably, the study population consisted mainly of ocular dominant MMP. SNP rs17203398 is located intronically in the *β-galactocerebrosidase* (*GALC*) gene on chromosome 14 (Sadik et al. 2014). The most established pathologic association between the *GALC* gene is the homozygous deletion that causes Krabbe's disease (Hill et al. 2013). Although, β-galactocerebrosidase dysfunction results in a basal proinflammatory lymphocytic state and is copy number dependent, how this particular SNP modulates MMP pathology is unclear (Formichi et al. 2007; Liu et al. 2011).

The second associated SNP was rs9936045, located on chromosome 16 between the genes

Cancer susceptibility candidate 16 (CASC16) and *Chromatin-helicase DNA binding protein (CHD9)*. The significance of this intergenic SNP on gene expression, and whether these genes are pathogenically involved in MMP is not currently known (Sadik et al. 2014).

3.4 Epidermolysis Bullosa Acquisita

Epidermolysis bullosa acquisita (EBA) is a rare autoimmune blistering disease presenting clinically with mucocutaneous blisters and erosions (Amber et al. 2018b; Ludwig 2013). Autoantibodies against collagen VII (COLVII), specifically the NC1 domain, are characteristic and bind to anchoring fibrils at the dermal–epidermal junction (DEJ) (Amber et al. 2018b; Koga et al. 2018). Several subtypes are recognized with many presenting with clinical features reminiscent of other AIBD as well as dystrophic epidermolysis bullosa (DEB), an inherited condition characterized by mutations in the gene encoding for COLVII, *COL7A1* (Koga et al. 2018).

The incidence of EBA is reported to be less than 0.5 per million annually (Amber et al. 2018b; Kridin 2018b). Although, it may present at any age with reports ranging from 1 to 94 years, its incidence peaks during the second and seventh decade of life (Amber et al. 2018b; Koga et al. 2018). Due to the low prevalence of this disease few investigations into the genetic contributions in humans have been conducted relative to the previously discussed AIBD. Here we highlight those studies.

3.4.1 HLA Genes

Investigations into genetic associations and EBA are particularly sparse which may be attributed to the low prevalence of this acquired disease. Currently, the literature only has four studies regarding links between unique HLA class II genes and the development of EBA which will be briefly discussed here. The HLA-DR2 allele, which corresponds to DRB1*15, was significantly elevated in black Americans of African descent (Gammon et al. 1988). Korean patients with the DRB1*13 have a genetic predisposition to EBA (Lee et al. 1996). French individuals of sub-Saharan African origins had significant associations with DRB1*15:03. Those with West Indian ethnic roots did not have a greater prevalence of the DRB1*15:03 allele, however, this observation may be attributable to the small patient study population (Zumelzu et al. 2011). Each patient bearing the DRB1*15:03 allele additionally was found to harbor the DQB1*06:02 allele, which is known to be in linkage disequilibrium with DRB1*15:03 (Zumelzu et al. 2011).

3.4.2 Collagen VII

Several reports exist on the development of EBA in DEB patients (Guerra et al. 2018; Hayashi et al. 2016). DEB and EBA are both subepidermal blistering diseases with similar clinical presentations but significant differences in pathogenic origins as DEB is an inherited disorder while EBA is an acquired autoimmune disease (Amber et al. 2018b). Dominant and recessive mutations in the *COL7A1* gene, which codes for COLVII are responsible for the genetically inherited structural instability in the anchoring fibrils of DEB patients which is subtyped into a dominant and recessive type (Vorobyev et al. 2017). Detection of anti-COLVII antibodies in recessive DEB (RDEB) has been identified in over 50% of patients (Pendaries et al. 2010; Tampoia et al. 2013; Woodley et al. 2014). However, due to lack of characteristic immunofluorescent findings consistent with EBA; IgG, or C3 in a μ-serrated pattern at the DEJ, these antibodies are considered non-pathogenic and patients with these antibodies largely do not develop EBA (Pendaries et al. 2010; Tampoia et al. 2013; Vodegel et al. 2004; Woodley et al. 2014). Genetic studies across 3 generations of dominant DEB (DDEB) in a Japanese family identified a recurrent heterozygous missense mutation c.7868G > A (p. Gly2623Asp) in the *COL7A1* gene of all afflicted individuals (Hayashi et al. 2016). This mutation has been correlated with a mild form of DEB (Sawamura et al. 2006). Curiously, the eldest genotyped patient developed went on to develop EBA.

Case reports concerning an Italian patient with a mild, nails-only RDEB who developed EBA in adulthood identified novel mutations in *COLVII gene*. Heterozygous missense mutations identified were c.410G > A (p.Arg137Gln) and c.3674C > T (p.Ala1225_Gln1241del) (Guerra et al. 2018). This arginine to glycine substitution corresponds to a conserved residue in the NC1 domain (Colombatti and Bonaldo 1991). The 3674C > T mutation results in a 17 amino acid deletion due to exon skipping and is postulated to disturb the formation of cystine knots which may favor partial unfolding of the triple helix (Wegener et al. 2014). The direct contributions of these mutations to the development of EBA can only be speculated. However, reports similar to this in the literature with EBA development in DEB families suggest a yet unidentified genetic predisposition (Noe et al. 2008). It is important to recognize that individuals with DEB may also be predisposed to EBA through environmental factors rather than these reported genetic variants. Thus, consideration of this related autoimmune disease is important when a DEB patient experiences worsening symptoms later in life.

4 Conclusions

Autoimmune blistering diseases represent a diverse group of antigen direct autoantibody-mediated diseases. While much remains to be elucidated regarding the pathogenesis of these diseases, it is apparent that genetic predisposition plays a significant role. With improvements and improved access to advanced genomic techniques, identifying key genetic predispositions may provide insight into the pathogenesis of each disease.

References

Abida O, Zitouni M, Kallel-Sellami M, Mahfoudh N, Kammoun A, Ben Ayed M, Masmoudi A, Mokni M, Fezzaa B, Ben Osman A, Kammoun MR, Turki H, Makni H, Gilbert D, Joly P, Tron F, Makni S, Masmoudi H, Pemphigus F-TGfSaRo (2009) Tunisian endemic pemphigus foliaceus is associated with the HLA-DR3 gene: anti-desmoglein 1 antibody-positive healthy subjects bear protective alleles. Br J Dermatol 161:522–527

Ahmed AR, Kaveri S (2018) Reversing autoimmunity combination of rituximab and intravenous immunoglobulin. Front Immunol 9:1189

Ahmed AR, Konqui A, Park MS, Tiwari JL, Terasaki PI (1984) DR antigens in bullous pemphigoid. Arch Dermatol 120:795

Ahmed AR, Yunis EJ, Khatri K, Wagner R, Notani G, Awdeh Z, Alper CA (1990) Major histocompatibility complex haplotype studies in Ashkenazi Jewish patients with pemphigus vulgaris. Proc Natl Acad Sci U S A 87:7658–7662

Ahmed AR, Foster S, Zaltas M, Notani G, Awdeh Z, Alper CA, Yunis EJ (1991) Association of DQw7 (DQB1*0301) with ocular cicatricial pemphigoid. Proc Natl Acad Sci U S A 88:11579–11582

Alpsoy E, Akman-Karakas A, Uzun S (2015) Geographic variations in epidemiology of two autoimmune bullous diseases: pemphigus and bullous pemphigoid. Arch Dermatol Res 307:291–298

Altun E, Yayli S, Toraman B, Arica DA, Kalay E, Selcuk LB, Bahadir S (2017) HLA-E*0101/0103X is associated with susceptibility to pemphigus vulgaris: a case-control study. Acta Dermatovenerol Croat 25:189–194

Amagai M, Klaus-Kovtun V, Stanley JR (1991) Autoantibodies against a novel epithelial cadherin in pemphigus vulgaris, a disease of cell adhesion. Cell 67:869–877

Amber KT, Korta DZ, de Feraudy S, Grando SA (2017) Vesiculobullous eruption in a patient receiving psoralen ultraviolet A (PUVA) treatment for prurigo nodules: a case of PUVA-aggravated pemphigoid nodularis. Clin Exp Dermatol 42:833–835

Amber KT, Maglie R, Solimani F, Eming R, Hertl M (2018a) Targeted therapies for autoimmune bullous diseases: current status. Drugs 78:1527–1548

Amber KT, Murrell DF, Schmidt E, Joly P, Borradori L (2018b) Autoimmune subepidermal bullous diseases of the skin and mucosae: clinical features, diagnosis, and management. Clin Rev Allergy Immunol 54:26–51

Amber KT, Valdebran M, Grando SA (2018c) Non-desmoglein antibodies in patients with pemphigus vulgaris. Front Immunol 9:1190

Amber KT, Valdebran M, Grando SA (2018d) Paraneoplastic autoimmune multiorgan syndrome (PAMS): beyond the single phenotype of paraneoplastic pemphigus. Autoimmun Rev 17:1002–1010

Ameglio F, D'Auria L, Bonifati C, Ferraro C, Mastroianni A, Giacalone B (1998) Cytokine pattern in blister fluid and serum of patients with bullous pemphigoid: relationships with disease intensity. Br J Dermatol 138:611–614

Anan T, Shimizu F, Hatano Y, Okamoto O, Katagiri K, Fujiwara S (2011) Paraneoplastic pemphigus associated with corneal perforation and cutaneous alternariosis: a case report and review of cases treated with rituximab. J Dermatol 38:1084–1089

Anhalt GJ, Labib RS, Voorhees JJ, Beals TF, Diaz LA (1982) Induction of pemphigus in neonatal mice by passive transfer of IgG from patients with the disease. N Engl J Med 306:1189–1196

Aoki V, Rivitti EA, Diaz LA, Research CGoFS (2015) Update on fogo selvagem, an endemic form of pemphigus foliaceus. J Dermatol 42:18–26

Aoki-Ota M, Kinoshita M, Ota T, Tsunoda K, Iwasaki T, Tanaka S, Koyasu S, Nishikawa T, Amagai M (2006) Tolerance induction by the blockade of CD40/CD154 interaction in pemphigus vulgaris mouse model. J Invest Dermatol 126:105–113

Arundhathi S, Ragunatha S, Mahadeva KC (2013) A cross-sectional study of clinical, histopathological and direct immunofluorescence spectrum of vesiculobullous disorders. J Clin Diagn Res 7:2788–2792

Augusto DG, Lobo-Alves SC, Melo MF, Pereira NF, Petzl-Erler ML (2012) Activating KIR and HLA Bw4 ligands are associated to decreased susceptibility to pemphigus foliaceus, an autoimmune blistering skin disease. PLoS One 7:e39991

Banfield CC, Wojnarowska F, Allen J, George S, Venning VA, Welsh KI (1998) The association of HLA-DQ7 with bullous pemphigoid is restricted to men. Br J Dermatol 138:1085–1090

Barańska M, Rychlik-Sych M, Skrętkowicz J, Dudarewicz M, Dziankowska-Bartkowiak B, Owczarek J, Waszczykowska E (2017) Genotype and haplotype analysis of ABCB1 at 1236, 2677 and 3435 among systemic sclerosis patients. Autoimmunity 50:277–282

Bassuny WM, Ihara K, Sasaki Y, Kuromaru R, Kohno H, Matsuura N, Hara T (2003) A functional polymorphism in the promoter/enhancer region of the FOXP3/Scurfin gene associated with type 1 diabetes. Immunogenetics 55:149–156

Baum S, Sakka N, Artsi O, Trau H, Barzilai A (2014) Diagnosis and classification of autoimmune blistering diseases. Autoimmun Rev 13:482–489

Ben Jmaa M, Abida O, Bahloul E, Toumi A, Khlif S, Fakhfakh R, Elloumi N, Sellami K, Masmoudi A, Turki H, Masmoudi H (2017) Role of FOXP3 gene polymorphism in the susceptibility to Tunisian endemic Pemphigus Foliaceus. Immunol Lett 184:105–111

Bhanusali DG, Sachdev A, Rahmanian A, Gerlach JA, Tong JC, Seiffert-Sinha K, Sinha AA (2013) HLA-E*0103X is associated with susceptibility to Pemphigus vulgaris. Exp Dermatol 22:108–112

Birol A, Anadolu RY, Tutkak H, Gürgey E (2002) HLA-class 1 and class 2 antigens in Turkish patients with pemphigus. Int J Dermatol 41:79–83

Boggon TJ, Murray J, Chappuis-Flament S, Wong E, Gumbiner BM, Shapiro L (2002) C-cadherin ectodomain structure and implications for cell adhesion mechanisms. Science 296:1308–1313

Borthwick GM, Sunderland CA, Holmes RC, Black MM, Stirrat GM (1984) Abnormal expression of HLA-DR antigen in the placenta of a patient with pemphigoid gestationis. J Reprod Immunol 6:393–396

Brandt O, Rafei D, Podstawa E, Niedermeier A, Jonkman MF, Terra JB, Hein R, Hertl M, Pas HH, Muller R (2012) Differential IgG recognition of desmoglein 3 by paraneoplastic pemphigus and pemphigus vulgaris sera. J Invest Dermatol 132:1738–1741

Brochado MJ, Nascimento DF, Campos W, Deghaide NH, Donadi EA, Roselino AM (2016) Differential HLA class I and class II associations in pemphigus foliaceus and pemphigus vulgaris patients from a prevalent Southeastern Brazilian region. J Autoimmun 72:19–24

Büdinger L, Borradori L, Yee C, Eming R, Ferencik S, Grosse-Wilde H, Merk HF, Yancey K, Hertl M (1998) Identification and characterization of autoreactive T cell responses to bullous pemphigoid antigen 2 in patients and healthy controls. J Clin Invest 102:2082–2089

Bumiller-Bini V, Cipolla GA, de Almeida RC, Petzl-Erler ML, Augusto DG, Boldt ABW (2018) Sparking fire under the skin? Answers from the association of complement genes with pemphigus foliaceus. Front Immunol 9:695

Caillot F, Derambure C, Berkani N, Riou G, Maho-Vaillant M, Calbo S, Joly P, Musette P (2018) Long-term increase of Kcnn4 potassium channel surface expression on B cells in pemphigus patients after rituximab treatment. J Invest Dermatol 138:2666–2668

Calvanico NJ, Martins CR, Diaz LA (1991) Characterization of pemphigus foliaceus antigen from human epidermis. J Invest Dermatol 96:815–821

Camargo CM, Augusto DG, Petzl-Erler ML (2016) Differential gene expression levels might explain association of LAIR2 polymorphisms with pemphigus. Hum Genet 135:233–244

Camporeale A, Poli V (2012) IL-6, IL-17 and STAT3: a holy trinity in auto-immunity? Front Biosci (landmark Ed) 17:2306–2326

Capon F, Bharkhada J, Cochrane NE, Mortimer NJ, Setterfield JF, Reynaert S, Black MM, Vaughan RW, Trembath RC, Harman KE (2006) Evidence of an association between desmoglein 3 haplotypes and pemphigus vulgaris. Br J Dermatol 154:67–71

Carrozzo M, Fasano ME, Broccoletti R, Carbone M, Cozzani E, Rendine S, Roggero S, Parodi A, Gandolfo S (2001) HLA-DQB1 alleles in Italian patients with mucous membrane pemphigoid predominantly affecting the oral cavity. Br J Dermatol 145:805–808

Carrozzo M, Dametto E, Fasano ME, Broccoletti R, Carbone M, Rendine S, Amoroso A (2014) Interleukin-4RA gene polymorphism is associated with oral mucous membrane pemphigoid. Oral Dis 20:275–280

Chagury AA, Sennes LU, Gil JM, Kalil J, Rodrigues H, Rosales CB, Miziara ID (2018) HLA-C*17, DQB1*03:01, DQA1*01:03 and DQA1*05:05 alleles associated to bullous pemphigoid in Brazilian population. Ann Dermatol 30:8–12

Chan LS, Wang T, Wang XS, Hammerberg C, Cooper KD (1994) High frequency of HLA-

DQB1*0301 allele in patients with pure ocular cicatricial pemphigoid. Dermatology 189(Suppl 1):99–101

Chan LS, Hammerberg C, Cooper KD (1997) Significantly increased occurrence of HLA-DQB1*0301 allele in patients with ocular cicatricial pemphigoid. J Invest Dermatol 108:129–132

Chan PT, Ohyama B, Nishifuji K, Yoshida K, Ishii K, Hashimoto T, Amagai M (2010) Immune response towards the amino-terminus of desmoglein 1 prevails across different activity stages in nonendemic pemphigus foliaceus. Br J Dermatol 162:1242–1250

Chang YT, Liu HN, Yu CW, Lin MW, Huang CH, Chen CC, Liu MT, Lee DD, Wang WJ, Tsai SF (2006) Cytokine gene polymorphisms in bullous pemphigoid in a Chinese population. Br J Dermatol 154:79–84

Cheema GS, Roschke V, Hilbert DM, Stohl W (2001) Elevated serum B lymphocyte stimulator levels in patients with systemic immune-based rheumatic diseases. Arthritis Rheum 44:1313–1319

Chernyavsky A, Amber KT, Agnoletti AF, Wang C, Grando SA (2019) Synergy among non-desmoglein antibodies contributes to the immunopathology of desmoglein antibody-negative pemphigus vulgaris. J Biol Chem

Chiu YW, Chen YD, Hua TC, Wu CH, Liu HN, Chang YT (2017) Comorbid autoimmune diseases in patients with pemphigus: a nationwide case-control study in Taiwan. Eur J Dermatol 27:375–381

Cho MJ, Ellebrecht CT, Payne AS (2015) The dual nature of interleukin-10 in pemphigus vulgaris. Cytokine 73:335–341

Cipolla GA, Park JK, de Oliveira LA, Lobo-Alves SC, de Almeida RC, Farias TD, DeS L, Malheiros D, Lavker RM, Petzl-Erler ML (2016) A 3'UTR polymorphism marks differential KLRG1 mRNA levels through disruption of a miR-584-5p binding site and associates with pemphigus foliaceus susceptibility. Biochim Biophys Acta 1859:1306–1313

Colliou N, Picard D, Caillot F, Calbo S, Le Corre S, Lim A, Lemercier B, Le Mauff B, Maho-Vaillant M, Jacquot S, Bedane C, Bernard P, Caux F, Prost C, Delaporte E, Doutre MS, Dreno B, Franck N, Ingen-Housz-Oro S, Chosidow O, Pauwels C, Picard C, Roujeau JC, Sigal M, Tancrede-Bohin E, Templier I, Eming R, Hertl M, D'Incan M, Joly P, Musette P (2013) Long-term remissions of severe pemphigus after rituximab therapy are associated with prolonged failure of desmoglein B cell response. Sci Transl Med 5:175ra130

Colombatti A, Bonaldo P (1991) The superfamily of proteins with von Willebrand factor type A-like domains: one theme common to components of extracellular matrix, hemostasis, cellular adhesion, and defense mechanisms. Blood 77:2305–2315

Das N, Biswas B, Khera R (2013) Membrane-bound complement regulatory proteins as biomarkers and potential therapeutic targets for SLE. Adv Exp Med Biol 735:55–81

Davies A, Lachmann PJ (1993) Membrane defence against complement lysis: the structure and biological properties of CD59. Immunol Res 12:258–275

de Graauw E, Sitaru C, Horn M, Borradori L, Yousefi S, Simon HU, Simon D (2017) Evidence for a role of eosinophils in blister formation in bullous pemphigoid. Allergy 72:1105–1113

De Sena Nogueira Maehara L, De-Souza-Santana FC, Porro AM, Marcos EVC, Ura S, Nolte IM, Pas HH, Jonkman MF, Tomimori J (2018) HLA class II alleles of susceptibility and protection in Brazilian and Dutch pemphigus foliaceus. Br J Dermatol 178:e212–e214

Deckert M, Kubar J, Bernard A (1992) CD58 and CD59 molecules exhibit potentializing effects in T cell adhesion and activation. J Immunol 148:672–677

Delgado JC, Turbay D, Yunis EJ, Yunis JJ, Morton ED, Bhol K, Norman R, Alper CA, Good RA, Ahmed R (1996) A common major histocompatibility complex class II allele HLA-DQB1* 0301 is present in clinical variants of pemphigoid. Proc Natl Acad Sci U S A 93:8569–8571

Denfeld RW, Hollenbaugh D, Fehrenbach A, Weiss JM, von Leoprechting A, Mai B, Voith U, Schöpf E, Aruffo A, Simon JC (1996) CD40 is functionally expressed on human keratinocytes. Eur J Immunol 26:2329–2334

Di Zenzo G, Di Lullo G, Corti D, Calabresi V, Sinistro A, Vanzetta F, Didona B, Cianchini G, Hertl M, Eming R, Amagai M, Ohyama B, Hashimoto T, Sloostra J, Sallusto F, Zambruno G, Lanzavecchia A (2012) Pemphigus autoantibodies generated through somatic mutations target the desmoglein-3 cis-interface. J Clin Invest 122:3781–3790

Di Zenzo G, Amber KT, Sayar BS, Müller EJ, Borradori L (2016) Immune response in pemphigus and beyond: progresses and emerging concepts. Semin Immunopathol 38:57–74

Drouet M, Delpuget-Bertin N, Vaillant L, Chauchaix S, Boulanger MD, Bonnetblanc JM, Bernard P (1998) HLA-DRB1 and HLA-DQB1 genes in susceptibility and resistance to cicatricial pemphigoid in French Caucasians. Eur J Dermatol 8:330–333

Eberhard Y, Burgos E, Gagliardi J, Vullo CM, Borosky A, Pesoa S, Serra HM (2005) Cytokine polymorphisms in patients with pemphigus. Arch Dermatol Res 296:309–313

Eming R, Hennerici T, Bäcklund J, Feliciani C, Visconti KC, Willenborg S, Wohde J, Holmdahl R, Sønderstrup G, Hertl M (2014) Pathogenic IgG antibodies against desmoglein 3 in pemphigus vulgaris are regulated by HLA-DRB1*04:02-restricted T cells. J Immunol 193:4391–4399

Esmaili N, Mortazavi H, Chams-Davatchi C, Daneshpazhooh M, Damavandi MR, Aryanian Z, Amirzargar AA (2013) Association between HLA-DQB1*03:01 and Bullous pemphigoid in Iranian patients. Iran J Immunol 10:1–9

Etesami I, Seirafi H, Ghandi N, Salmani H, Arabpour M, Nasrollahzadeh A, Teimourpour A, Daneshpazhooh M, Keramatipour M (2018) The association between ST18 gene polymorphism and severe pemphigus disease among Iranian population. Exp Dermatol 27:1395–1398

Fang H, Shao S, Cao T, Lei J, Dang E, Zhang J, Wang G (2016) Increased expression of NLRP3 inflammasome components and interleukin-18 in patients with bullous pemphigoid. J Dermatol Sci 83:116–123

Fang H, Shen S, Zheng X, Dang E, Zhang J, Shao S, Qiao P, Li Q, Wang H, Li C, Sun L, Wang G (2018) Association of HLA class I and class II alleles with bullous pemphigoid in Chinese Hans. J Dermatol Sci 89:258–262

Farias TDJ, Augusto DG, de Almeida RC, Malheiros D, Petzl-Erler ML (2019) Screening the full leucocyte receptor complex genomic region revealed associations with pemphigus that might be explained by gene regulation. Immunology 156:86–93

Farkas I, Baranyi L, Ishikawa Y, Okada N, Bohata C, Budai D, Fukuda A, Imai M, Okada H (2002) CD59 blocks not only the insertion of C9 into MAC but inhibits ion channel formation by homologous C5b–8 as well as C5b–9. J Physiol 539:537–545

Feinstein A, Yorav S, Movshovitz M, Schewach-Millet M (1991) Pemphigus in families. Int J Dermatol 30:347–351

Firooz A, Mazhar A, Ahmed AR (1994) Prevalence of autoimmune diseases in the family members of patients with pemphigus vulgaris. J Am Acad Dermatol 31:434–437

Formichi P, Radi E, Battisti C, Pasqui A, Pompella G, Lazzerini PE, Laghi-Pasini F, Leonini A, Di Stefano A, Federico A (2007) Psychosine-induced apoptosis and cytokine activation in immune peripheral cells of Krabbe patients. J Cell Physiol 212:737–743

Funakoshi T, Lunardon L, Ellebrecht CT, Nagler AR, O'Leary CE, Payne AS (2012) Enrichment of total serum IgG4 in patients with pemphigus. Br J Dermatol 167:1245–1253

Futei Y, Amagai M, Sekiguchi M, Nishifuji K, Fujii Y, Nishikawa T (2000) Use of domain-swapped molecules for conformational epitope mapping of desmoglein 3 in pemphigus vulgaris. J Invest Dermatol 115:829–834

Futei Y, Amagai M, Hashimoto T, Nishikawa T (2003) Conformational epitope mapping and IgG subclass distribution of desmoglein 3 in paraneoplastic pemphigus. J Am Acad Dermatol 49:1023–1028

Gammon WR, Heise ER, Burke WA, Fine JD, Woodley DT, Briggaman RA (1988) Increased frequency of HLA-DR2 in patients with autoantibodies to epidermolysis bullosa acquisita antigen: evidence that the expression of autoimmunity to type VII collagen is HLA class II allele associated. J Invest Dermatol 91:228–232

Gao Y, Zhang Q (1999) Polymorphisms of the GSTM1 and CYP2D6 genes associated with susceptibility to lung cancer in Chinese. Mutat Res 444:441–449

Gao XH, Winsey S, Li G, Barnardo M, Zhu XJ, Chen HD, Song F, Zhai N, Fuggle S, Wojnarowska F (2002) HLA-DR and DQ polymorphisms in bullous pemphigoid from northern China. Clin Exp Dermatol 27:319–321

Gao L, Li K, Li F, Li H, Liu L, Wang L, Zhang Z, Gao T, Liu Y (2010) Polymorphisms in the FOXP3 gene in Han Chinese psoriasis patients. J Dermatol Sci 57:51–56

García-González E, Castro-Llamas J, Karchmer S, Zúñiga J, de Oca DM, Ambaz M, Bolaños R, Granados J (1999) Class II major histocompatibility complex typing across the ethnic barrier in pemphigoid gestationis. A study in Mexicans. Int J Dermatol 38:46–51

Gazit E, Slomov Y, Goldberg I, Brenner S, Loewenthal R (2004) HLA-G is associated with pemphigus vulgaris in Jewish patients. Hum Immunol 65:39–46

Geng L, Wang Y, Zhai N, Lu YN, Song FJ, Chen HD (2005) Association between pemphigus vulgaris and human leukocyte antigen in Han nation of northeast China. Chin Med Sci J 20:166–170

Getsios S, Huen AC, Green KJ (2004) Working out the strength and flexibility of desmosomes. Nat Rev Mol Cell Biol 5:271–281

Gibson WT, Walter MA, Ahmed AR, Alper CA, Cox DW (1994) The immunoglobulin heavy chain and disease association: application to pemphigus vulgaris. Hum Genet 94:675–683

Gil JM, Weber R, Rosales CB, Rodrigues H, Sennes LU, Kalil J, Chagury A, Miziara ID (2017) Study of the association between human leukocyte antigens (HLA) and pemphigus vulgaris in Brazilian patients. Int J Dermatol 56:557–562

Gołab-Janowska M, Honczarenko K, Gawrońska-Szklarz B, Potemkowski A (2007) CYP2D6 gene polymorphism as a probable risk factor for Alzheimer's disease and Parkinson's disease with dementia. Neurol Neurochir Pol 41:113–121

González-Escribano MF, Jiménez G, Walter K, Montes M, Perez-Bernal AM, Rodríguez MR, Conejo-Mir JS, Núñez-Roldán A (1998) Distribution of HLA class II alleles among Spanish patients with pemphigus vulgaris. Tissue Antigens 52:275–278

Gorter A, Meri S (1999) Immune evasion of tumor cells using membrane-bound complement regulatory proteins. Immunol Today 20:576–582

Grando SA, Bystryn JC, Chernyavsky AI, Frusić-Zlotkin M, Gniadecki R, Lotti R, Milner Y, Pittelkow MR, Pincelli C (2009) Apoptolysis: a novel mechanism of skin blistering in pemphigus vulgaris linking the apoptotic pathways to basal cell shrinkage and suprabasal acantholysis. Exp Dermatol 18:764–770

Groh V, Wu J, Yee C, Spies T (2002) Tumour-derived soluble MIC ligands impair expression of NKG2D and T-cell activation. Nature 419:734–738

Groom J, Kalled SL, Cutler AH, Olson C, Woodcock SA, Schneider P, Tschopp J, Cachero TG, Batten M, Wheway J, Mauri D, Cavill D, Gordon TP, Mackay CR, Mackay F (2002) Association of BAFF/BLyS overexpression and altered B cell differentiation with Sjögren's syndrome. J Clin Invest 109:59–68

Guerra L, Condorelli AG, Fortugno P, Calabresi V, Pedicelli C, Di Zenzo G, Castiglia D (2018)

Epidermolysis bullosa (EB) acquisita in an adult patient with previously unrecognized mild dystrophic EB and biallelic COL7A1 mutations. Acta Derm Venereol 98:411–415

Guilabert A, Lozano F, Iranzo P, Suárez-Casasús B, Martinez-De Pablo I, Julià M, Mascaró JM (2011) A case of aggressive bullous pemphigoid associated with the defective functional variant of Fc gamma receptor IIb: implications for pathogenesis? J Am Acad Dermatol 65:1062–1063

Haase O, Alneebari R, Eldarouti MA, Abd El Hady M, Dorgham D, El-Nabarawy E, El Din Mahmoud SB, Mosaad El Sayed H, Darwish M, Abbas F, Salah S, Mosaad Y, El-Chennawi F, Al Mongy S, Abdelaziz AM, Abd El Gaber S, Hertl M, Eming R, Recke A, Möller S, Schmidt E, Zillikens D, Ibrahim S (2015) Association with HLA-DRB1 in Egyptian and German pemphigus vulgaris patients. Tissue Antigens 85:283–286

Haider N, Neuman R, Foster CS, Ahmed AR (1992) Report on the sequence of DQB1*0301 gene in ocular cicatricial pemphigoid patients. Curr Eye Res 11:1233–1238

Harfouch E, Daoud S (2014) Allelic variation in HLA-DRB1* loci in Syrian pemphigus vulgaris patients. Int J Dermatol 53:1460–1463

Hashimoto K, Miki Y, Nakata S, Matsuyama M (1977) HLA-A10 in pemphigus among Japanese. Arch Dermatol 113:1518–1519

Hayashi R, Natsuga K, Watanabe M, Iwata H, Shinkuma S, Ito A, Masui Y, Ito M, Shimomura Y (2016) Epidermolysis bullosa acquisita develops in dominant dystrophic epidermolysis bullosa. J Invest Dermatol 136:320–323

Heelan K, Mahar AL, Walsh S, Shear NH (2015) Pemphigus and associated comorbidities: a cross-sectional study. Clin Exp Dermatol 40:593–599

Hershey GK, Friedrich MF, Esswein LA, Thomas ML, Chatila TA (1997) The association of atopy with a gain-of-function mutation in the alpha subunit of the interleukin-4 receptor. N Engl J Med 337:1720–1725

Hertl M, Jedlickova H, Karpati S, Marinovic B, Uzun S, Yayli S, Mimouni D, Borradori L, Feliciani C, Ioannides D, Joly P, Kowalewski C, Zambruno G, Zillikens D, Jonkman MF (2015) Pemphigus. S2 guideline for diagnosis and treatment–guided by the European Dermatology Forum (EDF) in cooperation with the European Academy of Dermatology and Venereology (EADV). J Eur Acad Dermatol Venereol 29:405–414

Heupel WM, Zillikens D, Drenckhahn D, Waschke J (2008) Pemphigus vulgaris IgG directly inhibit desmoglein 3-mediated transinteraction. J Immunol 181:1825–1834

Hill CH, Graham SC, Read RJ, Deane JE (2013) Structural snapshots illustrate the catalytic cycle of β-galactocerebrosidase, the defective enzyme in Krabbe disease. Proc Natl Acad Sci U S A 110:20479–20484

Hines C (1978) Vitamins. Absorption and malabsorption. Arch Intern Med 138:619–621

Hirose M, Schilf P, Benoit S, Eming R, Gläser R, Homey B, Kunz M, Nebel A, Peitsch WK, Pföhler C, Sárdy M, Schreiber S, Zillikens D, Schmidt E, Ibrahim SM, Group GAGS (2015) Polymorphisms in the mitochondrially encoded ATP synthase 8 gene are associated with susceptibility to bullous pemphigoid in the German population. Exp Dermatol 24:715–717

Hofmann SC, Juratli HA, Eming R (2018) Bullous autoimmune dermatoses. J Dtsch Dermatol Ges 16:1339–1358

Hübner F, Setterfield J, Recke A, Zillikens D, Schmidt E, Dart J, Ibrahim S, 2009 MSG (2018) HLA alleles in British Caucasians with mucous membrane pemphigoid. Eye (Lond) 32:1540–1541

Hviid TV, Hylenius S, Rørbye C, Nielsen LG (2003) HLA-G allelic variants are associated with differences in the HLA-G mRNA isoform profile and HLA-G mRNA levels. Immunogenetics 55:63–79

Intong LR, Murrell DF (2011) Pemphigoid gestationis: pathogenesis and clinical features. Dermatol Clin 29 (447–452):ix

Ishii K, Lin C, Siegel DL, Stanley JR (2008) Isolation of pathogenic monoclonal anti-desmoglein 1 human antibodies by phage display of pemphigus foliaceus autoantibodies. J Invest Dermatol 128:939–948

Jacobson EM, Concepcion E, Oashi T, Tomer Y (2005) A Graves' disease-associated Kozak sequence single-nucleotide polymorphism enhances the efficiency of CD40 gene translation: a case for translational pathophysiology. Endocrinology 146:2684–2691

Javor J, Chmurova N, Parnicka Z, Ferencik S, Grosse-Wilde H, Buc M, Svecova D (2010) TNF-alpha and IL-10 gene polymorphisms show a weak association with pemphigus vulgaris in the Slovak population. J Eur Acad Dermatol Venereol 24:65–68

Jeannin P, Delneste Y, Lecoanet-Henchoz S, Gauchat JF, Ellis J, Bonnefoy JY (1997) CD86 (B7–2) on human B cells. A functional role in proliferation and selective differentiation into IgE- and IgG4-producing cells. J Biol Chem 272:15613–15619

Jefferis R, Lefranc MP (2009) Human immunoglobulin allotypes: possible implications for immunogenicity. Mabs 1:332–338

Joly P, Mouquet H, Roujeau JC, D'Incan M, Gilbert D, Jacquot S, Gougeon ML, Bedane C, Muller R, Dreno B, Doutre MS, Delaporte E, Pauwels C, Franck N, Caux F, Picard C, Tancrede-Bohin E, Bernard P, Tron F, Hertl M, Musette P (2007) A single cycle of rituximab for the treatment of severe pemphigus. N Engl J Med 357:545–552

Joly P, Richard C, Gilbert D, Courville P, Chosidow O, Roujeau JC, Beylot-Barry M, D'incan M, Martel P, Lauret P, Tron F (2000) Sensitivity and specificity of clinical, histologic, and immunologic features in the diagnosis of paraneoplastic pemphigus. J Am Acad Dermatol 43:619–626

Kalantari-Dehaghi M, Chen Y, Deng W, Chernyavsky A, Marchenko S, Wang PH, Grando SA (2013) Mechanisms of mitochondrial damage in keratinocytes by pemphigus vulgaris antibodies. J Biol Chem 288:16916–16925

Kaplan I, Hodak E, Ackerman L, Mimouni D, Anhalt GJ, Calderon S (2004) Neoplasms associated with paraneoplastic pemphigus: a review with emphasis on nonhematologic malignancy and oral mucosal manifestations. Oral Oncol 40:553–562

Katzenelson V, David M, Zamir R, Mellibovsky J, Idises C, Sandbank M (1990) Familial pemphigus vulgaris. Dermatologica 181:48–50

Kawasaki A, Tsuchiya N, Fukazawa T, Hashimoto H, Tokunaga K (2002) Analysis on the association of human BLYS (BAFF, TNFSF13B) polymorphisms with systemic lupus erythematosus and rheumatoid arthritis. Genes Immun 3:424–429

Kelly SE, Black MM, Fleming S (1989) Pemphigoid gestationis: a unique mechanism of initiation of an autoimmune response by MHC class II molecules? J Pathol 158:81–82

Kemler R (1993) From cadherins to catenins: cytoplasmic protein interactions and regulation of cell adhesion. Trends Genet 9:317–321

Khan SW, Iftikhar N, Ahmed TA, Bashir M (2015) HLA-DR alleles in Pakistani patients of pemphigus vulgaris. J Coll Physicians Surg Pak 25:233–236

Köck J, Kreher S, Lehmann K, Riedel R, Bardua M, Lischke T, Jargosch M, Haftmann C, Bendfeldt H, Hatam F, Mashreghi MF, Baumgrass R, Radbruch A, Chang HD (2014) Nuclear factor of activated T cells regulates the expression of interleukin-4 in Th2 cells in an all-or-none fashion. J Biol Chem 289:26752–26761

Koga H, Prost-Squarcioni C, Iwata H, Jonkman MF, Ludwig RJ, Bieber K (2018) Epidermolysis bullosa acquisita: the 2019 update. Front Med (lausanne) 5:362

Konttinen YT, Ceponis A, Meri S, Vuorikoski A, Kortekangas P, Sorsa T, Sukura A, Santavirta S (1996) Complement in acute and chronic arthritides: assessment of C3c, C9, and protectin (CD59) in synovial membrane. Ann Rheum Dis 55:888–894

Kopp TI, Andersen V, Tjonneland A, Vogel U (2015) Polymorphisms in ATP-binding cassette transporter genes and interaction with diet and life style factors in relation to colorectal cancer in a Danish prospective case-cohort study. Scand J Gastroenterol 50:1469–1481

Korman NJ, Eyre RW, Klaus-Kovtun V, Stanley JR (1989) Demonstration of an adhering-junction molecule (plakoglobin) in the autoantigens of pemphigus foliaceus and pemphigus vulgaris. N Engl J Med 321:631–635

Koulu L, Kusumi A, Steinberg MS, Klaus-Kovtun V, Stanley JR (1984) Human autoantibodies against a desmosomal core protein in pemphigus foliaceus. J Exp Med 160:1509–1518

Kridin K (2018a) Emerging treatment options for the management of pemphigus vulgaris. Ther Clin Risk Manag 14:757–778

Kridin K (2018b) Subepidermal autoimmune bullous diseases: overview, epidemiology, and associations. Immunol Res 66:6–17

Kridin K, Ludwig RJ (2018) The growing incidence of bullous pemphigoid: overview and potential explanations. Front Med (lausanne) 5:220

Kridin K, Zelber-Sagi S, Khamaisi M, Cohen AD, Bergman R (2016) Remarkable differences in the epidemiology of pemphigus among two ethnic populations in the same geographic region. J Am Acad Dermatol 75:925–930

Kridin K, Sagi SZ, Bergman R (2017) Mortality and cause of death in patients with pemphigus. Acta Derm Venereol 97:607–611

Kridin K, Shihade W, Bergman R (2019) Mortality in patients with bullous pemphigoid: a retrospective cohort study, systematic review and meta-analysis. Acta Derm Venereol 99:72–77

Kumar R, Goswami R, Agarwal S, Israni N, Singh SK, Rani R (2007) Association and interaction of the TNF-alpha gene with other pro- and anti-inflammatory cytokine genes and HLA genes in patients with type 1 diabetes from North India. Tissue Antigens 69:557–567

Kwok WW, Domeier ME, Johnson ML, Nepom GT, Koelle DM (1996) HLA-DQB1 codon 57 is critical for peptide binding and recognition. J Exp Med 183:1253–1258

Langan SM, Smeeth L, Hubbard R, Fleming KM, Smith CJ, West J (2008) Bullous pemphigoid and pemphigus vulgaris—incidence and mortality in the UK: population based cohort study. BMJ 337:a180

Laskaris G, Sklavounou A, Stavrou A, Stavropoulou K (1989) Familial pemphigus vulgaris with oral manifestations affecting two Greek families. J Oral Pathol Med 18:49–53

Lee YH, Bae SC (2017) Association between functional CYP2D6 polymorphisms and susceptibility to autoimmune diseases: a meta-analysis. Immunol Invest 46:109–122

Lee CW, Kim SC, Han H (1996) Distribution of HLA class II alleles in Korean patients with epidermolysis bullosa acquisita. Dermatology 193:328–329

Lee E, Lendas KA, Chow S, Pirani Y, Gordon D, Dionisio R, Nguyen D, Spizuoco A, Fotino M, Zhang Y, Sinha AA (2006) Disease relevant HLA class II alleles isolated by genotypic, haplotypic, and sequence analysis in North American Caucasians with pemphigus vulgaris. Hum Immunol 67:125–139

Lee J, Bloom R, Amber KT (2015) A systematic review of patients with mucocutaneous and respiratory complications in paraneoplastic autoimmune multiorgan syndrome: castleman's disease is the predominant malignancy. Lung 193:593–596

Li N, Aoki V, Hans-Filho G, Rivitti EA, Diaz LA (2003) The role of intramolecular epitope spreading in the

pathogenesis of endemic pemphigus foliaceus (fogo selvagem). J Exp Med 197:1501–1510
Li Y, Hofmann M, Wang Q, Teng L, Chlewicki LK, Pircher H, Mariuzza RA (2009) Structure of natural killer cell receptor KLRG1 bound to E-cadherin reveals basis for MHC-independent missing self recognition. Immunity 31:35–46
Li S, Zhang Q, Wang P, Li J, Ni J, Wu J, Liang Y, Leng RX, Pan HF, Ye DQ (2018) Association between HLA-DQB1 polymorphisms and pemphigus vulgaris: a meta-analysis. Immunol Invest 47:101–112
Liu Q, Bu DF, Li D, Zhu XJ (2008) Genotyping of HLA-I and HLA-II alleles in Chinese patients with paraneoplastic pemphigus. Br J Dermatol 158:587–591
Liu Y, Gibson J, Wheeler J, Kwee LC, Santiago-Turla CM, Akafo SK, Lichter PR, Gaasterland DE, Moroi SE, Challa P, Herndon LW, Girkin CA, Budenz DL, Richards JE, Allingham RR, Hauser MA (2011) GALC deletions increase the risk of primary open-angle glaucoma: the role of Mendelian variants in complex disease. PLoS One 6: e27134
Lobo-Alves SC, Augusto DG, Magalhães WCS, Tarazona-Santos E, Lima-Costa MF, Barreto ML, Horta BL, de Almeida RC, Petzl-Erler ML (2019) Long non-coding RNA polymorphisms influence susceptibility to endemic pemphigus foliaceus. Br J Dermatol
Loiseau P, Lecleach L, Prost C, Lepage V, Busson M, Bastuji-Garin S, Roujeau JC, Charron D (2000) HLA class II polymorphism contributes to specify desmoglein derived peptides in pemphigus vulgaris and pemphigus foliaceus. J Autoimmun 15:67–73
Lombardi ML, Mercuro O, Ruocco V, Lo Schiavo A, Lombari V, Guerrera V, Pirozzi G, Manzo C (1999) Common human leukocyte antigen alleles in pemphigus vulgaris and pemphigus foliaceus Italian patients. J Invest Dermatol 113:107–110
Lopez-Pajares V, Qu K, Zhang J, Webster DE, Barajas BC, Siprashvili Z, Zarnegar BJ, Boxer LD, Rios EJ, Tao S, Kretz M, Khavari PA (2015) A LncRNA-MAF:MAFB transcription factor network regulates epidermal differentiation. Dev Cell 32:693–706
Ludwig RJ (2013) Clinical presentation, pathogenesis, diagnosis, and treatment of epidermolysis bullosa acquisita. ISRN Dermatol 2013:812029
Malheiros D, Petzl-Erler ML (2009) Individual and epistatic effects of genetic polymorphisms of B-cell co-stimulatory molecules on susceptibility to pemphigus foliaceus. Genes Immun 10:547–558
Malheiros D, Panepucci RA, Roselino AM, Araújo AG, Zago MA, Petzl-Erler ML (2014) Genome-wide gene expression profiling reveals unsuspected molecular alterations in pemphigus foliaceus. Immunology 143:381–395
Marchenko S, Chernyavsky AI, Arredondo J, Gindi V, Grando SA (2010) Antimitochondrial autoantibodies in pemphigus vulgaris: a missing link in disease pathophysiology. J Biol Chem 285:3695–3704
Merk HF (2009) Drug skin metabolites and allergic drug reactions. Curr Opin Allergy Clin Immunol 9:311–315
Mimouni D, Bar H, Gdalevich M, Katzenelson V, David M (2008) Pemphigus–analysis of epidemiological factors in 155 patients. J Eur Acad Dermatol Venereol 22:1232–1235
Minagawa A, Arakura F, Koga H, Tokuda Y, Hashimoto T, Okuyama R (2015) An immunogenetic study of bullous pemphigoid with mucosal involvement in two siblings. Eur J Dermatol 25:186–188
Miyagawa S, Niizeki H, Yamashina Y, Kaneshige T (2002) Genotyping for HLA-A, B and C alleles in Japanese patients with pemphigus: prevalence of Asian alleles of the HLA-B15 family. Br J Dermatol 146:52–58
Mondino BJ, Brown SI, Rabin BS (1978) HLA antigens in ocular cicatricial pemphigoid. Br J Ophthalmol 62:265–267
Mondino BJ, Brown SI, Rabin BS (1979) HLA antigens in ocular cicatricial pemphigoid. Arch Ophthalmol 97:479
Monleón I, Martínez-Lorenzo MJ, Anel A, Lasierra P, Larrad L, Piñeiro A, Naval J, Alava MA (2000) CD59 cross-linking induces secretion of APO2 ligand in overactivated human T cells. Eur J Immunol 30:1078–1087
Moore PA, Belvedere O, Orr A, Pieri K, LaFleur DW, Feng P, Soppet D, Charters M, Gentz R, Parmelee D, Li Y, Galperina O, Giri J, Roschke V, Nardelli B, Carrell J, Sosnovtseva S, Greenfield W, Ruben SM, Olsen HS, Fikes J, Hilbert DM (1999) BLyS: member of the tumor necrosis factor family and B lymphocyte stimulator. Science 285:260–263
Moravvej H, Tabatabaei-Panah PS, Ebrahimi E, Esmaeili N, Ghaderian SMH, Ludwig RJ, Akbarzadeh R (2018) TNF-α -308G/a gene polymorphism in bullous pemphigoid and alopecia areata. Hum Antibodies 26:201–207
Mortazavi H, Amirzargar AA, Esmaili N, Toofan H, Ehsani AH, Hosseini SH, Rezaei N (2013) Association of human leukocyte antigen class I antigens in Iranian patients with pemphigus vulgaris. J Dermatol 40:244–248
Mosaad YM, Fathy H, Fawzy Z, El-Saied MA (2012) Tumor necrosis factor-α-308 G>A and interleukin-6-174 G>C promoter polymorphisms and pemphigus. Hum Immunol 73:560–565
Mostafa MI, Hassib NF, Nemat AH (2010) Oral mucous membrane pemphigoid in a 6-year-old boy: diagnosis, treatment and 4 years follow-up. Int J Paediatr Dent 20:76–79
Mostafa MI, Zarouk WA, El-Kamah GY (2011) Class II alleles HLA-DQB1*0301 among a seven-membered Egyptian family of a child with oral pemphigoid. Bratisl Lek Listy 112:591–594
Mota P, Silva HC, Soares MJ, Pego A, Loureiro M, Cordeiro CR, Regateiro FJ (2015) Genetic polymorphisms of phase I and phase II metabolic enzymes as modulators of lung cancer susceptibility. J Cancer Res Clin Oncol 141:851–860

Murrell DF, Marinovic B, Caux F, Prost C, Ahmed R, Wozniak K, Amagai M, Bauer J, Beissert S, Borradori L, Culton D, Fairley JA, Fivenson D, Jonkman MF, Marinkovich MP, Woodley D, Zone J, Aoki V, Bernard P, Bruckner-Tuderman L, Cianchini G, Venning V, Diaz L, Eming R, Grando SA, Hall RP, Hashimoto T, Herrero-Gonzalez JE, Hertl M, Joly P, Karpati S, Kim J, Chan Kim S, Korman NJ, Kowalewski C, Lee SE, Rubenstein DR, Sprecher E, Yancey K, Zambruno G, Zillikens D, Doan S, Daniel BS, Werth VP (2015) Definitions and outcome measures for mucous membrane pemphigoid: recommendations of an international panel of experts. J Am Acad Dermatol 72:168–174

Nagar B, Overduin M, Ikura M, Rini JM (1996) Structural basis of calcium-induced E-cadherin rigidification and dimerization. Nature 380:360–364

Nagel A, Hertl M, Eming R (2009) B-cell-directed therapy for inflammatory skin diseases. J Invest Dermatol 129:289–301

Nanda A, Al-Saeed K, Dvorak R, Al-Muzairai I, Al-Sabah H, Al-Arbash M, Alsaleh QA (2003) Clinicopathological features and HLA tissue typing in pemphigoid gestationis patients in Kuwait. Clin Exp Dermatol 28:301–306

Nguyen VT, Ndoye A, Bassler KD, Shultz LD, Shields MC, Ruben BS, Webber RJ, Pittelkow MR, Lynch PJ, Grando SA (2001) Classification, clinical manifestations, and immunopathological mechanisms of the epithelial variant of paraneoplastic autoimmune multiorgan syndrome: a reappraisal of paraneoplastic pemphigus. Arch Dermatol 137:193–206

Noe MH, Chen M, Woodley DT, Fairley JA (2008) Familial epidermolysis bullosa acquisita. Dermatol Online J 14:2

Nose A, Tsuji K, Takeichi M (1990) Localization of specificity determining sites in cadherin cell adhesion molecules. Cell 61:147–155

Nousari HC, Deterding R, Wojtczack H, Aho S, Uitto J, Hashimoto T, Anhalt GJ (1999) The mechanism of respiratory failure in paraneoplastic pemphigus. N Engl J Med 340:1406–1410

Okazaki A, Miyagawa S, Yamashina Y, Kitamura W, Shirai T (2000) Polymorphisms of HLA-DR and -DQ genes in Japanese patients with bullous pemphigoid. J Dermatol 27:149–156

Okuyama R, Tagami H, Aiba S (2008) Notch signaling: its role in epidermal homeostasis and in the pathogenesis of skin diseases. J Dermatol Sci 49:187–194

Orlov MD, Chernyavsky AI, Arredondo J, Grando SA (2006) Synergistic actions of pemphigus vulgaris IgG, Fas-ligand and tumor necrosis factor-alpha during induction of basal cell shrinkage and acantholysis. Autoimmunity 39:557–562

Oyama N, Setterfield JF, Powell AM, Sakuma-Oyama Y, Albert S, Bhogal BS, Vaughan RW, Kaneko F, Challacombe SJ, Black MM (2006) Bullous pemphigoid antigen II (BP180) and its soluble extracellular domains are major autoantigens in mucous membrane pemphigoid: the pathogenic relevance to HLA class II alleles and disease severity. Br J Dermatol 154:90–98

Parameswaran A, Attwood K, Sato R, Seiffert-Sinha K, Sinha AA (2015) Identification of a new disease cluster of pemphigus vulgaris with autoimmune thyroid disease, rheumatoid arthritis and type I diabetes. Br J Dermatol 172:729–738

Park SW, Lomri N, Simeoni LA, Fruehauf JP, Mechetner E (2003) Analysis of P-glycoprotein-mediated membrane transport in human peripheral blood lymphocytes using the UIC2 shift assay. Cytometry A 53:67–78

Park O, Grishina I, Leung PS, Gershwin ME, Prindiville T (2005) Analysis of the Foxp3/scurfin gene in Crohn's disease. Ann N Y Acad Sci 1051:218–228

Párnická Z, Švecová D, Javor J, Shawkatová I, Buc M (2013) High susceptibility to pemphigus vulgaris due to HLA-DRB1*14:54 in the Slovak population. Int J Immunogenet 40:471–475

Patsatsi A, Kyriakou A, Werth VP (2018) Bullous pemphigoid in adolescence. Pediatr Dermatol

Payne AS, Ishii K, Kacir S, Lin C, Li H, Hanakawa Y, Tsunoda K, Amagai M, Stanley JR, Siegel DL (2005) Genetic and functional characterization of human pemphigus vulgaris monoclonal autoantibodies isolated by phage display. J Clin Invest 115:888–899

Pendaries V, Gasc G, Titeux M, Leroux C, Vitezica ZG, Mejía JE, Décha A, Loiseau P, Bodemer C, Prost-Squarcioni C, Hovnanian A (2010) Immune reactivity to type VII collagen: implications for gene therapy of recessive dystrophic epidermolysis bullosa. Gene Ther 17:930–937

Piovezan BZ, Petzl-Erler ML (2013) Both qualitative and quantitative genetic variation of MHC class II molecules may influence susceptibility to autoimmune diseases: the case of endemic pemphigus foliaceus. Hum Immunol 74:1134–1140

Piscopo R, Romano M, Maria AD, Vinciguerra R, Vinciguerra P (2018) Ocular onset of paraneoplastic pemphigus presenting as hyperemic conjunctivitis and massive bilateral eyelid ulceration: a case report and literature review. Ocul Immunol Inflamm 26:265–268

Rabelo DF, Nguyen T, Caufield BA, Ahmed AR (2014) Mucous membranepemphigoid in two half-sisters. The potential roles of autoantibodies to β4 integrin subunits and HLA-DQβ1*0301. J Dermatol Case Rep 8:9–12

Rashid KA, Gürcan HM, Ahmed AR (2006) Antigen specificity in subsets of mucous membrane pemphigoid. J Invest Dermatol 126:2631–2636

Raux G, Gilbert D, Joly P, Daveau M, Martel P, Christ M, Tron F (2000) Association of KM genotype with bullous pemphigoid. J Autoimmun 14:79–82

Recke A, Sitaru C, Vidarsson G, Evensen M, Chiriac MT, Ludwig RJ, Zillikens D (2010) Pathogenicity of IgG subclass autoantibodies to type VII collagen: induction of dermal-epidermal separation. J Autoimmun 34:435–444

Recke A, Vidarsson G, Ludwig RJ, Freitag M, Möller S, Vonthein R, Schellenberger J, Haase O, Görg S, Nebel A, Flachsbart F, Schreiber S, Lieb W, Gläser R, Benoit S, Sárdy M, Eming R, Hertl M, Zillikens D, König IR, Schmidt E, Ibrahim S, Group GAGS (2015) Allelic and copy-number variations of FcγRs affect granulocyte function and susceptibility for autoimmune blistering diseases. J Autoimmun 61:36–44

Recke A, Konitzer S, Lemcke S, Freitag M, Sommer NM, Abdelhady M, Amoli MM, Benoit S, El-Chennawy F, Eldarouti M, Eming R, Gläser R, Günther C, Hadaschik E, Homey B, Lieb W, Peitsch WK, Pföhler C, Robati RM, Saeedi M, Sárdy M, Sticherling M, Uzun S, Worm M, Zillikens D, Ibrahim S, Vidarsson G, Schmidt E, Group GAGS (2018) The p.Arg435His variation of IgG3 with high affinity to FcRn is associated with susceptibility for pemphigus vulgaris-analysis of four different ethnic cohorts. Front Immunol 9:1788

Rinn JL, Chang HY (2012) Genome regulation by long noncoding RNAs. Annu Rev Biochem 81:145–166

Rock B, Labib RS, Diaz LA (1990) Monovalent Fab' immunoglobulin fragments from endemic pemphigus foliaceus autoantibodies reproduce the human disease in neonatal Balb/c mice. J Clin Invest 85:296–299

Roy M, Waldschmidt T, Aruffo A, Ledbetter JA, Noelle RJ (1993) The regulation of the expression of gp39, the CD40 ligand, on normal and cloned CD4+ T cells. J Immunol 151:2497–2510

Rychlik-Sych M, Baranska M, Waszczykowska E, Torzecka JD, Zebrowska A, Skretkowicz J (2013) Genetic polymorphisms of CYP2D6 oxidation in patients with autoimmune bullous diseases. Postepy Dermatol Alergol 30:211–217

Rychlik-Sych M, Barańska M, Wojtczak A, Skrętkowicz J, Żebrowska A, Waszczykowska E (2015) The impact of the CYP2D6 gene polymorphism on the risk of pemphigoid. Int J Dermatol 54:1396–1401

Rychlik-Sych M, Barańska M, Dudarewicz M, Skrętkowicz J, Żebrowska A, Owczarek J, Waszczykowska E (2017) ABCB1 gene is associated with the risk of bullous pemphigoid in a polish population. J Dtsch Dermatol Ges 15:499–505

Rychlik-Sych M, Barańska M, Dudarewicz M, Skrętkowicz J, Żebrowska A, Woźniacka A, Owczarek J, Orszulak-Michalak D, Waszczykowska E (2018) Haplotypes of ABCB1 1236C >T (rs1128503), 2677G >T/A (rs2032582), and 3435C >T (rs1045642) in patients with bullous pemphigoid. Arch Dermatol Res 310:515–522

Sadik CD, Lima AL, Zillikens D (2016) Pemphigoid gestationis: Toward a better understanding of the etiopathogenesis. Clin Dermatol 34:378–382

Sadik CD, Bischof J, van Beek N, Dieterich A, Benoit S, Sárdy M, Worm M, Meller S, Gläser R, Zillikens D, Homey B, Setterfield J, Minassian D, Schmidt E, Dart J, Ibrahim SM, 2014 Msg-, Group ABDS (2017) Genomewide association study identifies GALC as susceptibility gene for mucous membrane pemphigoid. Exp Dermatol 26:1214–1220

Sáenz-Cantele AM, Fernández-Mestre M, Montagnani S, Calebotta A, Balbas O, Layrisse Z (2007) HLA-DRB1*0402 haplotypes without DQB1*0302 in Venezuelan patients with pemphigus vulgaris. Tissue Antigens 69:318–325

Saha M, Harman K, Mortimer NJ, Binda V, Black MM, Kondeatis E, Vaughan R, Groves RW (2010) Pemphigus vulgaris in White Europeans is linked with HLA Class II allele HLA DRB1*1454 but not DRB1*1401. J Invest Dermatol 130:311–314

Saha M, Harman K, Mortimer NJ, Binda V, Black MM, Kondeatis E, Vaughan R, Groves RW (2018) Sporadic pemphigus foliaceus and class II human leucocyte antigen allele associations in the white British and Indo-Asian populations in the UK. Clin Exp Dermatol

Sajda T, Hazelton J, Patel M, Seiffert-Sinha K, Steinman L, Robinson W, Haab BB, Sinha AA (2016) Multiplexed autoantigen microarrays identify HLA as a key driver of anti-desmoglein and -non-desmoglein reactivities in pemphigus. Proc Natl Acad Sci U S A 113:1859–1864

Salviano-Silva A, Petzl-Erler ML, Boldt ABW (2017) CD59 polymorphisms are associated with gene expression and different sexual susceptibility to pemphigus foliaceus. Autoimmunity 50:377–385

Salviano-Silva A, Lobo-Alves S, Augusto D, Farias Della Justina T, Luiza Petzl-Erler M, Almeida R, Malheiros D (2018a) Immune-related long non-coding RNAs Polymorphisms associated with the endemic autoimmune disease pemphigus foliaceous. In: International Congress of genetics. Puerto Rico, City

Salviano-Silva A, Lobo-Alves SC, Almeida RC, Malheiros D, Petzl-Erler ML (2018b) Besides pathology: long non-coding RNA in cell and tissue homeostasis. Noncoding RNA 4

Sarig O, Bercovici S, Zoller L, Goldberg I, Indelman M, Nahum S, Israeli S, Sagiv N, Martinez de Morentin H, Katz O, Baum S, Barzilai A, Trau H, Murrell DF, Bergman R, Hertl M, Rosenberg S, Nöthen MM, Skorecki K, Schmidt E, Zillikens D, Darvasi A, Geiger D, Rosset S, Ibrahim SM, Sprecher E (2012) Population-specific association between a polymorphic variant in ST18, encoding a pro-apoptotic molecule, and pemphigus vulgaris. J Invest Dermatol 132:1798–1805

Sawamura D, Mochitomi Y, Kanzaki T, Nakamura H, Shimizu H (2006) Glycine substitution mutations by different amino acids at the same codon in COL7A1 cause different modes of dystrophic epidermolysis bullosa inheritance. Br J Dermatol 155:834–837

Schaller J, Feleke W, Haustein UF, Baldauf C, Kunze G (1991) HLA in bullous pemphigoid. The probable role of HLA-B7 as a marker for poor responders to immunosuppressive therapy. Int J Dermatol 30:36–38

Schmidt E, Zillikens D (2013) Pemphigoid diseases. Lancet 381:320–332

Schmidt E, Mittnacht A, Schömig H, Dummer R, Bröcker EB, Zillikens D (1996) Detection of IL-1 alpha, IL-1 beta and IL-1 receptor antagonist in blister fluid of bullous pemphigoid. J Dermatol Sci 11:142–147

Schmidt T, Sitaru C, Amber K, Hertl M (2014) BP180- and BP230-specific IgG autoantibodies in pruritic disorders of the elderly: a preclinical stage of bullous pemphigoid? Br J Dermatol 171:212–219

Schneider P, MacKay F, Steiner V, Hofmann K, Bodmer JL, Holler N, Ambrose C, Lawton P, Bixler S, Acha-Orbea H, Valmori D, Romero P, Werner-Favre C, Zubler RH, Browning JL, Tschopp J (1999) BAFF, a novel ligand of the tumor necrosis factor family, stimulates B cell growth. J Exp Med 189:1747–1756

Sekiguchi M, Futei Y, Fujii Y, Iwasaki T, Nishikawa T, Amagai M (2001) Dominant autoimmune epitopes recognized by pemphigus antibodies map to the N-terminal adhesive region of desmogleins. J Immunol 167:5439–5448

Setterfield J, Bhogal B, Black MM, McGibbon DH (1997) Dermatitis herpetiformis and bullous pemphigoid: a developing association confirmed by immunoelectron-microscopy. Br J Dermatol 136:253–256

Setterfield J, Theron J, Vaughan RW, Welsh KI, Mallon E, Wojnarowska F, Challacombe SJ, Black MM (2001) Mucous membrane pemphigoid: HLA-DQB1*0301 is associated with all clinical sites of involvement and may be linked to antibasement membrane IgG production. Br J Dermatol 145:406–414

Shams S, Amirzargar AA, Yousefi M, Rezaei N, Solgi G, Khosravi F, Ansaripour B, Moradi B, Nikbin B (2009) HLA class II (DRB, DQA1 and DQB1) allele and haplotype frequencies in the patients with pemphigus vulgaris. J Clin Immunol 29:175–179

Sharma P, Mao X, Payne AS (2007) Beyond steric hindrance: the role of adhesion signaling pathways in the pathogenesis of pemphigus. J Dermatol Sci 48:1–14

Shornick JK, Stastny P, Gilliam JN (1981) High frequency of histocompatibility antigens HLA-DR3 and DR4 in herpes gestations. J Clin Invest 68:553–555

Shornick JK, Stastny P, Gilliam JN (1983) Paternal histocompatibility (HLA) antigens and maternal anti-HLA antibodies in herpes gestationis. J Invest Dermatol 81:407–409

Shornick JK, Meek TJ, Nesbitt LT, Gilliam JN (1984) Herpes gestationis in blacks. Arch Dermatol 120:511–513

Shornick JK, Artlett CM, Jenkins RE, Briggs DC, Welsh KI, Garvey MP, Kelly SE, Black MM (1993) Complement polymorphism in herpes gestationis: association with C4 null allele. J Am Acad Dermatol 29:545–549

Shornick JK, Jenkins RE, Artlett CM, Briggs DC, Welsh KI, Kelly SE, Garvey MP, Black MM (1995) Class II MHC typing in pemphigoid gestationis. Clin Exp Dermatol 20:123–126

Simmonds MJ, Heward JM, Barrett JC, Franklyn JA, Gough SC (2006) Association of the BTNL2 rs2076530 single nucleotide polymorphism with Graves' disease appears to be secondary to DRB1 exon 2 position beta74. Clin Endocrinol (oxf) 65:429–432

Simpson LJ, Ansel KM (2015) MicroRNA regulation of lymphocyte tolerance and autoimmunity. J Clin Invest 125:2242–2249

Sivasankar B, Donev RM, Longhi MP, Hughes TR, Davies R, Cole DS, Morgan BP, Marchbank KJ (2007) CD59a deficient mice display reduced B cell activity and antibody production in response to T-dependent antigens. Mol Immunol 44:2978–2987

Skrętkowicz J, Barańska M, Kaczorowska A, Rychlik-Sych M (2011) Genetic polymorphisms of CYP2D6 oxidation in patients with systemic lupus erythematosus. Arch Med Sci 7:864–869

Slomov E, Loewenthal R, Korostishevsky M, Goldberg I, Brenner S, Gazit E (2005) Pemphigus vulgaris is associated with the transporter associated with antigen processing (TAP) system. Hum Immunol 66:1213–1222

Song WC (2006) Complement regulatory proteins and autoimmunity. Autoimmunity 39:403–410

Stanley JR, Koulu L, Klaus-Kovtun V, Steinberg MS (1986) A monoclonal antibody to the desmosomal glycoprotein desmoglein I binds the same polypeptide as human autoantibodies in pemphigus foliaceus. J Immunol 136:1227–1230

Stapleton NM, Andersen JT, Stemerding AM, Bjarnarson SP, Verheul RC, Gerritsen J, Zhao Y, Kleijer M, Sandlie I, de Haas M, Jonsdottir I, van der Schoot CE, Vidarsson G (2011) Competition for FcRn-mediated transport gives rise to short half-life of human IgG3 and offers therapeutic potential. Nat Commun 2:599

Stavropoulos PG, Zarafonitis G, Petridis A, Hashimoto T, Harman KE, Black MM (2001) Pemphigus vulgaris in two sisters. Acta Derm Venereol 81:149

Sun CC, Wu J, Wong TT, Wang LF, Chuan MT (2000) High levels of interleukin-8, soluble CD4 and soluble CD8 in bullous pemphigoid blister fluid. The relationship between local cytokine production and lesional T-cell activities. Br J Dermatol 143:1235–1240

Sun Y, Liu H, Wang Z, Fu X, Wang C, Mi Z, Sun L, Bao F, Yu G, Zhou G, Zhang F (2018) The HLA-DQB1*03:01 is associated with bullous pemphigoid in the han chinese population. J Invest Dermatol 138:1874–1877

Sun Y, Liu H, Yang B, Wang C, Foo JN, Bao F, Irwanto A, Yu G, Fu X, Wang Z, You J, Liu J, Zhou G, Zhang F (2019) Investigation of the predisposing factor of pemphigus and its clinical subtype through a genome-wide association and next generation sequence analysis. J Eur Acad Dermatol Venereol 33:410–415

Svecova D, Parnicka Z, Pastyrikova L, Urbancek S, Luha J, Buc M (2015) HLA DRB1* and DQB1* alleles are associated with disease severity in patients with pemphigus vulgaris. Int J Dermatol 54:168–173

Swanberg M, Lidman O, Padyukov L, Eriksson P, Akesson E, Jagodic M, Lobell A, Khademi M, Börjesson O, Lindgren CM, Lundman P, Brookes AJ, Kere J, Luthman H, Alfredsson L, Hillert J, Klareskog L, Hamsten A, Piehl F,

Olsson T (2005) MHC2TA is associated with differential MHC molecule expression and susceptibility to rheumatoid arthritis, multiple sclerosis and myocardial infarction. Nat Genet 37:486–494

Tampoia M, Bonamonte D, Filoni A, Garofalo L, Morgese MG, Brunetti L, Di Giorgio C, Annicchiarico G (2013) Prevalence of specific anti-skin autoantibodies in a cohort of patients with inherited epidermolysis bullosa. Orphanet J Rare Dis 8:132

Tanasilovic S, Popadic S, Medenica L, Popadic D (2017) Pemphigus vulgaris and pemphigus foliaceus determined by CD86 and CTLA4 polymorphisms. Clin Dermatol 35:236–241

Thoma-Uszynski S, Uter W, Schwietzke S, Schuler G, Borradori L, Hertl M (2006) Autoreactive T and B cells from bullous pemphigoid (BP) patients recognize epitopes clustered in distinct regions of BP180 and BP230. J Immunol 176:2015–2023

Thorne JE, Anhalt GJ, Jabs DA (2004) Mucous membrane pemphigoid and pseudopemphigoid. Ophthalmology 111:45–52

Tong JC, Tan TW, Sinha AA, Ranganathan S (2006) Prediction of desmoglein-3 peptides reveals multiple shared T-cell epitopes in HLA DR4- and DR6-associated pemphigus vulgaris. BMC Bioinformatics 7(Suppl 5):S7

Torzecka JD, Narbutt J, Sysa-Jedrzejowska A, Borowiec M, Ptasinska A, Woszczek G, Kowalski ML (2003) Tumour necrosis factor-alpha polymorphism as one of the complex inherited factors in pemphigus. Mediators Inflamm 12:303–307

Toumi A, Abida O, Ben Ayed M, Masmoudi A, Turki H, Masmoudi H (2013) Cytokine gene polymorphisms in Tunisian endemic pemphigus foliaceus: a possible role of il-4 variants. Hum Immunol 74:658–665

Tsunoda K, Ota T, Aoki M, Yamada T, Nagai T, Nakagawa T, Koyasu S, Nishikawa T, Amagai M (2003) Induction of pemphigus phenotype by a mouse monoclonal antibody against the amino-terminal adhesive interface of desmoglein 3. J Immunol 170:2170–2178

Tunca M, Musabak U, Sagkan RI, Koc E, Akar A (2010) Association of human leukocyte antigen class II alleles with pemphigus vulgaris in a Turkish population. J Dermatol 37:246–250

Ujiie H, Muramatsu K, Mushiroda T, Ozeki T, Miyoshi H, Iwata H, Nakamura A, Nomoto H, Cho KY, Sato N, Nishimura M, Ito T, Izumi K, Nishie W, Shimizu H (2018) HLA-DQB1*03:01 as a biomarker for genetic susceptibility to bullous pemphigoid induced by DPP-4 inhibitors. J Invest Dermatol 138:1201–1204

Uzun S, Durdu M, Akman A, Gunasti S, Uslular C, Memisoglu HR, Alpsoy E (2006) Pemphigus in the Mediterranean region of Turkey: a study of 148 cases. Int J Dermatol 45:523–528

Vaira F, Della Valle V, Fanoni D, Pontini P, Muratori S (2013) Bullous pemphigoid and dermatitis herpetiformis association: a genetic predisposition. J Dermatol 40:940–941

van den Berg CW, Cinek T, Hallett MB, Horejsi V, Morgan BP (1995) Exogenous glycosyl phosphatidylinositol-anchored CD59 associates with kinases in membrane clusters on U937 cells and becomes Ca(2+)-signaling competent. J Cell Biol 131:669–677

Veldman C, Stauber A, Wassmuth R, Uter W, Schuler G, Hertl M (2003) Dichotomy of autoreactive Th1 and Th2 cell responses to desmoglein 3 in patients with pemphigus vulgaris (PV) and healthy carriers of PV-associated HLA class II alleles. J Immunol 170:635–642

Venning VA, Taylor CJ, Ting A, Wojnarowska F (1989) HLA type in bullous pemphigoid, cicatricial pemphigoid and linear IgA disease. Clin Exp Dermatol 14:283–285

Venning VA, Dean D, Wojnarowska F (1992) Absence of expression of class II major histocompatibility complex determinants on keratinocytes in bullous pemphigoid. Br J Dermatol 126:463–467

V'lckova-Laskoska MT, Laskoski DS, Kamberova S, Caca-Biljanovska N, Volckova N (2007) Epidemiology of pemphigus in Macedonia: a 15-year retrospective study (1990–2004). Int J Dermatol 46:253–258

Vodegel RM, Jonkman MF, Pas HH, de Jong MC (2004) U-serrated immunodeposition pattern differentiates type VII collagen targeting bullous diseases from other subepidermal bullous autoimmune diseases. Br J Dermatol 151:112–118

Vodo D, Sarig O, Geller S, Ben-Asher E, Olender T, Bochner R, Goldberg I, Nosgorodsky J, Alkelai A, Tatarskyy P, Peled A, Baum S, Barzilai A, Ibrahim SM, Zillikens D, Lancet D, Sprecher E (2016) Identification of a functional risk variant for pemphigus vulgaris in the ST18 gene. PLoS Genet 12: e1006008

Vogel LA, Noelle RJ (1998) CD40 and its crucial role as a member of the TNFR family. Semin Immunol 10:435–442

Vorobyev A, Ludwig RJ, Schmidt E (2017) Clinical features and diagnosis of epidermolysis bullosa acquisita. Expert Rev Clin Immunol 13:157–169

Wang M, Liang L, Li L, Han K, Li Q, Peng Y, Peng X, Zeng K (2017) Increased miR-424-5p expression in peripheral blood mononuclear cells from patients with pemphigus. Mol Med Rep 15:3479–3484

Warren SJ, Arteaga LA, Rivitti EA, Aoki V, Hans-Filho G, Qaqish BF, Lin MS, Giudice GJ, Diaz LA (2003) The role of subclass switching in the pathogenesis of endemic pemphigus foliaceus. J Invest Dermatol 120:104–108

Weber R, Monteiro F, Preuhs-Filho G, Rodrigues H, Kalil J, Miziara ID (2011) HLA-DRB1*04:02, DRB1*08:04 and DRB1*14 alleles associated to pemphigus vulgaris in southeastern Brazilian population. Tissue Antigens 78:92–93

Wegener H, Paulsen H, Seeger K (2014) The cysteine-rich region of type VII collagen is a cystine knot with a new topology. J Biol Chem 289:4861–4869

Weisenseel P, Martin S, Partscht K, Messer G, Prinz JC (2007) Relevance of the low-affinity type of the Fcgamma-receptor IIIa-polymorphism in bullous pemphigoid. Arch Dermatol Res 299:163–164

Winsey S, Lonie L, Allen J, Bunce M, Marshall SE, Wojnarowska F (2004) Genetic variation in COL17A1 and the development of bullous pemphigoid. Exp Dermatol 13:140–147

Woodley DT, Cogan J, Wang X, Hou Y, Haghighian C, Kudo G, Keene DR, Chen M (2014) De novo anti-type VII collagen antibodies in patients with recessive dystrophic epidermolysis bullosa. J Invest Dermatol 134:1138–1140

Wucherpfennig KW, Yu B, Bhol K, Monos DS, Argyris E, Karr RW, Ahmed AR, Strominger JL (1995) Structural basis for major histocompatibility complex (MHC)-linked susceptibility to autoimmunity: charged residues of a single MHC binding pocket confer selective presentation of self-peptides in pemphigus vulgaris. Proc Natl Acad Sci U S A 92:11935–11939

Xiao Y, Lazaro AM, Masaberg C, Haagenson M, Vierra-Green C, Spellman S, Dakshanamurthy S, Ng J, Hurley CK (2009) Evaluating the potential impact of mismatches outside the antigen recognition site in unrelated hematopoietic stem cell transplantation: HLA-DRB1*1454 and DRB1*140101. Tissue Antigens 73:595–598

Yamagami J (2018) Recent advances in the understanding and treatment of pemphigus and pemphigoid. F1000Res 7

Yan L, Wang JM, Zeng K (2012) Association between HLA-DRB1 polymorphisms and pemphigus vulgaris: a meta-analysis. Br J Dermatol 167:768–777

Yang J, Siqueira MF, Behl Y, Alikhani M, Graves DT (2008) The transcription factor ST18 regulates proapoptotic and proinflammatory gene expression in fibroblasts. FASEB J 22:3956–3967

Yari F, Zavaran Hosseini A, Nemat Gorgani M, Khorramizadeh MR, Mansouri P, Kazemnejad A (2008) Expression of HLA-G in the skin of patients with pemphigus vulgaris. Iran J Allergy Asthma Immunol 7:7–12

Yu X, Wester-Rosenlöf L, Gimsa U, Holzhueter SA, Marques A, Jonas L, Hagenow K, Kunz M, Nizze H, Tiedge M, Holmdahl R, Ibrahim SM (2009) The mtDNA nt7778 G/T polymorphism affects autoimmune diseases and reproductive performance in the mouse. Hum Mol Genet 18:4689–4698

Yue Z, Fu X, Chen M, Wang Z, Wang C, Yang B, Zhou G, Liu H, Zhang F (2014) Lack of association between the single nucleotide polymorphism of ST18 and pemphigus in Chinese population. J Dermatol 41:353–354

Yunis JJ, Mobini N, Yunis EJ, Alper CA, Deulofeut R, Rodriguez A, Foster CS, Marcus-Bagley D, Good RA, Ahmed AR (1994) Common major histocompatibility complex class II markers in clinical variants of cicatricial pemphigoid. Proc Natl Acad Sci U S A 91:7747–7751

Zakka LR, Keskin DB, Reche P, Ahmed AR (2010) Relationship between target antigens and major histocompatibility complex (MHC) class II genes in producing two pathogenic antibodies simultaneously. Clin Exp Immunol 162:224–236

Zakka LR, Reche P, Ahmed AR (2011) Role of MHC Class II genes in the pathogenesis of pemphigoid. Autoimmun Rev 11:40–47

Zaltas MM, Ahmed R, Foster CS (1989) Association of HLA-DR4 with ocular cicatricial pemphigoid. Curr Eye Res 8:189–193

Zhang R, Liu Q, Liao Q, Zhao Y (2018a) CD59: a promising target for tumor immunotherapy. Future Oncol 14:781–791

Zhang SY, Zhou XY, Zhou XL, Zhang Y, Deng Y, Liao F, Yang M, Xia XY, Zhou YH, Yin DD, Ojaswi P, Hou QQ, Wang L, Zhang DY, Xia DM, Deng YQ, Ding L, Liu HJ, Yan W, Li MM, Ma WT, Ma JJ, Yu Q, Liu B, Yang L, Zhang W, Shu Y, Xu H, Li W (2018b) Subtype-specific inherited predisposition to pemphigus in the Chinese population. Br J Dermatol

Zhong X, Liu MY, Sun XH, Wei MJ (2016) Association between ABCB1 polymorphisms and haplotypes and Alzheimer's disease: a meta-analysis. Sci Rep 6:32708

Zitouni M, Martel P, Ben Ayed M, Raux G, Gilbert D, Joly P, Mokhtar I, Ridha Kamoun M, Turki H, Zahaf A, Mokni M, Ben Osman A, Masmoudi H, Makni S, Tron F (2002) Pemphigus is not associated with allotypic markers of immunoglobulin kappa. Genes Immun 3:50–52

Zivanovic D, Bojic S, Medenica L, Andric Z, Popadic D (2016) Human leukocyte antigen class II (DRB1 and DQB1) alleles and haplotypes frequencies in patients with pemphigus vulgaris among the Serbian population. HLA 87:367–374

Zumelzu C, Le Roux-Villet C, Loiseau P, Busson M, Heller M, Aucouturier F, Pendaries V, Lièvre N, Pascal F, Brette MD, Doan S, Charron D, Caux F, Laroche L, Petit A, Prost-Squarcioni C (2011) Black patients of African descent and HLA-DRB1*15:03 frequency overrepresented in epidermolysis bullosa acquisita. J Invest Dermatol 131:2386–2393

Immunogenetics of Lupus Erythematosus

Begüm Ünlü, Ümit Türsen, Navid Jabalameli, Fahimeh Abdollahimajd, and Fateme Rajabi

Abstract

Lupus erythematosus (LE) is a heterogeneous disease with a wide range of manifestations ranging from localized lesions in cutaneous lupus erythematosus (CLE) to severe disseminated disease in systemic lupus erythematosus (SLE).

Lupus results from a complex interaction between genetic and epigenetic backgrounds and environmental triggers that cause loss of tolerance to self-antigens and the formation of autoantibodies. Genetic susceptibility plays a key role in the pathogenesis of lupus erythematosus. In most cases, multiple common alleles with modest effect sizes are combined to result in the polygenic inheritance of the disease but monogenic variants of lupus have also been described. Genes from the innate and adaptive immune system along with genes involved in apoptosis and immunoglobulin clearance have been linked to SLE. This chapter aims to explore the functions of these genes and their contribution to the pathogenesis of the disease.

Keywords

Lupus · Cutaneous lupus · Immunogenetics · Single-nucleotide polymorphism · Pathogenesis

1 Introduction

The lupus erythematosus (LE) is a heterogeneous disease with a wide spectrum of signs and symptoms, ranging from localized lesions in cutaneous lupus erythematosus (CLE) to severe disseminated disease in systemic lupus erythematosus (SLE) (Castro et al. 2008; Grönhagen et al. 2011).

In SLE, the accumulation of pathogenic autoantibodies and immune complexes leads to organ-specific inflammation and damage (Hersh et al. 2016). While virtually any organ can be affected by SLE, the disease tends to involve the joints, the kidneys, the hematologic system, the central nervous system, and the skin more often than the others. Mucocutaneous involvement is

B. Ünlü · Ü. Türsen (✉)
Department of Dermatology, Mersin University, Mersin, Turkey
e-mail: utursen@mersin.edu.tr

N. Jabalameli · F. Rajabi
Network of Dermatology Research (NDR), Universal Scientific Education and Research Network (USERN), Tehran, Iran

F. Abdollahimajd
Skin Research Center, Shahid Beheshti University of Medical Sciences, Tehran, Iran

F. Rajabi
Center for Research & Training in Skin Diseases & Leprosy, Tehran University of Medical Sciences, Tehran, Iran

N. Rezaei and F. Rajabi (eds.), *The Immunogenetics of Dermatologic Diseases*, Advances in Experimental Medicine and Biology 1367,
https://doi.org/10.1007/978-3-030-92616-8_9

very common in SLE, affecting up to 75% of patients in the course of the disease and 25% at the time of diagnosis (Tebbe and Orfanos 1997). The most common form of cutaneous involvement is a butterfly-shaped rash on the nose and the malar region, followed by oral/nasal ulcers, photosensitivity, non-scarring alopecias, and scarring discoid lesions (Medlin et al. 2016). The incidence of SLE is reported to be between 0.3 and 23.2 in 100,000 person-years (Javinani et al. 2019). It primarily affects female patients similar to other autoimmune diseases (Castro et al. 2008).

CLE is a distinct form of lupus primarily diagnosed via histopathological assessment. It can occur in the setting of systemic involvement as a manifestation of SLE but more often is an independent skin-limited entity (Grönhagen et al. 2011; Hersh et al. 2016). The incidence of CLE is slightly higher than that of SLE and is around 4.3 in 100,000 person-years (Durosaro et al. 2009). There are three clinically and histologically diverse subtypes of CLE, acute cutaneous lupus (ACLE) (Fig. 1), subacute cutaneous lupus (SCLE) (Fig. 2), and chronic cutaneous lupus (CCLE) (Fig. 3) (Fernando et al. 2012; Petri et al. 2012). Table 1 summarizes the feature of each subtype and their rate of association with systemic symptoms.

2 The Pathogenesis of Lupus

Lupus results from a complex interaction between genetic and epigenetic backgrounds and environmental triggers that result in loss of tolerance to self-antigens and formation of autoantibodies directed against double-stranded DNA and/or small nuclear RNA-binding proteins. These antibodies form immune complexes that are deposited within organs and cause inflammation and tissue damage. The slower clearance of antibody complexes and cellular apoptotic debris perpetuates the inflammatory cycle (Ghodke-Puranik and Niewold 2013, 2015).

The most prominent environmental triggers of lupus are viral infections, drugs, smoking, and ultraviolet (UV) radiation (Castro et al. 2008; Ghodke-Puranik and Niewold 2015). Both UVA and UVB have been implicated in the pathogenesis of lupus. UV radiation causes apoptosis mainly in keratinocytes by promoting the formation of reactive oxygen species (ROS) and inducing DNA damage (Fig. 4) (Gruijl et al. 2001). The UVB-damaged DNA activates the intracellular nucleic acid-sensing elements and pattern recognition receptors (PRRs) such as stimulator of interferon genes (STINGs) that results in the promotion of type-1 interferon (IFN) secretion (Kemp et al. 2015). In the presence of high amounts of circulating type-1 IFN, the UV-radiated keratinocytes and Langerhans cells express high levels of IL-6, IL-1β, and TNF-α (Umare et al. 2014; Yu et al. 2013). This cytokine milieu triggers the recruitment of T-cells and creates a vicious inflammatory cycle that activates the adaptive immune response (Fig. 5) (Meller et al. 2005; Wolf et al. 2018). UV-induced apoptosis also evokes translocation of intracellular components such as Ro60, Ro59, and the interferon-inducible protein 16 (IFI16) into the cytoplasmic membrane (Costa et al. 2011; Seelig et al. 1994). The inherent slower clearance of apoptotic debris in individuals with lupus prolongs the exposure of these sequestered antigens to the immune system (Bijl et al. 2006; Herrmann et al. 1998; Reefman et al. 2006). This results in the formation of autoreactive CD8+ T-cells and autoantibodies directed against these immune-privileged components (Wolf et al. 2018). Anti-Ro antibodies (directed against Ro60 and Ro59) can promote inflammation by interfering with the functions of these two proteins (Jones 1992). The Ro60 protein is involved in the degradation of misfolded non-coding RNA molecules that can cause inflammation if accumulated within the cell and the Ro59 protein interacts with interferon regulatory factors (IRFs).

Viral infections such as Epstein–Barr virus (EBV), parvovirus B19, and cytomegalovirus (CMV) can also trigger lupus (Bourn et al. 2016). Viral nucleic acids activate the innate immune response via TLRs and produce massive amounts of IFNα. High levels of type-1 IFN could trigger an unbalanced inflammatory milieu that results in

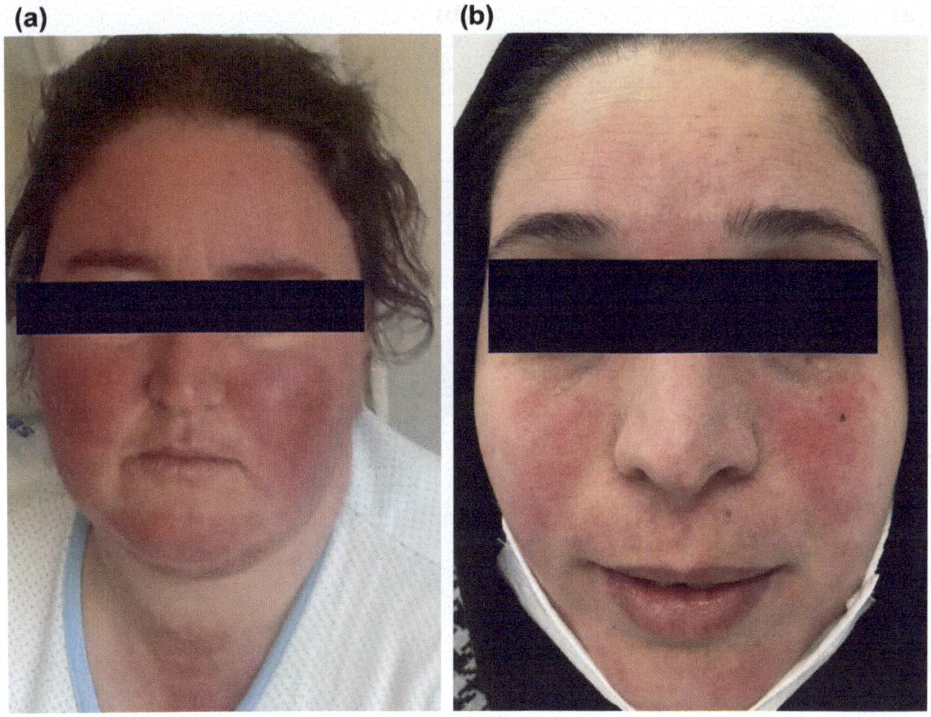

Fig. 1 Acute cutaneous lupus with malar rash (A and B)

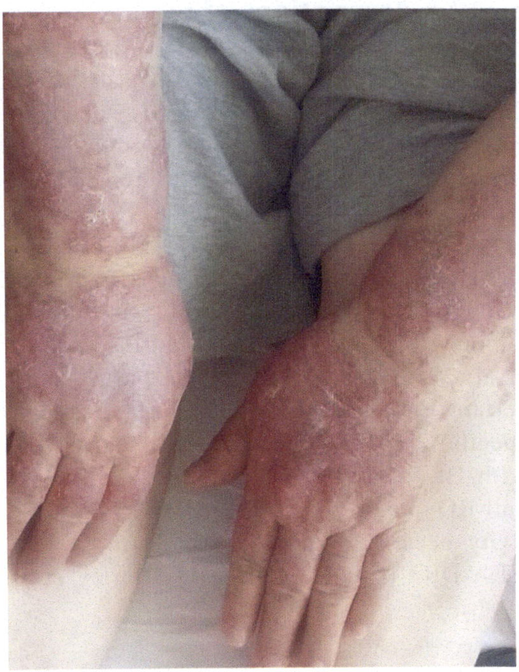

Fig. 2 Lesions of subacute cutaneous lupus erythematosus (SCLE)

autoimmunity in genetically vulnerable individuals (Rönnblom and Leonard 2019). Viral antigens can induce autoantibodies against dsDNA, Ro, and Sm through molecular mimicry and epitope spreading (Poole et al. 2006). EBV produces proteins that imitate the functions of Bcl-2, interleukin-10, and CD40. The BCL-2 homolog delays apoptosis. The IL-10 homolog reduces the expression of scavenger receptors on monocytes and inhibits apoptosis (Jog et al. 2018). The CD40 homolog promotes an aberrant B-cells immune response (Graham et al. 2010). The consequence of this functional mimicry is a lupus-like phenotype. Viral pathogens could also enhance the expression of autoimmunity loci within the host genome. EBV's main transcription factor, EBNA2, has been shown to occupy numerous genetic loci linked to autoimmune diseases (Harley et al. 2018).

The pathogenesis of drug-induced lupus is more complicated. Drugs can alter gene transcription by inhibiting DNA methylation as in SLE induced by hydralazine and procainamide (Richardson 2019).

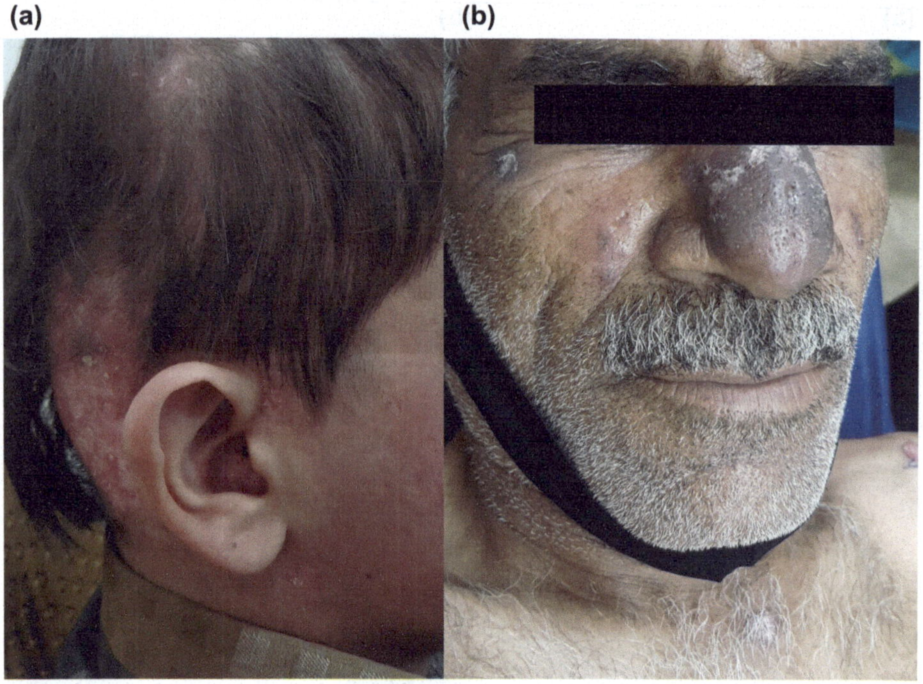

Fig. 3 Discoid lupus erythematosus (DLE) involving the face (A) and scalp (B)

They can also disrupt the balance of cytokine milieu toward an IFNα response as seen in biologic agents (Richardson 2019).

Genetic susceptibility plays a key role in the pathogenesis of lupus erythematosus. Familial aggregation and twin studies support this notion and several candidate susceptibility loci have been identified in case–control association studies(Alarcón-Segovia et al. 2005; Castro et al. 2008; Ghodke-Puranik and Niewold 2015). In most cases, multiple alleles with modest effect sizes are combined to result in the polygenic inheritance of the disease but monogenic variants of lupus have also been described (Alarcón-Segovia et al. 2005; Castro et al. 2008; Ghodke-Puranik and Niewold 2015).

Both human leukocyte antigen (HLA) regions and non-HLA susceptibility loci are associated with SLE. Table 2 summarizes the genes implicated in the pathogenesis of lupus based on their most relevant functions (Moser et al. 2009).

3 HLA Associations of Lupus

The class II HLAs (HLA-DR, -DQ, -DP) were the first genes to be linked to SLE and CLE susceptibility and they have shown the strongest association with different phenotypes of lupus in GWAS studies (Rönnblom et al. 2006). The HLA-DQA, HLA-DRB1, and HLA-DR3 are among the more consistent genotypes to confer susceptibility in different ethnic groups (Chung et al. 2011; Graham et al. 2002; Kunz et al. 2015). Furthermore, certain types of HLAs have been linked to specific lupus autoantibodies. Individuals with HLA-DQ1/ DQ2 are more likely to be anti-RO positive and anti-dsDNA seropositivity occurs more frequently in those with HLA-DR3 (Chung et al. 2011; Harley et al. 1986).

Table 1 Clinical and pathological findings in different subtypes of cutaneous lupus erythematosus and its association with systemic lupus (Grönhagen and Nyberg 2014; Merola and Moschella 2016)

Subtypes of cutaneous lupus erythematosus	Acute cutaneous lupus erythematosus (ACLE)	Subacute cutaneous lupus erythematosus (SCLE)	Chronic cutaneous lupus erythematosus (CCLE)
Clinical features	– Malar rash – Localized erythematous plaques provoked by sun exposure – Generalized maculopapular rash with photosensitivity sparing the knuckles – Variants: Bullous like lesions with toxic epidermal necrolysis features	– Annular or psoriasiform plaques – Photo-distributed but often spares the mid-face – Variants: • Poikilodermatous, • Erythrodermic, • Erythema multiforme-like (Rowell syndrome) • Neonatal lupus	– Discoid hyperkeratotic plaques with follicular plugging are associated with an atrophic telangiectatic scar in the head and neck – Variants: • Lupus erythematosus tumidus • Lupus profundus • Lupus panniculitis • Chilblain lupus erythematosus
Histological features	– Vacuolization of the basal layer – Lymphocytic infiltration at the dermo-epidermal junction and the superficial dermis – Mucin deposition within the dermis	– Vacuolization of the basal layer – Lymphocytic infiltration around the vessels and adnexa – Mucin deposition within the dermis – Follicular plugging and hyperkeratosis	– Basement membrane thickening – Follicular plugging and hyperkeratosis – Vacuolization of the basal layer – Lymphocytic infiltration around the vessels, the adnexa, and the dermo-epidermal junction – Mucin deposition within the dermis
Association with systemic lupus erythematosus	>90%	~50%	No association for lupus tumidus 5–10% for lupus panniculitis 5–10% in localized lesions 15–28% in generalized lesions

4 Non-HLA Associations of Lupus

4.1 The Innate Immunity-Related Genes

Activation of the innate immunity and production IFNα mark the initial steps in the pathogenesis of lupus. Individuals with SLE have higher baseline levels of circulating IFNα compared to normal healthy individuals (Castro et al. 2008; Niewold et al. 2007). Tissues affected by lupus also demonstrate a remarkable overexpression of genes that are involved in type-1 IFN signaling, production, and response (Castro et al. 2008; Ghodke-Puranik and Niewold 2015). In cutaneous lupus, the main source of IFNα is UV-damaged keratinocytes. UV-radiation promotes cellular stress, DNA damage, and apoptosis. Nucleic acid debris released from apoptotic cells can enter the cytosol of neighboring keratinocytes via liposome-based transfection and activate pattern recognition receptors (PRRs) such as cyclic GMP-AMP synthase (cGAS),

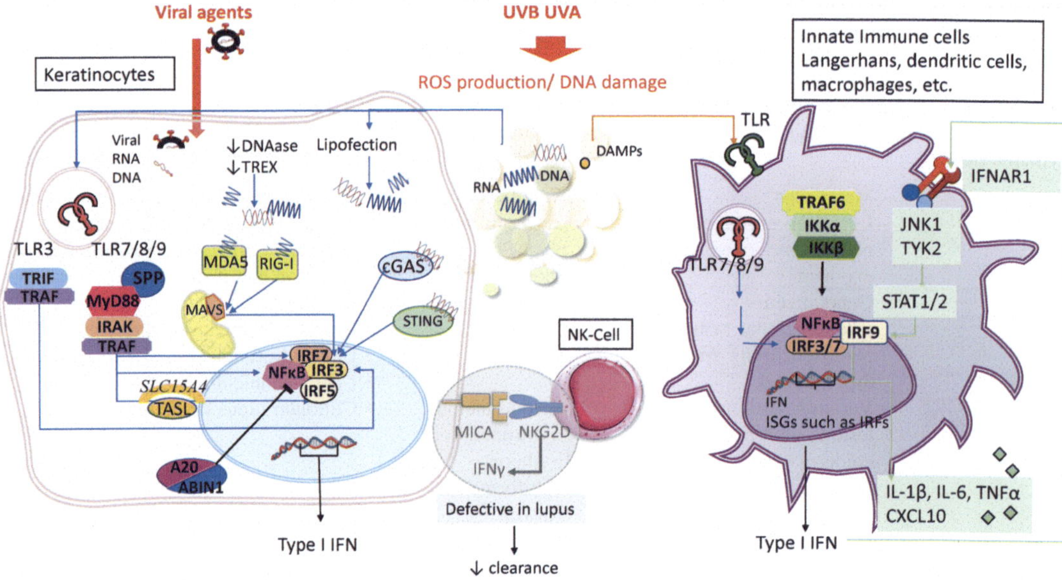

Fig. 4 The pathogenesis of lupus erythematosus and its susceptibility genes. The innate immune response is involved in the induction of the disease. Environmental triggers such as ultraviolet (UV) radiation and viruses activate toll-like receptors (TLRs) and other cytosolic pattern recognition receptors (PRRs) such as cGAS-STING, MDA5, and RIG-I to produce massive amounts of interferon (IFN) type I. The IFN, in turn, activates interferon-stimulated genes (ISGs) promoting the production of proinflammatory chemokines and cytokines such as interleukin-1 (IL-1), IL-6, and tumor necrosis factor α (TNFα). The sustained inflammation and the recruitment of the naïve T-cells initiate the adaptive immune response. A20 and ABIN1 are encoded by TNFAIP3 and TNIP1, respectively. DAMP, damage-associated molecular patterns. ROS, reactive oxygen species

STING, melanoma differentiation-associated protein 5 (MDA5), and retinoic acid-inducible gene I (RIG-I). DNAase deficiency could also lead to the build-up of nucleic acids within cells and can also engage PRRs. Through multiple subcellular signaling pathways activation of PRRs leads to transcription of type-1 IFN genes. The innate immune system is also involved in later steps ofof pathogenesis when autoimmune antinuclear antibodies have been formed. The release of nuclein acids from apoptotic cells enables the formation of antibody-nucleic acid complexes that are engulfed by CD32+ plasmacytoid dendritic cells (PDCs) and presented to endosomal Toll-like receptors (TLR3, TLR7, and TLR9) which prompt IFNα production. Though these pathways are triggered by environmental stress, the amount of IFN production is determined genetically (Castro et al. 2008; Kariuki and Niewold 2010; Niewold et al. 2007). Variations in genes encoding the PRRs such as MDA5 also known as interferon induced with helicase C domain 1 (IFIH) and TLRs and their downstream signaling elements such as IL-1 receptor-associated kinase (IRAK)-1, osteopontin (SPP), and interferon regulatory factors (IRFs) are involved in the IFN regulation and have been linked to SLE susceptibility (Castro et al. 2008). Polymorphisms in genes encoding some components of the PRR pathway, including IRAK4, MYD88, and the uncoordinated-93 homolog B1 (UNC93B), however, have not been linked to SLE (Isnardi et al. 2008).

The type-1 IFNs include IFNα, β, ε, ω, and κ. These IFNs bind to their specific receptors on the cell surfaces and activate Janus kinase1 (JAK1) and tyrosine kinase2 (TYK2), which together promote the phosphorylation and activation of signal transducer and activator of transcription (STAT) proteins. STAT1, STAT2, and IRF9 form a complex known as interferon-stimulated gene factor 3 (ISGF3) that is translocated to the

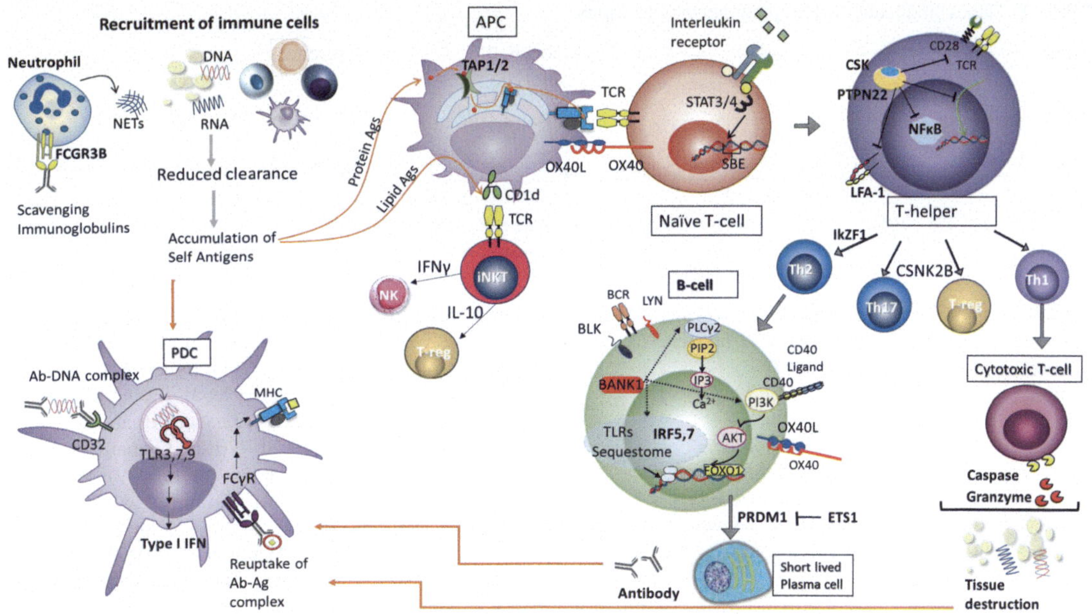

Fig. 5 The adaptive immune cells including different types of helper T-cells, B-cell, and plasma cells are involved in the establishment of the lupus erythematosus. The reduced clearance mechanisms that prolong the exposure of the immune system to self-antigens trigger the activation of the adaptive immune responses. NET, neutrophil extracellular traps; APC, antigen-presenting cells; PDC, plasmacytoid dendritic cells. iNKT, invariant natural killer T-cells

nucleus and initiates the transcription of IFN-inducible cytokine and chemokine genes by binding to the interferon-stimulated regulatory element (ISRE) in the promoter region of these genes (Kline and Kitagaki 2006; Rönnblom and Leonard 2019). To a lesser extent, JAK1/TYK2 also promotes the activation and dimerization of STAT3, 4, 5, and 6. These STAT hetero/homo dimers would then translocate to the nucleus and initiate the transcription of target genes by binding to the IFN-gamma-activated sequence (GAS) in their promoters (Asmana Ningrum 2014; Gao et al. 2004).

Polymorphisms within the genes that code components of the pathways downstream type-1 IFN signaling could potentially affect the responsiveness of the cells to IFNs and thus have an impact on the pathogenesis of lupus through regulating the intensity of the inflammatory and apoptotic cascades following IFN stimulation. Variations in genes encoding TYK2 and STAT4 have been linked to SLE susceptibility (Graham et al. 2011; Kaplan 2005; Tao et al. 2011).

The *IFIH1/MDA5* gene

IFIH1 (MDA5) is an innate immune receptor that detects intracytoplasmic dsRNAs (usually due to viral infections) and stimulates the production of type-1 IFN through promoting phosphorylation and activation of the IRFs (Kline and Kitagaki 2006). The rs1990760 variant of the *IFIH1* gene has been linked to multiple autoimmune diseases including lupus erythematosus (Ghodke-Puranik and Niewold 2013; Graham et al. 2011). This variant is a missense mutation that results in increased transcription of *IFIH1* (gain of function) in addition to increased levels of IFN and IFN-stimulated gene (ISG) expression (Ghodke-Puranik and Niewold 2013; Robinson et al. 2011). It is associated with higher anti-dsDNA antibodies in patients with SLE (Robinson et al. 2011). Recently, three additional *IFIH1* variants have been identified to confer risk for lupus erythematosus. These variants were also associated with increased autoantibody production, a higher rate of apoptosis, and extensive expression of inflammation-related genes (Molineros et al. 2013).

Table 2 Genes implicated in the pathogenesis of lupus

Gene			Associated phenotype	References
HLA genes		*A1, B7, B8,* *DQ2, DQA1, DQA2* *DR2, DR3, DRA, DRB1, DRB3, DRw52*	*DR2* and *DR3* with *CLE* *A1, B7, B8, DR2,* and *DR3* with DLE *A1, B8, DR3, DQ2,* and *DRw52* with SCLE	Millard and McGregor (2001), Fernando et al. (2007), Morris et al. (2012), Kunz et al. (2015), Chung et al. (2011), Hom et al. (2008), Han et al. (2009b)
Innate immunity-related genes	PRR pathways	***IFIH1: Interferon-induced with helicase C domain 1***[b] *TLR7, TLR8, TLR9: Toll-like receptor 7-9* *SPP: Osteopontin* ***ACP5: Acid phosphatase 5, tartrate-resistant***[a/b] *IRAK1: Interleukin-1 receptor-associated kinase 1* *IRF5, IRF7, IRF8: Intron regulatory factor 5 -8* *SLC15A4: Solute carrier family 15, member 4*	*IRF5* with both DLE and SCLE *TYK2* with DLE *SLC15A4* with DLE	Kurata et al. (2013), Kunz et al. (2015), Fernando et al. (2012), Fojtíková (2011), Sánchez et al. (2011), Harley et al. (2008b), Cui et al. (2013), Järvinen et al. (2010), Briggs et al. (2011), Graham et al. (2011), Gateva et al. (2009), Han et al. (2008), Kariuki et al. (2009a), He et al. (2010), Graham et al. (2008c), Wang et al. (2012), Chung et al. (2011), Han et al. (2009b), Sheng et al. (2011)
	NFκB pathway	***TNFAIP3: Tumor necrosis factor, alpha-induced protein 3***[b] *TNIP1: TNFAIP3-interacting protein 1* *UBE2L3: Ubiquitin-conjugating enzyme E2L 3* *PRKCB: Protein kinase C, beta* *TRIM39: Tripartite motif-containing protein 39* *RPP21: Ribonuclease P protein subunit 21*	*TRIM39/RPP21* with CLE *UBE2L3* with skin involvement in SLE *TNFAIP3* with malar rash in SLE	
	IFN pathway	*TYK2: Tyrosine kinase 2* *STAT4: Signal transducer and activator of transcription 4* *MICA: MHC class I chain-related A* *MICB: MHC class I chain-related B*	*TYK2* with DLE *STAT4* with DLE *MICB* with SCLE and cutaneous involvement in SLE	
DNA/RNA degradation Apoptosis		***DNASE1: Deoxyribonuclease 1***[b] ***DNASE1L3: Deoxyribonuclease 1 Like 3***[a] ***TREX1: Three prime repair exonuclease 1*** ***FAS, FASL***[b]	*TREX1* with chilblain lupus	Al-Mayouf et al. (2011), Harley et al. (2008b), Han et al. (2009b), Lu et al. (2012), Xiang et al. (2013)

(continued)

Table 2 (continued)

Gene			Associated phenotype	References
		ATG5: Autophagy-related 5		
Adaptive immunity-related genes	B-cells	*FcγRs: Fc fragment of IgG receptors* *MSH5: MutS homolog 5* ***IkZF1: IKAROS family zinc finger 1***[b] *RASGRP3: Ras guanyl-releasing protein 3* *BLK: B lymphocyte kinase* *BANK1: B-cell scaffold protein with ankyrin repeats* *LYN: Yamaguchi sarcoma viral oncogene* *PRDM1: PR domain zinc finger protein 1* *Ets-1: Ets-1 protein, or p54* *AFF1: AF4/FMR2 family member 1* *NCF2: Neutrophil cytosolic factor 2* *IL-21: Interleukin-21* *IL-10: Interleukin 10*	*FCGR2A* with DLE in the setting of SLE *FCGR3B* with malar rash *IkZF1* with CLE and cutaneous involvement in the setting of SLE *BANK1* with malar rash *Ets-1* with discoid lesions *IL-21* with cutaneous involvement in the setting of SLE	Harley et al. (2008b), Fernando et al. (2012), Kunz et al. (2015), Li et al. (2009), Sanchez et al. (2011), He et al. (2010), Han et al. (2009b), Lazarus et al. (1997) Harley et al. (2008b), Han et al. (2009b), Ramos et al. (2011), Kozyrev et al. (2008), Okada et al. (2012), Deng and Tsao (2010), Webb et al. (2009), Sullivan et al. (2000), Ruiz-Larrañaga et al. (2016)
	T-cells	*CSNK2B: Casein Kinase 2 subunit Beta* ***PTPN22: Protein tyrosine phosphatase non-receptor 22***[b] ***TNFSF4 (OX40L): Tumor necrosis factor superfamily, member 4*** *ILT3: Immunoglobulin-like transcript 3* *CD44: Cluster differentiation 44* *CTLA4: Cytotoxic T-lymphocyte antigen 4* *PDCD1: Programmed cell death 1*	CTLA4 with DLE	Kyogoku et al. (2004), Orru et al. (2009), Han et al. (2009b), Gateva et al. (2009), Lessard et al. (2011), Crispín et al. (2010), Jensen et al. (2012), Järvinen et al. (2010), Kailashiya et al. (2019)
Neutrophil/monocyte		*FCγR (3A, 3B, and 2B): Fc fragments of IgG low-affinity receptor* *ICAM-1*: Intracellular adhesion molecule-1 *ITGAM: Integrin Subunit Alpha M, also known as complement receptor-3 or CD11b*	Systemic	
Complement Immune complex clearance		*FCγR (3A, 3B, and 2B): Fc fragments of IgG low-affinity receptor*	C1q with DLE, SCLE	Harley et al. (2008b), Hom et al. (2008), Nath et al. (2008), Han et al. (2009b)

(continued)

Table 2 (continued)

Gene		Associated phenotype	References
	C1Q[a], ***C1R/C1S***[a] ***C2***[a] ***C4A/B***[b] *CFHR (1 and 3): Complement factor H related genes*	C2 with malar rash, discoid rash, photosensitivity	Truedsson et al. (2007), Zhao et al. (2011), Connolly and Hakonarson (2012), Deng and Tsao (2010), Braathen et al. (1986), Meyer et al. (1985), Millard and McGregor (2001)
Miscellaneous	*MUC21: Mucin 1* *PSORS1C1: Psoriasis susceptibility 1 candidate 1* *FLOT1: Flotillin-1* *VDR: Vitamin D receptor* *STK17a: Serine/threonine kinase 17a* *LY9: Lymphocyte antigen 9*	*MUC21, PSORS1C1, FLOT1, VDR, and STK17a* with CLE *LY9* with skin involvement in the setting of SLE	Wenzel (2019), Graham et al. (2008a), Monticielo et al. (2012), Ruiz-Larrañaga et al. (2016), Kunz et al. (2015), da Silva Fonseca et al. (2013)

[a]Linked to monogenic lupus with autosomal recessive mode of inheritance
[b]Linked to monogenic lupus with autosomal dominant mode of inheritance

The *TLR* genes

In lupus erythematosus, the TLR induction of IFNα occurs mainly after autoantibody production. That is when the nucleic acid-antibody complexes are endocytosed by pDCs. The single-stranded RNA (ssRNA) elements of these complexes bind with TLR7/8, the double-stranded RNAs (dsRNA) bind with TLR3, and the CpG DNAs activate TLR9. Indeed, in patients with SLE, the expression of *TLR7* correlates with anti-RNA titers while TLR9 expression is associated with anti-dsDNA titers (Chauhan et al. 2013). However, the role of TLR9 in the pathogenesis of SLE is more complex and both higher and lower expressions of this gene have been shown to cause/exacerbate lupus erythematosus (Celhar and Fairhurst 2014).

Genetic variations in the genes encoding these TLRs and their downstream signaling molecules have been shown to confer risk for lupus erythematosus. Multiple association studies and meta-analyses have suggested a link between the variants of the X-linked *TLR7* (rs3853839 in Asians and rs179008 in Africans), *TLR8* (rs3764879 in Caucasians), and *TLR9* (rs187084) genes and susceptibility to SLE (Lee et al. 2012, 2016).

The G-allele of the TLR7 rs3853839 is associated with higher levels of TLR7 and IFNα (Deng et al. 2013; Shen et al. 2010). The T-allele of the TLR7 rs179008 alters protein processing and is associated with a lower IFN response to viral infections that may secondarily predispose the carriers to SLE (Bordignon et al. 2013; Lee et al. 2012). The rs3764879 of the TLR8 gene is located near the translation start site thus may change its translation rate (Lee et al. 2012). The TLR9 rs187084 variant is located within the promoter region of the *TLR9* gene and could potentially influence gene expression levels (Hamann et al. 2006).

Moreover, the copy number variations (CNVs) of the *TLR7* gene can also confer risk for lupus erythematosus, especially the childhood-onset phenotype (Ortiz 2019). It has been demonstrated that females possessing more than two copies of the *TLR7* gene, and males with more than one copy (including individuals with an extra X chromosome, such as those with Klinefelter's syndrome) are at a higher risk for developing SLE (Dillon et al. 2012).

Though multiple small studies have been able to demonstrate associations between genetic variants of other TLRs and lupus erythematosus, these findings were not replicated in large-scale studies (Devarapu and Anders 2018).

The *IRAK1* gene

The *IRAK1* gene encodes a kinase downstream TLR signaling, which interacts with the myeloid differentiation primary response protein 88 (Myd88) and is thus involved in IFNα production. IRAK1 also controls the activation of the nuclear factor-kappa B (NFκB) pathway by acting both as an "on" and "off" switch. The *IRAK1* gene is located on chromosome Xq28, a locus that has been associated with SLE. Aside from the *IRAK1* gene, this locus also contains the *methyl CpG binding protein*-2 (*MECP2*) gene, which is a transcriptional regulator that controls the transcription of methylation-sensitive genes. The risk allele of the rs1059702 is associated with lower levels of MECP2 mRNA, which can lead to hypomethylation of IFN-regulated genes in T-cells and an amino acid substitution in IRAK1 protein that increases the NFκB activity (Jacob et al. 2009; Kaufman et al. 2013). Thus this risk allele contributes to SLE susceptibility by altering the functions of both of these genes.

The *SPP1* gene

The SPP1 gene encodes osteopontin, a 60 kDa complex protein residing in both intracellular and extracellular environments. Osteopontin mediates IFNα production by interacting with the MyD88 downstream of the TLR9 pathway and is thus involved in the pathogenesis of lupus erythematosus (Cao and Liu 2006). Some variants of the *SPP1* gene have been linked to high levels of IFN in patients with SLE (Forton et al. 2002; Kariuki et al. 2009a). Osteopontin is also involved in the pathogenesis of multiple autoimmune diseases by promoting IL-17 and B-cell differentiation (Clemente et al. 2016).

The ACP5 gene

The *acid phosphatase 5 (ACP5)* is another gene in the PRR pathway that has been linked to SLE. Missense mutations of the *ACP5* gene cause an autosomal recessive syndrome known as Spondyloenchondrodysplasia, which presents with skeletal dysplasia, neurological symptoms, and features of SLE such as arthritis, nephritis, cytopenias, and elevated levels of antinuclear and anti-dsDNA (Briggs et al. 2011; Lausch et al. 2011; Moser et al. 2009). Thus unlike most susceptibility loci that can induce lupus through polygenic interactions, *APC5* can also single-handedly cause monogenic lupus (Alperin et al. 2018). Moreover, it has been demonstrated that single allele loss-of-function mutations of the *ACP5* gene are more common in individuals with SLE compared with the normal population (An et al. 2017).

The *APC5* gene encodes an enzyme known as the tartrate-resistant acid phosphatase (TRAP). This metalloprotein enzyme is normally expressed in osteoclasts, macrophages, and dendritic cells and is responsible for the regulation of osteopontin (Ek-Rylander et al. 1994; Oddie et al. 2000).

It has been hypothesized that missense mutations of *ACP5* and downregulation of the TRAP protein would allow osteopontin to remain persistently activated. Hyperactivation of osteopontin promotes the production of IFNα through TLR9 and its downstream signaling pathways which in turn can induce SLE (Behrens and Graham 2011; Lausch et al. 2011). Consistent with this theory patients with Spondyloenchondrodysplasia have elevated levels of plasma IFNα and urine phosphorylated osteopontin.

The *IRF* genes

IRFs are a group of transcription factors that bind to interferon consensus sequence (ICS) present within the promoter region of IFNα and upstream interferon-inducible genes. Based on their pattern of dimerization they can act as both active and repressive complexes (Tamura et al. 2008). Most of the IRFs are activated downstream TLR signaling pathways and play an important role in IFNα induction (Honda et al. 2006; Kyogoku and Tsuchiya 2007). IRF3 and IRF7 are also activated by cytosolic RNA and DNA receptors such as IFIH1 (MDA5). IRF6 possesses a negative controlling role on cytokine production following TLR2 and 4 activations (Joly et al. 2016).

Genetic variations in three members of this family, *IRF5*, *IRF6*, and *IRF8* have shown an association with SLE in multiple studies (Chung et al. 2011; Graham et al. 2011; Han et al. 2009a). The *IRF5* has the most significant association with SLE among the members of the IRF family and is the only gene proven to be necessary for the induction of lupus in animal studies (Deng and Tsao 2010). The four main *IRF5* variants associated with lupus include a polymorphism within the promoter, two polymorphisms in the exons, and a three prime untranslated region (3′-UTR) polymorphism that results in a shorter more stable mRNA (Graham et al. 2007). The risk haplotypes composed of these four variants are accompanied by higher titers of anti-Ro, anti-La, and anti-dsDNA autoantibodies (Niewold et al. 2012). In several human SLE studies, some *IRF7* variants were associated with susceptibility to lupus erythematosus (Salloum et al. 2010). *IRF7* risk variants are associated with higher levels of circulating IFNα both through a cis-expression quantitative trait loci (eQTL) SNP promoting the *IRF7* expression and a trans-eQTL affecting the elements of type-1 IFN response (Lee et al. 2014; Salloum et al. 2010). Risk variants of *IRF8* result in higher IRF8 levels in B-cells of patients with SLE and have a significant association with anti-dsDNA antibodies (Chrabot et al. 2013).

The *solute carrier family 15, member 4* (*SLC15A4*) gene

SLC15A4 protein is an endolysosomal transporter that together with an adaptor protein named TASL mediates the recruitment of IRF5 and type-1 IFN production following TLR7/8/9 activation (Heinz et al. 2020). The SLC15A4 polymorphisms confer risk for SLE (Budarf et al. 2011; Han et al. 2009a; Zhang et al. 2016).

The NFκB pathway genes

The NF-κB is an inducible transcription factor involved in the regulation of genes encoding cytokines, chemokines, and other inflammatory molecules in both innate and adaptive immune responses. As mentioned earlier, aside from the usual IRF-dependent IFNα production, the PRRs such as TLRs are also capable of inducing interleukins (ILs) via the canonical NF-κB pathway (Liu et al. 2017; Sasai et al. 2010). Thus higher levels of NF-κB activity are expected in autoimmune inflammatory diseases.

This NF-κB pathway is regulated by a deubiquitinating enzyme, known as A20 encoded by the *tumor necrosis factor-alpha inducible protein3 (TNFAIP3)* gene and a polyubiquitin-binding protein known as A20-binding inhibitor of NF-κB activation1 (ABIN1) encoded by the *TNFAIP3-interacting protein1* (*TNIP1*) gene. Ubiquitination is the process of adding small polypeptides known as ubiquitin to target proteins. Ubiquitination alters the function, location, and degradation of proteins and is thus involved in a wide variety of cellular functions such as cell cycle progression, apoptosis, autophagy, antigen presentation, and immune responses (Pickart 2001; Sun and Chen 2004). ABIN1 facilitates the A20-mediated cleavage of polyubiquitin from NF-κB mediator proteins that results in their inactivation and degradation (G'Sell et al. 2015). Thus lower amounts of ABIN1 and A20 increase the activity of NF-κB.

Accordingly, loss-of-function polymorphisms within the *TNFAIP3* gene have been shown to confer the risk for SLE (Adrianto et al. 2011; Graham et al. 2008c). Polymorphisms within the promoter region of the *TNIP1* gene that has been linked to lupus susceptibility are also associated with lower expression levels of the gene (Gurevich et al. 2011; Han et al. 2009a; Zhang et al. 2013).

The *ubiquitin-conjugating enzyme E2L 3* (*UBE2L3*) gene encodes a protein involved in the degradation of TLRs and ubiquitination of NFκB precursors (Budarf et al. 2011; Chuang and Ulevitch 2004). As shown by multiple GWASs, genetic variations in this gene confer susceptibility to SLE (Han et al. 2009a; Harley et al. 2008a).

The *protein kinase C, beta* (*PRKCB*), is another SLE susceptibility gene (Budarf et al. 2011; Han et al. 2009a; Sheng et al. 2011). It is deemed essential for B-cell receptor (BCR) mediated activation of NFκB and thus plays an important role in SLE pathogenesis by increasing the survival of B-cells (Su et al. 2002).

Another NFκB-related susceptibility gene that has been linked to lupus is the *tripartite motif-containing protein 39* (*TRIM39*). The *TRIM39* gene is located near *ribonuclease P protein Subunit-21* (*RPP21*) gene and three susceptibility loci within this proximity have shown an association with lupus (Kunz et al. 2015).

The TRIM family is a group of ubiquitin-ligating (E3) enzymes that carry out the last step of the ubiquitination cascade (Tol et al. 2017). The TRIM family in particular is involved in the type-I interferon and NF-κB signaling pathways (Tol et al. 2017). TRIM39 down-regulates the NF-κB signaling pathways by stabilizing an NF-κB inhibitory protein (Suzuki et al. 2016). It also enhances apoptosis in response to DNA damage by stabilizing the enhancer of proapoptotic Bax protein (Huang et al. 2012). Furthermore, a TRIM39/RPP21 readthrough transcript is involved in the type-1 interferon response (Kurata et al. 2013). *RPP21* encodes a subunit of RNase P that inhibits the degradation of non-coding long RNAs. Accumulation of nucleic acids within the cells could active PRRs and promote the production of IFNs (Wilusz et al. 2012). Thus through multiple pathways, the polymorphisms within the *TRIM39* and *RPP21* genes can be involved in the pathogenesis of lupus.

The *STAT* and TYK2 genes

Tyrosine kinase 2 (TYK2) mediates IFNα receptors signaling that leads to increased production of interferon responsive genes. Genetic variants of the *TYK2* gene are associated with and higher levels of IFNα and have been shown to confer risk for SLE in meta-analyses and GWASs (Graham et al. 2011; Tao et al. 2011).

STAT4 is a signal transduction molecule that is activated by IFNα, IL-12, and IL-23. It is involved in innate immune responses and also mediates the differentiation of T-cell subtypes (especially Th17) (Korman et al. 2008). Polymorphisms in the *STAT4* gene have been implicated in the pathogenesis of several autoimmune diseases including SLE (Kaplan 2005). The SLE-associated risk variant of the *STAT4* gene has been shown to increase the sensitivity to IFNα signaling (concurrent lower serum IFNα and higher ISG expression) (Kariuki et al. 2009b). It is also more prevalent in individuals with a recalcitrant SLE with a higher frequency of lupus nephritis and higher titers of anti-dsDNA antibodies (Sanchez et al. 2011; Zheng et al. 2013).

4.2 The DNA/RNA Degradation and Apoptosis-Related Genes

As mentioned earlier, the apoptosis of keratinocytes and the release of intracellular proteins and nucleic acid components that activate the innate immune response mark the initial step in the pathogenesis of cutaneous lupus. It has been demonstrated that the accumulation of cellular debris and DNA/RNA particles due to insufficient and slower clearance could promote autoimmunity by increasing the chance of encountering PRRs such as TLRs, STING, RIG-I, and MDA5. Several enzymes are involved in DNA/RNA degradation including deoxyribonuclease-I that is encoded by *DNASE1*, deoxyribonuclease-gamma encoded by the *DNASE1L3*, and 3′->5′ DNA exonuclease encoded by *TREX1* have been linked to lupus susceptibility (Al-Mayouf et al. 2011; Namjou et al. 2011). DNASE1 is responsible for the degradation of extracellular nucleic acids such as neutrophil extracellular traps (NETs) that are released during neutrophil activation in response to pathogens. Genetic polymorphisms and single gene mutation of the *DNASE1* gene could lead to insufficient clearance of NETs. Prolonged exposure of the immune system to the sequestered DNA material present in NETs can cause autoimmunity (Garcia-Romo et al. 2011). *DNASE1* mutations cause familial forms of SLE (Al-Mayouf et al. 2011).

DNASE2 is responsible for the degradation of self-DNA in lysosomes. Thus, hypothetically its mutations could result in the breach of tolerance to self nucleic acids. Since DNASE2 mutations are lethal there is no clinical evidence to support this notion (Arneth 2019).

TREX1 is a type 3 DNASE that degrades intracytoplasmic nucleic acids. A single genetic mutation (D18N) within the *TREX1* gene could cause familial chilblain lupus (Lee-Kirsch et al. 2007, 2006; Yasutomo et al. 2001). This mutation significantly reduces the activity of this exonucleolytic enzyme, which in turn results in the accumulation of nucleic acids within the cell cytoplasm and through the activation PRRs triggers type-I interferon production and autoimmunity (Fiehn 2017; Jabalameli et al. 2021; Lee-Kirsch et al. 2007; Stetson et al. 2008).

Dysregulated apoptosis (both higher and lower rates) can promote autoimmunity. A higher rate of apoptosis would lead to relative inadequacy of apoptosis clearance mechanisms that lead to the accumulation of cellular debris and defective apoptosis could halt the elimination of autoreactive T-cells (Navratil and Ahearn 2000). Polymorphisms in genes encoding apoptosis-related proteins such as FAS, FASL, and autophagy-related-5 (ATG5) have been shown to confer risk for lupus (Lu et al. 2012).

FAS (CD95) is a transmembrane receptor that activates the caspase-dependent apoptosis pathways upon encountering its natural ligand (FASL) or monoclonal antibodies. Meta-analysis has revealed a significant association between *FAS* and *FASL* polymorphisms and lupus susceptibility in different populations (Lu et al. 2012). It has been suggested that these SNPs render autoreactive T-cells resistant to programmed cell death.

The *ATG5* encodes a protein that contributes to the autophagy process by allowing the binding of autophagosome to lysozyme and thus is involved in antigen presentation pathways (Tanida 2011). It also possesses a role in apoptosis activating caspases in the mitochondria (Yousefi et al. 2006). ATG5 suppresses the production of type 1 IFN responses by blocking MyD88 and NFκB (Inomata et al. 2013).

Multiple GWASs have identified associations between SLE and *ATG5* polymorphisms (Ciccacci et al. 2018; Harley et al. 2008a; Zhou et al. 2011). Lupus-related *ATG5* SNPs can promote the development of lupus through dysregulating the IFN production, antigen presentation, and apoptosis (Ye et al. 2018). It has been suggested that lupus-associated SNPs within the *ATG5* gene could affect the pathogenesis of the disease through its interaction with other genes (cis and trans-eQTLs) (Ye et al. 2018). Many genes associated with lupus and involved in the apoptosis pathways, NF-κB signaling, and IFN production are regulated by *ATG5* (Detecting genetic associations between ATG5 and lupus nephritis by trans-eQTL. 2015; Zhou et al. 2011).

The *MHC class I chain-related A* and *B* (*MICA*, *MICB*) genes are located near the HLA encoding genes on the short arm of the 6th chromosome. MICA and MICB are two ligands that are expressed on cellular surfaces alarming the buildup of intracellular oxidative stress (Groh et al. 1996; Valés-Gómez 2015; Yamamoto et al. 2001). These ligands interact with the NKG2D activating receptor on natural killer cells (NK-cells), which would lead to the destruction of the stressed cell by the innate immune system (Rajabi et al. 2018).

Genetic polymorphisms within the MICA and MICB genes have been linked to both systemic and cutaneous lupus along with multiple other autoimmune diseases (Gambelunghe et al. 2005; Kunz et al. 2015; Sanchez et al. 2006). The rs2844559, located ~27 kb proximal to *MICA*, and the rs3099844, ~15 kb proximal to the *MICB* are associated with CLE (Kunz et al. 2015). Eight MICA alleles have been described to date seven of which constitute trinucleotide microsatellite [GCT]n repeat polymorphisms (A4, A5, A6, A7, A8, A9, A10) in the exon 5 of the transmembrane segment region and one is a G insertion between the second and third repetitions (allele MICA-A5.1) (Ota et al. 1997; Rueda et al. 2002). The MICA A5, A5.1, and A9 alleles confer the risk for SLE development with the A9 allele associated with a higher risk for skin involvement in the setting of SLE (Fojtíková et al. 2011; Gambelunghe et al. 2005).

The aberrant expression and malfunction of the *MICA* and potentially *MICB* risk alleles alter their ability to engage with NKG2D receptors on NK-cells (Suemizu et al. 2002; Yoshida et al. 2011). It has been postulated that the reduced activation of the NK-cells would lead to impaired innate immune surveillance (Suemizu et al. 2002) and clearance of stressed and damaged cells which consequently increases the chances of autoimmunity through activation of the adaptive immune response (Park et al. 2009).

4.3 Genes Regulating the Adaptive Immune System

The type I IFNs, IL-6, IL-1β, and TNF-α. which are either directly released from UV radiated keratinocytes and Langerhans cells or are produced as a product of the activation of innate immunity, are considered primary cytokines that can initiate a cascade of cytokine release from other immune cells. The IFNα and IFN-inducible cytokines and chemokines attract and activate multiple cell lines including dendritic cells, neutrophils, macrophages, and subsets of B- and T-cells. High levels of type I IFN enhance antigen presentation by dendritic cells, promote NETosis by neutrophils, activate T-cells, and support B-cell survival, differentiation, and immunoglobulin class-switching (Blanco et al. 2001; Chang et al. 2015; Crow 2014).

The IFNα induces IP10/CXCL10 that can selectively recruit Th1 cells. These cells in turn produce massive amounts of IFNγ, which promotes the activity of cytotoxic T-cells and apoptosis of keratinocytes via granzyme B and caspase (Achtman and Werth 2015; Ohl 2011; Seery 2000). IL-6 promotes IL-17 and IL-21 secretion by Th17 cells, type 3 innate lymphoid cells (ILC3), and neutrophils (Martin et al. 2014). IL-17 is a powerful proinflammatory cytokine that can boost the production of autoantibodies in germinal centers, promote chemokine release and NETosis (Martin et al. 2014).

IFNα facilitates antigen presentation by dendritic cells. These cells uptake the apoptotic material such as nucleic acids and present them to naïve CD4+ T-cells that in turn could activate B-cells and promote Ab formation (Crow 2014). A subset of B-cells also expressing TLRs are activated following uptake of autoantigens (Pan et al. 2020). These cells would then migrate to the lymph nodes and through interaction with follicular helper T-cells (Tfh) form follicular germinal centers. The Tfh cells promote the proliferation and differentiation of autoreactive B-cell and increase antibody class-switching (Fig. 6) (Pan et al. 2020). Autoantibodies and antigens form immune complexes that could reach almost all organs through the bloodstream. The precipitation of Ag–Ab complexes results in inflammation and tissue destruction, which creates a vicious cycle by releasing more self-antigens. Though B-cells and autoantibodies play a major role in the pathogenesis of SLE, ACLE, and SCLE, they don't seem to have an essential role in the perpetuation of DLE (Hofmann et al. 2013a; Vital et al. 2015).

The stressed keratinocytes and other APCs can express lipid-based antigens such as apoptosis-derived oxidized lipid derivatives through special antigen-presenting molecules known as CD1d (non-classical MHC I). The CD1d/lipid antigen complex is recognized by TCRs in a subset of T-cells known as invariant natural killer T-cells (iNKTs). These cells can produce both immune-regulatory (IL-10) and immune-stimulatory cytokines (IFNγ, IL-17) (Chuang et al. 2012; Hofmann et al. 2013b; Kaer and Wu 2018). The iNKT cells have a dual effect on lupus. In CLE, the number of iNKT cells is increased and they are thought to contribute to the promotion of adaptive responses. While in SLE, iNKT cells are reduced and there is a negative correlation between the number and function of these cells and the autoantibodies titers that suggest a suppressive effect on autoreactive B-cells (Chuang et al. 2012; Hofmann et al. 2013b; Shen et al. 2015).

Defects in central and peripheral tolerance also contribute to the pathogenesis of lupus by allowing the autoreactive T- and B-cell to remain in the circulation (Achtman and Werth 2015; Cappione et al. 2005).

Genetic inheritance can affect many aspects of the adaptive immune response. Genetic polymorphisms could affect the threshold of BCR and TCR signaling, the tolerance regulation in the lymph nodes, thymus, and peripheral blood, the rate of Ig production and its class switching, and

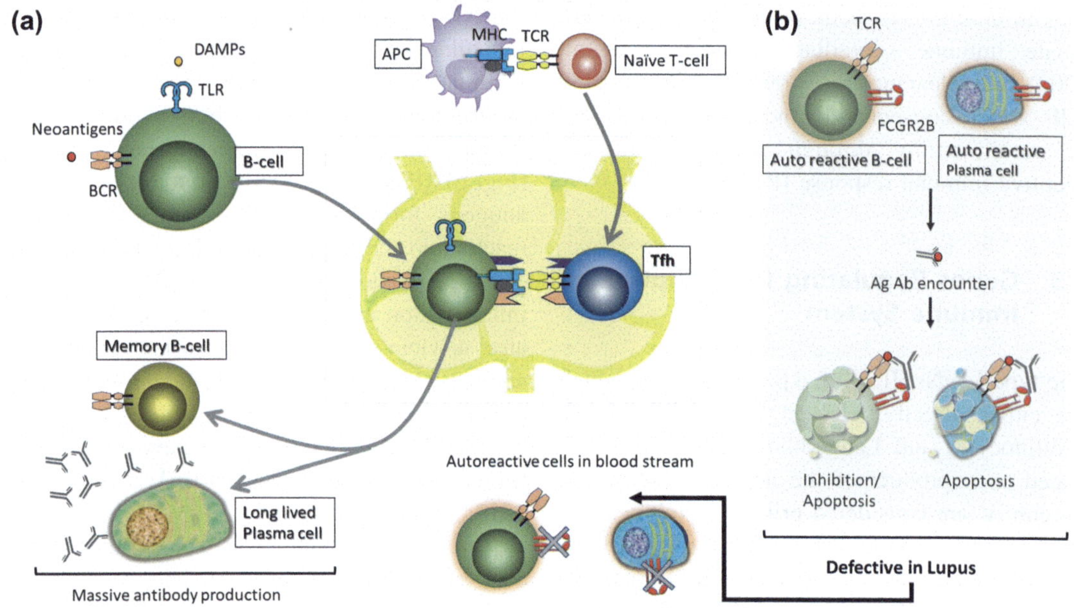

Fig. 6 Autoreactive B-cells play a major role in the pathogenesis of lupus. **a** A subset of B-cells that transit through the lymph nodes following the uptake of autoantigens can interact with follicular helper T-cells (Tfh) in the lymph node germinal centers. The output of this interaction is the formation of autoreactive memory B-cells and long-lasting plasma cells that can maintain a stronger immune response. **b** The expression of the inhibitory Fc receptor γ IIB which is a restrictive mechanism that keeps the production and function of autoreactive B-cells in check in the normal conditions is altered in lupus

the clearance of Ag–Ab complex (Jenks and Sanz 2009; Moulton and Tsokos 2011).

4.3.1 Humoral Immunity and B-cells

The *Fcγ receptor* genes

The Fcγ receptor family consists of several members (FcγRI, FcγRIIA, FcγRIIB, FcγRIIIA, FcγRIIIB, and FcγRIV) with different affinities toward the Fc segment of IgG (Nimmerjahn and Ravetch 2008). Expect for the FcγRIIB subtype that carries inhibitory intracellular motifs, the other members of the FcγR family relay an activating signal upon encountering IgG-Ag complexes. Fcγ receptors are expressed on most cells in the hematopoietic system and are involved in numerous immunological functions (Nimmerjahn and Ravetch 2006). The macrophages, neutrophils, and NK-cells mainly express activating Fcγ receptors that promote phagocytosis of IgG-opsonized pathogens, antibody-dependent cell-mediated cytotoxicity (ADCC), complement-mediated lysis, and cytokine secretion. Dendritic cells uptake IgG-Ag complexes with their Fcγ receptors and present their Ag peptides via MHC molecules (Roon 2007). B-cells and plasma-cell solely express the FcγRIIB. The inhibitory effects of this receptor promote apoptosis in plasma cells and modulate the activating signals transmitted by B-cell receptors (BCR) (Fig. 6) (Roon 2007). Thus a delicate immune balance is created by the simultaneous function of these activating and inhibitory receptors. Aberrant expression or genetic variations that alter the affinity of each of these receptors could easily unhinge this balance and provoke autoimmunity (Activating and inhibitory FcγRs in autoimmune disorders 2006). Multiple alleles of genes encoding FcγR family members have been linked to SLE.

Several GWASs in multiple ethnic groups have shown an association between a G-to-A variant in the *FCGR2A* gene (rs1801274) encoding the activating FcγRIIA and SLE susceptibility (Duits et al. 1995; Salmon et al. 1996;

Song et al. 1998). This was also confirmed by a meta-analysis that demonstrated a 1.3-fold increased risk for SLE in individuals carrying this risk allele (Karassa et al. 2002). This risk allele not only confers susceptibility to SLE but is also associated with SLE severity and the presence of renal involvement (Haseley et al. 1997). The G-to-A substitution results in the replacement of histidine by arginine at position 131 that reduces the affinity of the receptor towards IgG2 and decreases the pathogen clearance ability of phagocytes (Salmon et al. 1992).

Two SNPs on the *FCGR2B* gene encoding the inhibitory FcγRIIB have been linked to SLE susceptibility, rs1050501 in the Asian population and rs3219018 in the Caucasians (Blank et al. 2005; Kono et al. 2005; Li et al. 2009).

The T-to-C transition at nucleotide 775 in the 4th exon of the *FCGR2B* gene (rs1050501) results in the replacement of threonine by isoleucine at position 187 in the transmembrane domain of the receptor (Kyogoku et al. 2002; Li et al. 2003). The risk allele promotes autoimmunity by altering the receptor signaling and reducing the inhibitory strain on BCRs (Kono et al. 2005).

The G-to-C switch at position –343 in the promoter region of the *FCGR2B* gene (rs3219018) is associated with a reduced transcription rate of the receptor and thus could result in unbalanced activation of B-cells (Blank et al. 2005). A haplotype containing this SNP, − 386 C-120A, also confers susceptibility to SLE (Su et al. 2004b). Surprisingly, this haplotype is associated with an increased expression of the *FCGR2B* gene and higher activity of its corresponding protein. It has been suggested that this gain-of-function polymorphism could increase the risk of autoimmunity by altering the negative selection of autoreactive B-cells (Su et al. 2004a).

The T/G rs396991 SNP on the gene encoding the FcγRIIIA is also linked to SLE susceptibility (Li et al. 2009). The G allele corresponds to the placement of phenylalanine instead of valine at position 159 in the extracellular domain of the receptor. This amino acid substitution would decrease receptor affinity and thus reduce the clearance of the immune complexes by FcγRIIIA on scavenger cells. The accumulation of circulating immune complexes can cause SLE (Koene et al. 1997; Wu et al. 1997).

FcγRIIIB has two relatively common polymorphic forms, NA1 and NA2. Five nucleotides within exon 3 differ between the two variants (Salmon et al. 1992). Lower affinity toward IgG subtypes has been attributed to the NA2 allele that also confers risk for lupus in the Japanese population (Hatta et al. 1999; Li et al. 2009; Siriboonrit et al. 2003). The copy number variations (CNV) in the *FCGR3B* gene have also been linked to SLE in the Caucasian population (Morris et al. 2010; Willcocks et al. 2008). The *FCGR3B* copy number is directly proportional to gene expression and protein function. Thus, the lower *FcγRIIIb* CNV increases the risk of SLE by impairing immune complex clearance (Willcocks et al. 2008).

The *MSH5* gene

The *MutS protein homolog-5* (*MSH5*) is an MHC class III gene that is linked to susceptibility to SLE and CLE in three GWASs (Fernando et al. 2012; Kunz et al. 2015; Sánchez et al. 2011). The MSH5 protein binds with MSH4 and forms a heterodimer that acts as a scaffold for DNA recombination machinery and recognizes and resolves the Holliday junctions between the homologous DNA strands throughout meiosis (Snowden et al. 2004). Moreover, this complex is also involved in the immunoglobulin class-switch DNA recombination (CSR) in B-cells (Sekine et al. 2007). Genetic variations in *MSH5* that impair its binding to MSH4 protein are known to be associated with IgA deficiency (IgAD), common variable immune deficiency (CVID), and premature ovarian failure (Guo et al. 2017; Sekine et al. 2007). There is a significant association between these primary immunodeficiency syndromes and SLE (Grammatikos and Tsokos 2012). Though the precise mechanism involved is not fully understood it has been suggested that the insufficient clearance of pathogens may provoke autoimmunity through molecular mimicry (Guo et al. 2017).

The *IkZF1* gene

The rs2366293 and rs4917014 on the *IkZF1* gene are associated with susceptibility to SLE in the Chinese and Caucasian populations, respectively (Bentham et al. 2015; He et al. 2010). The risk allele of the rs2366293 SNP is associated with decreased gene expression. Individuals with SLE also demonstrated lower expression of IkZF1 mRNA (Honma et al. 1999; Hu et al. 2011). The *IkZF1* gene encodes a transcription factor known as the Ikaros, which belongs to the Ikaros zinc finger (IkZF) transcription factor family. Other members of this family include Helios (encoded by *IkZF2*), Aiolos (encoded by *IkZF3*), Eos (encoded by *IkZF4*), and Pegasus (encoded by *IkZF5*) (Kelley et al. 1998; Morgan et al. 1997; Perdomo et al. 2000). The IkZF family is involved in T-cell subset differentiation through interacting with cytokine-STAT pathways (Powell et al. 2019). The IkZF1 transcription factor has positive effects on the differentiation of Th2, Th17, Treg and a negative effect on the differentiation of Th1 (Powell et al. 2019). Ikaros is also involved in restraining a subset of B-cells linked to autoimmunity known as B1-cells (Macias-Garcia et al. 2016). This cell line is an element of the innate immune response since it spontaneously produces polyreactive IgM antibodies that can also bind to auto-antigens (Duan and Morel 2006). Ikaros mediates the class switching of the IgG2a, b, and c through its interaction with IRF5 (Fang et al. 2012; Sellars et al. 2009). The IgG glycosylation pattern which affects its stability and binding affinity is also regulated by the *IkZF1* gene (Lauc et al. 2013). The Ikaros controls the expression of *the IkZF3* gene encoding Aiolos (Ghadiri et al. 2007). The Aiolos has an essential role in the differentiation of B-cells and *IkZF3* knocked-out mice develop an autoimmune phenotype resembling SLE with spontaneous formation of autoantibodies (Wang et al. 1998). Thus through multiple hypothetical pathways, alteration in the expression and function of the IkZF1 due to genetic polymorphisms could promote SLE (Hu et al. 2011).

The *ras guanyl-releasing protein 3* (*RASGRP3*)

The rs13385731 and rs12612030 located within the intron of the *RASGRP3* gene confer susceptibility to lupus in the Chinese Han population (He et al. 2010; Singh et al. 2017). The overexpression of *RASGRP3* has been documented in SLE and is associated with disease severity (An et al. 2019). The *RASGRP3* gene is highly expressed in B-cells and is thought to regulate the activation of the Ras/Erk pathway downstream of BCR signaling (Coughlin et al. 2005). The Ras/Erk pathway is involved in the production of antibodies and cytokines such as IL-6 and TNFα (An et al. 2019; Coughlin et al. 2005; Liu et al. 2005). Thus, the overexpression of the *RASGRP3* could promote autoimmunity by increasing the sensitivity of the B-cells towards signals from autoreactive T-cells (Coughlin et al. 2006).

The *B-lymphoid tyrosine kinase* (*BLK*)

The rs13277113 of the *BLK* gene confers susceptibility to SLE in all ethnic groups and the rs2736340 and rs2248932 are associated with SLE in Caucasian and Asian populations (Fan et al. 2011a; Song and Lee 2017).

The rs13277113 is located in the shared promoter of *BLK* and *C8orf13* genes and its risk allele is associated with reduced expression of the former and increased expression of the later gene. The function of the *C8orf13* is unknown (Hom et al. 2008). The *BLK* gene encodes a non-receptor tyrosine kinase that belongs to the Src family and is highly expressed in B-cell lineage (Dymecki et al. 1990). The BLK protein is activated downstream the BCR signaling pathway and is involved in B-cell proliferation, maturation, and function (Samuelson et al. 2012; Texido et al. 2000).

There are several hypotheses regarding the effect of polymorphisms in the *BLK* gene and its role in autoimmunity. A study on rheumatoid arthritis has been able to show an increased sensitivity to BCR signaling in individuals carrying the risk alleles, which was also associated with enhanced interaction between B-cells and T-cells and a higher number of class-switched memory B-cells (Simpfendorfer et al. 2015). The is expected since BLK acts as a negative regulator of BCR signaling and the risk alleles are associated with reduced expression of *BLK* (Delgado-Vega et al. 2012; Zhang et al. 2020).

In a study of rare variants of *BLK*, it was demonstrated that rare mutant alleles that conferred susceptibility to SLE had lower kinase activity that resulted in insufficient suppression of the IRF5 dependent IFNβ production by B-cells following TLR7/8 stimulation (Jiang et al. 2019). Thus individuals carrying the risk alleles had higher expression of interferon-regulated genes (Jiang et al. 2019).

The lower *BLK* expression is associated with an increase in the population of innate B1 B-cells in peripheral blood and higher levels of anti-dsDNA (Wu et al. 2015). The B1 B-cells are linked to autoimmunity and are found in increased numbers in the tubulointerstitial infiltrates of lupus nephritis (Macias-Garcia et al. 2016) (Wu et al. 2015).

The *Lck/Yes-related novel protein tyrosine kinase* (*LYN*)

The *LYN* rs7829816 and rs2667978 polymorphisms confer susceptibility to SLE in European females and the rs6983130 is associated with SLE in both male and female individuals with European ancestry (Harley et al. 2008a; Lu et al. 2009). Patients with SLE demonstrate lower levels of *LYN* expression (Liossis et al. 2001).

The *LYN* gene encodes a member of the Src family that acts as a rheostat for B-cell surface proteins such as BCR, CD40, CD19, CD22, and CD32 (Campbell and Sefton 1992; Melissaropoulos and Liossis 2018; Ren et al. 1994; Xu et al. 2005). Though it acts in a non-binary manner and balances the threshold of signaling pathways, its inhibitory effects on BCR signaling are more prominent than its stimulatory signals (Lowell 2004). This has been confirmed through studies on *LYN* knocked-out mice that demonstrated enhanced BCR signaling that led to hyperproliferative responses (Xu et al. 2012). These *Lyn*$^{-/-}$ mice developed an autoimmune phenotype similar to SLE (Mayeux et al. 2015; Pore et al. 2018). It has been suggested that the increased sensitivity of the B-cells toward activating signals can impair the self/non-self selection process and allow the autoreactive B-cells to mature and induce autoimmunity (Lamagna et al. 2014; Zhang et al. 2020). Another path through which Lyn deficiency could increase the risk of autoimmunity is by impairing the regulation of IRF5-dependent production of type I IFN (Jiang et al. 2019).

The *B-cell scaffold protein with ankyrin repeats* (*BANK1*)

A meta-analysis of multiple studies on different populations has been able to identify rs10516487, rs17266594, and rs3733197 of the *BANK1* gene to confer susceptibility to SLE (Fan et al. 2011b).

The *BANK1* gene encodes a scaffold protein strictly expressed on B-cells. This protein is involved in the mobilization of calcium following B-cell stimulation (Georg et al. 2020).

The *BANK1* risk alleles alter the signaling pathways downstream of BCR, CD40, and TLR receptors. Reduced BCR and TLR signaling can impact the negative selection of autoreactive B-cells and thus promote autoimmunity (Wu et al. 2013, 2016).

The *BANK1* risk alleles cause a decrease in the phosphorylation rate of PLCγ2 and reduce the activity of AKT which in turn increases the expression of FOXO1 transcriptional factor. The FOXO1/AKT balance and the FOXO1 target genes are responsible for Ig class-switching, B-cell homing to lymph nodes, and maturation of memory B-cells (Dengler et al. 2008; Kerdiles et al. 2009; Omori et al. 2006; Yazdani et al. 2017). The increased number of memory B-cells could contribute to the expansion of autoreactive B-cells and cause autoimmunity (Dam et al. 2016).

Other low-frequency *BANK1* alleles associated with SLE can induce autoimmunity through enhanced B-cell production of type I IFN by altering the localization of BANK1 to sequestosomes, which in turn is associated with increased availability of IRF5, an IFN stimulator, in the nucleus (Jiang et al. 2019).

The *positive regulatory domain zinc finger protein-1* (*PRDM1*) and *Ets1*

The *PRDM1* gene encodes a protein known as Blimp-1 that regulates gene expression. Its target genes include *IFNβ*, *myc*, *MHC class II trans-activator*, *Pax-5*, and *CD23b* (Keller and Maniatis 1991; Lin et al. 2002, 1997; Piskurich et al. 2000). The repression of the four later genes is required for the differentiation of B-cells to plasma cells. Thus *PRDM1* is considered a cell fate determinant for B-cells (Györy et al. 2003). Increased plasma cell differentiation has been documented in lupus and patients with SLE have increased levels of Blimp-1 protein that also correlates with disease severity (Jacobi et al. 2003; Luo et al. 2013). Moreover, ectopic expression of the Blimp-1 protein can induce lupus-like autoimmune diseases by enhancing the plasma cell differentiation in premature B-cells (Bönelt et al. 2019). Thus, it is convincible that variations in the *PRDM1* gene could be involved in the pathogenesis of lupus (Jang et al. 2017).

Two SNPs within the *PRDM1* gene are associated with SLE in multiple ethnicities, rs548234 and rs6568431 (located in the intergenic region between *ATG5* and *BRDM1*) (Gateva et al. 2009; Taylor et al. 2011; Zhou et al. 2011).

The *Ets-1* encodes a transcription factor known as p54 that inhibits PRDM1 (John et al. 2008). It negatively regulates the differentiation of B-cells (Garrett-Sinha et al. 2016; Pan et al. 2011). It is also involved in the suppression of follicular Th2 cells by repressing the expression of BCL6, IL-4RA, and CXCR5 (Kim et al. 2018). Ets-1 negatively regulates the differentiation of Th17 cells that are implicated in the pathogenesis of many autoimmune diseases including SLE (Abou Ghanima et al. 2012; Moisan et al. 2007).

The deletion of the Ets-1 gene in B-cells and CD4+ T-cells could induce lupus-like autoimmune diseases in murine models (Kim et al. 2018; Wang et al. 2005a). Moreover, polymorphisms in the *Ets-1* gene that confer susceptibility to SLE are associated with reduced expression of *Ets-1* (Garrett-Sinha et al. 2016; Han et al. 2009a; Sullivan et al. 2000; Yang et al. 2010).

The *AF4/FMR2 family member 1 and 2* (*AFF1* and *AFF2*)

The *AFF1* polymorphisms show a significant association with SLE in Japanese, Chinese, and Iranians (Arabi et al. 2016; Cen et al. 2012; Okada et al. 2012a). Few studies have also documented an association between *AFF3* polymorphisms and SLE (Cen et al. 2012).

The *AFF1* encodes an RNA polymerase II regulator that encourages RNA elongation (Melko et al. 2011). The *AFF1* is expressed in CD4+ and CD19+ peripheral blood cells and deletion of the *AFF1* gene affects the development of both T- and B-cells by reducing the expression of CD4 and CD8 receptors on cells within the thymus and decreasing the number of premature and mature B-cells in the bone marrow (Isnard et al. 2000). Since *AFF1* genetic polymorphisms alter the gene expression levels, their association with autoimmunity seems reasonable.

The *Neutrophil cytosolic factor 2* (*NCF2*):

The *NCF2* gene encodes a subunit of NADPH oxidase, which is one of the main cellular systems for producing reactive oxygen species (ROS). Point mutations and genetic variations associated with reduced NADPH activity confer susceptibility to SLE (Armstrong et al. 2015; Jacob et al. 2012). The exact mechanism in which reduced NADPH activity could promote autoimmunity is not clear. However, it has been hypothesized that reduced ROS-mediated killing of the internalized microbes would allow the promotion of other compensatory cellular defense mechanisms through PRRs such as TLRs (Cachat et al. 2015; Holmdahl et al. 2016). This would lead to increased production of cytokines and IFNs that could promote autoimmunity by shifting the balance from innate responses to adaptive immune responses (Jacob et al. 2017). Increased expression of IFN-related genes has been documented in carriers of the *NCF2* risk allele (Jacob et al. 2017). Furthermore, ROS derivatives are involved in cell-to-cell signaling that can influence antigen presentation, immune regulation, B-cell differentiation, and antibody production (Jacob et al. 2017; Vené et al. 2010).

The interleukin encoding genes:
Polymorphisms in two interleukin encoding genes, *IL-10* and *IL-21* are associated with SLE susceptibility. Multiple SNPs and a microsatellite repeat polymorphisms in *IL-10* gene have been associated with SLE in different ethnic groups including, the rs3024505, -1082A/G, -3575 T/A, -2763C/A, -819 T/C, -592A/C, and -2849G/A (Gateva et al. 2009; Liu et al. 2013; Rianthavorn et al. 2013; Tian et al. 2014). IL-10 mainly functions as an immune-regulatory cytokine that suppresses T-cells, macrophages, and antigen-presenting cells but has a stimulatory effect on B-cells by promoting their differentiation and antibody production (Llorente et al. 1995). IL-10 plays an active role in the pathogenesis of SLE as demonstrated by high levels of IL-10 in sera of patients suffering from lupus and the amelioration of symptoms following the administration of IL-10 blocking antibodies (Godsell et al. 2016; Llorente et al. 2000; Park et al. 1998; Yao et al. 2016). Thus, polymorphisms that affect *IL-10* gene expression could hypothetically influence the pathogenesis of SLE (Rianthavorn et al. 2013).

The rs907715, rs2221903, and rs2055979 SNPs in the gene encoding IL-21 and rs3093301 SNP of *IL-21 receptor* gene are linked to SLE susceptibility in multiple ethnicities (Lan et al. 2014; Qi et al. 2015; Sawalha et al. 2008; Webb et al. 2009). For some of these SNPs, the risk allele is associated with higher levels of soluble IL-21 (Lan et al. 2014). IL-21 regulates B-cell function. It promotes both immune-regulatory and immune-stimulatory phenotypes in B-cells (Hagn et al. 2009; Mauri and Menon 2015; Sawalha et al. 2008). It is involved in the pathogenesisthe pathogenesis of SLE through promoting the differentiation of autoreactive plasma cells from an unusual subset of memory B-cell (CD11c+ T-bet+ B) (Wang et al. 2018) and down-regulating the T-reg differentiation (Kato and Perl 2018). Multiple studies have sown elevated levels of IL-21 and IL-21 secreting T-cells in sera of patients with SLE (Dolff et al. 2011; Nakou et al. 2013; Terrier et al. 2012) and IL-21 blockade has shown to be effective in reducing the SLE severity (Choi et al. 2017).

Other interleukin encoding genes have also been linked to SLE susceptibility, albeit with lesser evidence. These genes include *IL-1*, *IL-6*, and *IL-19* (Katkam et al. 2017; Lin et al. 2016; Zhu et al. 2021).

4.3.2 Cellular Immunity and T-cells

The CSNK2B gene

Another gene associated with cutaneous lupus is the *CSNK2B* gene. This gene is significantly overexpressed in the blood of individuals with cutaneous lupus and an SNP, rs9267531, located within the intronic region of this gene shows a strong link with cutaneous lupus (Dey-Rao and Sinha 2019; Kunz et al. 2015).

The CSNK2B is a regulatory subunit of the casein kinase II (CKII) that phosphorylates numerous proteins and is involved in many cellular functions such as the progression of the NF-κB and JAK/STAT pathways (Gibson and Benveniste 2018). The kinase activity of the CKII tetramer is attributed to two CK2α and 2α′ subunits that can also function independently. In the CKII tetramer, the CK2β unit confers substrate specificity and acts as a modulator (Gibson and Benveniste 2018). With the wide range of cell-specific functions attributed to the CKII enzyme and its subunits, the description of its precise role in the immune system and the pathogenesis of autoimmune diseases is rather difficult (Gibson and Benveniste 2018). It has been demonstrated that the CK2β is required for the maintenance of the suppressive effects of regulatory T-cells on Th2 cells (Ulges et al. 2015). On contrary, CK2β also promotes inflammation through unbalancing the Th17/ regulatory T-cell ratio (Ulges et al. 2015). The CK2α overexpression, independent of CK2β, is involved in the progression of lupus glomerulonephritis in rat models. The appliance of CK2α inhibitors reduces inflammation in this animal model (Yamada et al. 2005). The role of CK2β in the pathogenesis of CLE has not been investigated independently.

The *protein phosphatase non-receptor type 22* (*PTPN22*)

The *PTPN22* polymorphisms are one of the most prominent non-HLA genetic risk factors of SLE and multiple other autoimmune diseases (Fousteri et al. 2013). The association between the rs2476601 (R620W) SNP and SLE are more prominent in familial cases and those with European ancestry (Cui et al. 2013; Gateva et al. 2009; Harley et al. 2008a; Moser et al. 2009). Aside from this gain-of-function mutation (620 W), another loss-of-function variant of the *PTPN22* gene, the R263Q, has been described to have protective effects against SLE (Orru et al. 2009).

The *PTPN22* gene encodes a tyrosine phosphatase mainly expressed by immune cells which regulate signaling pathways downstream TCR, BCR, and TLRs. The PTPN22 enhances TLR signaling and thus promotes IFN production in innate immune cells. It inhibits the activation of NF-κB and MAPK downstream intracellular PRRs in monocytes and macrophages. PTPN22 has negative effects on TCR signaling by interfering with the functions of the Src family of kinases (Fousteri et al. 2013). The risk allele of the *PTPN22* gene, 620 W, increases the kinase activity of the protein but rather than suppressing the immune response, its overall effect on the immune system is stimulatory (Fousteri et al. 2013). It has been hypothesized that this might be attributed to the altered negative selection of autoreactive T-cells in the thymus due to ineffective TCR signaling or reduced efficacy of T-regs in suppressing effector T-cells (Mustelin et al. 2019; Vang et al. 2013, 2007). The effects of the *PTPN22* risk allele on B-cells are not fully understood but an increase in the number of CD27+ IgM− IgD+ autoreactive memory B-cells has been documented in carriers of the risk allele (Habib et al. 2012).

The *tumor necrosis factor superfamily member 4* (*TNFSF4*)

The TNFSF4 gene encodes a co-stimulatory surface molecule also known as OX40L or CD252 that is usually expressed by antigen-presenting cells. This ligand engages with TNFSFR4 (OX40, CD154) on activated CD4+/CD8+ T-cells and promotes the development of memory T-cells, and suppresses IL-10-producing regulatory cells (Cortini et al. 2017; Farres et al. 2011; Soroosh et al. 2006). The OX40L is also expressed on B-cells and is stimulated by CD+ 4 OX40+ T-cells. This would lead to an increase in the proliferation of B-cell and the production of immunoglobulins (Stüber and Strober 1996). The rs2205960 SNP upstream *TNFSF4* gene is linked to SLE susceptibility in multiple ethnicities (Graham et al. 2008b; Gupta et al. 2018). The risk allele and haplotype are associated with a higher gene transpiration rate that could escalate the T-cell B-cell interaction and thus promote autoimmunity (Graham et al. 2008b).

Immunoglobulin-like transcript 3 (ILT3)

ILT3 and ILT4 are among the main tolerogenic receptors expressed on antigen-presenting cells (APC). These immunosuppressive surface receptors are capable of inducing tyrosine phosphorylation and thus inhibiting the downstream signaling pathways that lead to the secretion of proinflammatory cytokines, chemokines, and co-stimulatory molecules from APCs (Suciu-Foca and Cortesini 2007; Vlad et al. 2010). Through cell-to-cell signaling, ILTs promote APC-induced differentiation of CD4+ T-regs and CD8+ suppressor T-cells (Suciu-Foca and Cortesini 2007; Vlad et al. 2010). The soluble form of ILT3 linked to mutated IgG1 Fc (ILT3-Fc) is also capable of promoting an antigen-specific regulatory phenotype in T-cells through targeting miRNAs (Vlad and Suciu-Foca 2012). ILT3 and ILT4 expression on APCs is promoted in response to IL-10, cyclooxygenase (COX) inhibitors, vitamin-D analogs, rapamycin, and HLA-G (Ristich et al. 2005; Rosborough et al. 2014; Vlad et al. 2010). IFNα and β also stimulate the expression of ILT3 on dendritic cells creating a negative feedback pathway that regulates type I IFN production. Antigen-specific CD8+ suppressor T-cells also promote ILT3/4 expression on APCs and thus a positive feedback loop is created that perpetuates tolerance (Vlad et al. 2010).

Two loss-of-function polymorphisms of *ILT3*, rs11540761, and rs1048801, were found to be associated with SLE susceptibility in a case-control study (Jensen et al. 2012). These polymorphisms were associated with increased levels of IFN and TNFα (Jensen et al. 2012). The role of ILTs in tthe pathogenesis of SLE was further clarified by a study demonstrating a reduced number of ILT4 expressing dendritic cells in patients with SLE compared to normal individuals (Guerra-de Blas et al. 2016).

The *Cytotoxic T-lymphocyte antigen-4* (*CTLA4*) gene

The CTLA4 (CD152) is an immune checkpoint receptor that binds to B7-1 (CD80)/B7-2 (CD86) on APCs and acts as a rheostat for controlling the unleashed activity of T-cells following TCR-MHC interaction (Jago et al. 2004). It is homologous to CD28 in its binding partners but rather than co-stimulation, it relays a negative signal that inhibits IL-2 production and cell-cycle progression (Krummel and Allison 1996; Oosterwegel et al. 1999). CTLA4 is also constitutively expressed by regulatory T-cells and contributes to their immunosuppressive activity (Takahashi et al. 2000).

Studies on CLTA4 null mice have been able to demonstrate its importance in autoimmunity (Chambers et al. 1997; Krummel and Allison 1996; Tivol et al. 1995). Selective deletion/inactivation of CTLA4 in regulatory T-cells results in the proliferation of autoreactive naïve T-cells in lymphoid tissue. Deletion/inactivation of CLTA4 in conventional T-cells results in infiltration and destruction of non-lymphoid tissue by autoreactive T-cells (Jain et al. 2010).

Genetic polymorphisms of the *CTLA4* gene are associated with multiple autoimmune diseases including SLE. The *CTLA4* rs231775 has been linked to SLE susceptibility in Asian populations (Iranian, Indian, and Japanese) (Barreto et al. 2004; Kailashiya et al. 2019; Lee et al. 2005). A haplotype of CTLA4 has also been linked to DLE (Järvinen et al. 2010). The most common allele to confers susceptibility to SLE causes an amino acid substitution in the leader sequence of CTLA4 protein and is thus associated with functional changes (Kailashiya et al. 2019; Lee et al. 2005).

Altered functions of CTLA4 have been documented in T-cells of SLE patients. These cells demonstrate reduced expression and function of CTLA4 upon CD28/CD3 co-stimulation (Jury et al. 2010). Moreover, Abatacept, a CTLA4–IgGFc1 fusion protein, has been successfully used in the treatment of SLE (Danion et al. 2016).

The *programmed cell death 1* (PDCD1) gene

The *PDCD1* gene encodes another inhibitory immune checkpoint receptor belonging to the B7/CD28 family also known as PD1 or CD279. It is expressed by activated T-cells and B-cells upon persistent antigen stimulation, NKT-cells, monocytes, and double-negative (CD4-CD8-) immature T-cells in the thymus (Agata et al. 1996; Keir et al. 2007a; Nishimura et al. 1996). Its ligands, PD1-L1, and PD1-L2 are constitutively expressed by APCs, macrophages, mast cells, B-cells, T-cells (mostly regulatory T-cells), and non-hematopoietic cells such as endothelial cells (Keir et al. 2007a). The binding of the PD1 and its ligands in the setting of persistent low TCR signaling inhibits T-cells activation and promotes apoptosis. PD1 enforces a greater inhibitory effect on T-cells than CTLA4 and also reduces the survival of T-cells by reducing the expression of Bcl-xL (Parry et al. 2005). In the thymus, the expression of PD1 ligands by the thymic cells contributes to both positive selection of reactive CD4+/CD8+ T-cells and negative selection of autoreactive T-cells (Blank et al. 2003; Keir et al. 2007b). PD1 is also involved in maintaining peripheral tolerance. PD1 is upregulated on T-cells following TCR-MHC interaction and limits effector T-cell proliferation and cytokine production (Francisco et al. 2010). In the presence of TGFβ, the PD1 stimulation deviates the path of naïve peripheral T-cells from becoming effector T-cells into adaptive T-regs (Francisco et al. 2010). The expression of PD1 ligands by non-hematopoietic cells such as endothelial cells helps in upholding immune privilege by inducing apoptosis in auto-reactive

T-cells that have been able to escape other tolerance mechanisms (Keir et al. 2006; Rodig et al. 2003).

The profound role of PD1 in maintaining self-tolerance has made it an interesting subject to study in autoimmune diseases. It has been shown that PD-1 knocked-out mice develop a lupus-like disease with glomerulonephritis and high levels of autoantibodies (Nishimura et al. 1999; Wang et al. 2005b). However, there is a lot of discrepancy in the studies evaluating the PD1 expression in SLE (Curran et al. 2019).

The *PDCD1* gene was among the first genes to be linked to SLE by positional cloning approaches and linkage studies (Magnusson et al. 2000). The results of case-control studies on *PDCD1* SNPs, however, were diverse (Gao et al. 2017). An intron 3 SNP, PD1.3, was found by multiple studies to confer risk for SLE in Mexicans and Caucasians (Gao et al. 2017; Lee et al. 2009; Liu et al. 2009). The PD1.3A allele is associated with alterations in the transcription factor binding site and thus might result in lower expression of PD1 (Suarez-Gestal et al. 2008). An SNP in the fifth intron, PD1.5, has been linked to SLE susceptibility in Europeans (Lee et al. 2009). A recent meta-analysis has been able to show the protective effect of the A allele of PD1.6 against SLE development that was not detected in any of the previous studies (Francisco et al. 2010).

The *CD44* gene

The CD44 is a transmembrane glycoprotein with multiple isoforms arising from alternative splicing of its encoding gene and glycosylation with different molecules (Goldstein and Butcher 1990). CD44 is capable of interacting with multiple ligands such as hyaluronan, collagen, and matrix metalloproteinases (MPPs). The engagement of CD44 on the surface of immune cells with its ligands activates a multitude of downstream signaling pathways that result in cell migration, adhesion, proliferation, production of cytokines, and maturation of dendritic cells (Jordan et al. 2015; Rafi et al. 1997; Siegelman et al. 1999; Termeer et al. 2002).

CD44 plays a pivotal role in the pathogenesis of SLE as apparent from studies demonstrating amelioration of the lupus nephritis following inhibition of CD44 in murine models (Sela et al. 2005; Weber 2004). Some isoforms of CD44 are increased on T-cells of individuals with SLE and their presence is associated with disease severity (Crispín et al. 2010; Estess et al. 1998). Conversely, in patients with SLE, the expression of CD44 on monocytes and macrophages is reduced resulting in the accumulation of apoptotic cells (Cairns et al. 2001). Thus it seems that CD44 could contribute to autoimmunity following diverse pathways through distinct isoforms on different cells (Yung and Chan 2012).

Two SNPs near the *CD44* gene, rs2732552, and rs387619, are related to SLE susceptibility in multiple ethnicities but their effect on the expression of CD44 remains to be elucidated (Lessard et al. 2011).

4.4 Genes Involved in the Regulation of Neutrophils and Monocytes

The *Intercellular adhesion molecule-1* (*ICAM-1*)

ICAM-1 (also known as CD54) is a cell-to-cell adhesion glycoprotein expressed by a variety of cells including endothelial and immune cells. It binds to integrins including CD11a/CD18 also known as lymphocyte-function associated antigens-1 (LFA-1), CD11b/CD18, fibrinogen, and bacterial and viral components (Stolpe and Saag 1996). The extracellular part of ICAM-1 with its ligand-binding domains is cleaved to soluble ICAM-1 (s-ICAM-1), which is detectable in plasma. The s-ICAM-1 levels are determined by the rate of gene expression and proteolysis (Stolpe and Saag 1996). ICAM-1 is involved in immune responses. Its expression on endothelial cells facilitates the transmigration of the activated immune cell. It enhances antigen presentation by attracting the MHC molecules to the contact pole of the cell surface. ICAM-1 also acts as a co-stimulatory molecule for T-cell activation (Lebedeva et al. 2005).

High levels of s-ICAM-1 have been detected in patients with SLE (Guo Liu et al. 2020). Multiple polymorphisms located within the *ICAM* gene complex are associated with SLE susceptibility. However, none of them affect transcription levels and thus their exact role in the pathogenesis of SLE remains to be elucidated (Kim et al. 2012; Ruiz-Larrañaga et al. 2016).

The *Integrin Subunit Alpha M* (*ITGAM*)
The ITGAM (CD11b) is a protein subunit of the integrin family of transmembrane obligatory heterodimers. It partners with integrin β2 (CD18) to form αMβ2 (CD11b/CD18) integrin also known as the complement receptor-3 (CR3) or macrophage-1 antigen (Mac-1) (Solovjov et al. 2005). Integrins facilitate cell-to-cell and cell-to-matrix adhesion and are involved in signal transduction that regulates the cell cycle, migration, and spreading (Giancotti and Ruoslahti 1999; Hynes 2002). The αMβ2 is expressed on the surface of immune cells and binds to ICAM-1, inactive complement component 3 (iC3b), fibrinogen, and Factor X (Solovjov et al. 2005). It possesses both immune-regulatory and immune-stimulatory roles. It promotes the effector function of some receptors such as CD14, dectin, and FCγR. The enhances leukocyte recruitment, phagocytosis, degranulation, and ROS production (Rosetti and Mayadas 2016). It has inhibitory effects on BCR, TLRs, FCγRIIA, IFNα receptors, and induces a tolerogenic response in dendritic cells (Rosetti and Mayadas 2016). The dual function of CD11b is also reflected in murine studies demonstrating both exacerbation and amelioration of autoimmune inflammation following the deletion/inhibition of CD11b (Han et al. 2010; Kevil et al. 2004; Rosetti et al. 2012; Tang et al. 1997).

Several SNPs in the *ITGAM* gene have been shown to confer susceptibility to SLE in GWASs and meta-analyses (Han et al. 2009b; Hom et al. 2008). The risk allele of rs1143678 and rs1143683 are associated with a reduced capacity of CD18 to bind complement and FcγR on neutrophils and thus reduce the phagocytic capacity of neutrophils and clearance of apoptotic debris (Zhou et al. 2013). They are also associated with reduced inhibitory effects on BCR signaling and thus could promote B-cell-mediated inflammation (Chung et al. 2011; Ding et al. 2013; Khan et al. 2018). The effects of the risk allele of rs1143679 on ligand binding are not well explained but it has been suggested that it may reduce the binding capacity to ligands in the presence of the sheering force of blood flow and thus result in weaker signal transduction (Rosetti and Mayadas 2016).

4.5 Complement and Immune Complex Clearance Genes

The complement system is involved in the maintenance of self-tolerance by rapidly clearing autoantibody-containing immune complexes and apoptotic cells via opsonization. Complements, precisely C1q promote the phagocytosis of NETs, which is mainly composed of DNA material. SLE is associated with overactive NETosis and thus insufficient clearance of NET material could easily lead to the accumulation of NET products (Salemme et al. 2019). NETs could exacerbate the innate immune response and IFN production by entangling TLRs (Farrera and Fadeel 2013; Lande et al. 2011). Much like apoptotic cells, prolonged exposure of the immune system to nucleic acids of NET structures, as a source of self-antigens, could provoke autoimmunity (Hakkim et al. 2010). Complements also interact with B- and T-cells (Leffler et al. 2014). C4 may be involved in the negative selection of autoreactive B-cells (Chatterjee et al. 2013). Cleaved components of C3 (C3d) can attach to T-cells and alter the Ca^{++} influx in a way that promotes the release of cytokines. The number of C3d+ T-cells is higher in patients with SLE (Borschukova et al. 2012). The complement receptor type-1 is expressed on erythrocytes, lymphocytes (both B- and T-cells), macrophages, and eosinophils (Khera and Das 2009). It binds to C3b, C4b, and Mannose-binding-lectin (MBL) and thus acts as a regulator for classic, alternative, and lectin pathways (Khera and Das 2009). The expression of CR1 on erythrocytes allows them to act as scavenger cells and uptake C3b/C4b bound immune complexes from the bloodstream (Yoshida et al. 1986). When expressed on macrophages, it acts in synergism with FCγRs and enhances phagocytosis of Ig/complement-opsonized particles (Ehlenberger and Nussenzweig 1977). It also regulates B- and T-cell responses (Erdei et al. 2003; Rødgaard et al. 1995). Complement Factor H (FH) is involved in the protection of self-cells from accidental complement activation by assuming an active conformation when bonded to surfaces of self-cells. The active form of FH accelerates the decay of C3-convertase and promotes the Factor I mediated C3b cleavage (Herbert et al. 2015). FH is also involved in balancing the immune activation upon clearance of apoptotic debris. It facilitates phagocytosis while simultaneously inhibiting cytokine release (Leffler et al. 2010; Mihlan et al. 2009). Both dysfunction of FH and lower levels of FH have been reported in patients with SLE and lupus nephritis (Wang et al. 2012a, 2016). Moreover, homozygous loss-of-function mutations in the genes encoding complement components cause monogenic SLE.

More than 90% of the individuals homozygous for non-functional alleles of the C1Q gene (Causing C1q deficiency or C1q functional defects) eventually develop SLE (Manderson et al. 2004). The heterozygous individuals don't seem to be affected (Manderson et al. 2004) but an SNP associated with reduced C1q levels was found to confer susceptibility to SCLE (Racila et al. 2003).

C1r and C1s deficiencies are very rare but are also associated with features of lupus in over 60% of the cases (Arason et al. 2010; Traustadottir et al. 2002). The genes encoding the C1s and C1r proteins are in close linkage and most individuals with C1r deficiency also have lower levels of C1s (Lipsker and Hauptmann 2010; Loos and Heinz 1986). At least two individuals with isolated C1s deficiency have been described to date both of which developed a lupus-like disease at a very young age (Dragon-Durey et al. 2001; Inoue et al. 1998).

C4 is encoded by two separate genes, *C4A* and *C4B*, closely located on a tandem within the MHCIII region. More than 70% of individuals homozygous for non–functional alleles on the C4A gene (but not C4B) develop lupus (Moser et al. 2009; Traustadottir et al. 2002).

Only 10-30% of individuals with homozygous *C2* deficiencies develop SLE (Macedo and Isaac 2016). *C2* heterozygous individuals do not develop lupus and account for up to 2% of the normal Caucasian population (Moser et al. 2009; Pickering et al. 2000; Sullivan et al. 1994).

Polymorphisms in the genes encoding mannose-binding lectin (MBL) are also associated with SLE. SNPs that are associated with increased expression of MBL have a protective effect against developing SLE and those associated with lower levels of MBL confer susceptibility to lupus (Davies et al. 1997; Garred et al. 1999; Ip et al. 1998).

C3 deficiency is very rare only described in about 27 patients 6 of which developed lupus (Lipsker and Hauptmann 2010).

Though *CR1* loss-of-function mutations have not been described to date, polymorphisms resulting in structural modifications have been linked to SLE (Nath et al. 2005). The functional significance of these structural changes is not known (Nath et al. 2005).

Polymorphisms in genes encoding FH and genes encoding factor H-related proteins (FHR 1-5) are associated with SLE susceptibility. The risk alleles were shown to have either reduced binding affinity or reduced gene expression, which would result in altered apoptosis clearance (Tan et al. 2017; Wang et al. 2016; Zhao et al. 2011b).

The effects of complements on SLE development have been confirmed through animal studies. Deletion/inactivation of *C4*, *C1q*, and *FH* in murine models lead to the development of auto-antibodies and in some cases glomerulonephritis (Bao et al. 2011; Botto et al. 1998; Manderson et al. 2004; Paul et al. 2002). Moreover, transfusion of plasma in SLE patients suffering from C1q deficiency ameliorates the symptoms (Mehta et al. 2010).

4.6 Genes with Miscellaneous Functions

Three SNPs in the *MUC21* gene, rs114090659, rs118044183, and rs3094084, have been linked to SLE and cutaneous lupus by three separate GWASs (Bentham et al. 2015; Kunz et al. 2015; Lessard et al. 2016). This gene encodes the protein part of a membrane-bound glycoprotein belonging to the mucin family (Itoh et al. 2008). It is mainly expressed in the lungs, thymus, gastrointestinal tract, and testis (Joshi et al. 2015). Though transmembrane mucins can relay pro-and anti-inflammatory signals by their cytoplasmic tails, the precise role of MUC21 in the pathogenesis of lupus remains unknown (Bose and Mukherjee 2020).

The *psoriasis susceptibility 1 candidate 1* (*PSORS1C1*) gene, a major psoriasis susceptibility gene has also been linked to both cutaneous and systemic lupus (Ciccacci et al. 2014; Kunz et al. 2015). This gene is located near the MHC region of 6p21.3 and has an overlap with *corneodesmosin* (*CDSN*) and *psoriasis susceptibility 1 candidate 2* (*PSORS1C2*) genes (Holm et al. 2003). Though the precise function of this gene is not known, it has been shown that downregulation of *PSORS1C1* expression would lead to lower levels of IL-17 and IL-1β (Sun et al. 2013).

The *FLOT1* gene encodes Flotillin-1, a caveolae-associated protein that is involved in vesicular trafficking, cell-to-cell adhesion, signal transduction, and cell migration by modulating the cell cytoskeleton (Bickel et al. 1997; Bodin et al. 2014; Kwiatkowska et al. 2020). Flotillin-1 is involved in TCR recycling after endocytosis and arranging the membrane pouch that contains TCR and its co-stimulatory transmembrane receptors at immunological synapses (Redpath et al. 2019; Slaughter et al. 2003). It is also involved in forming adherens junctions by providing a scaffold that allows for multiple cadherin molecules to form a collection (Bodin et al. 2014). Flotillin-1 is required for neutrophil chemotaxis and uropod formation in polarized T-cells that allow for T-cell migration (Giri et al. 2007; Ludwig et al. 2010). However, *FLOT1* deletion on CD8 + T-cells has minor effects on the overall T-cell functions and thus its contribution to autoimmunity remains to be elucidated (Ficht et al. 2019).

Another SLE-related gene is the *MAS1L* which encodes a proto-oncogene-like receptor with unknown functions (Kunz et al. 2015; Martínez-Bueno and Alarcón-Riquelme 2019).

Polymorphisms in the *vitamin D receptor* (*VDR*) gene have been linked to lupus by multiple case-control studies but meta-analysis has failed to confirm these findings (Bae and Lee 2018; Azevêdo et al. 2013; Lee et al. 2011; Monticielo et al. 2012). The vitamin D receptor acts as a ligand-induced transcription factor with multiple effects in different parts of the immune system (Chun et al. 2014). It promotes T-regs and Th2 responses while inhibiting Th1 and Th17 differentiation and cytokine production (Chun et al. 2014). Thus, alteration in VDR signaling hypothetically could exacerbate autoimmunity (Chun et al. 2014). However, the effects of *VDR* risk alleles on the transcriptional functions of this receptor remain unclear (Bizzaro et al. 2017).

The *serine/threonine kinase 17a* (*STK17a*) gene product is a DNA repair protein that promotes apoptosis. It has been linked to SLE in a single case-control study but its functional relevance is unknown (Silva Fonseca et al. 2013).

The *lymphocyte antigen 9* (*LY9*) gene has been linked to SLE susceptibility in multiple case-control studies (Graham et al. 2008a; Ruiz-Larrañaga et al. 2016). LY9 belongs to the signaling lymphocyte activation molecule family (SLAMF) and it is designated as SLAMF3 (CD229) (Schwartzberg et al. 2009). Most members of SLAMF are self-ligand receptors expressed on the surface of innate and adaptive immune cells that facilitate the adhesion and communication between cells (Veillette 2010). The functions of SLAMF are mediated through a family of intracytoplasmic adapter proteins known as SLAM-associated proteins (SAPs) (Schwartzberg et al. 2009). In the presence of SAP, SLAMF receptors relay positive signals (Veillette 2010). In the absence of SAP, the signals from SLAMFs are mainly inhibitory

(Veillette 2010). This occurs physiologically in B-cells, mast cells, and neutrophils that have a very low expression of SAP (Veillette 2010). Thus considering the functions of these proteins, it is not surprising that alterations in their structure and function could invoke autoimmunity (Kumar et al. 2006; Wandstrat et al. 2004). As such, it has been demonstrated that both *LY9* and *SLAMF4* (*2B4*) deletion are associated with loss of tolerance to self-DNA and autoimmunity in mice models (Brown et al. 2011; Salort et al. 2013). The precise scenario in which LY9 deficiency contributes to the formation of autoantibodies is unclear but LY9 increases IFNγ production by CD4+ T-cells and directs isotype switching toward more potent IgG2 (Salort et al. 2013).

5 Epigenetic Influences

Changes in epigenetic modifications can impact the expression and function of genes involved in SLE pathogenesis. These modifications include DNA methylation, histone acetylation, histone ubiquitination, and histone phosphorylation. Several factors such as ultraviolet light, pharmaceutical agents, aging, and altered expression of certain microRNAs can change the epigenetic landscape of DNA (Hedrich and Tsokos 2011). Epigenetic modifications of type 1 IFN genes leading to immune dysregulation have been documented in SLE (Absher et al. 2013; Ghodke-Puranik and Niewold 2015; Hedrich and Tsokos 2011).

6 Conclusion

SLE is a complex multifactorial autoimmune disease with many environmental triggers. Genetics plays a major role in the pathogenesis of SLE and cutaneous lupus. Multiple GWAS and case–control studies have been able to demonstrate the effects of common alleles on susceptibility to SLE. Genetic studies on familial cases of lupus have provided valuable information on the contribution of rare alleles and mutations to the development of lupus. However, there is still a substantial shortage in genetic studies of cutaneous lupus and its subtypes.

References

Abou Ghanima AT, Elolemy GG, Ganeb SS, Abo Elazem A, Abdelgawad ER (2012) Role of T helper 17 cells in the pathogenesis of systemic lupus erythematosus. Egypt J Immunol 19:25–33

Absher DM, Li X, Waite LL, Gibson A, Roberts K, Edberg J, Chatham WW, Kimberly RP (2013) Genome-wide DNA methylation analysis of systemic lupus erythematosus reveals persistent hypomethylation of interferon genes and compositional changes to CD4+ T-cell populations. PLoS Genet 9:e1003678

Achtman JC, Werth VP (2015) Pathophysiology of cutaneous lupus erythematosus. Arthritis Res Therapy 17:1–10

Adrianto I, Wen F, Templeton A, Wiley G, King JB, Lessard CJ, Bates JS, Hu Y, Kelly JA, Kaufman KM (2011) Association of a functional variant downstream of TNFAIP3 with systemic lupus erythematosus. Nat Genet 43:253–258

Agata Y, Kawasaki A, Nishimura H, Ishida Y, Tsubat T, Yagita H, Honjo T (1996) Expression of the PD-1 antigen on the surface of stimulated mouse T and B lymphocytes. Int Immunol 8:765–772

Al-Mayouf SM, Sunker A, Abdwani R, Al Abrawi S, Almurshedi F, Alhashmi N, Al Sonbul A, Sewairi W, Qari A, Abdallah E (2011) Loss-of-function variant in DNASE1L3 causes a familial form of systemic lupus erythematosus. Nat Genet 43:1186–1188

Alarcón-Segovia D, Alarcón-Riquelme ME, Cardiel MH, Caeiro F, Massardo L, Villa AR, Pons-Estel BA, Eritematoso GLdEdL (2005) Familial aggregation of systemic lupus erythematosus, rheumatoid arthritis, and other autoimmune diseases in 1,177 lupus patients from the GLADEL cohort. Arthritis Rheum 52:1138–1147

Alperin JM, Ortiz-Fernández L, Sawalha AH (2018) Monogenic lupus: a developing paradigm of disease. Front Immunol 9:2496

An J, Briggs TA, Dumax-Vorzet A, Alarcón-Riquelme ME, Belot A, Beresford M, Bruce IN, Carvalho C, Chaperot L, Frostegård J (2017) Tartrate-resistant acid phosphatase deficiency in the predisposition to systemic lupus erythematosus. Arthritis Rheumatol 69:131–142

An X-J, Xia Y, Li J, Dong L-Y, Wang Y-J, Yang J, Li Y, Shen C, Zhang Y-M, Yang M (2019) RasGRP3 in peripheral blood mononuclear cells is associated with disease activity and implicated in the development of systemic lupus erythematosus. Am J Transl Res 11:1800

Arabi E, Garshasbi M, Jamshidi A, Khalesi R, Ahmadzadeh N, Akbarian M, Mahmoudi M (2016)

Association study of AFF1 gene polymorphism (rs340630) with Iranian systemic lupus erythematosus patients. Acta Reumatol Port 41

Arason G, Jorgensen G, Ludviksson B (2010) Primary immunodeficiency and autoimmunity: lessons from human diseases. Scand J Immunol 71:317–328

Armstrong DL, Eisenstein M, Zidovetzki R, Jacob CO (2015) Systemic lupus erythematosus-associated neutrophil cytosolic factor 2 mutation affects the structure of NADPH oxidase complex. J Biol Chem 290:12595–12602

Arneth BM (2019) Systemic lupus erythematosus and DNA degradation and elimination defects. Front Immunol 10:1697

Asmana Ningrum R (2014) Human interferon alpha-2b: a therapeutic protein for cancer treatment. Scientifica

Bae S-C, Lee YH (2018) Vitamin D receptor FokI, TaqI, and ApaI polymorphisms and susceptibility to systemic lupus erythematosus: an updated meta-analysis. Clin Rheumatol 37:1529–1537

Bao L, Haas M, Quigg RJ (2011) Complement factor H deficiency accelerates development of lupus nephritis. J Am Soc Nephrol 22:285–295

Barreto M, Santos E, Ferreira R, Fesel C, Fontes MF, Pereira C, Martins B, Andreia R, Viana JF, Crespo F (2004) Evidence for CTLA4 as a susceptibility gene for systemic lupus erythematosus. Eur J Hum Genet 12:620–626

Behrens TW, Graham RR (2011) TRAPing a new gene for autoimmunity. Nat Genet 43:90–91

Bentham J, Morris DL, Graham DSC, Pinder CL, Tombleson P, Behrens TW, Martín J, Fairfax BP, Knight JC, Chen L (2015) Genetic association analyses implicate aberrant regulation of innate and adaptive immunity genes in the pathogenesis of systemic lupus erythematosus. Nat Genet 47:1457–1464

Bickel PE, Scherer PE, Schnitzer JE, Oh P, Lisanti MP, Lodish HF (1997) Flotillin and epidermal surface antigen define a new family of caveolae-associated integral membrane proteins. J Biol Chem 272:13793–13802

Bijl M, Reefman E, Horst G, Limburg PC, Kallenberg CG (2006) Reduced uptake of apoptotic cells by macrophages in systemic lupus erythematosus: correlates with decreased serum levels of complement. Ann Rheum Dis 65:57–63

Bizzaro G, Antico A, Fortunato A, Bizzaro N (2017) Vitamin D and autoimmune diseases: is vitamin D receptor (VDR) polymorphism the culprit. Isr Med Assoc J 19:438–443

Blanco P, Palucka AK, Gill M, Pascual V, Banchereau J (2001) Induction of dendritic cell differentiation by IFN-α in systemic lupus erythematosus. Science 294:1540–1543

Blank C, Brown I, Marks R, Nishimura H, Honjo T, Gajewski TF (2003) Absence of programmed death receptor 1 alters thymic development and enhances generation of CD4/CD8 double-negative TCR-transgenic T cells. J Immunol 171:4574–4581

Blank MC, Stefanescu RN, Masuda E, Marti F, King PD, Redecha PB, Wurzburger RJ, Peterson MG, Tanaka S, Pricop L (2005) Decreased transcription of the human FCGR2B gene mediated by the-343 G/C promoter polymorphism and association with systemic lupus erythematosus. Hum Genet 117:220–227

Bodin S, Planchon D, Morris ER, Comunale F, Gauthier-Rouvière C (2014) Flotillins in intercellular adhesion–from cellular physiology to human diseases. J Cell Sci 127:5139–5147

Bönelt P, Wöhner M, Minnich M, Tagoh H, Fischer M, Jaritz M, Kavirayani A, Garimella M, Karlsson MC, Busslinger M (2019) Precocious expression of Blimp1 in B cells causes autoimmune disease with increased self-reactive plasma cells. EMBO J 38:1–19

Bordignon M, Bargagli E, Agostini C, Cinetto F, Baldo V, Alaibac M, Rottoli P (2013) TLR7 Gln11Leu single nucleotide polymorphism in patients with sarcoidosis. Sarcoidosis, Vasculitis, Diffuse Lung Dis off J WASOG 30:157

Borschukova O, Paz Z, Ghiran I, Liu C, Kao A, Manzi S, Ahearn J, Tsokos G (2012) Complement fragment C3d is colocalized within the lipid rafts of T cells and promotes cytokine production. Lupus 21:1294–1304

Bose M, Mukherjee P (2020) Microbe–MUC1 crosstalk in cancer-associated infections. Trends Mol Med 26:324–336

Botto M, Dell'Agnola C, Bygrave AE, Thompson EM, Cook HT, Petry F, Loos M, Pandolfi PP, Walport MJ (1998) Homozygous C1q deficiency causes glomerulonephritis associated with multiple apoptotic bodies. Nat Genet 19:56–59

Bourn R, Slight-Webb S, James J (2016) Infections in Early Systemic Lupus Erythematosus Pathogenesis. In: Systemic lupus erythematosus. Elsevier, pp 191–197

Braathen LR, Bratlie A, Teisberg P (1986) HLA genotypes in a family with a case of homozygous C2 deficiency and discoid lupus erythematosus. Acta Derm Venereol 66:419–422

Briggs TA, Rice GI, Daly S, Urquhart J, Gornall H, Bader-Meunier B, Baskar K, Baskar S, Baudouin V, Beresford MW (2011) Tartrate-resistant acid phosphatase deficiency causes a bone dysplasia with autoimmunity and a type I interferon expression signature. Nat Genet 43:127–131

Brown DR, Calpe S, Keszei M, Wang N, McArdel S, Terhorst C, Sharpe AH (2011) Cutting edge: an NK cell-independent role for Slamf4 in controlling humoral autoimmunity. J Immunol 187:21–25

Budarf M, Goyette P, Boucher G, Lian J, Graham R, Claudio J, Hudson T, Gladman D, Clarke A, Pope J (2011) A targeted association study in systemic lupus erythematosus identifies multiple susceptibility alleles. Genes Immun 12:51–58

Cachat J, Deffert C, Hugues S, Krause K-H (2015) Phagocyte NADPH oxidase and specific immunity. Clin Sci 128:635–648

Cairns A, Crockard A, McConnell J, Courtney P, Bell A (2001) Reduced expression of CD44 on monocytes and neutrophils in systemic lupus erythematosus: relations with apoptotic neutrophils and disease activity. Ann Rheum Dis 60:950–955

Campbell M, Sefton BM (1992) Association between B-lymphocyte membrane immunoglobulin and multiple members of the Src family of protein tyrosine kinases. Mol Cell Biol 12:2315–2321

Cao W, Liu Y-J (2006) Opn: key regulator of pDC interferon production. Nat Immunol 7:441–443

Cappione A, Anolik JH, Pugh-Bernard A, Barnard J, Dutcher P, Silverman G, Sanz I (2005) Germinal center exclusion of autoreactive B cells is defective in human systemic lupus erythematosus. J Clin Investig 115:3205–3216

Castro J, Balada E, Ordi-Ros J, Vilardell-Tarrés M (2008) The complex immunogenetic basis of systemic lupus erythematosus. Autoimmun Rev 7:345–351

Celhar T, Fairhurst A-M (2014) Toll-like receptors in systemic lupus erythematosus: potential for personalized treatment. Front Pharmacol 5:265

Cen H, Leng R-X, Wang W, Zhou M, Feng C-C, Chen G-M, Li R, Pan H-F, Li X-P, Ye D-Q (2012) Association of AFF1 rs340630 and AFF3 rs10865035 polymorphisms with systemic lupus erythematosus in a Chinese population. Immunogenetics 64:935–938

Chambers CA, Sullivan TJ, Allison JP (1997) Lymphoproliferation in CTLA-4–deficient mice is mediated by costimulation-dependent activation of CD4+ T cells. Immunity 7:885–895

Chang N-H, Li TT, Kim JJ, Landolt-Marticorena C, Fortin PR, Gladman DD, Urowitz MB, Wither JE (2015) Interferon-α induces altered transitional B cell signaling and function in Systemic Lupus Erythematosus. J Autoimmun 58:100–110

Chatterjee P, Agyemang AF, Alimzhanov MB, Degn S, Tsiftsoglou SA, Alicot E, Jones SA, Ma M, Carroll MC (2013) Complement C 4 maintains peripheral B-cell tolerance in a myeloid cell dependent manner. Eur J Immunol 43:2441–2450

Chauhan SK, Singh VV, Rai R, Rai M, Rai G (2013) Distinct autoantibody profiles in systemic lupus erythematosus patients are selectively associated with TLR7 and TLR9 upregulation. J Clin Immunol 33:954–964

Choi J-Y, Seth A, Kashgarian M, Terrillon S, Fung E, Huang L, Wang LC, Craft J (2017) Disruption of pathogenic cellular networks by IL-21 blockade leads to disease amelioration in murine lupus. J Immunol 198:2578–2588

Chrabot BS, Kariuki SN, Zervou MI, Feng X, Arrington J, Jolly M, Boumpas DT, Reder AT, Goulielmos GN, Niewold TB (2013) Genetic variation near IRF8 is associated with serologic and cytokine profiles in systemic lupus erythematosus and multiple sclerosis. Genes Immun 14:471–478

Chuang T-H, Ulevitch RJ (2004) Triad3A, an E3 ubiquitin-protein ligase regulating Toll-like receptors. Nat Immunol 5:495–502

Chuang Y-P, Wang C-H, Wang N-C, Chang D-M, Sytwu H-K (2012) Modulatory function of invariant natural killer T cells in systemic lupus erythematosus. Clin Dev Immunol 2012

Chun RF, Liu PT, Modlin RL, Adams JS, Hewison M (2014) Impact of vitamin D on immune function: lessons learned from genome-wide analysis. Front Physiol 5:151

Chung SA, Taylor KE, Graham RR, Nititham J, Lee AT, Ortmann WA, Jacob CO, Alarcón-Riquelme ME, Tsao BP, Harley JB (2011) Differential genetic associations for systemic lupus erythematosus based on anti–dsDNA autoantibody production. PLoS Genet 7:e1001323

Ciccacci C, Perricone C, Alessandri C, Latini A, Politi C, Delunardo F, Pierdominici M, Conti F, Novelli G, Ortona E (2018) Evaluation of ATG5 polymorphisms in Italian patients with systemic lupus erythematosus: contribution to disease susceptibility and clinical phenotypes. Lupus 27:1464–1469

Ciccacci C, Perricone C, Ceccarelli F, Rufini S, Di Fusco D, Alessandri C, Spinelli FR, Cipriano E, Novelli G, Valesini G (2014) A multilocus genetic study in a cohort of Italian SLE patients confirms the association with STAT4 gene and describes a new association with HCP5 gene. PLoS One 9:e111991

Clemente N, Raineri D, Cappellano G, Boggio E, Favero F, Soluri MF, Dianzani C, Comi C, Dianzani U, Chiocchetti A (2016) Osteopontin bridging innate and adaptive immunity in autoimmune diseases. J Immunol Res

Connolly JJ, Hakonarson H (2012) Role of cytokines in systemic lupus erythematosus: recent progress from GWAS and sequencing. BioMed Res Int

Cortini A, Ellinghaus U, Malik TH, Graham DSC, Botto M, Vyse TJ (2017) B cell OX40L supports T follicular helper cell development and contributes to SLE pathogenesis. Ann Rheum Dis 76:2095–2103

Costa S, Borgogna C, Mondini M, De Andrea M, Meroni P, Berti E, Gariglio M, Landolfo S (2011) Redistribution of the nuclear protein IFI16 into the cytoplasm of ultraviolet B-exposed keratinocytes as a mechanism of autoantigen processing. Br J Dermatol 164:282–290

Coughlin JJ, Stang SL, Dower NA, Stone JC (2005) RasGRP1 and RasGRP3 regulate B cell proliferation by facilitating B cell receptor-Ras signaling. J Immunol 175:7179–7184

Coughlin JJ, Stang SL, Dower NA, Stone JC (2006) The role of RasGRPs in regulation of lymphocyte proliferation. Immunol Lett 105:77–82

Crispín JC, Keenan BT, Finnell MD, Bermas BL, Schur P, Massarotti E, Karlson EW, Fitzgerald LM, Ergin S, Kyttaris VC (2010) Expression of CD44 variant isoforms CD44v3 and CD44v6 is increased on T cells from patients with systemic lupus erythematosus and is correlated with disease activity. Arthritis Rheum 62:1431–1437

Crow MK (2014) Type I interferon in the pathogenesis of lupus. J Immunol 192:5459–5468

Cui Y, Sheng Y, Zhang X (2013) Genetic susceptibility to SLE: recent progress from GWAS. J Autoimmun 41:25–33

Curran CS, Gupta S, Sanz I, Sharon E (2019) PD-1 immunobiology in systemic lupus erythematosus. J Autoimmun 97:1–9

da Silva Fonseca AM, de Azevedo SJ, Pancotto JAT, Donadi EA, Segat L, Crovella S, Sandrin-Garcia P (2013) Polymorphisms in STK17A gene are associated with systemic lupus erythematosus and its clinical manifestations. Gene 527:435–439

Dam EM, Habib T, Chen J, Funk A, Glukhova V, Davis-Pickett M, Wei S, James R, Buckner JH, Cerosaletti K (2016) The BANK1 SLE-risk variants are associated with alterations in peripheral B cell signaling and development in humans. Clini Immunol 173:171–180

Danion F, Rosine N, Belkhir R, Gottenberg J, Hachulla E, Chatelus E, Pugnet G, Pers Y, Mariette X, Sibilia J (2016) Efficacy of abatacept in systemic lupus erythematosus: a retrospective analysis of 11 patients with refractory disease. Lupus 25:1440–1447

Davies E, Teh L, Ordi-Ros J, Snowden N, Hillarby M, Hajeer A, Donn R, Perez-Pemen P, Vilardell-Tarres M, Ollier W (1997) A dysfunctional allele of the mannose binding protein gene associates with systemic lupus erythematosus in a Spanish population. J Rheumatol 24:485–488

de Azevêdo SJ, Monteiro Fernandes K, Trés Pancotto J, Sotero Fragoso T, Donadi E, Crovella S, Sandrin-Garcia P (2013) Vitamin D receptor (VDR) gene polymorphisms and susceptibility to systemic lupus erythematosus clinical manifestations. Lupus 22:1110–1117

de Gruijl FR, van Kranen HJ, Mullenders LH (2001) UV-induced DNA damage, repair, mutations and oncogenic pathways in skin cancer. J Photochem Photobiol, B 63:19–27

de Salort J, Cuenca M, Terhorst C, Engel P, Romero X (2013) Ly9 (CD229) cell-surface receptor is crucial for the development of spontaneous autoantibody production to nuclear antigens. Front Immunol 4:225

Delgado-Vega AM, Dozmorov MG, Quirós MB, Wu Y-Y, Martínez-García B, Kozyrev SV, Frostegård J, Truedsson L, de Ramón E, González-Escribano MF (2012) Fine mapping and conditional analysis identify a new mutation in the autoimmunity susceptibility gene BLK that leads to reduced half-life of the BLK protein. Ann Rheum Dis 71:1219–1226

Deng Y, Tsao BP (2010) Genetic susceptibility to systemic lupus erythematosus in the genomic era. Nat Rev Rheumatol 6:683

Deng Y, Zhao J, Sakurai D, Kaufman KM, Edberg JC, Kimberly RP, Kamen DL, Gilkeson GS, Jacob CO, Scofield RH (2013) MicroRNA-3148 modulates allelic expression of toll-like receptor 7 variant associated with systemic lupus erythematosus. PLoS Genet 9:e1003336

Dengler HS, Baracho GV, Omori SA, Bruckner S, Arden KC, Castrillon DH, DePinho RA, Rickert RC (2008) Distinct functions for the transcription factor Foxo1 at various stages of B cell differentiation. Nat Immunol 9:1388–1398

Devarapu SK, Anders H-J (2018) Toll-like receptors in lupus nephritis. J Biomed Sci 25:35

Dey-Rao R, Sinha AA (2019) In silico analyses of skin and peripheral blood transcriptional data in cutaneous lupus reveals CCR2-A novel potential therapeutic target. Front Immunol 10:640

Dillon SP, Kurien BT, Li S, Bruner GR, Kaufman KM, Harley JB, Gaffney PM, Wallace DJ, Weisman MH, Scofield RH (2012) Sex chromosome aneuploidies among men with systemic lupus erythematosus. J Autoimmun 38:J129–J134

Ding C, Ma Y, Chen X, Liu M, Cai Y, Hu X, Xiang D, Nath S, Zhang H-g, Ye H (2013) Integrin CD11b negatively regulates BCR signalling to maintain autoreactive B cell tolerance. Nature Commun 4:1–13

Dolff S, Abdulahad WH, Westra J, Doornbos-van der Meer B, Limburg PC, Kallenberg CG, Bijl M (2011) Increase in IL-21 producing T-cells in patients with systemic lupus erythematosus. Arthritis Res Therapy 13:1–10

Dragon-Durey M-A, Quartier P, Frémeaux-Bacchi V, Blouin J, de Barace C, Prieur A-M, Weiss L, Fridman W-H (2001) Molecular basis of a selective C1s deficiency associated with early onset multiple autoimmune diseases. J Immunol 166:7612–7616

Duan B, Morel L (2006) Role of B-1a cells in autoimmunity. Autoimmun Rev 5:403–408

Duits AJ, Bootsma H, Derksen RH, Spronk PE, Kater L, Kallenberg CG, Capel PJ, Westerdaal NA, Spierenburg GT, Gmelig-Meyling FH (1995) Skewed distribution of IgG Fc receptor IIa (CD32) polymorphism is associated with renal disease in systemic lupus erythematosus patients. Arthritis Rheum 38:1832–1836

Durosaro O, Davis MD, Reed KB, Rohlinger AL (2009) Incidence of cutaneous lupus erythematosus, 1965–2005: a population-based study. Arch Dermatol 145:249–253

Dymecki SM, Niederhuber JE, Desiderio SV (1990) Specific expression of a tyrosine kinase gene, blk, in B lymphoid cells. Science 247:332–336

Ehlenberger AG, Nussenzweig V (1977) The role of membrane receptors for C3b and C3d in phagocytosis. J Exp Med 145:357–371

Ek-Rylander B, Flores M, Wendel M, Heinegård D, Andersson G (1994) Dephosphorylation of osteopontin and bone sialoprotein by osteoclastic tartrate-resistant acid phosphatase. Modulation of osteoclast adhesion in vitro. J Biol Chem 269:14853–14856

Erdei A, Prechl J, Isaák A, Molnár E (2003) Regulation of B-cell activation by complement receptors CD21 and CD35. Curr Pharm Des 9:1849–1860

Estess P, DeGrendele HC, Pascual V, Siegelman MH (1998) Functional activation of lymphocyte CD44 in peripheral blood is a marker of autoimmune disease activity. J Clin Investig 102:1173–1182

Fan Y, Tao J-H, Zhang L-P, Li L-H, Ye D-Q (2011a) Association of BLK (rs13277113, rs2248932) polymorphism with systemic lupus erythematosus: a meta-analysis. Mol Biol Rep 38:4445–4453

Fan Y, Tao JH, Zhang LP, Li LH, Ye DQ (2011b) The association between BANK1 and TNFAIP3 gene polymorphisms and systemic lupus erythematosus: a meta-analysis. Int J Immunogenet 38:151–159

Fang C, Roy S, Nielsen E, Paul M, Maul R, Paun A, Koentgen F, Raval F, Szomolanyi-Tsuda E, Pitha P (2012) Unique contribution of IRF-5-Ikaros axis to the B-cell IgG2a response. Genes Immun 13:421–430

Farrera C, Fadeel B (2013) Macrophage clearance of neutrophil extracellular traps is a silent process. J Immunol 191:2647–2656

Farres MN, Al-Zifzaf DS, Aly AA, Abd Raboh NM (2011) OX40/OX40L in systemic lupus erythematosus: association with disease activity and lupus nephritis. Ann Saudi Med 31:29–34

Fernando MM, Freudenberg J, Lee A, Morris DL, Boteva L, Rhodes B, Gonzalez-Escribano MF, Lopez-Nevot MA, Navarra SV, Gregersen PK (2012) Transancestral mapping of the MHC region in systemic lupus erythematosus identifies new independent and interacting loci at MSH5, HLA-DPB1 and HLA-G. Ann Rheum Dis 71:777–784

Fernando MM, Stevens CR, Sabeti PC, Walsh EC, McWhinnie AJ, Shah A, Green T, Rioux JD, Vyse TJ (2007) Identification of two independent risk factors for lupus within the MHC in United Kingdom families. PLoS Genet 3

Ficht X, Ruef N, Stolp B, Samson GP, Moalli F, Page N, Merkler D, Nichols BJ, Diz-Muñoz A, Legler DF (2019) In Vivo function of the lipid raft protein flotillin-1 during CD8+ T cell-mediated host surveillance. J Immunol 203:2377–2387

Fiehn C (2017) Familial Chilblain Lupus-What Can We Learn from Type I Interferonopathies? Curr Rheumatol Rep 19:61

Fojtíková M, Novota P, Čejková P, Pešičková S, Tegzová D, Černá M (2011) HLA class II, MICA and PRL gene polymorphisms: the common contribution to the systemic lupus erythematosus development in Czech population. Rheumatol Int 31:1195–1201

Forton A, Petri M, Goldman D, Sullivan K (2002) An osteopontin (SPP1) polymorphism is associated with systemic lupus erythematosus. Hum Mutat 19:459–459

Fousteri G, Liossis S-NC, Battaglia M (2013) Roles of the protein tyrosine phosphatase PTPN22 in immunity and autoimmunity. Clin Immunol 149:556–565

Francisco LM, Sage PT, Sharpe AH (2010) The PD-1 pathway in tolerance and autoimmunity. Immunol Rev 236:219–242

G'Sell RT, Gaffney PM, Powell DW (2015) ABIN1 a Physiological Inhibitor of NF-κB: a Molecular Switch for Inflammation and Autoimmunity. Arthritis Rheumatol (Hoboken, NJ) 67:2292

Gambelunghe G, Gerli R, Bartoloni Bocci E, Del Sindaco P, Ghaderi M, Sanjeevi C, Bistoni O, Bini V, Falorni A (2005) Contribution of MHC class I chain-related A (MICA) gene polymorphism to genetic susceptibility for systemic lupus erythematosus. Rheumatology 44:287–292

Gao B, Hong F, Radaeva S (2004) Host factors and failure of interferon-α treatment in hepatitis C virus. Hepatology 39:880–890

Gao J, Gai N, Wang L, Liu K, Liu X-H, Wei L-T, Tian T, Li S-L, Zheng Y, Deng Y-J (2017) Meta-analysis of programmed cell death 1 polymorphisms with systemic lupus erythematosus risk. Oncotarget 8:36885

Garcia-Romo GS, Caielli S, Vega B, Connolly J, Allantaz F, Xu Z, Punaro M, Baisch J, Guiducci C, Coffman RL (2011) Netting neutrophils are major inducers of type I IFN production in pediatric systemic lupus erythematosus. Sci Transl Med 3:73ra20–73ra20

Garred P, Madsen HO, Halberg P, Petersen J, Kronborg G, Svejgaard A, Andersen V, Jacobsen S (1999) Mannose-binding lectin polymorphisms and susceptibility to infection in systemic lupus erythematosus. Arthritis & Rheum off J Am Coll Rheumatol 42:2145–2152

Garrett-Sinha LA, Kearly A, Satterthwaite AB (2016) The role of the transcription factor Ets1 in lupus and other autoimmune diseases. Crit Rev™ Immunol 36

Gateva V, Sandling JK, Hom G, Taylor KE, Chung SA, Sun X, Ortmann W, Kosoy R, Ferreira RC, Nordmark G (2009) A large-scale replication study identifies TNIP1, PRDM1, JAZF1, UHRF1BP1 and IL10 as risk loci for systemic lupus erythematosus. Nat Genet 41:1228

Georg I, Díaz-Barreiro A, Morell M, Pey AL, Alarcón-Riquelme ME (2020) BANK1 interacts with TRAF6 and MyD88 in innate immune signaling in B cells. Cell Mol Immunol 17:954–965

Ghadiri A, Duhamel M, Fleischer A, Reimann A, Dessauge F, Rebollo A (2007) Critical function of Ikaros in controlling Aiolos gene expression. FEBS Lett 581:1605–1616

Ghodke-Puranik Y, Niewold TB (2013) Genetics of the type I interferon pathway in systemic lupus erythematosus. Int J Clin Rheumatol 8

Ghodke-Puranik Y, Niewold TB (2015) Immunogenetics of systemic lupus erythematosus: a comprehensive review. J Autoimmun 64:125–136

Giancotti FG, Ruoslahti E (1999) Integrin signaling. Science 285:1028–1033

Gibson SA, Benveniste EN (2018) Protein kinase CK2: An emerging regulator of immunity. Trends Immunol 39:82–85

Giri B, Dixit VD, Ghosh MC, Collins GD, Khan IU, Madara K, Weeraratna AT, Taub DD (2007) CXCL12-induced partitioning of flotillin-1 with lipid rafts plays a role in CXCR4 function. Eur J Immunol 37:2104–2116

Godsell J, Rudloff I, Kandane-Rathnayake R, Hoi A, Nold MF, Morand EF, Harris J (2016) Clinical associations of IL-10 and IL-37 in systemic lupus erythematosus. Sci Rep 6:1–10

Goldstein LA, Butcher EC (1990) Identification of mRNA that encodes an alternative form of H-CAM (CD44) in lymphoid and nonlymphoid tissues. Immunogenetics 32:389–397

Graham DC, Vyse T, Fortin P, Montpetit A, Cai Y, Lim S, McKenzie T, Farwell L, Rhodes B, Chad L (2008a) Association of LY9 in UK and Canadian SLE families. Genes Immun 9:93–102

Graham DSC, Graham RR, Manku H, Wong AK, Whittaker JC, Gaffney PM, Moser KL, Rioux JD, Altshuler D, Behrens TW (2008b) Polymorphism at the TNF superfamily gene TNFSF4 confers susceptibility to systemic lupus erythematosus. Nat Genet 40:83–89

Graham RR, Cotsapas C, Davies L, Hackett R, Lessard CJ, Leon JM, Burtt NP, Guiducci C, Parkin M, Gates C (2008c) Genetic variants near TNFAIP3 on 6q23 are associated with systemic lupus erythematosus. Nat Genet 40:1059–1061

Graham DSC, Morris DL, Bhangale TR, Criswell LA, Syvänen A-C, Rönnblom L, Behrens TW, Graham RR, Vyse TJ (2011) Association of NCF2, IKZF1, IRF8, IFIH1, and TYK2 with systemic lupus erythematosus. PLoS Genet 7:e1002341

Graham JP, Arcipowski KM, Bishop GA (2010) Differential B-lymphocyte regulation by CD40 and its viral mimic, latent membrane protein 1. Immunol Rev 237:226–248

Graham RR, Kyogoku C, Sigurdsson S, Vlasova IA, Davies LR, Baechler EC, Plenge RM, Koeuth T, Ortmann WA, Hom G (2007) Three functional variants of IFN regulatory factor 5 (IRF5) define risk and protective haplotypes for human lupus. Proc Natl Acad Sci 104:6758–6763

Graham RR, Ortmann WA, Langefeld CD, Jawaheer D, Selby SA, Rodine PR, Baechler EC, Rohlf KE, Shark KB, Espe KJ (2002) Visualizing human leukocyte antigen class II risk haplotypes in human systemic lupus erythematosus. Am J Hum Genet 71:543–553

Grammatikos AP, Tsokos GC (2012) Immunodeficiency and autoimmunity: lessons from systemic lupus erythematosus. Trends Mol Med 18:101–108

Groh V, Bahram S, Bauer S, Herman A, Beauchamp M, Spies T (1996) Cell stress-regulated human major histocompatibility complex class I gene expressed in gastrointestinal epithelium. Proc Natl Acad Sci 93:12445–12450

Grönhagen C, Fored C, Granath F, Nyberg F (2011) Cutaneous lupus erythematosus and the association with systemic lupus erythematosus: a population-based cohort of 1088 patients in Sweden. Br J Dermatol 164:1335–1341

Grönhagen CM, Nyberg F (2014) Cutaneous lupus erythematosus: An update. Ind Dermatol Online J 5:7

Guerra-de Blas PdC, Villaseñor-Talavera YS, Cruz-González DdJ, Baranda L, Doníz-Padilla L, Abud-Mendoza C, González-Amaro R, Monsiváis-Urenda AE (2016) Analysis of the expression and function of immunoglobulin-like transcript 4 (ILT4, LILRB2) in dendritic cells from patients with systemic lupus erythematosus. J Immunol Res

Guo Liu R-N, Cheng Q-Y, Zhou H-Y, Li B-Z, Ye D-Q (2020) Elevated blood and urinary ICAM-1 is a biomarker for systemic lupus erythematosus: a systematic review and meta-analysis. Immunol Invest 49:15–31

Guo T, Zhao S, Zhao S, Chen M, Li G, Jiao X, Wang Z, Zhao Y, Qin Y, Gao F (2017) Mutations in MSH5 in primary ovarian insufficiency. Hum Mol Genet 26:1452–1457

Gupta V, Kumar S, Pratap A, Singh R, Kumari R, Kumar S, Aggarwal A, Misra R (2018) Association of ITGAM, TNFSF4, TNFAIP3 and STAT4 gene polymorphisms with risk of systemic lupus erythematosus in a North Indian population. Lupus 27:1973–1979

Gurevich I, Zhang C, Francis N, Aneskievich BJ (2011) TNIP1, a retinoic acid receptor corepressor and A20-binding inhibitor of NF-κB, distributes to both nuclear and cytoplasmic locations. J Histochem Cytochem 59:1101–1112

Győry I, Fejér G, Ghosh N, Seto E, Wright KL (2003) Identification of a functionally impaired positive regulatory domain I binding factor 1 transcription repressor in myeloma cell lines. J Immunol 170:3125–3133

Habib T, Funk A, Rieck M, Brahmandam A, Dai X, Panigrahi AK, Prak ETL, Meyer-Bahlburg A, Sanda S, Greenbaum C (2012) Altered B cell homeostasis is associated with type I diabetes and carriers of the PTPN22 allelic variant. J Immunol 188:487–496

Hagn M, Schwesinger E, Ebel V, Sontheimer K, Maier J, Beyer T, Syrovets T, Laumonnier Y, Fabricius D, Simmet T (2009) Human B cells secrete granzyme B when recognizing viral antigens in the context of the acute phase cytokine IL-21. J Immunol 183:1838–1845

Hakkim A, Fürnrohr BG, Amann K, Laube B, Abed UA, Brinkmann V, Herrmann M, Voll RE, Zychlinsky A (2010) Impairment of neutrophil extracellular trap degradation is associated with lupus nephritis. Proc Natl Acad Sci 107:9813–9818

Hamann L, Glaeser C, Hamprecht A, Gross M, Gomma A, Schumann RR (2006) Toll-like receptor (TLR)-9 promotor polymorphisms and atherosclerosis. Clin Chim Acta 364:303–307

Han C, Jin J, Xu S, Liu H, Li N, Cao X (2010) Integrin CD11b negatively regulates TLR-triggered inflammatory responses by activating Syk and promoting degradation of MyD88 and TRIF via Cbl-b. Nat Immunol 11:734

Han J-W, Zheng H-F, Cui Y, Sun L-D, Ye D-Q, Hu Z, Xu J-H, Cai Z-M, Huang W, Zhao G-P (2009a) Genome-wide association study in a Chinese Han population identifies nine new susceptibility loci for systemic lupus erythematosus. Nat Genet 41:1234–1237

Han S, Guthridge JM, Harley IT, Sestak AL, Kim-Howard X, Kaufman KM, Namjou B, Deshmukh H, Bruner G, Espinoza LR (2008) Osteopontin and systemic lupus erythematosus association: a probable gene-gender interaction. PloS One 3

Han S, Kim-Howard X, Deshmukh H, Kamatani Y, Viswanathan P, Guthridge JM, Thomas K, Kaufman KM, Ojwang J, Rojas-Villarraga A (2009b)

Evaluation of imputation-based association in and around the integrin-α-M (ITGAM) gene and replication of robust association between a non-synonymous functional variant within ITGAM and systemic lupus erythematosus (SLE). Hum Mol Genet 18:1171–1180
Harley JB, Alarcón-Riquelme ME, Criswell LA, Jacob CO, Kimberly RP, Moser KL, Tsao BP, Vyse TJ, Langefeld CD (2008a) Genome-wide association scan in women with systemic lupus erythematosus identifies susceptibility variants in ITGAM, PXK, KIAA1542 and other loci. Nat Genet 40:204–210
Harley JB, Alarcón-Riquelme ME, Criswell LA, Jacob CO, Kimberly RP, Moser KL, Tsao BP, Vyse TJ, Langefeld CD, Genetics (2008b) Genome-wide association scan in women with systemic lupus erythematosus identifies susceptibility variants in ITGAM, PXK, KIAA1542 and other loci. Nat Genet 40:204
Harley JB, Chen X, Pujato M, Miller D, Maddox A, Forney C, Magnusen AF, Lynch A, Chetal K, Yukawa M (2018) Transcription factors operate across disease loci, with EBNA2 implicated in autoimmunity. Nat Genet 50:699–707
Harley JB, Reichlin M, Arnett FC, Alexander EL, Bias WB, Provost TT (1986) Gene interaction at HLA-DQ enhances autoantibody production in primary Sjogren's syndrome. Science 232:1145–1147
Haseley LA, Wisnieski JJ, Denburg MR, Michael-Grossman AR, Ginzler EM, Gourley MF, Hoffman JH, Kimberly RP, Salmon JE (1997) Antibodies to C1q in systemic lupus erythematosus: characteristics and relation to FcγRIIA alleles. Kidney Int 52:1375–1380
Hatta Y, Tsuchiya N, Ohashi J, Matsushita M, Fujiwara K, Hagiwara K, Juji T, Tokunaga K (1999) Association of Fcγ receptor IIIB, but not of Fcγ receptor IIA and IIIA, polymorphisms with systemic lupus erythematosus in Japanese. Genes Immun 1:53–60
He C, Liu Y, Cheng Y, Gao J, Pan T, Han J, Quan C, Sun L, Zheng H, Zuo X (2010) TNIP1, SLC15A4, ETS1, RasGRP3 and IKZF1 are associated with clinical features of systemic lupus erythematosus in a Chinese Han population. Lupus 19:1181–1186
Hedrich CM, Tsokos GC (2011) Epigenetic mechanisms in systemic lupus erythematosus and other autoimmune diseases. Trends Mol Med 17:714–724
Heinz LX, Lee J, Kapoor U, Kartnig F, Sedlyarov V, Papakostas K, César-Razquin A, Essletzbichler P, Goldmann U, Stefanovic A (2020) TASL is the SLC15A4-associated adaptor for IRF5 activation by TLR7–9. Nature 581:316–322
Herbert AP, Makou E, Chen ZA, Kerr H, Richards A, Rappsilber J, Barlow PN (2015) Complement evasion mediated by enhancement of captured factor H: implications for protection of self-surfaces from complement. J Immunol 195:4986–4998
Herrmann M, Voll RE, Zoller OM, Hagenhofer M, Ponner BB, Kalden JR (1998) Impaired phagocytosis of apoptotic cell material by monocyte-derived macrophages from patients with systemic lupus erythematosus. Arthritis Rheum 41:1241–1250
Hersh AO, Arkin LM, Prahalad S (2016) Immunogenetics of cutaneous lupus erythematosus. Curr Opin Pediatr 28:470
Hofmann S, Leandro M, Morris S, Isenberg D (2013a) Effects of rituximab-based B-cell depletion therapy on skin manifestations of lupus erythematosus–report of 17 cases and review of the literature. Lupus 22:932–939
Hofmann SC, Bosma A, Bruckner-Tuderman L, Vukmanovic-Stejic M, Jury EC, Isenberg DA, Mauri C (2013b) Invariant natural killer T cells are enriched at the site of cutaneous inflammation in lupus erythematosus. J Dermatol Sci 71:22–28
Holm SJ, Carlen LM, Mallbris L, Ståhle-Bäckdahl M, O'Brien KP (2003) Polymorphisms in the SEEK1 and SPR1 genes on 6p21. 3 associate with psoriasis in the Swedish population. Exp Dermatol 12:435–444
Holmdahl R, Sareila O, Olsson LM, Bäckdahl L, Wing K (2016) Ncf1 polymorphism reveals oxidative regulation of autoimmune chronic inflammation. Immunol Rev 269:228–247
Hom G, Graham RR, Modrek B, Taylor KE, Ortmann W, Garnier S, Lee AT, Chung SA, Ferreira RC, Pant PK (2008) Association of systemic lupus erythematosus with C8orf13–BLK and ITGAM–ITGAX. N Engl J Med 358:900–909
Honda K, Takaoka A, Taniguchi T (2006) Type I inteferon gene induction by the interferon regulatory factor family of transcription factors. Immunity 25:349–360
Honma Y, Kiyosawa H, Mori T, Oguri A, Nikaido T, Kanazawa K-y, Tojo M, Takeda J, Tanno Y, Yokoya S (1999) Eos: a novel member of the Ikaros gene family expressed predominantly in the developing nervous system. FEBS Lett 447:76–80
Hu W, Sun L, Gao J, Li Y, Wang P, Cheng Y, Pan T, Han J, Liu Y, Lu W (2011) Down-regulated expression of IKZF1 mRNA in peripheral blood mononuclear cells from patients with systemic lupus erythematosus. Rheumatol Int 31:819–822
Huang N-J, Zhang L, Tang W, Chen C, Yang C-S, Kornbluth S (2012) The Trim39 ubiquitin ligase inhibits APC/CCdh1-mediated degradation of the Bax activator MOAP-1. J Cell Biol 197:361–367
Hynes RO (2002) Integrins: bidirectional, allosteric signaling machines. Cell 110:673–687
Inomata M, Into T, Niida S, Murakami Y (2013) Atg5 regulates formation of MyD88 condensed structures and MyD88-dependent signal transduction. Biochem Biophys Res Commun 437:509–514
Inoue N, Saito T, Masuda R, Suzuki Y, Ohtomi M, Sakiyama H (1998) Selective complement C1s deficiency caused by homozygous four-base deletion in the C1s gene. Hum Genet 103:415–418
Ip W, Chan S, Lau C, Lau Y (1998) Association of systemic lupus erythematosus with promoter polymorphisms of the mannose-binding lectin gene. Arthritis Rheum 41:1663–1668

Isnard P, Coré N, Naquet P, Djabali M (2000) Altered lymphoid development in mice deficient for the mAF4 proto-oncogene. Blood, J Am Soc Hematol 96:705–710

Isnardi I, Ng Y-S, Srdanovic I, Motaghedi R, Rudchenko S, von Bernuth H, Zhang S-Y, Puel A, Jouanguy E, Picard C (2008) IRAK-4-and MyD88-dependent pathways are essential for the removal of developing autoreactive B cells in humans. Immunity 29:746–757

Itoh Y, Kamata-Sakurai M, Denda-Nagai K, Nagai S, Tsuiji M, Ishii-Schrade K, Okada K, Goto A, Fukayama M, Irimura T (2008) Identification and expression of human epiglycanin/MUC21: a novel transmembrane mucin. Glycobiology 18:74–83

Jabalameli N, Rajabi F, Firooz A, Rezaei N (2021) The overlap between genetic susceptibility to COVID-19 and skin diseases. Immunol Inv 1–8

Jacob CO, Eisenstein M, Dinauer MC, Ming W, Liu Q, John S, Quismorio FP, Reiff A, Myones BL, Kaufman KM (2012) Lupus-associated causal mutation in neutrophil cytosolic factor 2 (NCF2) brings unique insights to the structure and function of NADPH oxidase. Proc Natl Acad Sci 109:E59–E67

Jacob CO, Yu N, Yoo DG, Perez-Zapata LJ, Barbu EA, Kaplan MJ, Purmalek M, Pingel JT, Idol RA, Dinauer MC (2017) Haploinsufficiency of nadph oxidase subunit neutrophil cytosolic factor 2 is sufficient to accelerate full-blown lupus in nzm 2328 mice. Arthritis Rheumatol 69:1647–1660

Jacob CO, Zhu J, Armstrong DL, Yan M, Han J, Zhou XJ, Thomas JA, Reiff A, Myones BL, Ojwang JO (2009) Identification of IRAK1 as a risk gene with critical role in the pathogenesis of systemic lupus erythematosus. Proc Natl Acad Sci 106:6256–6261

Jacobi AM, Odendahl M, Reiter K, Bruns A, Burmester GR, Radbruch A, Valet G, Lipsky PE, Dörner T (2003) Correlation between circulating CD27high plasma cells and disease activity in patients with systemic lupus erythematosus. Arthritis Rheum 48:1332–1342

Jago C, Yates J, Olsen Saraiva Câmara N, Lechler R, Lombardi G (2004) Differential expression of CTLA-4 among T cell subsets. Clin Exp Immunol 136:463–471

Jain N, Nguyen H, Chambers C, Kang J (2010) Dual function of CTLA-4 in regulatory T cells and conventional T cells to prevent multiorgan autoimmunity. Proc Natl Acad Sci 107:1524–1528

Jang SH, Chen H, Gregersen PK, Diamond B, Kim SJ (2017) Kruppel-like factor4 regulates PRDM1 expression through binding to an autoimmune risk allele. JCI Insight 2

Järvinen TM, Hellquist A, Koskenmies S, Einarsdottir E, Koskinen LL, Jeskanen L, Berglind L, Panelius J, Hasan T, Ranki A (2010) Tyrosine kinase 2 and interferon regulatory factor 5 polymorphisms are associated with discoid and subacute cutaneous lupus erythematosus. Exp Dermatol 19:123–131

Javinani A, Ashraf-Ganjouei A, Aslani S, Jamshidi A, Mahmoudi M (2019) Exploring the etiopathogenesis of systemic lupus erythematosus: a genetic perspective. Immunogenetics 71:283–297

Jenks SA, Sanz I (2009) Altered B cell receptor signaling in human systemic lupus erythematosus. Autoimmun Rev 8:209–213

Jensen MA, Patterson KC, Kumar AA, Kumabe M, Franek BS, Niewold TB (2012) Functional genetic polymorphisms in ILT3 are associated with decreased surface expression on dendritic cells and increased serum cytokines in lupus patients. In: Arthritis research & therapy, vol 3. Springer, pp 1–28

Jiang SH, Athanasopoulos V, Ellyard JI, Chuah A, Cappello J, Cook A, Prabhu SB, Cardenas J, Gu J, Stanley M (2019) Functional rare and low frequency variants in BLK and BANK1 contribute to human lupus. Nat Commun 10:1–12

Jog NR, Chakravarty EF, Guthridge JM, James JA (2018) Epstein Barr virus interleukin 10 suppresses anti-inflammatory phenotype in human monocytes. Front Immunol 9:2198

John SA, Clements JL, Russell LM, Garrett-Sinha LA (2008) Ets-1 regulates plasma cell differentiation by interfering with the activity of the transcription factor Blimp-1. J Biol Chem 283:951–962

Joly S, Rhea L, Volk P, Moreland JG, Dunnwald M (2016) Interferon regulatory factor 6 has a protective role in the host response to endotoxic shock. PloS One 11:e0152385

Jones S (1992) Ultraviolet radiation (UVR) induces cell-surface Ro/SSA antigen expression by human keratinocytes in vitro: a possible mechanism for the UVR induction of cutaneous lupus lesions. Br J Dermatol 126:546–553

Jordan AR, Racine RR, Hennig MJ, Lokeshwar VB (2015) The role of CD44 in disease pathophysiology and targeted treatment. Front Immunol 6:182

Joshi S, Kumar S, Bafna S, Rachagani S, Wagner K-U, Jain M, Batra SK (2015) Genetically engineered mucin mouse models for inflammation and cancer. Cancer Metastasis Rev 34:593–609

Jury EC, Flores-Borja F, Kalsi HS, Lazarus M, Isenberg DA, Mauri C, Ehrenstein MR (2010) Abnormal CTLA-4 function in T cells from patients with systemic lupus erythematosus. Eur J Immunol 40:569–578

Kailashiya V, Sharma HB, Kailashiya J (2019) Role of CTLA4 A49G polymorphism in systemic lupus erythematosus and its geographical distribution. J Clin Pathol 72:659–662

Kaplan MH (2005) STAT4. Immunol Res 31:231–241

Karassa FB, Trikalinos TA, Ioannidis JP (2002) Role of the Fcγ receptor IIa polymorphism in susceptibility to systemic lupus erythematosus and lupus nephritis: a meta-analysis. Arthritis Rheum off J Am Coll Rheumatol 46:1563–1571

Kariuki S, Moore J, Kirou K, Crow M, Utset T, Niewold T (2009a) Age-and gender-specific modulation of serum osteopontin and interferon-α by osteopontin genotype in systemic lupus erythematosus. Genes Immun 10:487–494

Kariuki SN, Kirou KA, MacDermott EJ, Barillas-Arias L, Crow MK, Niewold TB (2009b) Cutting edge: autoimmune disease risk variant of STAT4 confers increased sensitivity to IFN-α in lupus patients in vivo. J Immunol 182:34–38

Kariuki SN, Niewold TB (2010) Genetic regulation of serum cytokines in systemic lupus erythematosus. Transl Res 155:109–117

Katkam S, Rajasekhar L, Kumaraswami K, Kutala V (2017) Association of IL-6-174 G> C polymorphism with the risk of SLE among south Indians: evidence from case–control study and meta-analysis. Lupus 26:1491–1501

Kato H, Perl A (2018) The IL-21-mTOR axis blocks Treg differentiation and function by suppression of autophagy in patients with systemic lupus erythematosus. Arthritis Rheumatol (Hoboken, NJ) 70:427

Kaufman KM, Zhao J, Kelly JA, Hughes T, Adler A, Sanchez E, Ojwang JO, Langefeld CD, Ziegler JT, Williams AH (2013) Fine mapping of Xq28: both MECP2 and IRAK1 contribute to risk for systemic lupus erythematosus in multiple ancestral groups. Ann Rheum Dis 72:437–444

Keir ME, Francisco LM, Sharpe AH (2007a) PD-1 and its ligands in T-cell immunity. Curr Opin Immunol 19:309–314

Keir ME, Freeman GJ, Sharpe AH (2007b) PD-1 regulates self-reactive CD8+ T cell responses to antigen in lymph nodes and tissues. J Immunol 179:5064–5070

Keir ME, Liang SC, Guleria I, Latchman YE, Qipo A, Albacker LA, Koulmanda M, Freeman GJ, Sayegh MH, Sharpe AH (2006) Tissue expression of PD-L1 mediates peripheral T cell tolerance. J Exp Med 203:883–895

Keller AD, Maniatis T (1991) Identification and characterization of a novel repressor of beta-interferon gene expression. Genes Dev 5:868–879

Kelley CM, Ikeda T, Koipally J, Avitahl N, Wu L, Georgopoulos K, Morgan BA (1998) Helios, a novel dimerization partner of Ikaros expressed in the earliest hematopoietic progenitors. Curr Biol 8:508-S501

Kemp MG, Lindsey-Boltz LA, Sancar A (2015) UV light potentiates STING (stimulator of interferon genes)-dependent innate immune signaling through deregulation of ULK1 (Unc51-like kinase 1). J Biol Chem 290:12184–12194

Kerdiles YM, Beisner DR, Tinoco R, Dejean AS, Castrillon DH, DePinho RA, Hedrick SM (2009) Foxo1 links homing and survival of naive T cells by regulating L-selectin, CCR7 and interleukin 7 receptor. Nat Immunol 10:176–184

Kevil CG, Hicks MJ, He X, Zhang J, Ballantyne CM, Raman C, Schoeb TR, Bullard DC (2004) Loss of LFA-1, but not Mac-1, protects MRL/MpJ-Faslpr mice from autoimmune disease. Am J Pathol 165:609–616

Khan SQ, Khan I, Gupta V (2018) CD11b activity modulates pathogenesis of lupus nephritis. Front Med 5:52

Khera R, Das N (2009) Complement Receptor 1: disease associations and therapeutic implications. Mol Immunol 46:761–772

Kim CJ, Lee C-G, Jung J-Y, Ghosh A, Hasan SN, Hwang S-M, Kang H, Lee C, Kim G-C, Rudra D (2018) The transcription factor Ets1 suppresses T follicular helper type 2 cell differentiation to halt the onset of systemic lupus erythematosus. Immunity 49:1034–1048. e1038

Kim K, Brown EE, Choi C-B, Alarcón-Riquelme ME, Kelly JA, Glenn SB, Ojwang JO, Adler A, Lee H-S, Boackle SA (2012) Variation in the ICAM1–ICAM4–ICAM5 locus is associated with systemic lupus erythematosus susceptibility in multiple ancestries. Ann Rheum Dis 71:1809–1814

Kline J, Kitagaki K (2006) Interferons

Koene HR, Kleijer M, Algra J, Roos D, Kr EG, von dem Borne A, de Haas M (1997) FcγRIIIa-158V/F polymorphism influences the binding of IgG by natural killer cell FcγRIIIa, independently of the FcγRIIIa-48L/R/H phenotype. Blood, J Am Soc Hematol 90:1109–1114

Kono H, Kyogoku C, Suzuki T, Tsuchiya N, Honda H, Yamamoto K, Tokunaga K, Honda Z-I (2005) FcγRIIB Ile232Thr transmembrane polymorphism associated with human systemic lupus erythematosus decreases affinity to lipid rafts and attenuates inhibitory effects on B cell receptor signaling. Hum Mol Genet 14:2881–2892

Korman BD, Kastner DL, Gregersen PK, Remmers EF (2008) STAT4: genetics, mechanisms, and implications for autoimmunity. Curr Allergy Asthma Rep 8:398–403

Kozyrev SV, Abelson A-K, Wojcik J, Zaghlool A, Reddy MPL, Sanchez E, Gunnarsson I, Svenungsson E, Sturfelt G, Jönsen A (2008) Functional variants in the B-cell gene BANK1 are associated with systemic lupus erythematosus. Nat Genet 40:211

Krummel MF, Allison JP (1996) CTLA-4 engagement inhibits IL-2 accumulation and cell cycle progression upon activation of resting T cells. J Exp Med 183:2533–2540

Kumar KR, Li L, Yan M, Bhaskarabhatla M, Mobley AB, Nguyen C, Mooney JM, Schatzle JD, Wakeland EK, Mohan C (2006) Regulation of B cell tolerance by the lupus susceptibility gene Ly108. Science 312:1665–1669

Kunz M, König IR, Schillert A, Kruppa J, Ziegler A, Grallert H, Müller-Nurasyid M, Lieb W, Franke A, Ranki A (2015) Genome-wide association study identifies new susceptibility loci for cutaneous lupus erythematosus. Exp Dermatol 24:510–515

Kurata R, Tajima A, Yonezawa T, Inoko H (2013) TRIM39R, but not TRIM39B, regulates type I interferon response. Biochem Biophys Res Commun 436:90–95

Kwiatkowska K, Matveichuk OV, Fronk J, Ciesielska A (2020) Flotillins: at the intersection of protein Spalmitoylation and lipid-mediated signaling. Int J Mol Sci 21:2283

Kyogoku C, Dijstelbloem HM, Tsuchiya N, Hatta Y, Kato H, Yamaguchi A, Fukazawa T, Jansen MD, Hashimoto H, van de Winkel JG (2002) Fcγ receptor gene polymorphisms in Japanese patients with systemic lupus erythematosus: contribution of FCGR2B to genetic susceptibility. Arthritis Rheum 46:1242–1254

Kyogoku C, Ortmann WA, Lee A, Selby S, Carlton VE, Chang M, Ramos P, Baechler EC, Batliwalla FM, Novitzke J (2004) Genetic association of the R620W polymorphism of protein tyrosine phosphatase PTPN22 with human SLE. Am J Hum Genet 75:504–507

Kyogoku C, Tsuchiya N (2007) A compass that points to lupus: genetic studies on type I interferon pathway. Genes Immun 8:445–455

Lamagna C, Hu Y, DeFranco AL, Lowell CA (2014) B cell–specific loss of Lyn kinase leads to autoimmunity. J Immunol 192:919–928

Lan Y, Luo B, Wang J-L, Jiang Y-W, Wei Y-S (2014) The association of interleukin-21 polymorphisms with interleukin-21 serum levels and risk of systemic lupus erythematosus. Gene 538:94–98

Lande R, Ganguly D, Facchinetti V, Frasca L, Conrad C, Gregorio J, Meller S, Chamilos G, Sebasigari R, Riccieri V (2011) Neutrophils activate plasmacytoid dendritic cells by releasing self-DNA–peptide complexes in systemic lupus erythematosus. Sci Trans Med 3:73ra19–73ra19

Lauc G, Huffman JE, Pučić M, Zgaga L, Adamczyk B, Mužinić A, Novokmet M, Polašek O, Gornik O, Krištić J (2013) Loci associated with N-glycosylation of human immunoglobulin G show pleiotropy with autoimmune diseases and haematological cancers. PLoS Genet 9:e1003225

Lausch E, Janecke A, Bros M, Trojandt S, Alanay Y, De Laet C, Hübner CA, Meinecke P, Nishimura G, Matsuo M (2011) Genetic deficiency of tartrate-resistant acid phosphatase associated with skeletal dysplasia, cerebral calcifications and autoimmunity. Nat Genet 43:132–137

Lazarus M, Hajeer A, Turner D, Sinnott P, Worthington J, Ollier W, Hutchinson I (1997) Genetic variation in the interleukin 10 gene promoter and systemic lupus erythematosus. J Rheumatol 24:2314–2317

Lebedeva T, Dustin ML, Sykulev Y (2005) ICAM-1 co-stimulates target cells to facilitate antigen presentation. Curr Opin Immunol 17:251–258

Lee-Kirsch MA, Chowdhury D, Harvey S, Gong M, Senenko L, Engel K, Pfeiffer C, Hollis T, Gahr M, Perrino FW (2007) A mutation in TREX1 that impairs susceptibility to granzyme A-mediated cell death underlies familial chilblain lupus. J Mol Med 85:531–537

Lee-Kirsch MA, Gong M, Schulz H, Rüschendorf F, Stein A, Pfeiffer C, Ballarini A, Gahr M, Hubner N, Linné M (2006) Familial chilblain lupus, a monogenic form of cutaneous lupus erythematosus, maps to chromosome 3p. Am J Hum Genet 79:731–737

Lee MN, Ye C, Villani A-C, Raj T, Li W, Eisenhaure TM, Imboywa SH, Chipendo PI, Ran FA, Slowikowski K (2014) Common genetic variants modulate pathogen-sensing responses in human dendritic cells. Science 343

Lee Y, Woo J, Choi S, Ji J, Song G (2009) Association of programmed cell death 1 polymorphisms and systemic lupus erythematosus: a meta-analysis. Lupus 18:9–15

Lee YH, Bae S-C, Choi SJ, Ji JD, Song GG (2011) Associations between vitamin D receptor polymorphisms and susceptibility to rheumatoid arthritis and systemic lupus erythematosus: a meta-analysis. Mol Biol Rep 38:3643–3651

Lee YH, Choi S, Ji JD, Song GG (2016) Association between toll-like receptor polymorphisms and systemic lupus erythematosus: a meta-analysis update. Lupus 25:593–601

Lee YH, Harley JB, Nath SK (2005) CTLA-4 polymorphisms and systemic lupus erythematosus (SLE): a meta-analysis. Hum Genet 116:361–367

Lee YH, Lee HS, Choi SJ, Ji JD, Song GG (2012) Associations between TLR polymorphisms and systemic lupus erythematosus: a systematic review and meta-analysis. Clin Exp Rheumatol 30:262–265

Leffler J, Bengtsson AA, Blom AM (2014) The complement system in systemic lupus erythematosus: an update. Ann Rheum Dis 73:1601–1606

Leffler J, Herbert AP, Norström E, Schmidt CQ, Barlow PN, Blom AM, Martin M (2010) Annexin-II, DNA, and histones serve as factor H ligands on the surface of apoptotic cells. J Biol Chem 285:3766–3776

Lessard CJ, Adrianto I, Kelly JA, Kaufman KM, Grundahl KM, Adler A, Williams AH, Gallant CJ, Anaya J-M, Bae S-C (2011) Identification of a systemic lupus erythematosus susceptibility locus at 11p13 between PDHX and CD44 in a multiethnic study. Am J Hum Genet 88:83–91

Lessard CJ, Sajuthi S, Zhao J, Kim K, Ice JA, Li H, Ainsworth H, Rasmussen A, Kelly JA, Marion M (2016) Identification of a systemic lupus erythematosus risk locus spanning ATG16L2, FCHSD2, and P2RY2 in Koreans. Arthritis & Rheumatol 68:1197–1209

Li X, Ptacek TS, Brown EE, Edberg JC (2009) Fcγ receptors: structure, function and role as genetic risk factors in SLE. Genes Immun 10:380–389

Li X, Wu J, Carter RH, Edberg JC, Su K, Cooper GS, Kimberly RP (2003) A novel polymorphism in the Fcγ receptor IIB (CD32B) transmembrane region alters receptor signaling. Arthritis Rheum 48:3242–3252

Lin J, Qin H, Wang Y, Liang J, Xu J, Jh X (2016) Analysis of interleukin 19 serum levels and single nucleotide polymorphisms in systemic lupus erythematosus. Genet Mol Res 15

Lin K-I, Angelin-Duclos C, Kuo TC, Calame K (2002) Blimp-1-dependent repression of Pax-5 is required for

differentiation of B cells to immunoglobulin M-secreting plasma cells. Mol Cell Biol 22:4771–4780
Lin Y, Wong K-k, Calame K (1997) Repression of c-myc transcription by Blimp-1, an inducer of terminal B cell differentiation. Science 276:596–599
Liossis S-NC, Solomou EE, Dimopoulos M-A, Panayiotidis P, Mavrikakis MM, Sfikakis PP (2001) B-cell kinase lyn deficiency in patients with systemic lupus erythematosus. J Investig Med 49:157–165
Lipsker D, Hauptmann G (2010) Cutaneous manifestations of complement deficiencies. Lupus 19:1096–1106
Liu JL, Zhang FY, Liang YH, Xiao FL, Zhang SQ, Cheng YL, Yuan CD, Chen QP, Yang S, Zhang XJ (2009) Association between the PD1. 3A/G polymorphism of the PDCD1 gene and systemic lupus erythematosus in European populations: a meta-analysis. J Eur Acad Dermatol Venereol 23:425–432
Liu K, Liang C, Liang Z, Tus K, Wakeland EK (2005) Sle1ab mediates the aberrant activation of STAT3 and Ras-ERK signaling pathways in B lymphocytes. J Immunol 174:1630–1637
Liu P, Song J, Su H, Li L, Lu N, Yang R, Peng Z (2013) IL-10 gene polymorphisms and susceptibility to systemic lupus erythematosus: a meta-analysis. PLoS One 8:e69547
Liu T, Zhang L, Joo D, Sun S-C (2017) NF-κB signaling in inflammation. Signal Transduct Target Therapy 2:1–9
Llorente L, Richaud-Patin Y, García-Padilla C, Claret E, Jakez-Ocampo J, Cardiel MH, Alcocer-Varela J, Grangeot-Keros L, Alarcón-Segovia D, Wijdenes J (2000) Clinical and biologic effects of anti–interleukin-10 monoclonal antibody administration in systemic lupus erythematosus. Arthritis Rheum off J Am Coll Rheumatol 43:1790–1800
Llorente L, Zou W, Levy Y, Richaud-Patin Y, Wijdenes J, Alcocer-Varela J, Morel-Fourrier B, Brouet J-C, Alarcon-Segovia D, Galanaud P (1995) Role of interleukin 10 in the B lymphocyte hyperactivity and autoantibody production of human systemic lupus erythematosus. J Exp Med 181:839–844
Loos M, Heinz H-P (1986) Component deficiencies 1. The first component: Clq, Clr, Cls. Hereditary Acquir Complement Defic Anim Man 39:212–231
Lowell CA (2004) Src-family kinases: rheostats of immune cell signaling. Mol Immunol 41:631–643
Lu M-M, Ye Q-L, Feng C-C, Yang J, Zhang T, Li J, Leng R-X, Pan H-F, Yuan H, Ye D-Q (2012) Association of FAS gene polymorphisms with systemic lupus erythematosus: a case-control study and meta-analysis. Exp Therapeutic Med 4:497–502
Lu R, Vidal GS, Kelly JA, Delgado-Vega AM, Howard XK, Macwana SR, Dominguez N, Klein W, Burrell C, Harley IT (2009) Genetic associations of LYN with systemic lupus erythematosus. Genes Immun 10:397–403
Ludwig A, Otto GP, Riento K, Hams E, Fallon PG, Nichols BJ (2010) Flotillin microdomains interact with the cortical cytoskeleton to control uropod formation and neutrophil recruitment. J Cell Biol 191:771–781
Luo J, Niu X, Liu H, Zhang M, Chen M, Deng S (2013) Up-regulation of transcription factor Blimp1 in systemic lupus erythematosus. Mol Immunol 56:574–582
Macedo ACL, Isaac L (2016) Systemic lupus erythematosus and deficiencies of early components of the complement classical pathway. Front Immunol 7:55
Macias-Garcia A, Heizmann B, Sellars M, Marchal P, Dali H, Pasquali J-L, Muller S, Kastner P, Chan S (2016) Ikaros is a negative regulator of B1 cell development and function. J Biol Chem 291:9073–9086
Magnusson V, Lindqvist A-K, Castillejo-Lopez C, Kristjansdottir H, Steinsson K, Gröndal G, Sturfelt G, Truedsson L, Svenungsson E, Lundberg I (2000) Fine mapping of the SLEB2 locus involved in susceptibility to systemic lupus erythematosus. Genomics 70:307–314
Manderson AP, Botto M, Walport MJ (2004) The role of complement in the development of systemic lupus erythematosus. Annu Rev Immunol 22:431–456
Martin JC, Baeten DL, Josien R (2014) Emerging role of IL-17 and Th17 cells in systemic lupus erythematosus. Clin Immunol 154:1–12
Martínez-Bueno M, Alarcón-Riquelme ME (2019) Exploring impact of rare variation in systemic lupus erythematosus by a genome wide imputation approach. Front Immunol 10:258
Mauri C, Menon M (2015) The expanding family of regulatory B cells. Int Immunol 27:479–486
Mayeux J, Skaug B, Luo W, Russell LM, John S, Saelee P, Abbasi H, Li Q-Z, Garrett-Sinha LA, Satterthwaite AB (2015) Genetic interaction between Lyn, Ets1, and Btk in the control of antibody levels. J Immunol 195:1955–1963
Medlin JL, Hansen KE, Fitz SR, Bartels CM (2016) A systematic review and meta-analysis of cutaneous manifestations in late-versus early-onset systemic lupus erythematosus. In: Seminars in arthritis and rheumatism, vol 6. Elsevier, pp 691–697
Mehta P, Norsworthy PJ, Hall AE, Kelly SJ, Walport MJ, Botto M, Pickering MC (2010) SLE with C1q deficiency treated with fresh frozen plasma: a 10-year experience. Rheumatology 49:823–824
Melissaropoulos K, Liossis S-N (2018) Decreased CD22 expression and intracellular signaling aberrations in B cells of patients with systemic sclerosis. Rheumatol Int 38:1225–1234
Melko M, Douguet D, Bensaid M, Zongaro S, Verheggen C, Gecz J, Bardoni B (2011) Functional characterization of the AFF (AF4/FMR2) family of RNA-binding proteins: insights into the molecular pathology of FRAXE intellectual disability. Hum Mol Genet 20:1873–1885
Meller S, Winterberg F, Gilliet M, Müller A, Lauceviciute I, Rieker J, Neumann NJ, Kubitza R, Gombert M, Bünemann E (2005) Ultraviolet radiation–induced injury, chemokines, and leukocyte recruitment: an

amplification cycle triggering cutaneous lupus erythematosus. Arthritis Rheum 52:1504–1516

Merola JF, Moschella S (2016) Overview of cutaneous lupus erythematosus. UpToDate UpToDate, Waltham, MA(Accessed on September 20, 2015)

Meyer O, Hauptmann G, Tappeiner G, Ochs HD, Mascart-Lemone F (1985) Genetic deficiency of C4, C2 or C1q and lupus syndromes. Association with anti-Ro (SS-A) antibodies. Clin Exp Immunol 62:678–684

Mihlan M, Stippa S, Józsi M, Zipfel P (2009) Monomeric CRP contributes to complement control in fluid phase and on cellular surfaces and increases phagocytosis by recruiting factor H. Cell Death Differ 16:1630–1640

Millard T, McGregor J (2001a) Molecular genetics of cutaneous lupus erythematosus. Clin Exp Dermatol 26:184–191

Moisan J, Grenningloh R, Bettelli E, Oukka M, Ho I-C (2007) Ets-1 is a negative regulator of Th17 differentiation. J Exp Med 204:2825–2835

Molineros JE, Maiti AK, Sun C, Looger LL, Han S, Kim-Howard X, Glenn S, Adler A, Kelly JA, Niewold TB (2013) Admixture mapping in lupus identifies multiple functional variants within IFIH1 associated with apoptosis, inflammation, and autoantibody production. PLoS Genet 9:e1003222

Monticielo OA, de Mattos TT, Chies JAB, Brenol JCT, Xavier RM (2012) Vitamin D and polymorphisms of VDR gene in patients with systemic lupus erythematosus. Clin Rheumatol 31:1411–1421

Morgan B, Sun L, Avitahl N, Andrikopoulos K, Ikeda T, Gonzales E, Wu P, Neben S, Georgopoulos K (1997) Aiolos, a lymphoid restricted transcription factor that interacts with Ikaros to regulate lymphocyte differentiation. The EMBO J 16:2004–2013

Morris DL, Roberts AL, Witherden AS, Tarzi R, Barros P, Whittaker JC, Cook TH, Aitman TJ, Vyse TJ (2010) Evidence for both copy number and allelic (NA1/NA2) risk at the FCGR3B locus in systemic lupus erythematosus. Eur J Hum Genet 18:1027–1031

Morris DL, Taylor KE, Fernando MM, Nititham J, Alarcón-Riquelme ME, Barcellos LF, Behrens TW, Cotsapas C, Gaffney PM, Graham RR (2012) Unraveling multiple MHC gene associations with systemic lupus erythematosus: model choice indicates a role for HLA alleles and non-HLA genes in Europeans. Am J Hum Genet 91:778–793

Moser KL, Kelly JA, Lessard CJ, Harley JB (2009) Recent insights into the genetic basis of systemic lupus erythematosus. Genes Immun 10:373–379

Moulton VR, Tsokos GC (2011) Abnormalities of T cell signaling in systemic lupus erythematosus. Arthritis Res Therapy 13:1–10

Mustelin T, Bottini N, Stanford SM (2019) The contribution of PTPN22 to rheumatic disease. Arthritis Rheumatol 71:486–495

Nakou M, Papadimitraki ED, Fanouriakis A, Bertsias GK, Choulaki C, Goulidaki N, Sidiropoulos P, Boumpas DT (2013) Interleukin-21 is increased in active systemic lupus erythematosus patients and contributes to the generation of plasma B cells. Clin Exp Rheumatol 31:172–179

Namjou B, Kothari PH, Kelly JA, Glenn SB, Ojwang JO, Adler A, Alarcón-Riquelme ME, Gallant CJ, Boackle SA, Criswell LA (2011) Evaluation of the TREX1 gene in a large multi-ancestral lupus cohort. Genes Immun 12:270–279

Nath SK, Han S, Kim-Howard X, Kelly JA, Viswanathan P, Gilkeson GS, Chen W, Zhu C, McEver RP, Kimberly RP (2008) A nonsynonymous functional variant in integrin-α M (encoded by ITGAM) is associated with systemic lupus erythematosus. Nat Genet 40:152

Nath SK, Harley JB, Lee YH (2005) Polymorphisms of complement receptor 1 and interleukin-10 genes and systemic lupus erythematosus: a meta-analysis. Hum Genet 118:225

Navratil JS, Ahearn JM (2000) Apoptosis and autoimmunity: complement deficiency and systemic lupus erythematosus revisited. Curr Rheumatol Rep 2:32–38

Niewold T, Hua J, Lehman T, Harley J, Crow M (2007) High serum IFN-α activity is a heritable risk factor for systemic lupus erythematosus. Genes Immun 8:492–502

Niewold TB, Kelly JA, Kariuki SN, Franek BS, Kumar AA, Kaufman KM, Thomas K, Walker D, Kamp S, Frost JM (2012) IRF5 haplotypes demonstrate diverse serological associations which predict serum interferon alpha activity and explain the majority of the genetic association with systemic lupus erythematosus. Ann Rheum Dis 71:463–469

Nimmerjahn F (2006) Activating and inhibitory FcγRs in autoimmune disorders. In: Springer seminars in immunopathology, vol 4. Springer, pp 305–319

Nimmerjahn F, Ravetch JV (2006) Fcγ receptors: old friends and new family members. Immunity 24:19–28

Nimmerjahn F, Ravetch JV (2008) Fcγ receptors as regulators of immune responses. Nat Rev Immunol 8:34–47

Nishimura H, Agata Y, Kawasaki A, Sato M, Imamura S, Minato N, Yagita H, Nakano T, Honjo T (1996) Developmentally regulated expression of the PD-1 protein on the surface of double-negative (CD4–CD8–) thymocytes. Int Immunol 8:773–780

Nishimura H, Nose M, Hiai H, Minato N, Honjo T (1999) Development of lupus-like autoimmune diseases by disruption of the PD-1 gene encoding an ITIM motif-carrying immunoreceptor. Immunity 11:141–151

Oddie G, Schenk G, Angel N, Walsh N, Guddat L, De Jersey J, Cassady A, Hamilton S, Hume D (2000) Structure, function, and regulation of tartrate-resistant acid phosphatase. Bone 27:575–584

Ohl K, Tenbrock K (2011) Inflammatory cytokines in systemic lupus erythematosus. J Biomed Biotechnol 2011

Okada Y, Shimane K, Kochi Y, Tahira T, Suzuki A, Higasa K, Takahashi A, Horita T, Atsumi T, Ishii T (2012) A genome-wide association study identified

AFF1 as a susceptibility locus for systemic lupus eyrthematosus in Japanese. PLoS Genet 8:e1002455

Omori SA, Cato MH, Anzelon-Mills A, Puri KD, Shapiro-Shelef M, Calame K, Rickert RC (2006) Regulation of class-switch recombination and plasma cell differentiation by phosphatidylinositol 3-kinase signaling. Immunity 25:545–557

Oosterwegel MA, Greenwald RJ, Mandelbrot DA, Lorsbach RB, Sharpe AH (1999) CTLA-4 and T cell activation. Curr Opin Immunol 11:294–300

Orru V, Tsai SJ, Rueda B, Fiorillo E, Stanford SM, Dasgupta J, Hartiala J, Zhao L, Ortego-Centeno N, D'Alfonso S (2009) A loss-of-function variant of PTPN22 is associated with reduced risk of systemic lupus erythematosus. Hum Mol Genet 18:569–579

Ortiz G (2019) Association of TLR7 copy number variation with susceptibility to childhood-onset systemic lupus erythematosus in Mexican population

Ota M, Katsuyama Y, Mizuki N, Ando H, Furihata K, Ono S, Pivetti-Pezzi P, Tabbara K, Palimeris G, Nikbin B (1997) Trinucleotide repeat polymorphism within exon 5 of the MICA gene (MHC class I chain-related gene A): allele frequency data in the nine population groups Japanese, Northern Han, Hui, Uygur, Kazakhstan, Iranian, Saudi Arabian, Greek and Italian. Tissue Antigens 49:448–454

Pan H-F, Leng R-X, Tao J-H, Li X-P, Ye D-Q (2011) Ets-1: a new player in the pathogenesis of systemic lupus erythematosus? Lupus 20:227–230

Pan L, Lu M-P, Wang J-H, Xu M, Yang S-R (2020) Immunological pathogenesis and treatment of systemic lupus erythematosus. World J Pediatr 16:19–30

Park Y, Lee S, Kim D, Lee J, Lee C, Song C (1998) Elevated interleukin-10 levels correlated with disease activity in systemic lupus erythematosus. Clin Exp Rheumatol 16:283–288

Park YW, Kee SJ, Cho YN, Lee EH, Lee HY, Kim EM, Shin MH, Park JJ, Kim TJ, Lee SS (2009) Impaired differentiation and cytotoxicity of natural killer cells in systemic lupus erythematosus. Arthritis Rheum off J Am Coll Rheumatol 60:1753–1763

Parry RV, Chemnitz JM, Frauwirth KA, Lanfranco AR, Braunstein I, Kobayashi SV, Linsley PS, Thompson CB, Riley JL (2005) CTLA-4 and PD-1 receptors inhibit T-cell activation by distinct mechanisms. Mol Cell Biol 25:9543–9553

Paul E, Pozdnyakova OO, Mitchell E, Carroll MC (2002) Anti-DNA autoreactivity in C4-deficient mice. Eur J Immunol 32:2672–2679

Perdomo J, Holmes M, Chong B, Crossley M (2000) Eos and pegasus, two members of the Ikaros family of proteins with distinct DNA binding activities. J Biol Chem 275:38347–38354

Petri M, Orbai AM, Alarcón GS, Gordon C, Merrill JT, Fortin PR, Bruce IN, Isenberg D, Wallace DJ, Nived O (2012) Derivation and validation of the systemic lupus international collaborating clinics classification criteria for systemic lupus erythematosus. Arthritis Rheum 64:2677–2686

Pickart CM (2001) Mechanisms underlying ubiquitination. Ann Rev Biochem 70

Pickering M, Botto M, Taylor P, Lachmann P, Walport M (2000) Systemic lupus erythematosus, complement deficiency, and apoptosis. Adv Immunol 76:226–324

Piskurich JF, Lin K-I, Lin Y, Wang Y, Ting JP-Y, Calame K (2000) BLIMP-1 mediates extinction of major histocompatibility class II transactivator expression in plasma cells. Nat Immunol 1:526–532

Poole BD, Scofield RH, Harley JB, James JA (2006) Epstein-Barr virus and molecular mimicry in systemic lupus erythematosus. Autoimmunity 39:63–70

Pore D, Huang E, Dejanovic D, Parameswaran N, Cheung MB, Gupta N (2018) Cutting edge: deletion of Ezrin in B cells of lyn-deficient mice downregulates lupus pathology. J Immunol 201:1353–1358

Powell MD, Read KA, Sreekumar BK, Oestreich KJ (2019) Ikaros zinc finger transcription factors: regulators of cytokine signaling pathways and CD4+ T helper cell differentiation. Front Immunol 10:1299

Qi J, Qi J, Xiang L, Nie G (2015) Association between IL-21 polymorphism and systemic lupus erythematosus: a meta-analysis. Genet Mol Res 14:603

Racila D, Sontheimer C, Sheffield A, Wisnieski J, Racila E, Sontheimer R (2003) Homozygous single nucleotide polymorphism of the complement C1QA gene is associated with decreased levels of C1q in patients with subacute cutaneous lupus erythematosus. Lupus 12:124–132

Rafi A, Nagarkatti M, Nagarkatti PS (1997) Hyaluronate-CD44 interactions can induce murine B-cell activation. Blood J Am Soc Hematol 89:2901–2908

Rajabi F, Drake L, Senna M, Rezaei N (2018) Alopecia areata: a review of disease pathogenesis. Br J Dermatol 179:1033–1048

Ramos PS, Williams AH, Ziegler JT, Comeau ME, Guy RT, Lessard CJ, Li H, Edberg JC, Zidovetzki R, Criswell LA (2011) Genetic analyses of interferon pathway–related genes reveal multiple new loci associated with systemic lupus erythematosus. Arthritis Rheum 63:2049–2057

Redpath GM, Ecker M, Kapoor-Kaushik N, Vartoukian H, Carnell M, Kempe D, Biro M, Ariotti N, Rossy J (2019) Flotillins promote T cell receptor sorting through a fast Rab5–Rab11 endocytic recycling axis. Nat Commun 10:1–14

Reefman E, Kuiper H, Jonkman MF, Limburg PC, Kallenberg CG, Bijl M (2006) Skin sensitivity to UVB irradiation in systemic lupus erythematosus is not related to the level of apoptosis induction in keratinocytes. Rheumatology 45:538–544

Ren CL, Morio T, Fu SM, Geha RS (1994) Signal transduction via CD40 involves activation of lyn kinase and phosphatidylinositol-3-kinase, and phosphorylation of phospholipase C gamma 2. J Exp Med 179:673–680

Rianthavorn P, Chokedeemeeboon C, Deekajorndech T, Suphapeetiporn K (2013) Interleukin-10 promoter polymorphisms and expression in Thai children with juvenile systemic lupus erythematosus. Lupus 22:721–726

Richardson BC (2019) Drug-induced lupus erythematosus. In: Dubois' lupus erythematosus and related syndromes. Elsevier, pp 377–388

Ristich V, Liang S, Zhang W, Wu J, Horuzsko A (2005) Tolerization of dendritic cells by HLA-G. Eur J Immunol 35:1133–1142

Robinson T, Kariuki SN, Franek BS, Kumabe M, Kumar AA, Badaracco M, Mikolaitis RA, Guerrero G, Utset TO, Drevlow BE (2011) Autoimmune disease risk variant of IFIH1 is associated with increased sensitivity to IFN-α and serologic autoimmunity in lupus patients. J Immunol 187:1298–1303

Rødgaard A, Thomsen S, Bendixen G, Bendtzen K (1995) Increased expression of complement receptor type 1 (CR1, CD35) on human peripheral blood T lymphocytes after polyclonal activation in vitro. Immunol Res 14:69

Rodig N, Ryan T, Allen JA, Pang H, Grabie N, Chernova T, Greenfield EA, Liang SC, Sharpe AH, Lichtman AH (2003) Endothelial expression of PD-L1 and PD-L2 down-regulates CD8+ T cell activation and cytolysis. Eur J Immunol 33:3117–3126

Rönnblom L, Eloranta ML, Alm GV (2006) The type I interferon system in systemic lupus erythematosus. Arthritis Rheum off J Am Coll Rheumatol 54:408–420

Rönnblom L, Leonard D (2019) Interferon pathway in SLE: one key to unlocking the mystery of the disease. Lupus Sci Med 6:e000270

Rosborough BR, Hackstein H, Turnquist HR (2014) A window into immunosuppressant immunoregulation: recipient conversion to rapamycin increases potentially tolerogenic immune cells. Kidney Int 85:743–745

Rosetti F, Mayadas TN (2016) The many faces of Mac-1 in autoimmune disease. Immunol Rev 269:175–193

Rosetti F, Tsuboi N, Chen K, Nishi H, Ernandez T, Sethi S, Croce K, Stavrakis G, Alcocer-Varela J, Gómez-Martin D (2012) Human lupus serum induces neutrophil-mediated organ damage in mice that is enabled by Mac-1 deficiency. J Immunol 189:3714–3723

Rueda B, Pascual M, López-Nevot M, Gonzalez E, Martín J (2002) A new allele within the transmembrane region of the human MICA gene with seven GCT repeats. Tissue Antigens 60:526–528

Ruiz-Larrañaga O, Migliorini P, Uribarri M, Czirják L, Alcaro MC, Del Amo J, Iriondo M, Manzano C, Escorza-Treviño S, Estonba A (2016) Genetic association study of systemic lupus erythematosus and disease subphenotypes in European populations. Clin Rheumatol 35:1161–1168

Salemme R, Peralta LN, Meka SH, Pushpanathan N, Alexander JJ (2019) The role of NETosis in systemic lupus erythematosus. J Cell Immunol 1:33

Salloum R, Franek BS, Kariuki SN, Rhee L, Mikolaitis RA, Jolly M, Utset TO, Niewold TB (2010) Genetic variation at the IRF7/PHRF1 locus is associated with autoantibody profile and serum interferon-α activity in lupus patients. Arthritis Rheum off J Am Coll Rheumatol 62:553–561

Salmon JE, Edberg JC, Brogle NL, Kimberly RP (1992) Allelic polymorphisms of human Fc gamma receptor IIA and Fc gamma receptor IIIB. Independent mechanisms for differences in human phagocyte function. J Clin Investig 89:1274–1281

Salmon JE, Millard S, Schachter LA, Arnett FC, Ginzler EM, Gourley MF, Ramsey-Goldman R, Peterson M, Kimberly RP (1996) Fc gamma RIIA alleles are heritable risk factors for lupus nephritis in African Americans. J Clin Investig 97:1348–1354

Samuelson EM, Laird RM, Maue AC, Rochford R, Hayes SM (2012) Blk haploinsufficiency impairs the development, but enhances the functional responses, of MZ B cells. Immunol Cell Biol 90:620–629

Sánchez E, Comeau ME, Freedman BI, Kelly JA, Kaufman KM, Langefeld CD, Brown EE, Alarcón GS, Kimberly RP, Edberg JC (2011) Identification of novel genetic susceptibility loci in African American lupus patients in a candidate gene association study. Arthritis Rheum 63:3493–3501

Sanchez E, Nadig A, Richardson BC, Freedman BI, Kaufman KM, Kelly JA, Niewold TB, Kamen DL, Gilkeson GS, Ziegler JT (2011) Phenotypic associations of genetic susceptibility loci in systemic lupus erythematosus. Ann Rheum Dis 70:1752–1757

Sanchez E, Torres B, Vilches J, Lopez-Nevot M, Ortego-Centeno N, Jimenez-Alonso J, Gonzalez-Gay M, de Ramon E, Sanchez-Roman J, Nunez-Roldan A (2006) No primary association of MICA polymorphism with systemic lupus erythematosus. Rheumatology 45:1096–1100

Sasai M, Linehan MM, Iwasaki A (2010) Bifurcation of Toll-like receptor 9 signaling by adaptor protein 3. Science 329:1530–1534

Sawalha AH, Kaufman KM, Kelly JA, Adler AJ, Aberle T, Kilpatrick J, Wakeland EK, Li Q-Z, Wandstrat AE, Karp D (2008) Genetic association of interleukin-21 polymorphisms with systemic lupus erythematosus. Ann Rheum Dis 67:458–461

Schwartzberg PL, Mueller KL, Qi H, Cannons JL (2009) SLAM receptors and SAP influence lymphocyte interactions, development and function. Nat Rev Immunol 9:39–46

Seelig HP, Ehrfeld H, Renz M (1994) Interferon-γ–inducible protein p16. a new target of antinuclear antibodies in patients with systemic lupus erythematosus. Arthritis Rheum off J Am Coll Rheumatol 37:1672–1683

Seery JP (2000) IFN-γ transgenic mice: clues to the pathogenesis of systemic lupus erythematosus? Arthritis Res Ther 2:1–4

Sekine H, Ferreira RC, Pan-Hammarström Q, Graham RR, Ziemba B, De Vries SS, Liu J, Hippen K, Koeuth T, Ortmann W (2007) Role for Msh5 in the regulation of Ig class switch recombination. Proc Natl Acad Sci 104:7193–7198

Sela U, Mauermann N, Hershkoviz R, Zinger H, Dayan M, Cahalon L, Liu JP, Mozes E, Lider O

(2005) The inhibition of autoreactive T cell functions by a peptide based on the CDR1 of an anti-DNA autoantibody is via TGF-β-mediated suppression of LFA-1 and CD44 expression and function. J Immunol 175:7255–7263

Sellars M, Reina-San-Martin B, Kastner P, Chan S (2009) Ikaros controls isotype selection during immunoglobulin class switch recombination. J Exp Med 206:1073–1087

Shen L, Zhang H, Caimol M, Benike CJ, Chakravarty EF, Strober S, Engleman EG (2015) Invariant natural killer T cells in lupus patients promote IgG and IgG autoantibody production. Eur J Immunol 45:612–623

Shen N, Fu Q, Deng Y, Qian X, Zhao J, Kaufman KM, Wu YL, Yu CY, Tang Y, Chen J-Y (2010) Sex-specific association of X-linked Toll-like receptor 7 (TLR7) with male systemic lupus erythematosus. Proc Natl Acad Sci 107:15838–15843

Sheng Y-J, Gao J-P, Li J, Han J-W, Xu Q, Hu W-L, Pan T-M, Cheng Y-L, Yu Z-Y, Ni C (2011) Follow-up study identifies two novel susceptibility loci PRKCB and 8p11. 21 for systemic lupus erythematosus. Rheumatology 50:682–688

Siegelman MH, DeGrendele HC, Estess P (1999) Activation and interaction of CD44 and hyaluronan in immunological systems. J Leukoc Biol 66:315–321

Simpfendorfer KR, Armstead BE, Shih A, Li W, Curran M, Manjarrez-Orduño N, Lee AT, Diamond B, Gregersen PK (2015) Autoimmune disease–associated haplotypes of BLK exhibit lowered thresholds for B cell activation and expansion of Ig class-switched B cells. Arthritis Rheumatol 67:2866–2876

Singh B, Borden P, Molineros J, Sun C, Looger L, Nath S (2017) Intronic variants of the B-cell proliferator RASGRP3 affect its expression, and might contribute to lupus risk. In: Arthritis & rheumatology. Wiley 111 River St, Hoboken 07030-5774, NJ USA

Siriboonrit U, Tsuchiya N, Sirikong M, Kyogoku C, Bejrachandra S, Suthipinittharm P, Luangtrakool K, Srinak D, Thongpradit R, Fujiwara K (2003) Association of Fcγ receptor IIb and IIIb polymorphisms with susceptibility to systemic lupus erythematosus in Thais. Tissue Antigens 61:374–383

Slaughter N, Laux I, Tu X, Whitelegge J, Zhu X, Effros R, Bickel P, Nel A (2003) The flotillins are integral membrane proteins in lipid rafts that contain TCR-associated signaling components: implications for T-cell activation. Clin Immunol 108:138–151

Snowden T, Acharya S, Butz C, Berardini M, Fishel R (2004) hMSH4-hMSH5 recognizes holiday junctions and forms a meiosis-specific sliding clamp that embraces homologous chromosomes. Mol Cell 15:437–451

Solovjov DA, Pluskota E, Plow EF (2005) Distinct roles for the α and β subunits in the functions of integrin αMβ2. J Biol Chem 280:1336–1345

Song G, Lee Y (2017) Association between BLK polymorphisms and susceptibility to SLE. Zeitschrift Für Rheumatol 76:176–182

Song YW, Han CW, Kang SW, Baek HJ, Lee EB, Shin CH, Hahn BH, Tsao BP (1998) Abnormal distribution of Fcγ receptor type IIa polymorphisms in Korean patients with systemic lupus erythematosus. Arthritis Rheum off J Am Col Rheumatol 41:421–426

Soroosh P, Ine S, Sugamura K, Ishii N (2006) OX40-OX40 ligand interaction through T cell-T cell contact contributes to CD4 T cell longevity. J Immunol 176:5975–5987

Stetson DB, Ko JS, Heidmann T, Medzhitov R (2008) Trex1 prevents cell-intrinsic initiation of autoimmunity. Cell 134:587–598

Stüber E, Strober W (1996) The T cell-B cell interaction via OX40-OX40L is necessary for the T cell-dependent humoral immune response. J Exp Med 183:979–989

Su K, Li X, Edberg JC, Wu J, Ferguson P, Kimberly RP (2004a) A promoter haplotype of the immunoreceptor tyrosine-based inhibitory motif-bearing FcγRIIb alters receptor expression and associates with autoimmunity. II. Differential binding of GATA4 and Yin-Yang1 transcription factors and correlated receptor expression and function. J Immunol 172:7192–7199

Su K, Wu J, Edberg JC, Li X, Ferguson P, Cooper GS, Langefeld CD, Kimberly RP (2004b) A promoter haplotype of the immunoreceptor tyrosine-based inhibitory motif-bearing FcγRIIb alters receptor expression and associates with autoimmunity. I. Regulatory FCGR2B polymorphisms and their association with systemic lupus erythematosus. J Immunol 172:7186–7191

Su TT, Guo B, Kawakami Y, Sommer K, Chae K, Humphries LA, Kato RM, Kang S, Patrone L, Wall R (2002) PKC-β controls IκB kinase lipid raft recruitment and activation in response to BCR signaling. Nat Immunol 3:780–786

Suarez-Gestal M, Ferreiros-Vidal I, Ortiz J, Gomez-Reino J, Gonzalez A (2008) Analysis of the functional relevance of a putative regulatory SNP of PDCD1, PD1. 3, associated with systemic lupus erythematosus. Genes Immun 9:309–315

Suciu-Foca N, Cortesini R (2007) Central role of ILT3 in the T suppressor cell cascade. Cell Immunol 248:59–67

Suemizu H, Radosavljevic M, Kimura M, Sadahiro S, Yoshimura S, Bahram S, Inoko H (2002) A basolateral sorting motif in the MICA cytoplasmic tail. Proc Natl Acad Sci 99:2971–2976

Sullivan K, Petri M, Schmeckpeper B, McLean R, Winkelstein J (1994) Prevalence of a mutation causing C2 deficiency in systemic lupus erythematosus. J Rheumatol 21:1128–1133

Sullivan KE, Piliero LM, Dharia T, Goldman D, Petri MA (2000) 3′ polymorphisms of ETS1 are associated with different clinical phenotypes in SLE. Hum Mutat 16:49–53

Sun H, Xia Y, Wang L, Wang Y, Chang X (2013) PSORS1C1 may be involved in rheumatoid arthritis. Immunol Lett 153:9–14

Sun L, Chen ZJ (2004) The novel functions of ubiquitination in signaling. Curr Opin Cell Biol 16:119–126

Suzuki M, Watanabe M, Nakamaru Y, Takagi D, Takahashi H, Fukuda S, Hatakeyama S (2016) TRIM39 negatively regulates the NFκB-mediated signaling pathway through stabilization of Cactin. Cell Mol Life Sci 73:1085–1101

Takahashi T, Tagami T, Yamazaki S, Uede T, Shimizu J, Sakaguchi N, Mak TW, Sakaguchi S (2000) Immunologic self-tolerance maintained by CD25+ CD4+ regulatory T cells constitutively expressing cytotoxic T lymphocyte–associated antigen 4. J Exp Med 192:303–310

Tamura T, Yanai H, Savitsky D, Taniguchi T (2008) The IRF family transcription factors in immunity and oncogenesis. Annu Rev Immunol 26:535–584

Tan M, Hao J, Chu H, Wang F, Song D, Zhu L, Yu F, Li Y, Song Y, Zhao M (2017) Genetic variants in FH are associated with renal histopathologic subtypes of lupus nephritis: a large cohort study from China. Lupus 26:1309–1317

Tang T, Rosenkranz A, Assmann KJ, Goodman MJ, Gutierrez-Ramos J-C, Carroll MC, Cotran RS, Mayadas TN (1997) A role for Mac-1 (CDIIb/CD18) in immune complex–stimulated neutrophil function in vivo: Mac-1 deficiency abrogates sustained Fcγ receptor–dependent neutrophil adhesion and complement-dependent proteinuria in acute glomerulonephritis. J Exp Med 186:1853–1863

Tanida I (2011) Autophagosome formation and molecular mechanism of autophagy. Antioxid Redox Signal 14:2201–2214

Tao J-H, Zou Y-F, Feng X-L, Li J, Wang F, Pan F-M, Ye D-Q (2011) Meta-analysis of TYK2 gene polymorphisms association with susceptibility to autoimmune and inflammatory diseases. Mol Biol Rep 38:4663–4672

Taylor KE, Chung SA, Graham RR, Ortmann WA, Lee AT, Langefeld CD, Jacob CO, Kamboh MI, Alarcón-Riquelme ME, Tsao BP (2011) Risk alleles for systemic lupus erythematosus in a large case-control collection and associations with clinical subphenotypes. PLoS Genet 7:e1001311

Tebbe B, Orfanos C (1997) Epidemiology and socioeconomic impact of skin disease in lupus erythematosus. Lupus 6:96–104

Termeer C, Benedix F, Sleeman J, Fieber C, Voith U, Ahrens T, Miyake K, Freudenberg M, Galanos C, Simon JC (2002) Oligosaccharides of Hyaluronan activate dendritic cells via toll-like receptor 4. J Exp Med 195:99–111

Terrier B, Costedoat-Chalumeau N, Garrido M, Geri G, Rosenzwajg M, Musset L, Klatzmann D, Saadoun D, Cacoub P (2012) Interleukin 21 correlates with T cell and B cell subset alterations in systemic lupus erythematosus. J Rheumatol 39:1819–1828

Texido G, Su I-h, Mecklenbräuker I, Saijo K, Malek SN, Desiderio S, Rajewsky K, Tarakhovsky A (2000) The B-cell-specific Src-family kinase Blk is dispensable for B-cell development and activation. Mol Cell Biol 20:1227–1233

Tian G, Li J-L, Wang D-G, Zhou D (2014) Targeting IL-10 in auto-immune diseases. Cell Biochem Biophys 70:37–49

Tivol EA, Borriello F, Schweitzer AN, Lynch WP, Bluestone JA, Sharpe AH (1995) Loss of CTLA-4 leads to massive lymphoproliferation and fatal multiorgan tissue destruction, revealing a critical negative regulatory role of CTLA-4. Immunity 3:541–547

Traustadottir KH, Sigfusson A, Steinsson K, Erlendsson K (2002) C4A deficiency and elevated level of immune complexes: the mechanism behind increased susceptibility to systemic lupus erythematosus. J Rheumatol 29:2359–2366

Truedsson L, Bengtsson AA, Sturfelt G (2007) Complement deficiencies and systemic lupus erythematosus. Autoimmunity 40:560–566

Ulges A, Klein M, Reuter S, Gerlitzki B, Hoffmann M, Grebe N, Staudt V, Stergiou N, Bohn T, Brühl T-J (2015) Protein kinase CK2 enables regulatory T cells to suppress excessive TH 2 responses in vivo. Nat Immunol 16:267–275

Umare V, Pradhan V, Nadkar M, Rajadhyaksha A, Patwardhan M, Ghosh KK, Nadkarni AH (2014) Effect of proinflammatory cytokines (IL-6, TNF-α, and IL-1β) on clinical manifestations in Indian SLE patients. Mediat Inflamm

Valés-Gómez M (2015) The impact of glycosylphosphatidyl-inositol anchored MICA alleles on novel NKG2D-based therapies. Front Immunol 6

Van de Stolpe A, Van der Saag P (1996) Intercellular adhesion molecule-1. J Mol Med 74:13–33

Van Kaer L, Wu L (2018) Therapeutic potential of invariant natural killer T cells in autoimmunity. Front Immunol 9:519

van Roon JA (2007) Activating and inhibitory Fcγ receptors in rheumatoid arthritis: from treatment to targeted therapies. BioMed Central

Van Tol S, Hage A, Giraldo MI, Bharaj P, Rajsbaum R (2017) The TRIMendous role of TRIMs in virus–host interactions. Vaccines 5:23

Vang T, Landskron J, Viken MK, Oberprieler N, Torgersen KM, Mustelin T, Tasken K, Tautz L, Rickert RC, Lie BA (2013) The autoimmune-predisposing variant of lymphoid tyrosine phosphatase favors T helper 1 responses. Hum Immunol 74:574–585

Vang T, Miletic AV, Bottini N, Mustelin T (2007) Protein tyrosine phosphatase PTPN22 in human autoimmunity. Autoimmunity 40:453–461

Veillette A (2010) SLAM-family receptors: immune regulators with or without SAP-family adaptors. Cold Spring Harb Perspect Biol 2:a002469

Vené R, Delfino L, Castellani P, Balza E, Bertolotti M, Sitia R, Rubartelli A (2010) Redox remodeling allows and controls B-cell activation and differentiation. Antioxid Redox Signal 13:1145–1155

Vital EM, Wittmann M, Edward S, Md Yusof MY, MacIver H, Pease CT, Goodfield M, Emery P (2015) Brief report: responses to rituximab suggest B cell–

independent inflammation in cutaneous systemic lupus erythematosus. Arthritis Rheumatol 67:1586–1591

Vlad G, Chang C-C, Colovai AI, Vasilescu ER, Cortesini R, Suciu-Foca N (2010) Membrane and soluble ILT3 are critical to the generation of T suppressor cells and induction of immunological tolerance. Int Rev Immunol 29:119–132

Vlad G, Suciu-Foca N (2012) Induction of antigen-specific human T suppressor cells by membrane and soluble ILT3. Exp Mol Pathol 93:294–301

Wandstrat AE, Nguyen C, Limaye N, Chan AY, Subramanian S, Tian X-H, Yim Y-S, Pertsemlidis A, Garner HR Jr, Morel L (2004) Association of extensive polymorphisms in the SLAM/CD2 gene cluster with murine lupus. Immunity 21:769–780

Wang D, John SA, Clements JL, Percy DH, Barton KP, Garrett-Sinha LA (2005a) Ets-1 deficiency leads to altered B cell differentiation, hyperresponsiveness to TLR9 and autoimmune disease. Int Immunol 17:1179–1191

Wang F-m, Yu F, Tan Y, Song D, Zhao M-h (2012a) Serum complement factor H is associated with clinical and pathological activities of patients with lupus nephritis. Rheumatology 51:2269–2277

Wang F, Song D, Pang Y, Song Y, Yu F, Zhao M (2016) The dysfunctions of complement factor H in lupus nephritis. Lupus 25:1328–1340

Wang J-H, Avitahl N, Cariappa A, Friedrich C, Ikeda T, Renold A, Andrikopoulos K, Liang L, Pillai S, Morgan BA (1998) Aiolos regulates B cell activation and maturation to effector state. Immunity 9:543–553

Wang J, Yoshida T, Nakaki F, Hiai H, Okazaki T, Honjo T (2005b) Establishment of NOD-Pdcd1-/-mice as an efficient animal model of type I diabetes. Proc Natl Acad Sci 102:11823–11828

Wang S, Adrianto I, Wiley GB, Lessard CJ, Kelly JA, Adler AJ, Glenn SB, Williams AH, Ziegler JT, Comeau ME (2012b) A functional haplotype of UBE2L3 confers risk for systemic lupus erythematosus. Genes Immun 13:380–387

Wang S, Wang J, Kumar V, Karnell JL, Naiman B, Gross PS, Rahman S, Zerrouki K, Hanna R, Morehouse C (2018) IL-21 drives expansion and plasma cell differentiation of autoreactive CD11c hi T-bet+ B cells in SLE. Nat Commun 9:1–14

Webb R, Merrill JT, Kelly JA, Sestak A, Kaufman KM, Langefeld CD, Ziegler J, Kimberly RP, Edberg JC, Ramsey-Goldman R (2009) A polymorphism within IL21R confers risk for systemic lupus erythematosus. Arthritis Rheum off J Am Coll Rheumatol 60:2402–2407

Weber GF (2004) The absence of CD44 ameliorates Faslpr/lpr disease. Autoimmunity 37:1–8

Wenzel J (2019) Cutaneous lupus erythematosus: new insights into pathogenesis and therapeutic strategies. Nat Rev Rheumatol 15:519–532

Willcocks LC, Lyons PA, Clatworthy MR, Robinson JI, Yang W, Newland SA, Plagnol V, McGovern NN, Condliffe AM, Chilvers ER (2008) Copy number of FCGR3B, which is associated with systemic lupus erythematosus, correlates with protein expression and immune complex uptake. J Exp Med 205:1573–1582

Wilusz JE, JnBaptiste CK, Lu LY, Kuhn C-D, Joshua-Tor L, Sharp PA (2012) A triple helix stabilizes the 3′ ends of long noncoding RNAs that lack poly (A) tails. Genes Dev 26:2392–2407

Wolf SJ, Estadt SN, Gudjonsson JE, Kahlenberg JM (2018) Human and murine evidence for mechanisms driving autoimmune photosensitivity. Front Immunol 9:2430

Wu J, Edberg JC, Redecha PB, Bansal V, Guyre PM, Coleman K, Salmon JE, Kimberly RP (1997) A novel polymorphism of FcgammaRIIIa (CD16) alters receptor function and predisposes to autoimmune disease. J Clin Investig 100:1059–1070

Wu Y-Y, Georg I, Díaz-Barreiro A, Varela N, Lauwerys B, Kumar R, Bagavant H, Castillo-Martín M, El Salem F, Marañón C (2015) Concordance of increased B1 cell subset and lupus phenotypes in mice and humans is dependent on BLK expression levels. J Immunol 194:5692–5702

Wu Y-Y, Kumar R, Dozmorov M, Haque M, Wren J, Castillejo-López C, Alarcón-Riquelme M (2013) BANK1 controls IL-6 secretion and a Type I interferon signature via a p38 and MNK1/2-eIF4E translation initiation pathway (P4060). Am Assoc Immnol

Wu Y-Y, Kumar R, Iida R, Bagavant H, Alarcon-Riquelme M (2016) BANK1 controls IgG production through TLR7-dependent STAT1 activation in a lupus model. Am Assoc Immnol

Xiang N, Li X-m, Wang G-s, Tao J-h, Li X-p (2013) Association of Fas gene polymorphisms with systemic lupus erythematosus: a meta-analysis. Mol Biol Rep 40:407–415

Xu Y, Harder KW, Huntington ND, Hibbs ML, Tarlinton DM (2005) Lyn tyrosine kinase: accentuating the positive and the negative. Immunity 22:9–18

Xu Y, Huntington ND, Harder KW, Nandurkar H, Hibbs ML, Tarlinton DM (2012) Phosphatidylinositol-3 kinase activity in B cells is negatively regulated by Lyn tyrosine kinase. Immunol Cell Biol 90:903–911

Yamada M, Katsuma S, Adachi T, Hirasawa A, Shiojima S, Kadowaki T, Okuno Y, Koshimizu T-a, Fujii S, Sekiya Y (2005) Inhibition of protein kinase CK2 prevents the progression of glomerulonephritis. Proc Natl Acad Sci 102:7736–7741

Yamamoto K, Fujiyama Y, Andoh A, Bamba T, Okabe H (2001) Oxidative stress increases MICA and MICB gene expression in the human colon carcinoma cell line (CaCo-2). Biochimica et Biophysica Acta (BBA)-General Subjects 1526:10–12

Yang W, Shen N, Ye DQ, Liu Q, Zhang Y, Qian XX, Hirankarn N, Ying D, Pan HF, Mok CC (2010) Genome-wide association study in Asian populations identifies variants in ETS1 and WDFY4 associated with systemic lupus erythematosus. PLoS Genet 6: e1000841

Yao Y, Wang J, Xin M, Li H, Liu B, Wang L, Wang L, Zhao L (2016) Balance between inflammatory and regulatory cytokines in systemic lupus erythematosus. Genet Mol Res 15:1–8

Yasutomo K, Horiuchi T, Kagami S, Tsukamoto H, Hashimura C, Urushihara M, Kuroda Y (2001) Mutation of DNASE1 in people with systemic lupus erythematosus. Nat Genet 28:313–314

Yazdani R, Ganjalikhani-Hakemi M, Esmaeili M, Abolhassani H, Vaeli S, Rezaei A, Sharifi Z, Azizi G, Rezaei N, Aghamohammadi A (2017) Impaired Akt phosphorylation in B-cells of patients with common variable immunodeficiency. Clin Immunol 175:124–132

Ye X, Zhou X-J, Zhang H (2018) Exploring the role of autophagy-related gene 5 (ATG5) yields important insights into autophagy in autoimmune/autoinflammatory diseases. Front Immunol 9:2334

Yoshida K, Komai K, Shiozawa K, Mashida A, Horiuchi T, Tanaka Y, Nose M, Hashiramoto A, Shiozawa S (2011) Role of the MICA polymorphism in systemic lupus erythematosus. Arthritis Rheum 63:3058–3066

Yoshida K, Yukiyama Y, Miyamoto T (1986) Interaction between immune complexes and C3b receptors on erythrocytes. Clin Immunol Immunopathol 39:213–221

Yousefi S, Perozzo R, Schmid I, Ziemiecki A, Schaffner T, Scapozza L, Brunner T, Simon H-U (2006) Calpain-mediated cleavage of Atg5 switches autophagy to apoptosis. Nat Cell Biol 8:1124–1132

Yu C, Chang C, Zhang J (2013) Immunologic and genetic considerations of cutaneous lupus erythematosus: a comprehensive review. J Autoimmun 41:34–45

Yung S, Chan TM (2012) The role of hyaluronan and CD44 in the pathogenesis of lupus nephritis. Autoimmune Dis

Zhang D-M, Cheng L-Q, Zhai Z-F, Feng L, Zhong B-Y, You Y, Zhang N, Song Z-Q, Yang X-C, Chen F-R (2013) Single-nucleotide polymorphism and haplotypes of TNIP1 associated with systemic lupus erythematosus in a Chinese Han population. J Rheumatol 40:1535–1544

Zhang M, Chen F, Zhang D, Zhai Z, Hao F (2016) Association study between SLC15A4 polymorphisms and haplotypes and systemic lupus erythematosus in a Han Chinese population. Genet Test Mol Biomark 20:451–458

Zhang X, Mei D, Zhang L, Wei W (2020) Src family protein kinase controls the fate of B cells in autoimmune diseases. Inflammation 1–11

Zhang YM, Cheng FJ, Zhou XJ, Qi YY, Hou P, Zhao MH, Zhang H (2015) Detecting genetic associations between ATG5 and lupus nephritis by trans-eQTL. J Immunol Res

Zhao J, Wu H, Khosravi M, Cui H, Qian X, Kelly JA, Kaufman KM, Langefeld CD, Williams AH, Comeau ME (2011) Association of genetic variants in complement factor H and factor H-related genes with systemic lupus erythematosus susceptibility. PLoS Genet 7

Zhao J, Wu H, Khosravi M, Cui H, Qian X, Kelly JA, Kaufman KM, Langefeld CD, Williams AH, Comeau ME (2011) Association of genetic variants in complement factor H and factor H-related genes with systemic lupus erythematosus susceptibility. PLoS Genet 7:e1002079

Zheng J, Yin J, Huang R, Petersen F, Yu X (2013) Meta-analysis reveals an association of STAT4 polymorphisms with systemic autoimmune disorders and anti-dsDNA antibody. Hum Immunol 74:986–992

Zhou X-j, Lu X-l, Lv J-c, Yang H-z, Qin L-x, Zhao M-h, Su Y, Li Z-g, Zhang H (2011) Genetic association of PRDM1-ATG5 intergenic region and autophagy with systemic lupus erythematosus in a Chinese population. Ann Rheum Dis 70:1330–1337

Zhou Y, Wu J, Kucik DF, White NB, Redden DT, Szalai AJ, Bullard DC, Edberg JC (2013) Multiple lupus-associated ITGAM variants alter Mac-1 functions on neutrophils. Arthritis Rheum 65:2907–2916

Zhu L, Chen P, Sun X, Zhang S (2021) Associations between polymorphisms in the IL-1 gene and the risk of rheumatoid arthritis and systemic lupus erythematosus: evidence from a meta-analysis. Int Arch Allergy Immunol 182:234–242

The Immunogenetics of Systemic Sclerosis

Begüm Ünlü, Ümit Türsen, Zeynab Rajabi,
Navid Jabalameli, and Fateme Rajabi

Abstract

Systemic sclerosis (SSc) is a rare disease with a prevalence ranging from 7 to 700 cases per million. Like with most autoimmune diseases, both environmental and genetic factors are involved in the pathogenesis of the SSc. Though the incidence of SSc in the family members of those affected and the concordance rate in twins is very low, inheritance is still the strongest risk factor of SSc. Thus, multiple studies have been conducted to identify the genes responsible for this inheritance including candidate gene association studies and genome-wide analyses. Variations and mutations in the genes encoding cytokines, adhesion molecules, and signaling proteins involved in the interaction between endothelial cells, fibroblasts, and immune cells have been found to be associated with SSc susceptibility. In this chapter, these genes and their contribution to the pathogenesis of the SSc are discussed in detail. These genes are categorized into five major groups of HLA genes, genes involved in the innate immune responses, genes affecting adaptive immune responses, genes with a role in the fibrogenesis pathways, and apoptosis, autophagy, and pyroptosis-related genes.

Keywords

Systemic sclerosis · Genetic polymorphisms · Susceptibility · Immunogenetics · Fibrosis

B. Ünlü · Ü. Türsen (✉)
Department of Dermatology, Mersin University, Mersin, Turkey
e-mail: utursen@mersin.edu.tr

Z. Rajabi
Tehran University of Medical Sciences, Tehran, Iran

N. Jabalameli · F. Rajabi
Network of Dermatology Research (NDR), Universal Scientific Education and Research Network (USERN), Tehran, Iran

F. Rajabi
Center for Research & Training in Skin Diseases & Leprosy, Tehran University of Medical Sciences, Tehran, Iran

1 Introduction

Systemic sclerosis (SSc) or scleroderma is a complex, chronic, recalcitrant autoimmune disease with heterogeneous clinical manifestations (Denton and Khanna 2017; Verhoeven et al. 2020). It is characterized by vascular damage and extensive fibrosis in the skin and internal organs (Denton and Khanna 2017). There are three main subgroups of SSc according to the extent of skin involvement and other clinical characteristics, limited cutaneous systemic sclerosis (lcSSc) also known as CREST syndrome, diffuse cutaneous systemic sclerosis (dcSSc), and sine scleroderma

N. Rezaei and F. Rajabi (eds.), *The Immunogenetics of Dermatologic Diseases*, Advances in Experimental Medicine and Biology 1367,
https://doi.org/10.1007/978-3-030-92616-8_10

(LeRoy et al. 1988). Individuals with lcSSc usually present with skin stiffening at the distal extremities associated with a long-lasting history of Raynaud's phenome (Fig. 1). The involvement of internal organs is usually limited to the upper portion of the gastrointestinal tract and pulmonary hypertension. The previously designated name of CREST syndrome is an acronym referring to the five most prominent features of lcSSc including calcinosis cutis, Raynaud's phenomenon, esophageal involvement (dysmotility that causes severe reflux), sclerodactyly, and telangiectasia (squared off capillary dilatations on the face, lips, and palms) (Adigun et al. 2020; LeRoy et al. 1988). The dcSSc is a more severe subtype with a robust progressive course and a pronounced involvement of internal organs. In dcSSc, skin sclerosis also affects the proximal extremity and trunk, and pulmonary fibrosis, renal crisis, and cardiac involvement are frequent features (Ostojić and Damjanov 2006). The sine scleroderma subtype presents with involvement of internal organs with fibrosis and vascular abnormalities accompanied by Raynaud's phenomenon without the skin sclerosis and sclerodactyly (Diab et al. 2014).

SSc is a rare disease with a prevalence ranging from 7 to 700 cases per million. This disease mostly affects middle-aged individuals and females (Mayes 1998).

Three major types of autoantibodies are present in SSc: anticentromeric antibody (ACA), anti-topoisomerase antibody (ATA) also known as anti-Scl-70, and anti-RNA polymerase III autoantibodies antibody (ARA). The autoantibody profile is different across ethnicities and disease phenotypes. The autoantibodies not only aid the diagnosis of the disease but also help in determining disease prognosis and involvement of specific organs (Hoogen et al. 2013). ACA is usually present in lcSSc with pulmonary hypertension while ATA is more common in individuals suffering from dcSSc with pulmonary fibrosis and ARA is associated with renal crisis in the setting of dcSSc (Nihtyanova and Denton 2010).

SSc is a multifactorial disease with a complex etiology like many other autoimmune diseases. Several environmental factors are blamed to be provocative agents including silica, organic solvents, epoxy resins, and pesticides (Rubio-Rivas et al. 2017). Many other chemical agents such as vinyl chloride and toxic oil could induce a scleroderma-like disorder (Black et al. 1983; Paz et al. 2001; Ward et al. 1976).

The genetic base of SSc was initially detected by epidemiological studies showing a higher incidence of the disease in the close relatives of those affected with SSc and reports on familial clusterings (Arnett et al. 2001; Englert et al.

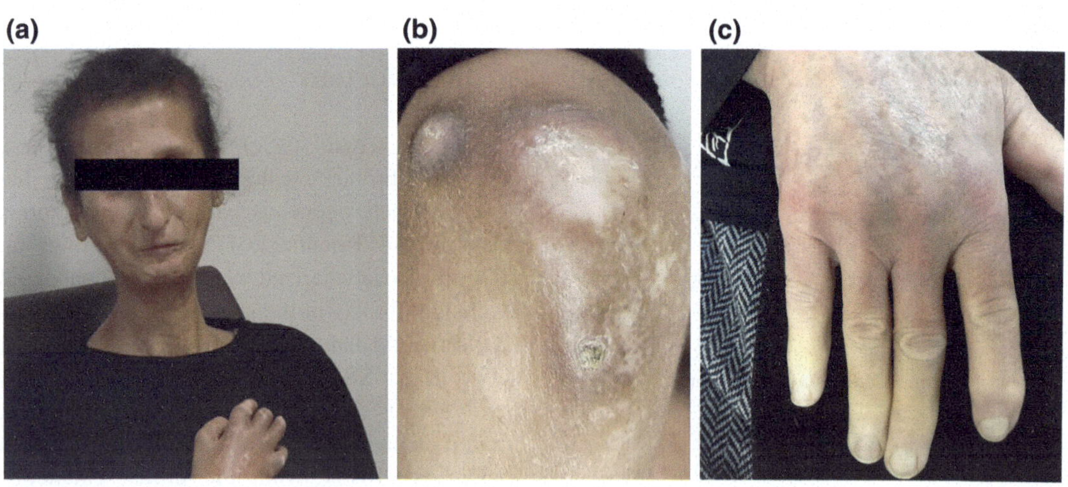

Fig. 1 Clinical features of systemic sclerosis. **a** General facial appearance. **b** Salt and pepper pigmentation and calcinosis cutis at the elbow. **c** Raynaud's phenomena

1999; Hudson et al. 2008; Koumakis et al. 2012; McGregor et al. 1988). The incidence of SSc is only about 1–1.6% in family members and the concordance in monozygotic and dizygotic twins is equally about 4% (Englert et al. 1999; Feghali-Bostwick et al. 2003). Still, inheritance is the strongest risk factor for developing SSc. Thus, multiple studies have been conducted to identify the genes responsible for this inheritance including candidate gene association studies and genome-wide analyses. In this chapter, we mainly discuss the results of these studies and their relevance to the pathogenesis of SSc.

2 The Pathogenesis of Systemic Sclerosis

The hallmark of SSc is extensive inflammation-induced fibrosis along with the altered function of vessels and endothelial cells (Fig. 2). The main The extensive fibrosis in SSc results from the accumulation of collagen I and III and extracellular matrix (ECM) components produced by a subset of cells known as myofibroblasts that either originate from tissue residing and bone marrow-derived circulating fibroblasts or epithelial/endothelial to mesenchymal transition (Jimenez 2013). The transforming growth factor β (TGFβ) is the most influential factor in the activation of fibroblasts and myofibroblasts. TGFβ exerts its effects through binding with the heterodimer receptor TGFβR1/2 and activating intracellular signaling molecules such as smad2/3. The smad complex forms a transcriptional factor that activates the expression of several genes including collagens (Varga and Pasche 2009). TGFβ also induces the expression of connective tissue growth factor (CTGF) and platelet-derived growth factor (PDGF) receptors on fibroblasts, which in turn help in sustaining a profibrotic phenotype by increasing the expression of basic fibroblast growth factor (bFGF) and forming an autocrine positive feedback loop (Leask et al. 2002; Yamakage et al. 1992). There are two sources for TGFβ, a latent form reserved within the connective tissue that is activated through interaction with integrins and matrix metalloproteinases (MMPs) and the more influential active form secreted by immune cells (Lafyatis 2014). Thus the immune cells might be considered the master regulator of fibrosis.

Besides fibrosis, inflammation induced by immune cells plays a dominant role in SSc associated vasculopathy with the altered functions of endothelial cells that are considered more influential in disease initiation and progression. Thus SSc is developed as a consequence of an interaction between fibroblasts, endothelial cells, and immune cells. However, compared to other autoimmune diseases, the role of immune cells in the pathogenesis of SSc is less prominent, which explains the modest effects of immunosuppressive treatments in this disease (Denton 2015).

Though the precise inciting event in the pathogenesis of SSc remains elusive, it has been suggested that the accumulation of reactive oxygen species (ROS) due to environmental stressors such as silica and organic solvents exceeding the buffering capacity of antioxidant machinery could trigger SSc by affecting the vascular tone regulation and endothelial cell integrity (Cooper et al. 2008; Hoy and Chambers 2020). ROS promotes vessel contraction by scavenging vasodilators such as nitric oxide (NO), increasing the production of contractile peptides and microRNAs (miRNAs), and changing calcium signaling within vascular smooth muscle cells (Chettimada et al. 2014; Dimmeler and Zeiher 2000; Moncada 1991; Touyz and Schiffrin 2004). The reaction between NO^- and ROS produces toxic peroxynitrite (NO_3^-) that is capable of destructing proteins by nitrosylation of their tyrosine molecules (Dooley et al. 2006). The ROS also oxidizes circulating low-density lipoproteins (LDLs), which in turn act as potent cytotoxic elements for endothelial cells (Blake et al. 1985). The injured endothelial cells have reduced nitric oxide and prostacyclin production and increased endothelin release further exacerbating vascular contraction and its accompanying hypoxia (Blake et al. 1985; Freedman et al. 1999; Matucci Cerinic and Kahaleh 2002; Romero et al. 2000). On the other hand, the tissue hypoxia resulting from vasoconstriction promotes the expression of hypoxia-

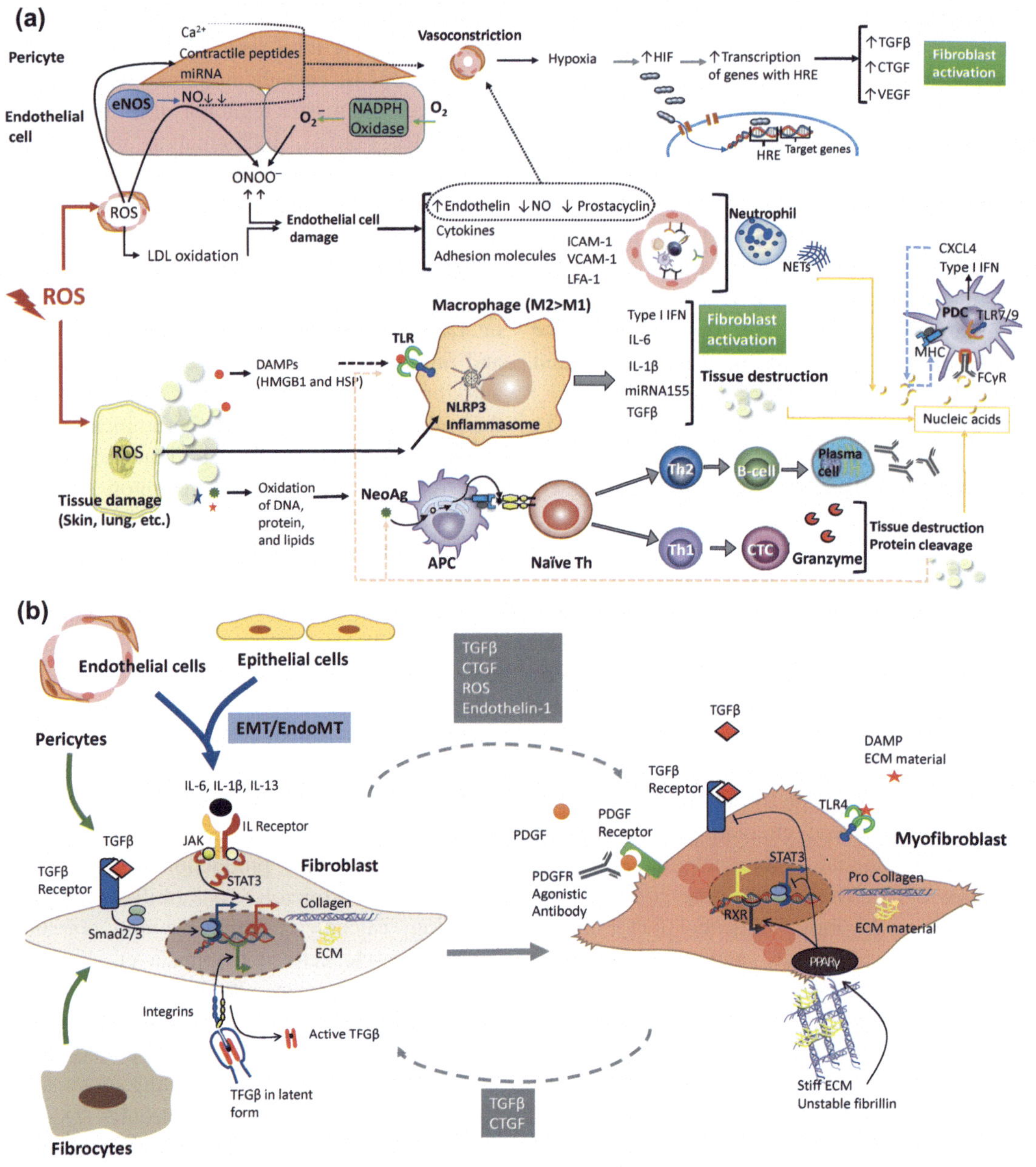

Fig. 2 The pathogenesis of systemic sclerosis (SSc). It has been suggested that reactive oxygen species (ROS) incite the disease by interfering with the regulation of vascular tone and promoting cellular damage. **a** The role of the immune system in the pathogenesis of SSc. **b** The pathways involving the fibroblasts and inflammation-induced fibrosis. HIF, hypoxia-inducible factor; HRE, hypoxia response element; ICAM-1, intercellular adhesion molecule-1; VCAM-1, vascular cell adhesion protein-1; LFA-1, lymphocyte function-associated antigen 1; NET, neutrophil extracellular traps; DAMP, damage-associated molecular patterns; HMGB1, high-mobility group box 1; HSP, heat shock protein; PDC, plasmacytoid dendritic cell; APC, antigen-presenting cell; CTCL, cytotoxic T-cell

inducible factor-1 α (HIF-1α) that in turn induces the expression of genes with hypoxia response element (HRE) at their promoters including TGFβ, CTGF, and vascular endothelial growth factor (VEGF) (Arbiser et al. 2002; Chora et al. 2017; Higgins et al. 2004; Kim and Byzova 2014; Kimura et al. 2000; Qian et al. 2015). These growth factors promote fibrosis and angiogenesis. Simulataneousy, VEGF activates NADPH to produce ROS which forms a positive feedback loop (Ushio-Fukai and Alexander 2004).

ROS is capable of activating the immune system via several mechanisms. It directly activates the NLRP3 inflammasome in innate immune cells such as macrophages and non-immune cells such as fibroblasts (Abais et al. 2015; Henderson and O'Reilly 2017; Zhang et al. 2018). The activated inflammasome promotes the expression of IL-1β and microRNA-155 (miR-155) (Artlett et al. 2017; Henderson and O'Reilly 2017). The miR-155, in turn, promotes the expression of TGFβ (Artlett et al. 2017). It provokes endothelial injury, which leads to the expression of adhesion molecules such as ICAM-1 on the cell surfaces and through interacting with lymphocyte function-associated antigen-1 (LFA-1) facilitates the migration of lymphocytes and leukocytes (Roebuck 1999). The damaged endothelial cells release damage-associated molecular patterns (DAMP) such as high mobility group box-1 (HMGB-1) and heat shock proteins (HSPs) that are sensed by toll-like receptors (TLRs) such TLR2 and TLR4 on the surface of innate immune cells such as macrophages (Ito et al. 2007; O'Reilly 2018; Ogawa et al. 2008). The activation of TLRs will in turn promote the release of type interferon (IFN) and inflammatory cytokines such as interleukin 1β (IL-1β), IL-6, and TGFβ (O'Reilly 2018). IL-6 is considered a profibrotic cytokine as it could both directly activate fibroblasts and indirectly induce the production of TGFβ (Denton et al. 2018; Khan et al. 2012). Since TGFβ is also capable of promoting IL-6 release, a self-perpetuating cycle is created that could make the fibroblast activation self-sufficient (Denton et al. 2018; Khan et al. 2012). The classically activated M1 macrophages play a major role in response to DAMPs by producing pro-inflammatory cytokines. Moreover, they further exacerbate the redox balance by actively producing ROS (Sica and Mantovani 2012). The M1 macrophages contribute to the fibrogenic mechanism recruiting fibrocytes with the help of CCL2 and facilitating the epithelial/endothelial to mesenchymal transition (EMT/EndoMT). However, M1 also possesses anti-fibrotic properties as it degrades the ECM with the help of MMPs (Braga et al. 2015; Cheng and Lovett 2003). Eventually, the ROS accumulation polarizes the macrophage differentiation towards the alternative M2 phenotype in an STAT6-dependent manner (Doridot et al. 2019; Frantz et al. 2018; Taroni et al. 2017; Zhang et al. 2013b). The M2 macrophages assist the fibrogenic pathway by producing massive amounts of TGFβ (Conway and Hughes 2012).

ROS can also activate the adaptive immune response by promoting the formation of neoantigens (Kurien et al. 2006). ROS-induced oxidation/peroxidation can modify the antigenic properties of intracellular proteins and lipids such as topoisomerases (Kavian et al. 2010; Servettaz et al. 2009). DNA somatic mutation and chromosomal instability evoked by ROS are other sources of neoantigens (Denton 2015; Emerit et al. 1997; Gopanenko et al. 2020). This is presumed to be the mechanism involved in the pathogenesis of bleomycin and taxane (docetaxel and paclitaxel) induced SSc, where oxidative stress increases the chromosomal breakage (Casciola-Rosen et al. 1997; Angelis et al. 2003). These neoantigens are released from apoptotic cells and uptaken and presented by dendritic cells and macrophages. Their interaction with T-cell receptors (TCRs) and B-cell receptors (BCRs) activates the adaptive immune responses. Further epitope spreading would then result in multiple other autoantibodies and further T-cell mediated tissue reactions (Kurien et al. 2006). The granzyme-mediated cell death by cytotoxic T-cells and natural killer cells (NK-cells) can also form neoantigens. Granzyme B is a serine protease that enables apoptosis by cleaving and activating several caspases. As a protease, it can also cleave other intracellular proteins and reveal new termini or induce conformational changes that by acting as novel antigenic epitopes can activate obscure TCR and BCRs upon their release from apoptotic cells (Casciola-Rosen et al. 1999; Schachna et al. 2002). This mechanism is involved in disease progression. For instance, SSc patients in an advanced stage suffering from ischemic digital loss have higher levels of autoantibodies against granzyme B cleaved centromeric fragments compared to controls with milder symptoms of early SSc (Schachna et al. 2002). The sensitivity of proteins to granzyme B cleavage is cell-specific which can explain the phenotype-specific immune responses (Ulanet et al. 2004). Interestingly, the granzyme B mediated cleavage of plasmin and plasminogen produces an anti-angiogenic protein known as tumstatin that is found to be elevated in sera of patients with SSc (Mulligan-Kehoe et al. 2007).

Most autoantibodies present in the sera of patients with SSc, however, do not have a significant effect on the pathogenesis of the disease and are simply present as byproducts. The very few antibodies effective in disease progression include anti-endothelial antibodies and agonistic antibodies against endothelin, PDGF, angiostatin, or their receptors (Kill et al. 2014; Svegliati et al. 2017).

Adaptive immune responses are associated with tissue destruction that further promotes inflammation, fibrosis, and hypoxia through multiple pathways. The release of extracellular components such as fibronectin, fibrinogen, and tenascin and inflammation-associated amyloid A activate TLR2 and TLR4 on the surface of both immune cells and fibroblasts promoting IL-6 production along with activation of fibroblast and collagen secretion (Bhattacharyya et al. 2014; Brandwein et al. 1984; Frasca and Lande 2020). The release of nucleic acid components from dying cells and neutrophil extracellular traps along with autoantibody complexes such as anti-topoisomerase activate intracellular TLRs such as TLR7, TLR8, and TLR9 in plasmacytoid dendritic cells (pDC) that produce massive amounts of IFNα (Eloranta et al. 2010; Frasca and Lande 2020; Kim et al. 2008). The pDCs also produce CXCL4. This chemokine can amplify the TLR3, TLR7/8, and TLR9 mediated responses by binding and forming immunogenic nanocrystallines with non-stimulatory self-DNA and -RNAs (Frasca and Lande 2020; Bon et al. 2014). It also stimulates the Th2 profibrotic cytokines, IL-4 and IL-13, and inhibits antifibrotic interferon γ (IFNγ) (Romagnani et al. 2005). The inflammatory milieu precisely the IL-6 also enhances fibrosis through up-regulating the differentiation of profibrotic T-helper 17 (Th17) cells (Denton 2015; Denton et al. 2018; Khanna et al. 2016).

Besides ROS, several other drugs, toxins, viruses, and cancers can also trigger SSc including the Ebstein Barr virus (EBV), parvovirus B19, cytomegalovirus (CMV), retrovirus, pentazocine, and cocaine (Efthymiou et al. 2019; Randone et al. 2008; Zakrzewska et al. 2019). The exact path through which these elements induce SSc is not fully understood but it has been suggested that antigen mimicry between the viral protein and self-antigens could be a source for breach in the self-tolerance as it has been described for retroviral antigens and topoisomerase (Maul et al. 1989). Moreover, EBV can infect both endothelial and fibroblast cells and its particles can activate TLRs and innate immune responses that can stimulate fibrogenic pathways and provoke transition to myofibroblasts (Farina et al. 2014; Frasca and Lande 2020). Cancer cells can have altered protein expression patterns such as increased presentation of silent or sequestered peptides that would stimulate the immune system in a manner that increases its sensitivity to the transient peripheral expression of the same set of antigens in tissues undergoing regeneration and thus promoting autoimmunity (Shah and Rosen 2011).

As mentioned earlier, the innate and adaptive immune responses promote the activation of myofibroblasts that are associated with increased expression of collagen and ECM. These myofibroblasts eventually become autonomous, which means they acquire a consistently active phenotype that does not require stimulation from the immune system. The path through which these cells become autonomous in the setting of SSc is a matter of debate. However, several hypotheses have been put forth. It has been suggested that genetic mutations or stable epigenetic changes (alteration in the methylation and acetylation pattern) in regulatory genes could give rise to fibroblast subpopulations with higher activity in a manner similar to proto-oncogenes in tumors (Jimenez et al. 2001; Wang et al. 2006b). Furthermore, the hypoxic and immunologic milieu can favor the dominance of naturally occurring hyperactive fibroblasts that are more susceptible to stimulatory signals and hypersensitive toward inhibitory feedback signals relayed by ECM and collagen through peroxisome proliferator-activated receptor γ (PPARγ) (Denton 2015). Alterations within the ECM such as stiffness and unstable fibrilins could also reduce the intensity of negative feedback loops and thus result in continuous fibroblast activity (Shiwen et al. 2015; Wallis et al. 2001).

3 The Immunogenetics of Systemic Sclerosis

Variations and mutations in the genes encoding cytokines, adhesion molecules, and signaling proteins discussed above could have major impacts on the pathogenesis of SSc and thus could affect an individual's susceptibility toward the disease. In the following sections, we discuss the genes implicated in the pathogenesis of SSc identified through candidate gene approaches and genome-wide association studies (Fig. 3).

3.1 The HLA Genes

Numerous candidate gene studies and at least six genome-wide association studies (GWAS) have been able to document associations between polymorphisms in genes encoding human leukocyte antigens (HLAs) and SSc (Chairta et al. 2017). Like most autoimmune diseases, SSc is more often associated with variation in major histocompatibility (MHC) class II encoding genes rather than MHC-I. From the twelve reported associations belonging to both MHC-II (HLA-DRB1, -DRB5, -DRA, -DMB, -DOA, -DQA1, -DQB1, -DPA1, -DPB1, and -DPB2) and MHC-I (HLA-B, and HLA-C) encoding genes the strongest associations were found for *HLA-DRB1*1104*, *HLA-DQA1*0501*, *HLA-DQB1*0301* haplotype, and *HLA-DQB1* and *HLA-DPB1* alleles which were repeated in multiple studies (Arnett et al. 2010; Chairta et al. 2017). The *HLADPB1*1301* and *HLA-DRB1*11* were also significantly associated with SSc especially in the subgroup of Caucasian patients with ATA autoantibodies (Gilchrist et al. 2001). In the Hispanic population, *HLA-DRB1*1104* and *HLA-DRB1*11* were shown to have a significant association with SSc in the ATA-positive subgroup (Reveille et al. 2001). *HLA-DQB1*0501*, *HLA-DQB1*26*, *HLA-DRB1*01*, *HLA-DRB1*04*, and *HLA-DRB1*08* alleles were associated with SSc in the ACA-positive subset of patients (Arnett et al. 2010; Gilchrist et al. 2001; Reveille et al. 2001). *HLA-DRB1*0404*, *HLA-DRB1*11*, and *HLA-DQB1*03* alleles were associated with SSc in anti-RNA polymerase III antibody-positive SSc patients (Arnett et al. 2010). *HLA-DRB1*0101*, *HLA-DQA1*0101*, and *HLADQB1*0501* alleles were found to negatively correlate with the risk of diseases progression (Vigone et al. 2015). In the African-American population, *HLA-DRB1*0804*, *HLA-DQA1*0501*, and *HLA-DQB1*0301* alleles were reported to be associated with SSc (Arnett et al. 2010). The *HLA-DRB1*08* is associated with anti-RNA-polymerase III antibody (ARA) positivity in SSc patients (Arnett et al. 2010).

Almost all genome-wide studies (GWAS and immunochip studies) were able to demonstrate an association between HLA alleles and SSc (Chairta et al. 2017). Multiple single nucleotide polymorphisms (SNPs) on the *HLA-DPB1* and *HLA-DPB2* were associated with SSc in a GWAS performed on a Korean population with further replication in Caucasians. Precisely, the *HLA-DPB1*1301* and *HLA-DPB1*0901* were the most strongly associated risk alleles in Korean SSc patients with ATA and ACA autoantibodies (Zhou et al. 2009). Two much larger GWA studies performed on European patients found the strongest SSc association signal to be

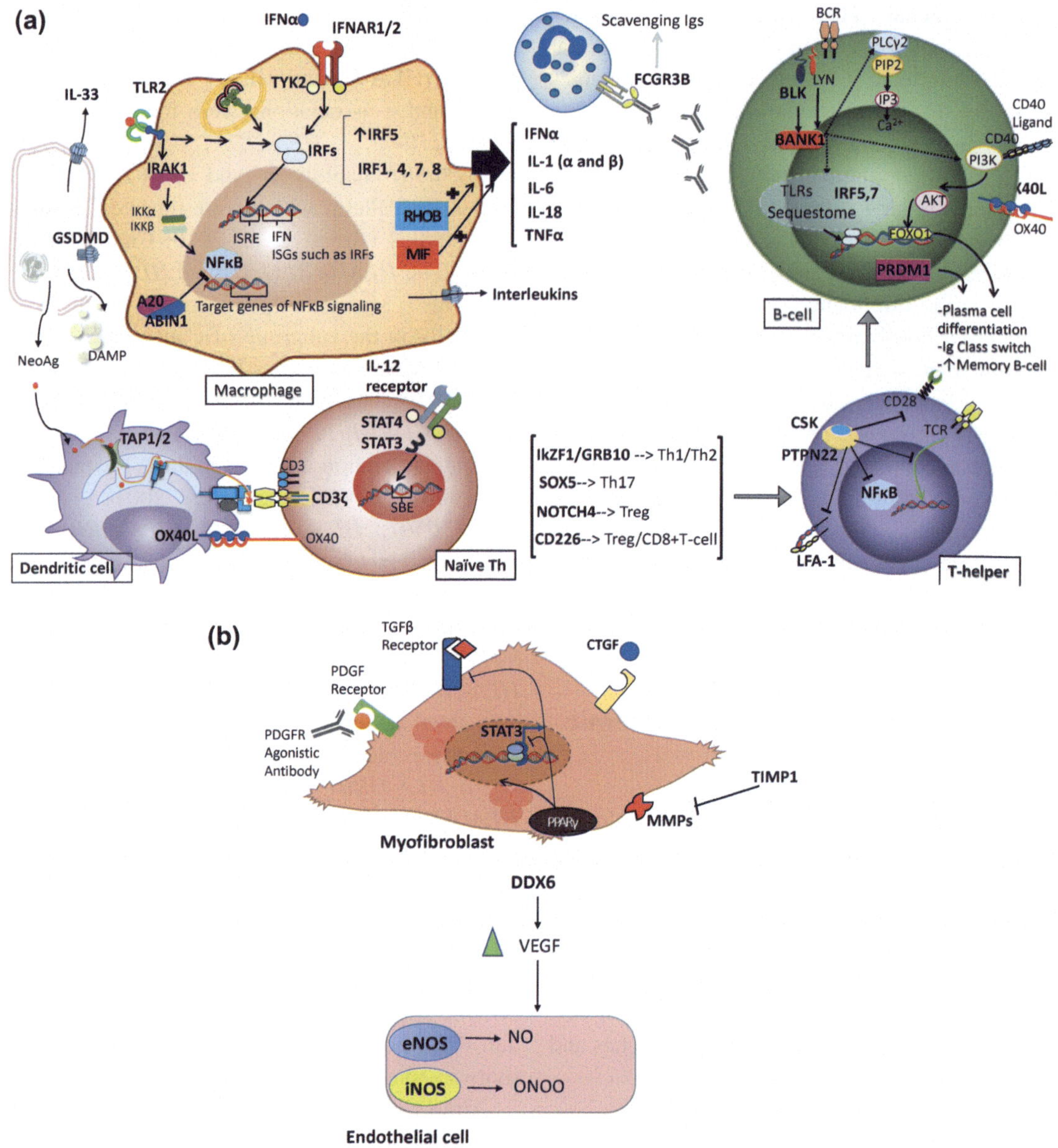

Fig. 3 Genes associated with susceptibility to systemic sclerosis. **a** Genes regulating immune function. A20 and ABIN1 are encoded by *TNFAIP3* and *TNIP1*, respectively **b** Genes with direct effects on fibroblasts and endothelial cells. ISRE, IFN-stimulated response element; ISG, IFN stimulated genes; SBE, stat biding element

located at *HLA-DQB1* (Allanore et al. 2011; Radstake et al. 2010). Subgroup analysis of GWAS based on the presence of different types of autoantibodies revealed a strong association signal located at *HLA-DQB1* for ACA-positive subgroup and multiple association signals located at *HLA-DPA1/DPB1* (presumably *HLA-DPB1*1301*), *HLA-DRA*, and *HLA-DQA1/DRB1* (likely *HLA-DRB1*1104*) in the ATA-positive patients (González-Serna et al. 2020; Gorlova et al. 2011).

An immunochip study by *Mayes et al.* reported that genetic variations causing amino acid substitutions at position 13 of HLA-DRB1 and position 69 of the HLA-DQα1 protein along with the rs12528892 and rs6933319 conferred risk for SSc in the subset of patients positive for ACA. The SNPs affecting the amino acids 67th and 85th of the HLA-DRB1 and the SNPs affecting the 76th and 96th amino acid of the HLA-DPB1 were associated with ATA-positive SSc (Mayes et al. 2014). These amino acids are either positioned at the binding pocket of the HLA molecule or affect the three-dimensional structures of these molecules in a way that affects antigen binding (Mayes et al. 2014). The association between SSc and the *HLA-DRB1* was also confirmed in another immunochip study on Australian patients (Zochling et al. 2014). A transethnic GWAS meta-analysis of Japanese and European patients found different association patterns between the two ethnic groups, which resulted in the modulation of the association signal in the pooled data analysis. The *HLA-DRA* was found to confer susceptibility to SSc in Japanese patients (Terao et al. 2017).

3.2 The Genes Involved in the Innate Immune Responses

The *interferon regulatory factor* (*IRF*) genes

Several reports have suggested that innate immunity may play a role in the pathogenesis of SSc (Bossini-Castillo et al. 2015). One of the prominent effectors of the innate immune responses is a family of transcription factors known as IRFs that not only enable the expression of type I IFNs (IFNα and β) following the activation of pattern recognition receptors such as TLRs (especially TLR3, TLR7/8, and TLR9) but also work downstream type I IFN receptors (IFNAR-1/IFNAR-2) to promote the expression of IFN stimulated genes (ISGs) (Lee and Ashkar 2018). The IRFs bind to specific DNA sequences at the promoter of the IFN gene and ISGs known as IFN regulatory element (IRE) or IFN-stimulated response element (ISRE) (Mogensen 2019). As IRFs can also bind to their own promoters and increase their own transcription, they can form a feed-forward cross-talk between TLR and IFN pathways by increasing the access to newly synthesized transcription factors (Barnes et al. 2002).

Nine different types of IRF have been described in humans thus far with slightly different functions and expression patterns in different cell lines (Antonczyk et al. 2019; Barnes et al. 2002).

The *IRF5* gene was the first member of this category to be associated with SSc by candidate gene studies in different ethnicities (Dieudé et al. 2009a; Ito et al. 2009). Quite interestingly, SNPs within *the IRF5-TNPO3* region (7q32) showed the strongest association peaks outside the HLA region in multiple SSc GWA and immunochip studies (Allanore et al. 2011; Gorlova et al. 2011; López-Isac et al. 2019; Mayes et al. 2014; Radstake et al. 2010; Zochling et al. 2014). The SNPs reported by candidate genes studies (rs2004640 at exon–intron border of exon 1B, rs2280714 in the intergenic segment between *IRF5* and *TNPO3* gene, and rs10954213 located at the 9th exon) are different from those reported by GWA studies (rs34381587, rs10488631, rs36073657, and rs12155080) (Dieudé et al. 2009a; Ito et al. 2009; López-Isac et al. 2019; Radstake et al. 2010; Zochling et al. 2014). This seems to be related to the fact that many of these SNPs are in linkage disequilibrium (LD). The *IRF5* polymorphisms have been also linked to multiple other autoimmune diseases including systemic lupus erythematosus (SLE). The risk alleles are thought to be associated with increased *IRF5* expression that could eventually boost the IFN production (Clark et al. 2013; Deng and Tsao 2010).

Genetic polymorphisms in other members of the IRF family have also been linked to SSc including *IRF1* (González-Serna et al. 2020), *IRF4* (López-Isac et al. 2016b; Radstake et al. 2010), *IRF7* (López-Isac et al. 2019), and *IRF8* (Gorlova et al. 2011; López-Isac et al. 2019). The first GWAS to link SNPs within the *EXOC2-IRF4* region (6p25) to SSc failed to confirm this association in the replication phase and thus regarded it as a false positive association due to allelic heterogeneity (Radstake et al. 2010). However, a later larger cross-disease GWAS meta-analysis of SSc and rheumatoid arthritis (RA), identified *IRF4* as a common susceptibility gene shared between the two diseases (López-Isac et al. 2016b).

The rs11642873 located near the *IRF8* gene (16q24.1) was identified as an SSc risk locus by a GWAS study and its association was further confirmed by a follow-up cohort (Gorlova et al. 2011). A large GWAS meta-analysis of SSc patients found another SNP (rs11117420) located at an intragenic region near the *IRF8* to have a genome-wide level of association with SSc (López-Isac et al. 2019). This study was also able to detect a peak association signal within the *CDHR5 -IRF7* region (11p15.5) (López-Isac et al. 2019).

IRF1 (5q31.1) was found to contain a shared susceptibility locus between SSc and Crohn's disease (González-Serna et al. 2020).

Though the functional implications of the described polymorphisms are not clear, it is not irrational to assume that they promote inflammation by amplifying the cross-talk between TLRs and IFNs either by increasing the levels of activators (IRF1, IRF3, IRF5, IRF7, and IRF9) or decreasing the transcription of repressors (IRF2 and IRF8) (Barnes et al. 2002; Tan et al. 2006; Wu and Assassi 2013).

The *signal transducer and activator of transcription* (*STAT*) genes

The STATs are another group of transcription factors that are classically activated by Janus kinases (JNK) and tyrosine kinases (TYK) downstream membrane-bound cytokine receptors. Seven STAT molecules have been described to date, STAT1, STAT2, STAT3, STAT4, STAT5 (A and B), and STAT6.

The STAT1 homodimers mediated the type II IFN (IFNγ) signaling by stimulating the transcription of genes with gamma interferon activation site (GAS) at their promoters. A complex containing a STAT1-STAT2 heterodimer and an IRF9 mediate type I interferon signaling by binding to ISRE at the gene promoters. The STAT3, STAT4, and STAT5 homodimer are activated downstream interleukin receptors and are translocated to the nucleus to activate the transcription of genes with STAT binding elements (SBEs) at their promoters (Mogensen 2019). Besides the membrane receptors, some cytoplasmic receptors with intrinsic kinase activities such as PDGF and FGF receptors, G-protein-coupled receptors, and non-receptor kinases such as MAPK can also activate the STAT molecules (Verhoeven et al. 2020).

The STAT4 mediates IL-12, IL-17, and IL-23 pro-inflammatory signaling and is thus essential in T- and NK-cells mediated production of IFN-γ and to a lesser extent IFN-α in the early stages of the innate immune response (Deng et al. 2004; Lee and Ashkar 2018). It is also involved in T helper 1 (Th1) and T helper 17 (Th17) differentiation in the adaptive immune responses (Nishikomori et al. 2002; Xu et al. 2011). Though STAT4 mediates the release of both antifibrotic IFN-γ and profibrotic tumor necrosis factor α (TNF α) and IL-6, its overall effects are in favor of the fibrogenic pathway as it has been demonstrated that *STAT4* knockout prevents fibrosis in mouse models (Avouac et al. 2011; Barnes and Agarwal 2011; Gurujeyalakshmi and Giri 1995).

The association between SSc and polymorphisms in the gene encoding STAT4 (located at 2q32-33) was first documented by several candidate gene studies with a fairly large number of participants and later was confirmed by almost all GWAS, immunochip, and meta-analyses across multiple ethnicities (Allanore et al. 2011; Dieudé et al. 2009b; Gorlova et al. 2011; López-Isac et al. 2019; Mayes et al. 2014; Radstake et al. 2010; Rueda et al. 2009a; Terao et al. 2017; Tsuchiya et al. 2009; Xu et al. 2016; Zochling et al. 2014). The *STAT4* has been linked to multiple other autoimmune diseases including SLE and Crohn's disease (González-Serna et al. 2020; Kariuki et al. 2009).

The *STAT3* gene was found to contain a shared association signal between SSc and Crohn's disease in cross-disease GWAS meta-analysis. The shared SNP was found to confer susceptibility to SSc and protection from Crohn's disease (González-Serna et al. 2020). The STAT3 mediates the IL-6 induction of collagen synthesis by fibroblasts (Duncan and Berman 1991; Khan et al. 2012;

Wang et al. 2020). It is also activated by IL-21, IL-22, and IL-23 upon receptor binding and is thus essential in Th17 differentiation and function which has been shown to have a prominent role in promoting fibrosis in SSc through increasing the expression of IL-6m RNA (Harris et al. 2007; Park et al. 2018). Moreover, in established fibrosis, the stiffness of the ECM can directly activate the JNK/STAT3 pathway through mechanoreceptors and further promote TGFβ and collagen synthesis without the need for external stimuli (Oh et al. 2018; Wang et al. 2020). This may partially explain the well-known fibroblast autonomy in SSc.

The non-receptor tyrosine kinase family

The non-receptor tyrosine kinases are a group of intracellular enzymes that interact with surface receptors and transmit extracellular signals to downstream effector pathways such as transcription factors. Approximately ten families of non-receptor tyrosine kinases have been described including Janus kinases (JNK), Src-family kinases, Btk kinases, and Syk tyrosine kinases. The Janus kinase family consists of ubiquitously expressed Jak1, Jak2, and Tyk2 along with Jak3 expressed by hematopoietic cells (Szilveszter et al. 2019).

The Janus kinase family members couple with cytokine and IFN dimeric receptors and sense conformational changes on these receptors upon ligand binding which would result in the phosphorylation of the receptor chains. The Janus kinases would then also phosphorylate the STAT molecules promoting their dimerization and translocation to the nucleus. Though Jak and Tyk molecules do not form actual dimers, they cooperate in pairs since their corresponding receptors are dimeric (Szilveszter et al. 2019).

The *TYK2* polymorphisms have been linked to susceptibility to multiple autoimmune diseases (Dendrou et al. 2016; Graham et al. 2011; Tao et al. 2011). SSc is not an exception and a candidate gene study, an immunochip analysis, and a cross-disease meta-analysis have confirmed the association of *TYK2* SNPs (rs2304256, rs34536443, rs12720356, and rs35018800) with SSc (González-Serna et al. 2020; López-Isac et al. 2016a; Mayes et al. 2014). These polymorphisms change the enzyme's expression rate and kinase activity affecting the pathways mediated by TYK2 including IFN, IL-12, and IL-23 signaling related to both innate and adaptive immune responses (Dendrou et al. 2016; Karaghiosoff et al. 2000; Shimoda et al. 2000).

The nuclear factor κB (NF-κB) pathway genes

The NF-κBs are a family of transcription factors that regulate the expression of various genes including cytokines and chemokines belonging to both innate and adaptive immune responses (Zhang et al. 2017). The five members of this family, NF-κB1, NF-κB2, RelA, RelB, and c-rel, form homo- and heterodimers with positive and negative regulatory effects on the expression of target genes (Miraghazadeh and Cook 2018). Inherently, the NF-κB proteins are in a latent inactive form bound to IκB. Multiple different types of signals transduced by surface receptors such as TLRs, TNF receptors, antigen receptors, CD40, and OX40 could activate NF-κB by facilitating the degradation of IκB by the IKK complex (Liu et al. 2017b; Sasai et al. 2010).

The A20 zinc finger enzyme, encoded by the *tumor necrosis factor-alpha inducible protein3* (*TNFAIP3*) gene and its binding partner ABIN1 encoded by the *TNFAIP3-interacting protein1* (*TNIP1*) gene are one of the main negative regulators of the NF-κB pathway. The A20/ABIN1 complex facilitates the degradation of NF-κB mediator proteins by changing the ubiquitin structure of these molecules (Jarosz et al. 2017). A20 protein itself is transcribed by NF-κB in response to the TNF receptor activation and thus is believed to be part of a negative feedback loop that restricts the intensity and the duration TNFα-induced inflammation (G'Sell et al. 2015).

Polymorphisms in genes encoding these proteins have been linked to SSc susceptibility by both candidate gene approaches and GWA studies. An SNP (rs230534) located within the promoter of the *NFKB1* gene (4q24) was found to be linked to SSc in a recent GWAS (López-Isac et al. 2019). Two candidate gene studies on Turkish/Iranian and Han Chinese populations were able to confirm this association for rs4648133 and rs1599961 SNPs, respectively (González-Serna et al. 2019; Liu et al. 2021). The *NFKB1* polymorphisms confer susceptibility to multiple other immune diseases in the Asian population (Zou et al. 2011). Moreover, *NFKB1* mutations can give rise to a Mendelian autoimmune syndrome characterized by thrombocytopenia, arthritis, pneumonia, and gastroenteritis (Wei et al. 2016).

The G allele of the rs5029939 SNP located at the intron 2 of the *TNFAIP3* gene (6q23.3) was found to confer susceptibility to SSc in a small case–control study in Europe patients (Dieude et al. 2010). Another SNP (rs2230926) corresponding to a missense amino acid substitution of *TNFAIP3* was found to be associated with SSc with a genome-wide level of significance in a multiethnic meta-analysis (Terao et al. 2017). Interestingly, an integrative study assessing the interaction between genetic and environmental factors showed that the rs58905141 SNP of the *TNFAIP3* gene was strongly associated with the expressions of ECM-related genes such as MMPs in silica exposed fibroblasts (Wei et al. 2016). The *TNFAIP3* polymorphisms and mutations have not only been linked to multiple autoimmune diseases but can also cause a Mendelian syndrome similar to Behcet's disease (Adrianto et al. 2011; Duncan et al. 2018; Graham et al. 2008b; Wei et al. 2016). Several SSc GWA studies have documented multiple strongly associated SNPs within the *TNIP1* gene (5q33), which were also confirmed through replication studies (Allanore et al. 2011; Bossini-Castillo et al. 2013; López-Isac et al. 2019). SNPs within the same LD block have also been linked to susceptibility to SLE and psoriasis (Gateva et al. 2009; Nair et al. 2009).

The altered expression of NF-κB pathway genes has been documented in both early and late lesions of SSc (Kessel et al. 2004; Lis-Święty et al. 2017). SSc tissue samples and SSc cultured fibroblasts demonstrate reduced *TNIP1* mRNA and protein expression compared to controls. Recombinant TNIP1 nullifies the effects of cytokines on collagen and ECM synthesis by fibroblasts confirming the role of NF-kB in inflammation-induced fibrosis (Allanore et al. 2011). The forced expression of A20 reduces the TGFβ-induced myofibroblast transformation and collagen expression in fibroblast cultures. Contrariwise, A20 knockdown enhances TGFβ-mediated fibrotic responses (Bhattacharyya et al. 2016). Thus, it is likely for the risk alleles of the *TNFAIP3* and *TNIP1* genes to be associated with reduced gene expression or protein function (Adrianto et al. 2011; Graham et al. 2008b; Gurevich et al. 2011; Han et al. 2009; Zhang et al. 2013a). The effects of the *NFKB1* variants are harder to determine since it is involved in many aspects of immunity from innate immune responses to the development of the thymus and functions of T-cells, B-cells, and T-regs (Miraghazadeh and Cook 2018).

The interleukin-1 receptor-associated kinases (IRAKs)

The IRAKs are a family of putative kinases that are activated down-stream IL-1 receptor and TLRs. They interact with a different range of molecules to regulate NFκB, MAPK, and to a lesser extent IRF and STAT pathways. Four members of this family, IRAK1, IRAK2, IRAK4, and IRKAM act as both "on" and "off" switches for the NFκB (Su et al. 2020). Polymorphisms in the genes encoding the members of the IRAK family (precisely *IRAK1*) have been linked to susceptibility to different autoimmune diseases including SLE and psoriasis (Chatzikyriakidou et al. 2010; Jacob et al. 2009; Kaufman et al. 2013).

Candidate gene studies in SSc have also found the T allele and the TT genotype of the *IRAK1* rs1059702 to confer risk to SSc development and presence of pulmonary fibrosis (Carmona et al. 2013; Dieude et al. 2011; Zhao et al. 2017). The exact functional consequence of the risk variant is not known. However, it has been demonstrated that the peripheral blood mononuclear cells (PBMCs) of SSc patients have lower *IRAK1* expression (Zilahi et al. 2012). Another SNP (rs17435) within the locus containing the *IRAK1* gene (Xq28), located at the *methyl CpG binding protein-2* (*MECP2*) gene shows an independent association with SSc (dcSSc) (Carmona et al. 2013). The MECP2 is a transcriptional regulator that controls the expression of methylation-sensitive genes. Low levels of MECP2 mRNA can increase the expression of ISGs due to hypomethylation (Kaufman et al. 2013).

The *RHOB* gene

The *RHOB* gene 2p24 which encodes a protein involved in cell signaling and protein trafficking harbors an SSc susceptibility loci identified through GWAS and confirmed by cohorts in multiple ethnicities (Allanore et al. 2011; Bossini-Castillo et al. 2013; Shu et al. 2014). It possesses several roles that may explain its involvement in the pathogenesis of SSc. It enables endothelial cell survival during vasculogenesis (Adini et al. 2003) and it positively regulates the production of IL-1β, IL-6, and TNFα in macrophages in response to hypoxia and TLR signaling (Huang et al. 2017; Liu et al. 2017a). Moreover, in animal models of RA and lupus, the knockout of the *RHOB* gene impedes autoantibody production (Mandik-Nayak et al. 2017).

The macrophage migration inhibitory factor (MIF) gene

The MIF is a pleiotropic cytokine with diverse functions. The extracellular MIF interacts with CD74, CD44 and induces proinflammatory cytokines, and promotes the survival and clonal expansion of T-cells. Intracellular MIF facilitates TLR and NLRP3 signaling (Wen et al. 2021). Thus it promotes both innate and adaptive immune responses (Denkinger et al. 2004; Donn et al. 2004; Illescas et al. 2018; Saeedi et al. 2013). It is also involved in the preservation of immune privilege by inhibiting NK-cells from attacking self-cells lacking MHC expression (Apte et al. 1998; Ito et al. 2005; Rajabi et al. 2018). Besides its role in the immune system, MIF is a powerful inducer of NO synthesis and fibroblast proliferation and function (Cunha et al. 1993; Mitchell et al. 1999).

The role of MIF in the pathogenesis of SSc was initially proposed by a study demonstrating higher tissue and circulating levels of MIF in the skin of patients with scleroderma and dcSSC, respectively (Selvi et al. 2003). Later on, several case–control candidate gene studies investigated the association of *MIF* polymorphisms with SSc susceptibility to find out whether its role in the pathogenesis of SSc is derived by genetic factors or cytokines and inflammation secondarily increase its expression. Two common polymorphisms have been described for the *MIF* gene, a short tandem repeat (STR) ($CATT_{5-8}$) at position -794 (rs5844572) and a G to C substitution (-173G > C) at the promoter (rs755622). The higher number of CATT repeats and the C allele of -173G > C SNP are associated with increased gene expression (Baugh et al. 2002; De Benedetti et al. 2003). The frequency of the C allele of *MIF* rs755622 was lower in the patients with lcSSc compared to those with dcSSc and controls and the C7 haplotype was lower in lcSSc patients compared to patients with dcSSc in a candidate gene study with 740 participants (Wu et al. 2006). Two subsequent studies with 7082 and 20,873 subjects from European ancestry reported a lower presentation of the C allele in lcSSc patients compared to controls and a higher frequency of the rs755622 C allele in dcSSc patients (especially in those with concomitant pulmonary arterial hypertension) (Bossini-Castillo et al. 2017, 2011b). The effect of the STR polymorphism was not assessed directly by these studies. However, since it is in high LD with the rs755622, the same direction of effects is expected for this polymorphism. These findings were replicated in a Mexican cohort, which was also able to demonstrate a correlation between the levels of MIF and the levels of inflammatory cytokines such as IL-1 and IL-6 (Baños-Hernández et al. 2019). Treatment with MIF antagonists has shown efficacy in reducing fibrosis induced by bleomycin in murine models making it a promising future drug in SSc (Günther et al. 2018).

The TLR genes

Variabilities in the *TLR* genes do not contribute much to the pathogenesis of SSc. A candidate gene study evaluating multiple *TLR* genes was only able to link a rare gain-of-function variant of *TLR2* gene to subcategories of SSc including dcSSc, ATA + SSc, and SSc with pulmonary arterial hypertension (Broen et al. 2012).

3.3 The Genes Involved in the Adaptive Immune Responses

The *CD247* gene

The *CD247* gene, located at 1q22–23 was initially reported to harbor an association signal for SSc by the second GWAS performed in SSc (Radstake et al. 2010). Thereafter, this finding was confirmed in almost all subsequent studies except for a cohort in the Han Chinese population (Allanore et al. 2011; Gorlova et al. 2011; López-Isac et al. 2019; Wang et al. 2014; Zochling et al. 2014). The gene has also been linked to susceptibility to SLE, RA, and autoimmune diabetes (Lundholm et al. 2010; Teruel et al. 2013; Warchoł et al. 2009).

The *CD247* encodes a protein involved in the assembly of the CD3-TCR complex known as CD3ζ (Call and Wucherpfennig 2004). This receptor complex plays a central role in the immune response after antigen triggering. The risk SNP of the *CD247* gene (rs2056626) located with the intronic region was shown to affect the gene transcription rate (López-Isac et al. 2016a). Perhaps genetic variants with reduced CD3-ζ expression can attenuate TCR affinity of naïve T-cells altering the proper T-reg development or allowing the autoreactive T to scape the thymic negative selection (Call and Wucherpfennig 2004; Deng et al. 2013).

The *protein phosphatase non-receptor type 22* (*PTPN22*) and the *C-Src kinase* (*CSK*) genes

The *PTPN22* encodes the lymphoid tyrosine phosphatase (LYP), which forms a complex with CSK, a tyrosine-protein kinase belonging to the Src family of non-receptor tyrosine kinases, and negatively regulates the TCR/CD3 signaling upon antigen stimulation (Fousteri et al. 2013). It exerts its inhibitory effects on multiple levels downstream of TCR signaling including on JNK2, LCK, CD28, and NF-κB (Begovich et al. 2004; Gjörloff-Wingren et al. 1999). This complex also negatively regulates the lymphocyte migration by inhibiting the LFA-1 (the binding partner of ICAM-1 on lymphocytes (Burn et al. 2016). The PTPN22 also directly inhibits BCR signaling (Negro et al. 2012). In macrophages, monocytes, and dendritic cells, the PTPN22 acts as a positive regulator of TLR-mediated type 1 IFN production and NLRP3-mediated IL-1β release but a negative regulator of NF-κB and MAPK activation downstream intracellular cytosolic pattern recognition receptors such as nucleotide-binding and oligomerization domain-containing type 1 or 2 (NOD1 and 2) (Spalinger et al. 2016, 2017, 2013a, 2013b; Wang et al. 2013). The PTPN22 modulates the macrophage polarization and favors the M2 differentiation over M1 (Chang et al. 2013).

The sets of functions attributed to PTPN22 make it an appealing factor in the pathogenesis of autoimmune diseases. Numerous studies have reported on the association of *PTPN22* polymorphisms with autoimmune diseases. Even though early on several small candidate-gene approaches failed to demonstrate a link between this gene and SSc susceptibility (Balada et al. 2006; Wipff et al. 2006) recent larger case–control studies and meta-analysis have shown the T allele of rs2476601 SNP (1858C > T) corresponding to arginine to tryptophan substitution at amino acid 620 (R620W) to confer susceptibility to SSc (Diaz-Gallo et al. 2011; Dieudé et al. 2008; Gourh et al. 2006; Lee et al. 2012). Moreover, this gene was identified as one of the shared susceptibility loci between SSc and RA in a cross-diseases GWAS (López-Isac et al. 2016b). The minor risk allele has different effects on the diverse functions of the PTPN22 protein possibly because of its interactions with CSK in some of these pathways (Armitage et al. 2021). The amino acid substitution enhances the effects of PTPN22 on TCR and BCR signaling (gain-of-function) altering the receptor affinity in naïve immune cells and allowing the autoreactive lymphocytes to escape the central tolerance. It also promotes pro-fibrotic M2 polarization (gain-of-function) but enhances T-cell migration (loss-of-function) (Armitage et al. 2021).

An intronic SNP (rs1378942) of the *CSK* gene showed a significant association with SSc in a GWAS and a GWAS follow-up (López-Isac et al. 2019; Martin et al. 2012a). Aside from the immunological consequences of *CSK* polymorphisms, it can also affect fibroblast function since the CSK protein also regulates the matrix-cell signaling in fibroblasts and thus affects fibroblast collagen production and its differentiation into myofibroblasts (Skhirtladze et al. 2008; Thannickal et al. 2003; Vittal et al. 2005).

The fate-determining genes

The *neurogenic locus notch homolog 4* (*NOTCH4*) encodes a transmembrane protein that regulates cell-to-cell interactions and determines the differentiation of keratinocytes (Lin et al. 2000; Powell et al. 1998). It is also involved in the function and differentiation of T-regs (Harb et al. 2021, 2020; Janghorban et al. 2018). *NOTCH4* gene harbors significantly enriched hotspots shared between multiple autoimmune diseases such as psoriasis, celiac disease, and type I diabetes (Jeck et al. 2012). Similarly, a GWAS and a candidate gene study in Han Chinese patients have found multiple SNPs within the *NOTCH4* gene to confer susceptibility to SSc (Gorlova et al. 2011; Zhou et al. 2019). Interestingly, a familial whole-genome sequencing study identified a very rare missense variant of this gene to cause SSc in three generations (Cardinale et al. 2016).

The CD226, also known as platelet and T-cell antigen 1 (PTA-1) and DNAX accessory molecule-1 (DNAM-1), is an immune cell surface receptor that is most commonly expressed by NK cells and T-cells. It is involved in the migration and differentiation of CD8+ T-cells and mediates the functions of NK cells. It also inhibits the suppressive effects of T-reg as it competes with the T-reg co-inhibitory receptor TIGIT over the same ligand (Huang et al. 2020; Lozano et al. 2012). Polymorphisms in the *CD226* gene have been linked to autoimmune diseases such as SLE and type I diabetes (Du et al. 2011; Mattana et al. 2014). As SSc and SLE share several susceptibility loci and NK cells and T-regs are involved in the pathogenesis of SSc, the *CD226* polymorphisms seemed an interesting gene to explore in SSc (Dieudé et al. 2011). However, two large candidate gene studies in European patients found conflicting results. While one identified the T allele of the rs763361 to confer risk for SSc, the other was only able to show a link between a haplotype containing the T allele (TCG haplotype of rs763361, rs34794968, rs727088) and pulmonary fibrosis in the setting of SSc (Bossini-Castillo et al. 2012b; Dieudé et al. 2011). Nonetheless, CD226 has a higher expression in the SSc-affected skin, and its knockout rescues the skin from bleomycin-induced fibrosis in mice models via decreasing the production of profibrotic cytokines such as TNFα and IL-6 (Avouac et al. 2013).

The *GRB10* gene encodes another adaptor molecule showing a genome-wide level of association with SSc (Gorlova et al. 2011). The GRB10 molecule is presumed to be involved in apoptosis pathways (Nantel et al. 1998). The lead SNP in this region also confers susceptibility to SLE but has been linked to *IKZF1* instead of *GRB10* according to the GRAIL analysis (Martin et al. 2013). The *IkZF1* encodes a transcription factor involved in the differentiation of helper T-cell subsets (Powell et al. 2019).

An SNP on the *SOX5* gene was shown to confer susceptibility to SSc in a large GWAS and a meta-analysis of GWAS and cohort data (Gorlova et al. 2011). This gene encodes a transcriptional factor involved in Th17 differentiation and cartilage formation (Lefebvre et al. 2001; Shi et al. 2018; Tian et al. 2021).

The *B-cell scaffold protein with ankyrin repeats* (*BANK1*) and the *B-lymphoid tyrosine kinase* (*BLK*) genes

The *BANK1* gene (4q24) encodes a B-cells expressed scaffold protein. This protein is involved in the multiple paths downstream of BCR, TLR, and CD40 signaling in B-cells. It facilitates the calcium mobilization by interacting with the PLC-γ2 after BCR stimulation; it triggers the FOXO1 transcription factor via the downregulation of PI3K/AKT-mediated pathway downstream CD40 signaling; it upregulates IRF7 transcription of IFN and inflammatory cytokines after TLR7 stimulation; and it represses the IRF5-induced IFN production by sequestering the TRAF6 (Georg et al. 2020; Gómez Hernández et al. 2021). The BLK protein, a B-cell expressed non-receptor tyrosine kinase belonging to the Src family, is involved in the BANK1's interaction with PLCγ2 (Dymecki et al. 1990; Berre et al. 2021; Samuelson et al. 2012; Texido et al. 2000).

Polymorphisms in both genes have been linked to susceptibility to multiple autoimmune diseases including SSc. Similar to other autoimmune diseases, the rare alleles of the *BANK1* rs3733197 and rs10516487 SNPs (A and T, respectively) were shown to confer protection against SSc and the T allele of the rs17266594 was shown to confer risk for dcSSc in candidate gene studies (Dieudé et al. 2009b; Fan et al. 2011b; Rueda et al. 2010).

Concerning the *BLK* gene, the A allele of rs13277113 SNP and the T allele of rs2736340 were shown to confer susceptibility to SSc in candidate gene studies, consistent with the findings in other autoimmune diseases such as SLE (Fan et al. 2011a; Ito et al. 2010; Song and Lee 2017).

The association between SSc and both genes was confirmed by a large cohort (Gorlova et al. 2011) and the *BLK* rs2736340 was found as susceptibility loci in large GWAS (López-Isac et al. 2019) and a shared loci between SSc and RA in a cross-disease GWAS (López-Isac et al. 2016b).

The autoimmune risk variants of the *BANK1* gene are associated with reduced phosphorylation rate of PLCγ2 and AKT, which enhances the activity of FOXO1 transcriptional factor contributing to the promotion of Ig class-switching and memory B-cell maturation (Dengler et al. 2008; Kerdiles et al. 2009; Omori et al. 2006; Yazdani et al. 2017). The increased number of memory B-cells could contribute to the expansion of autoreactive B-cells and cause autoimmunity (Dam et al. 2016). Other rarer *BANK1* variants (associated with SLE) increase the risk of autoimmunity by altering the effects of BANK1 on IRF5 and thus enhancing IFN production (Jiang et al. 2019).

The risk allele of the *BLK* is associated with reduced gene expression level and thus restricting its negative regulatory effect on BCR signaling, which could promote autoimmunity and inflammation (Delgado-Vega et al. 2012; Macias-Garcia et al. 2016; Simpfendorfer et al. 2015; Wu et al. 2015; Zhang et al. 2020).

The *tumor necrosis factor ligand superfamily member-4* (*TNFSF4*) gene

The *TNFSF4* encodes OX40 ligand (OX40L) or CD252 which is a co-stimulatory molecule expressed on the surface of a variety of immune cells facilitating multiple functions including the promotion of memory T-cells, suppression of IL-10, and proliferation of B-cell (Cortini et al. 2017; Farres et al. 2011; Soroosh et al. 2006; Stüber and Strober 1996). Genetic variations of the *TNFSF4* have been linked to autoimmunity in multiple ethnicities (Graham et al. 2008a; Gupta et al. 2018). Multiple SNPs (located within the intronic and regulatory segments) of the *TNFSF4* gene have been linked to SSc susceptibility in both candidate gene approaches and GWA studies (Bossini-Castillo et al. 2011a; Gorlova et al. 2011; Gourh et al. 2010; López-Isac et al. 2019). The risk allele and haplotypes alter the repressor binding element of the gene and thus increase its transcription which could eventually lead to autoimmunity by increasing the differentiation and function of T-cells and B-cells (Graham et al. 2008a).

The *Fc Fragment Of IgG Receptor IIIb* (*FCGR3B*) gene

The *FCGR3B* encodes a low-affinity FcRγ expressed by activated neutrophils. It is involved in the recruitment of neutrophils and purging of immune complexes from the bloodstream reducing the chances of other activating FCγRs to encounter immunoglobulin complexes. A copy number variations (CNV) have been described for the *FCGR3B* gene, which is associated with gene expression. A large case–control study on Caucasian European patients was able to show that CN of ≤ 1 conferred risk for SSc (McKinney et al. 2012). Lower copy numbers (≤ 2) have also been linked to other autoimmune diseases such as SLE and RA (Fanciulli et al. 2007; McKinney et al. 2010).

The *positive regulatory domain zinc finger protein-1* (*PRDM1*) gene

An SNP within the *PRDM1* gene (rs4134466) was shown to be associated with SSc in both Caucasian and Japanese populations (Mayes et al. 2014; Terao et al. 2017). The *PRDM1* encodes Blimp-1 a transcriptional repressor that targets *IFNβ* and *MHC class II trans-activator* along with several other genes (Keller and Maniatis 1991; Lin et al. 2002, 1997; Piskurich et al. 2000). It is a fate-determining protein in plasma cells differentiation (Györy et al. 2003). Polymorphisms in this gene have also been linked to SLE susceptibility and increased levels of Blimp-1 have also been shown to correlate with SLE severity (Bönelt et al. 2019; Gateva et al. 2009; Luo et al. 2013; Zhou et al. 2011). Albeit unlike the independent association of *PRDM1* and SSc, the SNPs associated with SLE are located in the intragenic region between *ATG5* and *PRDM1*.

The *transporter associated with antigen processing* (*TAP*) genes

The *TAP* genes encode two sets of proteins (TAP1 and TAP2) that form a heterodimer that is involved in the transportation of antigenic peptides into the lumen of the endoplasmic reticulum and their assembly on the MHC-I (Trowsdale et al. 1990). Variations in the *TAP1* and *TAP2* genes can change the peptide selection and thus influence the immune response (Lankat-Buttgereit and Tampé 2002; Powis et al. 1992; Qian et al. 2017). These polymorphisms are associated with an increased risk of psoriasis and RA among other autoimmune diseases (Qian et al. 2017; Witkowska-Tobo³a et al. 2004; Zhang et al. 2002). They have also shown weak associations with SSc susceptibility in candidate gene studies (Song et al. 2005). An SNP (rs17500468) affecting the expression rate of the *TAP2* gene was found to be associated with SSc in an immunochip study (Mayes et al. 2014).

The genes encoding IL-12 and IL-12 receptor subunits (IL-12RB1 and IL-12RB2)

An intragenic region (rs77583790 at 3q25) between the *SCHIP1* and *IL12A* genes was identified as an SSc susceptibility loci in an immunochip study (Mayes et al. 2014). The association of another non-coding SNP of *IL-12A* (rs589446) and SSc was found in a GWAS (López-Isac et al. 2019). The functional effects of these polymorphisms are not clear but they are presumed to have a role in gene expression rate. This might be relevant as elevated levels of IL-12 have been documented in patients suffering from SSc (Sato et al. 2000). Moreover, the *IL-12RB2* rs3790567 and rs3790566 SNPs and *IL-12RB1* rs2305743 were found to be associated with SSc susceptibility with genome-wide levels of significance (Bossini-Castillo et al. 2012a; López-Isac et al. 2019; Lopez-Isac et al. 2014; Radstake et al. 2010). *IL-12RB2* also harbors a shared susceptibility locus (rs6659932) between SSc and Crohn's disease (González-Serna et al. 2020). Interpreting the functional consequences of these polymorphisms is a bit complex as it may vary in different cell lines. All in all, it seems that the risk alleles are associated with increased expression of IL-12 receptor subunits which favor inflammatory pathways (González-Serna et al. 2020; Lopez-Isac et al. 2014).

The IL-12 possesses both innate and adaptive immune functions. It promotes NK-cell IFN production and cytotoxicity and drives the differentiation of Th1 cells (Caspi 1998). However, the relation between IL-12 and autoimmunity is more complex than it seems. Though higher levels of IL-12 have been documented in SSc, the administration of IL-12 may have beneficial effects in reducing fibrosis as it diverts the immune response from profibrotic Th2 towards Th1 (Banning et al. 2006; Matsushita et al. 2006; Tsuji-Yamada et al. 2001). Additionally, the *IL-12RB2* knockout is associated with a higher risk of humoral autoimmunity with unopposed IL-6 upregulation (Airoldi et al. 2005; Pistoia et al. 2009).

Other Cytokines and cytokine receptors

Candidate gene studies have been able to document the association of several cytokine and cytokine receptor genes with SSc. Albeit none were detected in GWAS and immunochip studies. The *IL-2RA* rs2104286 was linked to susceptibility to ACA + SSc by a large study in

European Caucasians (Martin et al. 2012b). The IL-2RA (CD25) mediates the immunosuppressive functions of T-regs by scavenging IL-2 and upregulating co-inhibitory molecules such as CTLA4 (Gasteiger and Kastenmuller 2012; Kastenmuller et al. 2011). The *IL-6* rs2069840 was linked to lcSSc and its GGC haplotype of rs2069827-rs1800795-rs2069840 was linked to SSc in European Caucasians (Cénit et al. 2012). This is not surprising since as discussed above IL-6 is one of the main drivers of inflammation-induced fibrosis. Candidate gene case–control studies have been able to link variation in genes encoding multiple members of the IL-1 family to SSc (Xu et al. 2019). The rs1800587 and the rs17561 SNPs of *IL-1α*, the rs1143634 and rs16944 of the *IL-1β*, the rs1946518 and rs187238 of *IL-18*, and the rs7044343, rs1157505, rs11792633, and rs1929992 of *IL-33* have been linked to SSc (Abtahi et al. 2015; Beretta et al. 2008; Huang et al. 2016; Hutyrová et al. 2004; Kawaguchi et al. 2003; Mattuzzi et al. 2007). The *IL-2* and *IL-21* genes are located within a 180 kb segment mapped at 4q27. Thus an SNP within one gene most likely affects the other as well (Parrish-Novak et al. 2000). The rs6822844 and rs907715 within this region have been linked to SSc susceptibility in a large cohort of patients from North America and Europe (Diaz-Gallo et al. 2013). *IL-13RA2* and *IL-10RB* variants have also been linked to SSc by two relatively small studies that cannot confidently be referred to Granel et al. (2006).

3.4 The Gene Involved in Fibrogenesis

The genes encoding growth factors

The *cellular communication network factor 2* (*CCN2*) gene located at 6q23.2 encodes the CTGF. As mentioned earlier this growth factor plays a major role in the pathogenesis of SSc and has thus been an interesting gene to explore. The GG genotype of the rs6918698 (-945 G/C) polymorphism was initially linked to SSc by a large candidate gene study, which was also able to demonstrate the functional significance of this variant. The replacement of guanine alters the transcriptional binding site for the gene suppressors and thus increases the transcriptional activity of the gene and promotes fibrosis (Fonseca et al. 2007). Although the gene showed a near-significant association with SSc susceptibility in a GWAS subsequent cohort and meta-analysis were not able to show an association (Rueda et al. 2009b; Zhou et al. 2009). It seems that the association is confined to a subpopulation of patients with specific disease characteristics (pulmonary fibrosis) and ethnic backgrounds (Asian) (Zhang et al. 2012; Zhao et al. 2017).

The data on the association of genetic polymorphisms in the *TGFβ* (β_1, β_2, and β_3) genes and SSc are diverse as small studies show marginal association but meta-analysis and larger studies do not show a significant link (Ohtsuka et al. 2002; Susol et al. 2000).

The MMPs and the tissue inhibitors of MMPs (TIMPs)

Since the ECM turnover depends on the delicate balance between the levels and functions of MMPs and TIMPs, they are interesting genetic candidates for SSc susceptibility. Though none of the genes encoding these proteins appeared in GWA and immunochip studies, small case–control studies have shown some interesting findings. The 6A allele of *MMP3* rs35068180 (insertion of adenosine at position 1171) of Marasini et al. (2001) and the A allele of the *MMP12* rs2276109 SNP conferred risk for SSc and lcSSc in two small case–control studies in Italy, respectively (Carmona et al. 2013; Marasini et al. 2001). However, investigations on variants of the genes encoding the MMP1, MMP2, MMP9, and MMP14 proteins did not show an overall association with SSc in Caucasians, African-Americans, and Hispanics (Johnson et al. 2001; Wipff et al. 2010). However, the GGA allele of the rs1799750 of the *MMP1* gene (insertion of guanine at position 1607) associated with increased transcription of the gene was shown to confer risk for lcSSc in Korean patients (Joung et al. 2008) and the CT genotype of the *MMP9* rs3918242 was shown to be associated with a lower risk of digital ulcers in male SSc patients (Skarmoutsou et al. 2011).

The *TIMP1* rs4898 SNP (+372 T > C) was linked to SSc susceptibility only in male patients (Indelicato et al. 2006) with the C allele and CC genotype conferring protection against SSc and formation of digital ulcers in females (Skarmoutsou et al. 2012).

The caveolin family

The caveolin family of proteins including caveolin-1, caveolin-2, and caveolin-3 help the formation of caveolae vesicles that mediate multiple cellular functions such as migration, signal transduction, and endocytosis (Salanueva et al. 2007). The caveolin-1 is also involved in the regulation of fibrogenic pathways through numerous mechanisms. It inhibits the Smad-2 and Smad-3 phosphorylation and Erk1/2 and Janus kinas activation downstream TGF-β signaling and thus reduces the production of collagen, SMA-α, and fibronectin production by fibroblasts (Razani et al. 2001; Wang et al. 2006a). Accordingly, the knockout of caveolin-1 encoding gene, *Cav1,* results in increased collagen production and thickened lung and skin tissue and a Cav1 overexpression rescues the tissue from bleomycin-induced fibrosis (Drab et al. 2001; Wang et al. 2006a). Furthermore, the skin and alveolar tissue from patients with SSc and the fibroblasts of patients with idiopathic pulmonary fibrosis show reduced expression of Cav-1 (Galdo et al. 2008; Wang et al. 2006a).

Aside from the mentioned fibrogenic pathway, caveolin-1 is also involved in the regulation of nitric oxide production by endothelial cells. Both over expression and deletion of *Cav-1* result in the reduced activity of endothelial nitric oxide synthetase (Feron and Kelly 2001; Sbaa et al. 2005). The caveolin-1-mediated inhibition of Erk1/2 can also affect the VEGF signaling and angiogenesis (Almeida 2017; Fang et al. 2007). Pericytes and bone marrow-derived mesenchymal stem cells from SSc patients demonstrate impaired expression and function of caveolin-1 that could promote fibrosis through the persistent activity of VEGF (Cipriani et al. 2014).

Involvement in the aforementioned mechanisms makes *Cav-1* an interesting candidate gene in SSc susceptibility. Two large cohorts of European patients revealed that the minor C allele of the *Cav-1* rs959173 corresponding to higher expression levels of this protein conferred protection against SSc (Manetti et al. 2012, 2013).

The nitric oxide synthetase (NOS) encoding genes

Three main types of NOS have been described in humans, *NOS1* encoding the neuronal NOS (nNOS), *NOS2* encoding inducible NOS (iNOS) expressed in endothelial and smooth muscle cells along with fibroblast, and *NOS3* encoding the endothelial NOS (eNOS) (Ignarro 1990). The eNOS controls the vascular tone by producing NO which is both a vasodilator and a ROS scavenger. As mentioned earlier in the pathogenesis of SSc, endothelial cell injury could reduce the basal levels of NO production by eNOS and lead to vasoconstriction, increased adhesion molecule expression, platelet activation, and intimal proliferation (Matucci Cerinic and Kahaleh 2002). This is backed up by multiple studies demonstrating either reduced levels of NO or eNOS in sera of patients with SSc (Freedman et al. 1999; Kahaleh and Fan 1998). As the disease progresses, the tissue hypoxia and the inflammation induce the iNOS shifting the NO production from eNOS to iNOS (Cotton et al. 1999). In a hypoxic setting, the interaction between ROS and NO produces cytotoxic peroxynitrite (NO_3^-) that can cause damage to proteins and lipids (Herrick and Cerinic 2001). Thus according to the stage of the disease, NO can be either protective or harmful (Matucci Cerinic and Kahaleh 2002).

The involvement of iNOS and eNOS in the pathogenesis of SSc has made them interesting to genetic studies. Two *NOS3* genetic variants with reduced eNOS activity, the aa genotype of a 27pb long variable number of tandem repeats (VNTR) polymorphism located at the 4th intron and the CC genotype of the rs2070744 (-786 T > C), have been shown to confer susceptibility to SSc in a candidate gene study (Sinici et al. 2010). The TC haplotype of rs1799983 (894G > T) and rs2070744 (-786 T > C) was shown to affect the hemorheology profile and increase susceptibility to SSc (Fatini et al. 2006). The polymorphisms in the *NOS2* gene did not show an association with SSc (Allanore et al. 2004).

The PPARγ encoding gene

The peroxisome proliferator-activated receptors (PPARs) are transcriptional factors that regulate gene expression by binding to the retinoid X receptor (RXR). The *PPARγ* gene was initially linked to SSc by a GWAS follow-up study (rs310746) (López-Isac et al. 2014). Subsequently, a candidate gene study in European patients found an association between another SNP (rs10865710) residing within the intronic segment of this gene and SSc (Marangoni et al. 2015). As mentioned earlier, the PPARγ mediates the inhibitory feedback signals relayed by ECM components (Denton 2015). Moreover, the PPARγ and TFGβ have a bidirectional inhibitory effect on one another. Thus, the reduced function or expression of PPARγ could unleash the fibroblasts from their negative regulators and perhaps explain their autonomy. Altered expression of PPARγ has been demonstrated in patients with SSc (Wei et al. 2008, 2010).

The *TREH/DDX6* region

The 11q23 region contains several GWAS susceptibility loci for SSc, one residing at the intragenic region between *trehalase* (*TREH*) and *DEAD-box RNA helicase 6* (*DDX6*) (rs7130875) and another within the *DDX6* intron (rs11217020) (López-Isac et al. 2019; Mayes et al. 2014). The *DDX6* gene is relevant to the pathogenesis of SSc as it regulates VEGF under hypoxic conditions (Vries et al. 2013).

The *Allograft inflammatory factor* (*AIF*) gene

The AIF encoding gene demonstrated a significant association with ACA + SSc by a candidate gene study and a suggestive association with SSc in a GWAS (Alkassab et al. 2007; Zhou et al. 2009). This gene is among the differentially expressed genes in SSc and graft-versus-host disease (GVHD) compared to normal skin and it is presumed to play a role in the inflammation-induced proliferation of vascular smooth muscles cells (Christmann et al. 2014; Mayes and Trojanowska 2007).

3.5 Genes Involved in Apoptosis, Autophagy, and Pyroptosis

The *Deoxyribonuclease 1-like 3* (*DNASE1L3*) gene

Several SNPs residing in the *DNASE1L3* gene (located at 3p14.3) or in linkage disequilibrium with its lead SNP (intronic *FLNB* and *PXK* SNPs) have been shown to confer susceptibility to SSc in immunochip and GWA studies (López-Isac et al. 2019; Martin et al. 2013; Mayes et al. 2014; Zochling et al. 2014). This gene encodes deoxyribonuclease-I, which degrades nucleic acid material such as those released in apoptosis or present in neutrophil extracellular traps (NETs) (Al-Mayouf et al. 2011; Errami et al. 2013; Namjou et al. 2011). The lead *DNASE1L3* SNP associated with SSc, the rs35677470, is a loss-of-function mutation that could cause autoimmunity by decreasing the clearance of self-DNA and thus prolonging its exposure to the immune system (Garcia-Romo et al. 2011; Ueki et al. 2009). *DNASE1* mutations and polymorphisms are also involved in the pathogenesis of SLE (Al-Mayouf et al. 2011).

Autophagy-related genes

Autophagy refers to the clearance and degradation process that enables the cells to get rid of damaged and unwanted material within the cytoplasm by encapsulating them within a phagosome vesicle and facilitating the fusion of this vesicle with the lysosomes. Autophagy enables the adaptation of cells to environmental stressors such as hypoxia, lower concentrations of growth factors, and oxidative stress (Inomata et al. 2013; Mizushima 2007; Yousefi et al. 2006). Thus it possesses diverse functions across different cell lines. In the immune system, it is involved in several aspects of antigen presentation, thymic selection, and cytokine production which if derailed could cause autoimmunity (Kuballa et al. 2012; Ye et al. 2018).

Polymorphisms in two genes involved in autophagy have been linked to SSc, the *autophagy-related 5* (*ATG5*) gene and the *ras-related protein Rab-2A* (*RAB2A*) gene (Lőrincz et al. 2017; Tanida 2011).

The link between *ATG5* variants and SSc was identified through immunochip and GWA studies (López-Isac et al. 2019; Mayes et al. 2014). *ATG5* has also been linked to RA and SLE susceptibility (López-Isac et al. 2016b; Lu et al. 2012).

The intergenic region between the *CDH7* and *RAB2A* gene was shown to confer the risk for SSc with genome-wide levels of significance (López-Isac et al. 2019; Radstake et al. 2010). CDH7 encodes an adhesion molecule belonging to the cadherin family (Luo et al. 2004). Since other autophagy-related genes such as *ATG5* have also been linked to SSc, the *RAB2A* gene seems more relevant to the pathogenesis of SSc.

The pyroptosis-related genes

The gasdermin family consists of six pore-forming proteins encoded by genes located at 17q21.1. These proteins are cleaved and activated by caspases downstream cytosolic pattern recognition receptors, TLRs, and TNF receptor signaling. The cleaved proteins form multiple pores at the cell surface that allow the release of proinflammatory cytokines and danger-associated molecules and facilitate cell lysis by increasing permeability (Broz et al. 2020). Genetic variations can alter the expression and function of the masterminds and have been linked to multiple autoimmune and immune-mediated diseases but their precise role in the pathogenesis of these diseases remains to be elucidated (Broz et al. 2020). The gasdermin-A (GSDMA) and gasdermin-B (GSDMB) encoding genes harbor two independent SSc susceptibility loci with a genome-wide level of significance (González-Serna et al. 2020; López-Isac et al. 2019; Terao et al. 2017). The GDSMA gene represents a shared susceptibility gene between SSc and Crohn's disease (González-Serna et al. 2020).

3.6 Genes with Miscellaneous Functions

The association between variation in the *PSORS1C1* gene located at 6p21.1 and SSc was identified through a GWAS and confirmed in replication studies. Its precise role in the pathogenesis of SSc is not clear (Allanore et al. 2011; Bossini-Castillo et al. 2013).

A 287 bp insertion/deletion (InDel) polymorphism of the *angiotensin-converting enzyme* (*ACE*) affecting the gene expression has also been linked to SSc by a small case–control study (Guiducci et al. 2006; Rigat et al. 1990). The link was not confirmed by a later larger study (Wipff et al. 2009).

4 Conclusion

Genetic studies have been able to elucidate some previously unknown aspects of SSc pathogenesis such as the involvement of autophagy and pyroptosis pathways. These studies have also changed the previous assumptions on the importance of fibrogenic pathways. Unlike the histopathological and clinical evidence that underestimated the involvement of the immune system in SSc induction and progression, genetic studies have shown substantial evidence for the contribution of the immune system (Table 1). Most of the SSc-associated genes are immune system regulators. This highlights the importance of inflammation-induced fibrosis in SSc.

Genome-wide screening of other types of polymorphisms such as insertion and deletion polymorphisms and CNVs may be able to further our knowledge on SSc by identifying new susceptibility genes.

Table 1 Non-HLA genes associated with systemic sclerosis (SSc)

	Gene	Associated phenotype*	References
Innate immunity-related genes	*IRF1, 4, 5, and 8: Intron regulatory factor 4, 5, and 8*	IRF5: lcSSc > dcSSC, ACA+ or ATA + subtypes IRF5: PF IRF8: lcSSC	Allanore et al. (2011), González-Serna et al. (2020), Gorlova et al. (2011), López-Isac et al. (2019, 2016b), Mayes et al. (2014), Radstake et al. (2010), Zochling et al. (2014), Gorlova et al. (2011), López-Isac et al. (2019), Zhao et al. (2017)
	STAT4 and STAT3: Signal transducer and activator of transcription 4 and 3	lcSSC, PF	Allanore et al. (2011), Dieudé et al. (2009b), Gorlova et al. (2011), López-Isac et al. (2019), Mayes et al. (2014), Radstake et al. (2010), Rueda et al. (2009a), Terao et al. (2017), Tsuchiya et al. (2009), Xu et al. (2016), Zhao et al. (2017), Zochling et al. (2014)
	TYK2	SSc	González-Serna et al. (2020), López-Isac et al. (2016a), Mayes et al. (2014)
	NFKB1	SSc	González-Serna et al. (2019), Liu et al. (2021), López-Isac et al. (2019)
	TNFAIP3: Tumor necrosis factor, alpha-induced protein 3	SSc	Dieude et al. (2010), Terao et al. (2017), Wei et al. (2016)
	TNIP1: TNFAIP3 interacting protein 1	SSc	Allanore et al. (2011), Bossini-Castillo et al. (2013), López-Isac et al. (2019)
	IRAK1: Interleukin-1 receptor-associated kinase 1 MECP2: Methyl CpG binding protein-2	PF, dsSSc	Carmona et al. (2013), Dieude et al. (2011), Zhao et al. (2017)
	MIF: Macrophage migration inhibitory factor	dcSSc, PAH	Baños-Hernández et al. (2019), Bossini-Castillo et al. (2017, 2011b), Wu et al. (2006)
	RHOB: ras homolog family member b	SSc	Allanore et al. (2011), Bossini-Castillo et al. (2013), Shu et al. (2014)
	TLR2: Toll-like receptor 2	dcSSc, ATA+, PAH	Broen et al. (2012)

(continued)

Table 1 (continued)

	Gene	Associated phenotype*	References
Adaptive Immunity	*CD247 (CD3ζ)*	lcSSc > dcSSc, ACA+, and ATA+	Allanore et al. (2011), Gorlova et al. (2011), López-Isac et al. (2019), Radstake et al. (2010), Wang et al. (2014), Zochling et al. (2014)
	PTPN22: Protein tyrosine phosphatase non-receptor 22	ATA+	Diaz-Gallo et al. (2011), Dieudé et al. (2008), Gourh et al. (2006), Lee et al. (2012)
	CSK: C-Scr kinases	SSc	López-Isac et al. (2019), Martin et al. (2012a)
	NOTHC: Neurogenic locus notch homolog 4	Familial SC	Cardinale et al. (2016), Gorlova et al. (2011), Zhou et al. (2019)
	CD226	dcSSc, ATA+, and PF	Bossini-Castillo et al. (2012b), Dieudé et al. (2011)
	IKZF1: IKAROS family zinc finger 1	lcSSc	Martin et al. (2013), Powell et al. (2019)
	SOX5: Sex determining region Y-box 5	ACA+, lcSSc	Gorlova et al. (2011)
	BLK: B-lymphoid tyrosine kinase	ACA+	Fan et al. (2011a), Ito et al. (2010), Song and Lee (2017), López-Isac et al. (2019, 2016b), Gorlova et al. (2011)
	BANK1: B cell scaffold protein with ankyrin repeats	dcSSc, ATA+	Dieudé et al. (2009b), Fan et al. (2011b), Gorlova et al. (2011), Rueda et al. (2010)
	TNFSF4 (OX40L): Tumor necrosis factor superfamily, member 4	lcSSc, ACA+	Bossini-Castillo et al. (2011a), Gorlova et al. (2011), Gourh et al. (2010), López-Isac et al. (2019)
	FcγRIIIb: Fc fragment of IgG receptor IIIb	SSc	McKinney et al. (2012)
	PRDM1: Positive regulatory domain zinc finger protein-1	SSc	Mayes et al. (2014), Terao et al. (2017)
	Tap2: Transporter associated with antigen processing	SSc	Mayes et al. (2014), Song et al. (2005)
	IL-12: Interleukin-12 IL-12RB: Interleukin-12 receptor B1 and B2	lcSSc, ACA+	Mayes et al. (2014), Bossini-Castillo et al. (2012a), López-Isac et al. (2014, 2019), Radstake et al. (2010), González-Serna et al. (2020)
	IL-2RA: Interleukin-2 receptor A	ACA+	Martin et al. (2012b)
	IL-6: Interleukin-6	lcSSc	Cénit et al. (2012)
	IL-1A: Interleukin-1A	SSc	Abtahi et al. (2015), Beretta et al. (2008), Huang et al.

(continued)

Table 1 (continued)

	Gene	Associated phenotype*	References
	IL-1B: Interleukin-1B *IL-18: Interleukin-18* *IL-33: Interleukin-33*		(2016), Hutyrová et al. (2004), Kawaguchi et al. (2003), Mattuzzi et al. (2007)
	VCAM1: Vascular cell adhesion protein 1 *CXCR2: CXC chemokine receptor 2*	SSc and lcSSc	Zochling et al. (2014)
Genes involved in Fibrogenesis	*CCN2: Cellular communication network factor-2 also known as CTGF*	ATA+, PF	Fonseca et al. (2007), Rueda et al. (2009b), Zhang et al. (2012), Zhao et al. (2017), Zhou et al. (2009)
	TIMP1: Tissue inhibitors of matrix metalloproteinase MMP3,9, and 12: Matrix metalloproteinases 3, 9, and 12	MMP12 linked to lcSSc	Indelicato et al. (2006), Skarmoutsou et al. (2012), Marasini et al. (2001), Carmona et al. (2013), Joung et al. (2008), Marasini et al. (2001)
	CAV1: Caveolin-1	SSc	Manetti et al. (2012, 2013)
	NOS3: Nitric oxide synthetase 3 or endothelial NOS	SSc	Sinici et al. (2010), Fatini et al. (2006)
	PPARG: Peroxisome proliferator-activated receptor γ	SSc	López-Isac et al. (2014), Marangoni et al. (2015)
	DDX6: DEAD-box RNA helicase 6	SSc	Bhattacharyya et al. (2014), Bossini-Castillo et al. (2012a)
	AIF: Allograft inflammatory factor	ACA+	Alkassab et al. (2007), Zhou et al. (2009)
Apoptosis/Autophagy/Pyroptosis	*DNASE1L3: Deoxyribonuclease 1 Like 3**	ACA+, lcSSc	López-Isac et al. (2019), Martin et al. (2013), Mayes et al. (2014), Zochling et al. (2014)
	RAB2A-CHD7 *ATG5: Autophagy0related 5*	SSc SSc	López-Isac et al. (2019), Luo et al. (2004), Radstake et al. (2010), López-Isac et al. (2019, 2016b), Lu et al. (2012), Mayes et al. (2014)
	GSDMA: Gasdermin-A *GSDMB: Gasdermin-B*	lcSSc	López-Isac et al. (2019), Terao et al. (2017)
	GRB10: Growth factor receptor-bound protein 10	lcSSc	Gorlova et al. (2011)

(continued)

Table 1 (continued)

	Gene	Associated phenotype*	References
Genes with miscellaneous functions	*PSORS1C1: Psoriasis susceptibility 1 candidate 1*	SSc	Allanore et al. (2011), Bossini-Castillo et al. (2013)
	RPL41/ESYT1: Ribosomal protein L41/ Extended synaptotagmin 1	dcSSc	Gorlova et al. (2011)
	KIAA0319L	lcSSc	Zochling et al. (2014)
	JAZF1: Juxtaposed with another zinc finger protein 1	SSc	Zochling et al. (2014)
	DGKQ: Diacylglycerol kinase theta	SSc	Mayes et al. (2014), Zochling et al. (2014)
	NAB1: NGFI-A binding protein 1	SSc	López-Isac et al. (2019)
	*ARHGAP31: Rho GTPase Activating Protein 31***	SSc	López-Isac et al. (2019)
	NUP85-GRB2: Nucleoporin 85/Growth factor receptor bound protein 2	SSc	López-Isac et al. (2019)
	TSPAN32/CD81-AS1: Tetraspanin 32/CD81 Antisense RNA 1	SSc	López-Isac et al. (2019)
	GTF2I: General transcription factor IIi	SSc	Liu et al. (2021)
	ACE: Angiotensin-converting enzyme	SSc	Guiducci et al. (2006), Rigat et al. (1990), Wipff et al. (2009)

References

Abais JM, Xia M, Zhang Y, Boini KM, Li P-L (2015) Redox regulation of NLRP3 inflammasomes: ROS as trigger or effector? Antioxid Redox Signal 22:1111–1129

Abtahi S, Farazmand A, Mahmoudi M, Ashraf-Ganjouei A, Javinani A, Nazari B, Kavosi H, Amirzargar A, Jamshidi A, Gharibdoost F (2015) IL-1 A rs1800587, IL-1 B rs1143634 and IL-1 R 1 rs2234650 polymorphisms in I ranian patients with systemic sclerosis. Int J Immunogenet 42:423–427

Adigun R, Goyal A, Bansal P, Hariz A (2020) Systemic sclerosis (CREST syndrome). StatPearls [Internet]

Adini I, Rabinovitz I, Sun JF, Prendergast GC, Benjamin LE (2003) RhoB controls Akt trafficking and stage-specific survival of endothelial cells during vascular development. Genes Dev 17:2721–2732

Adrianto I, Wen F, Templeton A, Wiley G, King JB, Lessard CJ, Bates JS, Hu Y, Kelly JA, Kaufman KM (2011) Association of a functional variant downstream of TNFAIP3 with systemic lupus erythematosus. Nat Genet 43:253–258

Airoldi I, Di Carlo E, Cocco C, Sorrentino C, Fais F, Cilli M, D'Antuono T, Colombo MP, Pistoia V (2005) Lack of Il12rb2 signaling predisposes to spontaneous autoimmunity and malignancy. Blood 106:3846–3853

Alkassab F, Gourh P, Tan F, McNearney T, Fischbach M, Ahn C, Arnett F, Mayes M (2007) An allograft inflammatory factor 1 (AIF1) single nucleotide polymorphism (SNP) is associated with anticentromere antibody positive systemic sclerosis. Rheumatology 46:1248–1251

Allanore Y, Borderie D, Lemaréchal H, Ekindjian OG, Kahan A (2004) Lack of association of eNOS (G894T) and p22phox NADPH oxidase subunit (C242T) polymorphisms with systemic sclerosis in a cohort of French Caucasian patients. Clin Chim Acta 350:51–55

Allanore Y, Saad M, Dieudé P, Avouac J, Distler JH, Amouyel P, Matucci-Cerinic M, Riemekasten G, Airo P, Melchers I (2011) Genome-wide scan identifies TNIP1, PSORS1C1, and RHOB as novel risk loci for systemic sclerosis. PLoS Genet 7:e1002091

Al-Mayouf SM, Sunker A, Abdwani R, Al Abrawi S, Almurshedi F, Alhashmi N, Al Sonbul A, Sewairi W, Qari A, Abdallah E (2011) Loss-of-function variant in DNASE1L3 causes a familial form of systemic lupus erythematosus. Nat Genet 43:1186–1188

Antonczyk A, Krist B, Sajek M, Michalska A, Piaszyk-Borychowska A, Plens-Galaska M, Wesoly J, Bluyssen HA (2019) Direct inhibition of IRF-dependent transcriptional regulatory mechanisms associated with disease. Front Immunol 10:1176

Apte RS, Sinha D, Mayhew E, Wistow G, Niederkorn J (1998) Cutting edge: role of macrophage migration inhibitory factor in inhibiting NK cell activity and preserving immune privilege. J Immunol 160:5693–5696

Arbiser JL, Petros J, Klafter R, Govindajaran B, McLaughlin ER, Brown LF, Cohen C, Moses M, Kilroy S, Arnold RS (2002) Reactive oxygen generated by Nox1 triggers the angiogenic switch. Proc Natl Acad Sci 99:715–720

Armitage LH, Wallet MA, Mathews CE (2021) Influence of PTPN22 allotypes on innate and adaptive immune function in health and disease. Front Immunol 12

Arnett FC, Cho M, Chatterjee S, Aguilar MB, Reveille JD, Mayes MD (2001) Familial occurrence frequencies and relative risks for systemic sclerosis (scleroderma) in three United States cohorts. Arthritis Rheum Off J Am Coll Rheumatol 44:1359–1362

Arnett FC, Gourh P, Shete S, Ahn CW, Honey RE, Agarwal SK, Tan FK, McNearney T, Fischbach M, Fritzler MJ (2010) Major histocompatibility complex (MHC) class II alleles, haplotypes and epitopes which confer susceptibility or protection in systemic sclerosis: analyses in 1300 Caucasian, African-American and Hispanic cases and 1000 controls. Ann Rheum Dis 69:822–827

Artlett CM, Sassi-Gaha S, Hope JL, Feghali-Bostwick CA, Katsikis PD (2017) Mir-155 is overexpressed in systemic sclerosis fibroblasts and is required for NLRP3 inflammasome-mediated collagen synthesis during fibrosis. Arthritis Res Ther 19:1–8

Avouac J, Fürnrohr BG, Tomcik M, Palumbo K, Zerr P, Horn A, Dees C, Akhmetshina A, Beyer C, Distler O (2011) Inactivation of the transcription factor STAT-4 prevents inflammation-driven fibrosis in animal models of systemic sclerosis. Arthritis Rheum 63:800–809

Avouac J, Elhai M, Tomcik M, Ruiz B, Friese M, Piedavent M, Colonna M, Bernhardt G, Kahan A, Chiocchia G (2013) Critical role of the adhesion receptor DNAX accessory molecule-1 (DNAM-1) in the development of inflammation-driven dermal fibrosis in a mouse model of systemic sclerosis. Ann Rheum Dis 72:1089–1098

Balada E, Simeon-Aznar C, Serrano-Acedo S, Martinez-Lostao L, Selva-O Callaghan A, Fonollosa-Pla V, Vilardell-Tarrés M (2006) Lack of association of the PTPN22 gene polymorphism R620W with systemic sclerosis. Clin Exp Rheumatol 24:321

Banning U, Krutmann J, Körholz D (2006) The role of IL-4 and IL-12 in the regulation of collagen synthesis by fibroblasts. Immunol Invest 35:199–207

Baños-Hernández CJ, Navarro-Zarza JE, Bucala R, Hernández-Bello J, Parra-Rojas I, Ramírez-Dueñas MG, García-Arellano S, Hernández-Palma LA, Machado-Sulbarán AC, Muñoz-Valle JF (2019) Macrophage migration inhibitory factor polymorphisms are a potential susceptibility marker in systemic sclerosis from southern Mexican population: association with MIF mRNA expression and cytokine profile. Clin Rheumatol 38:1643–1654

Barnes J, Agarwal SK (2011) Targeting STAT4 in systemic sclerosis: a promising new direction. Exp Rev Clin Immunol 7:445–448

Barnes B, Lubyova B, Pitha PM (2002) On the role of IRF in host defense. J Interferon Cytokine Res 22:59–71

Baugh J, Chitnis S, Donnelly S, Monteiro J, Lin X, Plant B, Wolfe F, Gregersen P, Bucala R (2002) A functional promoter polymorphism in the macrophage migration inhibitory factor (MIF) gene associated with disease severity in rheumatoid arthritis. Genes Immun 3:170–176

Begovich AB, Carlton VE, Honigberg LA, Schrodi SJ, Chokkalingam AP, Alexander HC, Ardlie KG, Huang Q, Smith AM, Spoerke JM (2004) A missense single-nucleotide polymorphism in a gene encoding a protein tyrosine phosphatase (PTPN22) is associated with rheumatoid arthritis. Am J Hum Genet 75:330–337

Beretta L, Cappiello F, Moore JH, Barili M, Greene CS, Scorza R (2008) Ability of epistatic interactions of cytokine single-nucleotide polymorphisms to predict susceptibility to disease subsets in systemic sclerosis patients. Arthritis Care Res Off J Am Coll Rheumatol 59:974–983

Bhattacharyya S, Wang W, Graham LVD, Varga J (2016) A20 suppresses canonical Smad-dependent fibroblast activation: novel function for an endogenous inflammatory modulator. Arthritis Res Ther 18:1–10

Bhattacharyya S, Tamaki Z, Wang W, Hinchcliff M, Hoover P, Getsios S, White ES, Varga J (2014) FibronectinEDA promotes chronic cutaneous fibrosis through Toll-like receptor signaling. Sci Transl Med 6:232ra250–232ra250

Black C, Walker A, Catoggio L, Welsh K, Bernstein R, McGregor A, Jones JL (1983) Genetic susceptibility to scleroderma-like syndrome induced by vinyl chloride. Lancet 321:53–55

Blake D, Winyard P, Scott D, Brailsford S, Blann A, Lunec J (1985) Endothelial cell cytotoxicity in inflammatory vascular diseases—the possible role of oxidised lipoproteins. Ann Rheum Dis 44:176–182

Bönelt P, Wöhner M, Minnich M, Tagoh H, Fischer M, Jaritz M, Kavirayani A, Garimella M, Karlsson MC, Busslinger M (2019) Precocious expression of Blimp1 in B cells causes autoimmune disease with increased self-reactive plasma cells. EMBO J 38:1–19

Bossini-Castillo L, Broen JC, Simeon CP, Beretta L, Vonk MC, Ortego-Centeno N, Espinosa G, Carreira P, Camps MT, Navarrete N (2011a) A replication study confirms the association of TNFSF4 (OX40L) polymorphisms with systemic sclerosis in a large European cohort. Ann Rheum Dis 70:638–641

Bossini-Castillo L, Simeon CP, Beretta L, Vonk MC, Callejas-Rubio JL, Espinosa G, Carreira P, Camps MT, Rodríguez-Rodríguez L, Rodríguez-Carballeira M (2011b) Confirmation of association of the macrophage migration inhibitory factor gene with systemic sclerosis in a large European population. Rheumatology 50:1976–1981

Bossini-Castillo L, Martin J-E, Broen J, Gorlova O, Simeón CP, Beretta L, Vonk MC, Luis Callejas J, Castellví I, Carreira P (2012a) A GWAS follow-up study reveals the association of the IL12RB2 gene with systemic sclerosis in Caucasian populations. Hum Mol Genet 21:926–933

Bossini-Castillo L, Simeon CP, Beretta L, Broen JC, Vonk MC, Ríos-Fernández R, Espinosa G, Carreira P, Camps MT, Castillo MJ (2012b) A multicenter study confirms CD226 gene association with systemic sclerosis-related pulmonary fibrosis. Arthritis Res Ther 14:1–7

Bossini-Castillo L, Martin JE, Broen J, Simeon CP, Beretta L, Gorlova OY, Vonk MC, Ortego-Centeno N, Espinosa G, Carreira P (2013) Confirmation of TNIP1 but not RHOB and PSORS1C1 as systemic sclerosis risk factors in a large independent replication study. Ann Rheum Dis 72:602–607

Bossini-Castillo L, López-Isac E, Martín J (2015) Immunogenetics of systemic sclerosis: defining heritability, functional variants and shared-autoimmunity pathways. J Autoimmun 64:53–65

Bossini-Castillo L, Campillo-Davó D, López-Isac E, Carmona FD, Simeon CP, Carreira P, Callejas-Rubio JL, Castellví I, Fernández-Nebro A, Rodríguez-Rodríguez L (2017) An MIF promoter polymorphism is associated with susceptibility to pulmonary arterial hypertension in diffuse cutaneous systemic sclerosis. J Rheumatol 44:1453–1457

Braga TT, Agudelo JSH, Camara NOS (2015) Macrophages during the fibrotic process: M2 as friend and foe. Front Immunol 6:602

Brandwein SR, Medsger T, Skinner M, Sipe J, Rodnan G, Cohen A (1984) Serum amyloid A protein concentration in progressive systemic sclerosis (scleroderma). Ann Rheum Dis 43:586–589

Broen J, Bossini-Castillo L, Van Bon L, Vonk MC, Knaapen H, Beretta L, Rueda B, Hesselstrand R, Herrick A, Worthington J (2012) A rare polymorphism in the gene for Toll-like receptor 2 is associated with systemic sclerosis phenotype and increases the production of inflammatory mediators. Arthritis Rheum 64:264–271

Broz P, Pelegrin P, Shao F (2020) The gasdermins, a protein family executing cell death and inflammation. Nat Rev Immunol 20:143–157

Burn GL, Cornish GH, Potrzebowska K, Samuelsson M, Griffié J, Minoughan S, Yates M, Ashdown G, Pernodet N, Morrison VL (2016) Superresolution imaging of the cytoplasmic phosphatase PTPN22 links integrin-mediated T cell adhesion with autoimmunity. Sci Signal 9:ra99-ra99

Call ME, Wucherpfennig KW (2004) Molecular mechanisms for the assembly of the T cell receptor—CD3 complex. Mol Immunol 40:1295–1305

Cardinale CJ, Li D, Tian L, Connolly JJ, March ME, Hou C, Wang F, Snyder J, Kim CE, Chiavacci RM (2016) Association of a rare NOTCH4 coding variant with systemic sclerosis: a family-based whole exome sequencing study. BMC Musculoskelet Disord 17:1–6

Carmona FD, Cénit MC, Diaz-Gallo L-M, Broen JC, Simeón CP, Carreira PE, Callejas-Rubio J-L, Fonollosa V, López-Longo FJ, González-Gay MA (2013) New insight on the Xq28 association with systemic sclerosis. Ann Rheum Dis 72:2032–2038

Casciola-Rosen L, Wigley F, Rosen A (1997) Scleroderma autoantigens are uniquely fragmented by metal-catalyzed oxidation reactions: implications for pathogenesis. J Exp Med 185:71–80

Casciola-Rosen L, Andrade F, Ulanet D, Wong WB, Rosen A (1999) Cleavage by granzyme B is strongly predictive of autoantigen status: implications for initiation of autoimmunity. J Exp Med 190:815–826

Caspi RR (1998) IL-12 in autoimmunity. Clin Immunol Immunopathol 88:4–13

Cénit MC, Simeón CP, Vonk MC, Callejas-Rubio JL, Espinosa G, Carreira P, Blanco FJ, Narvaez J, Tolosa C, Román-Ivorra JA (2012) Influence of the IL6 gene in susceptibility to systemic sclerosis. J Rheumatol 39:2294–2302

Chairta P, Nicolaou P, Christodoulou K (2017) Genomic and genetic studies of systemic sclerosis: a systematic review. Hum Immunol 78:153–165

Chang H-H, Miaw S-C, Tseng W, Sun Y-W, Liu C-C, Tsao H-W, Ho I-C (2013) PTPN22 modulates macrophage polarization and susceptibility to dextran sulfate sodium-induced colitis. J Immunol 191:2134–2143

Chatzikyriakidou A, Voulgari P, Georgiou I, Drosos A (2010) The role of microRNA-146a (miR-146a) and its target IL-1R-associated kinase (IRAK1) in psoriatic arthritis susceptibility. Scand J Immunol 71:382–385

Cheng S, Lovett DH (2003) Gelatinase A (MMP-2) is necessary and sufficient for renal tubular cell

epithelial-mesenchymal transformation. Am J Pathol 162:1937–1949
Chettimada S, Ata H, Rawat DK, Gulati S, Kahn AG, Edwards JG, Gupte SA (2014) Contractile protein expression is upregulated by reactive oxygen species in aorta of Goto-Kakizaki rat. Am J Physiol Heart Circ Physiol 306:H214–H224
Chora I, Romano E, Manetti M, Mazzotta C, Costa R, Machado V, Cortez A, Bruni C, Lepri G, Guiducci S (2017) Evidence for a derangement of the microvascular system in patients with a very early diagnosis of systemic sclerosis. J Rheumatol 44:1190–1197
Christmann RB, Sampaio-Barros P, Stifano G, Borges CL, De Carvalho CR, Kairalla R, Parra ER, Spira A, Simms R, Capellozzi VL (2014) Association of interferon-and transforming growth factor β-regulated genes and macrophage activation with systemic sclerosis-related progressive lung fibrosis. Arthritis Rheumatol 66:714–725
Cipriani P, Di Benedetto P, Capece D, Zazzeroni F, Liakouli V, Ruscitti P, Pantano I, Berardicurti O, Carubbi F, Alesse E (2014) Impaired Cav-1 expression in SSc mesenchymal cells upregulates VEGF signaling: a link between vascular involvement and fibrosis. Fibrogenesis Tissue Repair 7:1–14
Clark DN, Read RD, Mayhew V, Petersen SC, Argueta LB, Stutz LA, Till RE, Bergsten SM, Robinson BS, Baumann DG (2013) Four promoters of IRF5 respond distinctly to stimuli and are affected by autoimmune-risk polymorphisms. Front Immunol 4:360
Conway B, Hughes J (2012) Cellular orchestrators of renal fibrosis. QJM Int J Med 105:611–615
Cooper GS, Gilbert KM, Greidinger EL, James JA, Pfau JC, Reinlib L, Richardson BC, Rose NR (2008) Recent advances and opportunities in research on lupus: environmental influences and mechanisms of disease. Environ Health Perspect 116:695–702
Cortini A, Ellinghaus U, Malik TH, Graham DSC, Botto M, Vyse TJ (2017) B cell OX40L supports T follicular helper cell development and contributes to SLE pathogenesis. Ann Rheum Dis 76:2095–2103
Cotton SA, Herrick AL, Jayson MI, Freemont AJ (1999) Endothelial expression of nitric oxide synthases and nitrotyrosine in systemic sclerosis skin. J Pathol 189:273–278
Cunha FQ, Weiser WY, David JR, Moss DW, Moncada S, Liew F (1993) Recombinant migration inhibitory factor induces nitric oxide synthase in murine macrophages. J Immunol 150:1908–1912
Dam EM, Habib T, Chen J, Funk A, Glukhova V, Davis-Pickett M, Wei S, James R, Buckner JH, Cerosaletti K (2016) The BANK1 SLE-risk variants are associated with alterations in peripheral B cell signaling and development in humans. Clin Immunol 173:171–180
de Almeida CJG (2017) Caveolin-1 and caveolin-2 can be antagonistic partners in inflammation and beyond. Front Immunol 8:1530
de Vries S, Naarmann-de Vries IS, Urlaub H, Lue H, Bernhagen J, Ostareck DH, Ostareck-Lederer A (2013) Identification of DEAD-box RNA helicase 6 (DDX6) as a cellular modulator of vascular endothelial growth factor expression under hypoxia. J Biol Chem 288:5815–5827
De Angelis R, Bugatti L, Cerioni A, Del Medico P, Filosa G (2003) Diffuse scleroderma occurring after the use of paclitaxel for ovarian cancer. Clin Rheumatol 22:49–52
De Benedetti et al., 2003De Benedetti F, Meazza C, Vivarelli M, Rossi F, Pistorio A, Lamb R, Lunt M, Thomson W, Group BPRS, Ravelli A (2003) Functional and prognostic relevance of the—173 polymorphism of the macrophage migration inhibitory factor gene in systemic-onset juvenile idiopathic arthritis. Arthritis Rheum 48:1398–1407
de la Paz MP, Philen RM, Borda IA (2001) Toxic oil syndrome: the perspective after 20 years. Epidemiol Rev 23:231–247
Delgado-Vega AM, Dozmorov MG, Quirós MB, Wu Y-Y, Martínez-García B, Kozyrev SV, Frostegård J, Truedsson L, de Ramón E, González-Escribano MF (2012) Fine mapping and conditional analysis identify a new mutation in the autoimmunity susceptibility gene BLK that leads to reduced half-life of the BLK protein. Ann Rheum Dis 71:1219–1226
Dendrou CA, Cortes A, Shipman L, Evans HG, Attfield KE, Jostins L, Barber T, Kaur G, Kuttikkatte SB, Leach OA (2016) Resolving TYK2 locus genotype-to-phenotype differences in autoimmunity. Sci Transl Med 8:363ra149–363ra149
Deng Y, Tsao BP (2010) Genetic susceptibility to systemic lupus erythematosus in the genomic era. Nat Rev Rheumatol 6:683
Deng JC, Zeng X, Newstead M, Moore TA, Tsai WC, Thannickal VJ, Standiford TJ (2004) STAT4 is a critical mediator of early innate immune responses against pulmonary Klebsiella infection. J Immunol 173:4075–4083
Deng G-M, Beltran J, Chen C, Terhorst C, Tsokos GC (2013) T cell CD3ζ deficiency enables multiorgan tissue inflammation. J Immunol 191:3563–3567
Dengler HS, Baracho GV, Omori SA, Bruckner S, Arden KC, Castrillon DH, DePinho RA, Rickert RC (2008) Distinct functions for the transcription factor Foxo1 at various stages of B cell differentiation. Nat Immunol 9:1388–1398
Denkinger CM, Metz C, Fingerle-Rowson G, Denkinger MD, Forsthuber T (2004) Macrophage migration inhibitory factor and its role in autoimmune diseases. Arch Immunol Ther Exp (warsz) 52:389–400
Denton CP (2015) Pathogenesis of systemic sclerosis (scleroderma). UpToDate http://www.update.com/contents/pathogensis-of-systemic-sclerosis-scleroderma. Accessed 27
Denton CP, Khanna D (2017) Systemic sclerosis. Lancet 390:1685–1699
Denton CP, Ong VH, Xu S, Chen-Harris H, Modrusan Z, Lafyatis R, Khanna D, Jahreis A, Siegel J, Sornasse T (2018) Therapeutic interleukin-6 blockade reverses

transforming growth factor-beta pathway activation in dermal fibroblasts: insights from the faSScinate clinical trial in systemic sclerosis. Ann Rheum Dis 77:1362–1371

Diab et al., 2014Diab S, Dostrovsky N, Hudson M, Tatibouet S, Fritzler MJ, Baron M, Khalidi N, Group CSR (2014) Systemic sclerosis sine scleroderma: a multicenter study of 1417 subjects. J Rheumatol 41:2179–2185

Diaz-Gallo L, Gourh P, Broen J, Simeon C, Fonollosa V, Ortego-Centeno N, Agarwal S, Vonk M, Coenen M, Riemekasten G (2011) Analysis of the influence of PTPN22 gene polymorphisms in systemic sclerosis. Ann Rheum Dis 70:454–462

Diaz-Gallo L-M, Simeon CP, Broen JC, Ortego-Centeno N, Beretta L, Vonk MC, Carreira PE, Vargas S, Román-Ivorra JA, González-Gay MA (2013) Implication of IL-2/IL-21 region in systemic sclerosis genetic susceptibility. Ann Rheum Dis 72:1233–1238

Dieudé P, Guedj M, Wipff J, Avouac J, Hachulla E, Diot E, Granel B, Sibilia J, Cabane J, Meyer O (2008) The PTPN22 620W allele confers susceptibility to systemic sclerosis: findings of a large case-control study of European Caucasians and a meta-analysis. Arthritis Rheum Off J Am Coll Rheumatol 58:2183–2188

Dieudé P, Guedj M, Wipff J, Avouac J, Fajardy I, Diot E, Granel B, Sibilia J, Cabane J, Mouthon L (2009a) Association between the IRF5 rs2004640 functional polymorphism and systemic sclerosis: a new perspective for pulmonary fibrosis. Arthritis Rheum 60:225–233

Dieudé P, Wipff J, Guedj M, Ruiz B, Melchers I, Hachulla E, Riemekasten G, Diot E, Hunzelmann N, Sibilia J (2009b) BANK1 is a genetic risk factor for diffuse cutaneous systemic sclerosis and has additive effects with IRF5 and STAT4. Arthritis Rheum Off J Am Coll Rheumatol 60:3447–3454

Dieudé P, Guedj M, Truchetet M-E, Wipff J, Revillod L, Riemekasten G, Matucci-Cerinic M, Melchers I, Hachulla E, Airo P (2011) Association of the CD226 Ser307 variant with systemic sclerosis: evidence of a contribution of costimulation pathways in systemic sclerosis pathogenesis. Arthritis Rheum 63:1097–1105

Dieude P, Guedj M, Wipff J, Ruiz B, Riemekasten G, Matucci-Cerinic M, Melchers I, Hachulla E, Airo P, Diot E (2010) Association of the TNFAIP3 rs5029939 variant with systemic sclerosis in the European Caucasian population. Ann Rheum Dis 69:1958–1964

Dieude P, Bouaziz M, Guedj M, Riemekasten G, Airo P, Mueller M, Cusi D, Matucci-Cerinic M, Melchers I, Koenig W (2011) Evidence of the contribution of the X chromosome to systemic sclerosis susceptibility: association with the functional IRAK1 196Phe/532Ser haplotype. Arthritis Rheum 63:3979–3987

Dimmeler S, Zeiher AM (2000) Reactive oxygen species and vascular cell apoptosis in response to angiotensin II and pro-atherosclerotic factors. Regul Pept 90:19–25

Donn RP, Plant D, Jury F, Richards HL, Worthington J, Ray DW, Griffiths CE (2004) Macrophage migration inhibitory factor gene polymorphism is associated with psoriasis. J Investig Dermatol 123:484–487

Dooley A, Gao B, Bradley N, Abraham D, Black C, Jacobs M, Bruckdorfer K (2006) Abnormal nitric oxide metabolism in systemic sclerosis: increased levels of nitrated proteins and asymmetric dimethylarginine. Rheumatology 45:676–684

Doridot L, Jeljeli M, Chêne C, Batteux F (2019) Implication of oxidative stress in the pathogenesis of systemic sclerosis via inflammation, autoimmunity and fibrosis. Redox Biol 25:101122

Drab M, Verkade P, Elger M, Kasper M, Lohn M, Lauterbach B, Menne J, Lindschau C, Mende F, Luft FC (2001) Loss of caveolae, vascular dysfunction, and pulmonary defects in caveolin-1 gene-disrupted mice. Science 293:2449–2452

Du Y, Tian L, Shen L, Wang F, Yu L, Song Y, Zhu J, Du R (2011) Association of the CD226 single nucleotide polymorphism with systemic lupus erythematosus in the Chinese Han population. Tissue Antigens 77:65–67

Duncan MR, Berman B (1991) Stimulation of collagen and glycosaminoglycan production in cultured human adult dermal fibroblasts by recombinant human interleukin 6. J Investig Dermatol 97:686–692

Duncan CJ, Dinnigan E, Theobald R, Grainger A, Skelton AJ, Hussain R, Willet JD, Swan DJ, Coxhead J, Thomas MF (2018) Early-onset autoimmune disease due to a heterozygous loss-of-function mutation in TNFAIP3 (A20). Ann Rheum Dis 77:783–786

Dymecki SM, Niederhuber JE, Desiderio SV (1990) Specific expression of a tyrosine kinase gene, blk, in B lymphoid cells. Science 247:332–336

Efthymiou G, Dardiotis E, Liaskos C, Marou E, Scheper T, Meyer W, Daponte A, Daoussis D, Hadjigeorgiou G, Bogdanos DP (2019) A comprehensive analysis of antigen-specific antibody responses against human cytomegalovirus in patients with systemic sclerosis. Clin Immunol 207:87–96

Eloranta M-L, Franck-Larsson K, Lövgren T, Kalamajski S, Rönnblom A, Rubin K, Alm GV, Rönnblom L (2010) Type I interferon system activation and association with disease manifestations in systemic sclerosis. Ann Rheum Dis 69:1396–1402

Emerit I, Filipe P, Meunier P, Auclair C, Freitas J, Deroussent A, Gouyette A, Fernandes A (1997) Clastogenic activity in the plasma of scleroderma patients: a biomarker of oxidative stress. Dermatology 194:140–146

Englert H, Small-McMahon J, Chambers P, O'Connor H, Davis K, Manolios N, White R, Dracos G, Brooks P (1999) Familial risk estimation in systemic sclerosis. Aust N Z J Med 29:36–41

Errami Y, Naura AS, Kim H, Ju J, Suzuki Y, El-Bahrawy AH, Ghonim MA, Hemeida RA, Mansy MS, Zhang J (2013) Apoptotic DNA fragmentation may be a cooperative activity between caspase-activated deoxyribonuclease and the poly (ADP-ribose) polymerase-regulated DNAS1L3, an endoplasmic reticulum-localized endonuclease that translocates to the nucleus during apoptosis. J Biol Chem 288:3460–3468

Fan Y, Tao J-H, Zhang L-P, Li L-H, Ye D-Q (2011a) Association of BLK (rs13277113, rs2248932) polymorphism with systemic lupus erythematosus: a meta-analysis. Mol Biol Rep 38:4445–4453

Fan Y, Tao JH, Zhang LP, Li LH, Ye DQ (2011b) The association between BANK1 and TNFAIP3 gene polymorphisms and systemic lupus erythematosus: a meta-analysis. Int J Immunogenet 38:151–159

Fanciulli M, Norsworthy PJ, Petretto E, Dong R, Harper L, Kamesh L, Heward JM, Gough SC, de Smith A, Blakemore AI (2007) FCGR3B copy number variation is associated with susceptibility to systemic, but not organ-specific, autoimmunity. Nat Genet 39:721–723

Fang K, Fu W, Beardsley AR, Sun X, Lisanti MP, Liu J (2007) Overexpression of caveolin-1 inhibits endothelial cell proliferation by arresting the cell cycle at G0/G1 phase. Cell Cycle 6:199–204

Farina A, Cirone M, York M, Lenna S, Padilla C, Mclaughlin S, Faggioni A, Lafyatis R, Trojanowska M, Farina GA (2014) Epstein-Barr virus infection induces aberrant TLR activation pathway and fibroblast–myofibroblast conversion in scleroderma. J Investig Dermatol 134:954–964

Farres MN, Al-Zifzaf DS, Aly AA, Abd Raboh NM (2011) OX40/OX40L in systemic lupus erythematosus: association with disease activity and lupus nephritis. Ann Saudi Med 31:29–34

Fatini C, Mannini L, Sticchi E, Rogai V, Guiducci S, Conforti ML, Cinelli M, Pignone AM, Bolli P, Abbate R (2006) Hemorheologic profile in systemic sclerosis: role of NOS3− 786T> C and 894G> T polymorphisms in modulating both the hemorheologic parameters and the susceptibility to the disease. Arthritis Rheum Off J Am Coll Rheumatol 54:2263–2270

Feghali-Bostwick C, Medsger TA Jr, Wright TM (2003) Analysis of systemic sclerosis in twins reveals low concordance for disease and high concordance for the presence of antinuclear antibodies. Arthritis Rheum Off J Am Coll Rheumatol 48:1956–1963

Feron O, Kelly RA (2001) The caveolar paradox: suppressing, inducing, and terminating eNOS signaling. Am Heart Assoc, City

Fonseca C, Lindahl GE, Ponticos M, Sestini P, Renzoni EA, Holmes AM, Spagnolo P, Pantelidis P, Leoni P, McHugh N (2007) A polymorphism in the CTGF promoter region associated with systemic sclerosis. N Engl J Med 357:1210–1220

Fousteri G, Liossis S-NC, Battaglia M (2013) Roles of the protein tyrosine phosphatase PTPN22 in immunity and autoimmunity. Clin Immunol 149:556–565

Frantz C, Pezet S, Avouac J, Allanore Y (2018) Soluble CD163 as a potential biomarker in systemic sclerosis. Disease markers 2018

Frasca L, Lande R (2020) Toll-like receptors in mediating pathogenesis in systemic sclerosis. Clin Exp Immunol 201:14–24

Freedman RR, Girgis R, Mayes MD (1999) Endothelial and adrenergic dysfunction in Raynaud's phenomenon and scleroderma. J Rheumatol 26:2386–2388

G'Sell RT, Gaffney PM, Powell DW (2015) ABIN1 a physiological inhibitor of NF-κB: a molecular switch for inflammation and autoimmunity. Arthritis Rheumatol (Hoboken, NJ) 67:2292

Galdo FD, Sotgia F, de Almeida CJ, Jasmin JF, Musick M, Lisanti MP, Jiménez SA (2008) Decreased expression of caveolin 1 in patients with systemic sclerosis: crucial role in the pathogenesis of tissue fibrosis. Arthritis Rheum 58:2854–2865

Garcia-Romo GS, Caielli S, Vega B, Connolly J, Allantaz F, Xu Z, Punaro M, Baisch J, Guiducci C, Coffman RL (2011) Netting neutrophils are major inducers of type I IFN production in pediatric systemic lupus erythematosus. Sci Transl Med 3:73ra20

Gasteiger G, Kastenmuller W (2012) Foxp3+ regulatory T-cells and IL-2: the Moirai of T-cell fates? Front Immunol 3:179

Gateva V, Sandling JK, Hom G, Taylor KE, Chung SA, Sun X, Ortmann W, Kosoy R, Ferreira RC, Nordmark G (2009) A large-scale replication study identifies TNIP1, PRDM1, JAZF1, UHRF1BP1 and IL10 as risk loci for systemic lupus erythematosus. Nat Genet 41:1228–1233

Georg I, Díaz-Barreiro A, Morell M, Pey AL, Alarcón-Riquelme ME (2020) BANK1 interacts with TRAF6 and MyD88 in innate immune signaling in B cells. Cell Mol Immunol 17:954–965

Gilchrist F, Bunn C, Foley P, Lympany P, Black C, Welsh K, Du Bois R (2001) Class II HLA associations with autoantibodies in scleroderma: a highly significant role for HLA-DP. Genes Immun 2:76–81

Gjörloff-Wingren A, Saxena M, Williams S, Hammi D, Mustelin T (1999) Characterization of TCR-induced receptor-proximal signaling events negatively regulated by the protein tyrosine phosphatase PEP. Eur J Immunol 29:3845–3854

Gómez Hernández G, Morell M, Alarcón-Riquelme ME (2021) The role of BANK1 in B cell signaling and disease. Cells 10:1184

González-Serna D, López-Isac E, Yilmaz N, Gharibdoost F, Jamshidi A, Kavosi H, Poursani S, Farsad F, Direskeneli H, Saruhan-Direskeneli G (2019) Analysis of the genetic component of systemic sclerosis in Iranian and Turkish populations through a genome-wide association study. Rheumatology 58:289–298

González-Serna D, Ochoa E, López-Isac E, Julià A, Degenhardt F, Ortego-Centeno N, Radstake TR, Franke A, Marsal S, Mayes MD (2020) A cross-disease meta-GWAS identifies four new susceptibility loci shared between systemic sclerosis and Crohn's disease. Sci Rep 10:1–11

Gopanenko AV, Kosobokova EN, Kosorukov VS (2020) Main strategies for the identification of neoantigens. Cancers 12:2879

Gorlova O, Martin J-E, Rueda B, Koeleman BP, Ying J, Teruel M, Diaz-Gallo L-M, Broen JC, Vonk MC, Simeon CP (2011) Identification of novel genetic markers associated with clinical phenotypes of systemic sclerosis through a genome-wide association strategy. PLoS Genet 7:e1002178

Gourh P, Tan FK, Assassi S, Ahn CW, McNearney TA, Fischbach M, Arnett FC, Mayes MD (2006) Association of the PTPN22 R620W polymorphism with anti-topoisomerase I—and anticentromere antibody—positive systemic sclerosis. Arthritis Rheum Off J Am Coll Rheumatol 54:3945–3953

Gourh P, Arnett FC, Tan FK, Assassi S, Divecha D, Paz G, McNearney T, Draeger H, Reveille JD, Mayes MD (2010) Association of TNFSF4 (OX40L) polymorphisms with susceptibility to systemic sclerosis. Ann Rheum Dis 69:550–555

Graham DSC, Graham RR, Manku H, Wong AK, Whittaker JC, Gaffney PM, Moser KL, Rioux JD, Altshuler D, Behrens TW (2008a) Polymorphism at the TNF superfamily gene TNFSF4 confers susceptibility to systemic lupus erythematosus. Nat Genet 40:83–89

Graham RR, Cotsapas C, Davies L, Hackett R, Lessard CJ, Leon JM, Burtt NP, Guiducci C, Parkin M, Gates C (2008b) Genetic variants near TNFAIP3 on 6q23 are associated with systemic lupus erythematosus. Nat Genet 40:1059–1061

Graham DSC, Morris DL, Bhangale TR, Criswell LA, Syvänen A-C, Rönnblom L, Behrens TW, Graham RR, Vyse TJ (2011) Association of NCF2, IKZF1, IRF8, IFIH1, and TYK2 with systemic lupus erythematosus. PLoS Genet 7:e1002341

Granel B, Allanore Y, Chevillard C, Arnaud V, Marquet S, Weiller P-J, Durand J-M, Harlé J-R, Grange C, Frances Y (2006) IL13RA2 gene polymorphisms are associated with systemic sclerosis. J Rheumatol 33:2015–2019

Guiducci S, Fatini C, Georgountzos A, Sticchi E, Cinelli M, Kaloudi O, Rogai V, Melchiorre D, Pignone A, Vlachoyannopoulos P (2006) Etrurians vs Greeks: may ACE I/D polymorphism be still considered as a marker of susceptibility to SSc? Clin Exp Rheumatol 24:432

Günther S, Bordenave J, Hua-Huy T, Nicco C, Cumont A, Thuillet R, Tu L, Quatremarre T, Guilbert T, Jalce G (2018) Macrophage migration inhibitory factor (MIF) inhibition in a murine model of bleomycin-induced pulmonary fibrosis. Int J Mol Sci 19:4105

Gupta V, Kumar S, Pratap A, Singh R, Kumari R, Kumar S, Aggarwal A, Misra R (2018) Association of ITGAM, TNFSF4, TNFAIP3 and STAT4 gene polymorphisms with risk of systemic lupus erythematosus in a North Indian population. Lupus 27:1973–1979

Gurevich I, Zhang C, Francis N, Aneskievich BJ (2011) TNIP1, a retinoic acid receptor corepressor and A20-binding inhibitor of NF-κB, distributes to both nuclear and cytoplasmic locations. J Histochem Cytochem 59:1101–1112

Gurujeyalakshmi G, Giri S (1995) Molecular mechanisms of antifibrotic effect of interferon gamma in bleomycin-mouse model of lung fibrosis: downregulation of TGF-β and procollagen I and III gene expression. Exp Lung Res 21:791–808

Györy I, Fejér G, Ghosh N, Seto E, Wright KL (2003) Identification of a functionally impaired positive regulatory domain I binding factor 1 transcription repressor in myeloma cell lines. J Immunol 170:3125–3133

Han J-W, Zheng H-F, Cui Y, Sun L-D, Ye D-Q, Hu Z, Xu J-H, Cai Z-M, Huang W, Zhao G-P (2009) Genome-wide association study in a Chinese Han population identifies nine new susceptibility loci for systemic lupus erythematosus. Nat Genet 41:1234–1237

Harb H, Stephen-Victor E, Crestani E, Benamar M, Massoud A, Cui Y, Charbonnier L-M, Arbag S, Baris S, Cunnigham A (2020) A regulatory T cell Notch4–GDF15 axis licenses tissue inflammation in asthma. Nat Immunol 21:1359–1370

Harb H, Benamar M, Lai PS, Contini P, Griffith JW, Crestani E, Schmitz-Abe K, Chen Q, Fong J, Marri L (2021) Notch4 signaling limits regulatory T-cell-mediated tissue repair and promotes severe lung inflammation in viral infections. Immunity

Harris TJ, Grosso JF, Yen H-R, Xin H, Kortylewski M, Albesiano E, Hipkiss EL, Getnet D, Goldberg MV, Maris CH (2007) Cutting edge: an in vivo requirement for STAT3 signaling in TH17 development and TH17-dependent autoimmunity. J Immunol 179:4313–4317

Henderson J, O'Reilly S (2017) Inflammasome lights up in systemic sclerosis. BioMed Central, City

Herrick A, Cerinic MM (2001) The emerging problem of oxidative stress and the role of antioxidants in systemic sclerosis. Clin Exp Rheumatol 19:4–8

Higgins DF, Biju MP, Akai Y, Wutz A, Johnson RS, Haase VH (2004) Hypoxic induction of Ctgf is directly mediated by Hif-1. Am J Physiol Renal Physiol 287:F1223–F1232

Hoy RF, Chambers DC (2020) Silica-related diseases in the modern world. Allergy 75:2805–2817

Huang X-L, Wu G-C, Wang Y-J, Yang X-K, Yang G-J, Tao J-H, Duan Y, Yan J-W, Li X-P, Ye D-Q (2016) Association of interleukin-1 family cytokines single nucleotide polymorphisms with susceptibility to systemic sclerosis: an independent case-control study and a meta-analysis. Immunol Res 64:1041–1052

Huang G, Su J, Zhang M, Jin Y, Wang Y, Zhou P, Lu J (2017) RhoB regulates the function of macrophages in the hypoxia-induced inflammatory response. Cell Mol Immunol 14:265–275

Huang Z, Qi G, Miller JS, Zheng SG (2020) CD226: an emerging role in immunologic diseases. Front Cell Dev Biol 8:564

Hudson M, Rojas-Villarraga A, Coral-Alvarado P, López-Guzmán S, Mantilla RD, Chalem P, Baron M, Anaya J-M, Group CSR, (2008) Polyautoimmunity and familial autoimmunity in systemic sclerosis. J Autoimmun 31:156–159

Hutyrová B, Lukác J, Bosák V, Buc M, du Bois R, Petrek M (2004) Interleukin 1alpha single-nucleotide polymorphism associated with systemic sclerosis. J Rheumatol 31:81–84

Ignarro LJ (1990) Biosynthesis and metabolism of endothelium-derived nitric oxide. Annu Rev Pharmacol Toxicol 30:535–560

Illescas O, Gomez-Verjan JC, García-Velázquez L, Govezensky T, Rodriguez-Sosa M (2018) Macrophage migration inhibitory factor-173 G/C polymorphism: a global meta-analysis across the disease spectrum. Front Genet 9:55

Indelicato M, Chiarenza V, Libra M, Malaponte G, Bevelacqua V, Marchini M, McCubrey JA, Stivala F, Scorza R, Mazzarino MC (2006) Analysis of TIMP-1 gene polymorphisms in Italian sclerodermic patients. J Clin Lab Anal 20:173–176

Inomata M, Into T, Niida S, Murakami Y (2013) Atg5 regulates formation of MyD88 condensed structures and MyD88-dependent signal transduction. Biochem Biophys Res Commun 437:509–514

Ito T, Ito N, Saathoff M, Stampachiacchiere B, Bettermann A, Bulfone-Paus S, Takigawa M, Nickoloff BJ, Paus R (2005) Immunology of the human nail apparatus: the nail matrix is a site of relative immune privilege. J Investig Dermatol 125:1139–1148

Ito I, Fukazawa J, Yoshida M (2007) Post-translational methylation of high mobility group box 1 (HMGB1) causes its cytoplasmic localization in neutrophils. J Biol Chem 282:16336–16344

Ito I, Kawaguchi Y, Kawasaki A, Hasegawa M, Ohashi J, Hikami K, Kawamoto M, Fujimoto M, Takehara K, Sato S (2009) Association of a functional polymorphism in the IRF5 region with systemic sclerosis in a Japanese population. Arthritis Rheum Off J Am Coll Rheumatol 60:1845–1850

Ito I, Kawaguchi Y, Kawasaki A, Hasegawa M, Ohashi J, Kawamoto M, Fujimoto M, Takehara K, Sato S, Hara M (2010) Association of the FAM167A–BLK region with systemic sclerosis. Arthritis Rheum 62:890–895

Jacob CO, Zhu J, Armstrong DL, Yan M, Han J, Zhou XJ, Thomas JA, Reiff A, Myones BL, Ojwang JO (2009) Identification of IRAK1 as a risk gene with critical role in the pathogenesis of systemic lupus erythematosus. Proc Natl Acad Sci 106:6256–6261

Janghorban M, Xin L, Rosen JM, Zhang XH-F (2018) Notch signaling as a regulator of the tumor immune response: to target or not to target? Front Immunol 9:1649

Jarosz M, Olbert M, Wyszogrodzka G, Młyniec K, Librowski T (2017) Antioxidant and anti-inflammatory effects of zinc. Zinc-dependent NF-Kb signaling. Inflammopharmacology 25:11–24

Jeck WR, Siebold AP, Sharpless NE (2012) a meta-analysis of GWAS and age-associated diseases. Aging Cell 11:727–731

Jiang SH, Athanasopoulos V, Ellyard JI, Chuah A, Cappello J, Cook A, Prabhu SB, Cardenas J, Gu J, Stanley M (2019) Functional rare and low frequency variants in BLK and BANK1 contribute to human lupus. Nat Commun 10:1–12

Jimenez SA, Gaidarova S, Saitta B, Sandorfi N, Herrich DJ, Rosenbloom JC, Kucich U, Abrams WR, Rosenbloom J (2001) Role of protein kinase C-δ in the regulation of collagen gene expression in scleroderma fibroblasts. J Clin Investig 108:1395–1403

Jimenez SA (2013) Role of endothelial to mesenchymal transition in the pathogenesis of the vascular alterations in systemic sclerosis. International scholarly research notices

Johnson R, Reveille J, McNearney T, Fischbach M, Friedman A, Ahn C, Arnett F, Tan F (2001) Lack of association of a functionally relevant single nucleotide polymorphism of matrix metalloproteinase-1 promoter with systemic sclerosis (scleroderma). Genes Immun 2:273–275

Joung C-I, Na Y-I, Shin E-S, Sung Y-K, Yoo D-H, Jun J-B (2008) The single nucleotide polymorphisms of matrix metalloproteinase-1 in patients with systemic sclerosis. Rheumatol Int 28:1183–1185

Kahaleh B, Fan P-S (1998) Down regulation of nitric oxide synthase gene in microvascular endothelial cells from lesional scleroderma: assessment by quantitative RT-PCR and possible role for cytotoxic T-cells. Arthritis Rheum 41

Karaghiosoff M, Neubauer H, Lassnig C, Kovarik P, Schindler H, Pircher H, McCoy B, Bogdan C, Decker T, Brem G (2000) Partial impairment of cytokine responses in Tyk2-deficient mice. Immunity 13:549–560

Kariuki SN, Kirou KA, MacDermott EJ, Barillas-Arias L, Crow MK, Niewold TB (2009) Cutting edge: autoimmune disease risk variant of STAT4 confers increased sensitivity to IFN-α in lupus patients in vivo. J Immunol 182:34–38

Kastenmuller W, Gasteiger G, Subramanian N, Sparwasser T, Busch DH, Belkaid Y, Drexler I, Germain RN (2011) Regulatory T cells selectively control CD8+ T cell effector pool size via IL-2 restriction. J Immunol 187:3186–3197

Kaufman KM, Zhao J, Kelly JA, Hughes T, Adler A, Sanchez E, Ojwang JO, Langefeld CD, Ziegler JT, Williams AH (2013) Fine mapping of Xq28: both MECP2 and IRAK1 contribute to risk for systemic lupus erythematosus in multiple ancestral groups. Ann Rheum Dis 72:437–444

Kavian N, Servettaz A, Mongaret C, Wang A, Nicco C, Chéreau C, Grange P, Vuiblet V, Birembaut P, Diebold MD (2010) Targeting ADAM-17/notch signaling abrogates the development of systemic sclerosis in a murine model. Arthritis Rheum 62:3477–3487

Kawaguchi Y, Tochimoto A, Ichikawa N, Harigai M, Hara M, Kotake S, Kitamura Y, Kamatani N (2003) Association of IL1A gene polymorphisms with susceptibility to and severity of systemic sclerosis in the Japanese population. Arthritis Rheum 48:186–192

Keller AD, Maniatis T (1991) Identification and characterization of a novel repressor of beta-interferon gene expression. Genes Dev 5:868–879

Kerdiles YM, Beisner DR, Tinoco R, Dejean AS, Castrillon DH, DePinho RA, Hedrick SM (2009) Foxo1 links homing and survival of naive T cells by regulating L-selectin, CCR7 and interleukin 7 receptor. Nat Immunol 10:176–184
Kessel A, Rosner I, Rozenbaum M, Zisman D, Sagiv A, Shmuel Z, Sabo E, Toubi E (2004) Increased CD8+ T cell apoptosis in scleroderma is associated with low levels of NF-κB. J Clin Immunol 24:30–36
Khan K, Xu S, Nihtyanova S, Derrett-Smith E, Abraham D, Denton CP, Ong VH (2012) Clinical and pathological significance of interleukin 6 overexpression in systemic sclerosis. Ann Rheum Dis 71:1235–1242
Khanna D, Denton CP, Jahreis A, van Laar JM, Frech TM, Anderson ME, Baron M, Chung L, Fierlbeck G, Lakshminarayanan S (2016) Safety and efficacy of subcutaneous tocilizumab in adults with systemic sclerosis (faSScinate): a phase 2, randomised, controlled trial. Lancet 387:2630–2640
Kill A, Tabeling C, Undeutsch R, Kühl AA, Günther J, Radic M, Becker MO, Heidecke H, Worm M, Witzenrath M (2014) Autoantibodies to angiotensin and endothelin receptors in systemic sclerosis induce cellular and systemic events associated with disease pathogenesis. Arthritis Res Ther 16:1–12
Kim Y-W, Byzova TV (2014) Oxidative stress in angiogenesis and vascular disease. Blood J Am Soc Hematol 123:625–631
Kim D, Peck A, Santer D, Patole P, Schwartz SM, Molitor JA, Arnett FC, Elkon KB (2008) Induction of interferon-α by scleroderma sera containing autoantibodies to topoisomerase I: association of higher interferon-α activity with lung fibrosis. Arthritis Rheum Off J Am Coll Rheumatol 58:2163–2173
Kimura H, Weisz A, Kurashima Y, Hashimoto K, Ogura T, D'Acquisto F, Addeo R, Makuuchi M, Esumi H (2000) Hypoxia response element of the human vascular endothelial growth factor gene mediates transcriptional regulation by nitric oxide: control of hypoxia-inducible factor-1 activity by nitric oxide. Blood J Am Soc Hematol 95:189–197
Koumakis E, Dieudé P, Avouac J, Kahan A, Allanore Y (2012) Familial autoimmunity in systemic sclerosis—results of a French-based case-control family study. J Rheumatol 39:532–538
Kuballa P, Nolte WM, Castoreno AB, Xavier RJ (2012) Autophagy and the immune system. Annu Rev Immunol 30:611–646
Kurien BT, Hensley K, Bachmann M, Scofield RH (2006) Oxidatively modified autoantigens in autoimmune diseases. Free Radical Biol Med 41:549–556
Lafyatis R (2014) Transforming growth factor β—at the centre of systemic sclerosis. Nat Rev Rheumatol 10:706–719
Lankat-Buttgereit B, Tampé R (2002) The transporter associated with antigen processing: function and implications in human diseases. Physiol Rev 82:187–204
Le Berre L, Chesneau M, Danger R, Dubois F, Chaussabel D, Garand M, Brouard S (2021) Connection of BANK1, tolerance, regulatory B cells, and apoptosis: perspectives of a reductionist investigation. Front Immunol 12:58
Leask A, Holmes A, Abraham DJ (2002) Connective tissue growth factor: a new and important player in the pathogenesis of fibrosis. Curr Rheumatol Rep 4:136–142
Lee AJ, Ashkar AA (2018) The dual nature of type I and type II interferons. Front Immunol 9:2061
Lee YH, Choi SJ, Ji JD, Song GG (2012) The association between the PTPN22 C1858T polymorphism and systemic sclerosis: a meta-analysis. Mol Biol Rep 39:3103–3108
Lefebvre V, Behringer R, De Crombrugghe B (2001) L-Sox5, Sox6 and Sox9 control essential steps of the chondrocyte differentiation pathway. Osteoarthr Cartil 9:S69–S75
LeRoy EC, Black C, Fleischmajer R, Jablonska S, Krieg T, Medsger T Jr, Rowell N, Wollheim F (1988) Scleroderma (systemic sclerosis): classification, subsets and pathogenesis. J Rheumatol 15:202–205
Lin Y, Wong K-k, Calame K (1997) Repression of c-myc transcription by Blimp-1, an inducer of terminal B cell differentiation. Science 276:596–599
Lin M-H, Leimeister C, Gessler M, Kopan R (2000) Activation of the Notch pathway in the hair cortex leads to aberrant differentiation of the adjacent hair-shaft layers. Development 127:2421–2432
Lin K-I, Angelin-Duclos C, Kuo TC, Calame K (2002) Blimp-1-dependent repression of Pax-5 is required for differentiation of B cells to immunoglobulin M-secreting plasma cells. Mol Cell Biol 22:4771–4780
Lis-Święty A, Gola J, Mazurek U, Brzezińska-Wcisło L (2017) Transcriptional activity of nuclear factor κB family genes in patients with systemic sclerosis. Ann Clin Lab Sci 47:306–309
Liu S, Huang L, Lin Z, Hu Y, Chen R, Wang L, Shan Y (2017a) RhoB induces the production of proinflammatory cytokines in TLR-triggered macrophages. Mol Immunol 87:200–206
Liu T, Zhang L, Joo D, Sun S-C (2017b) NF-κB signaling in inflammation. Signal Transduct Target Ther 2:1–9
Liu C, Yan S, Chen H, Wu Z, Li L, Cheng L, Li H, Li Y (2021) Association of GTF2I, NFKB1, and TYK2 regional polymorphisms with systemic sclerosis in a Chinese Han population. Front Immunol 12:2457
López-Isac E, Bossini-Castillo L, Simeon CP, Egurbide MV, Alegre-Sancho JJ, Callejas JL, Roman-Ivorra JA, Freire M, Beretta L, Santaniello A (2014) A genome-wide association study follow-up suggests a possible role for PPARG in systemic sclerosis susceptibility. Arthritis Res Ther 16:1–8
López-Isac E, Campillo-Davo D, Bossini-Castillo L, Guerra SG, Assassi S, Simeón CP, Carreira P, Ortego-Centeno N, de la Peña PG, Beretta L (2016a) Influence of TYK2 in systemic sclerosis susceptibility:

a new locus in the IL-12 pathway. Ann Rheum Dis 75:1521–1526

López-Isac E, Martín JE, Assassi S, Simeón CP, Carreira P, Ortego-Centeno N, Freire M, Beltrán E, Narváez J, Alegre-Sancho JJ (2016b) Brief report: IRF4 newly identified as a common susceptibility locus for systemic sclerosis and rheumatoid arthritis in a cross-disease meta-analysis of genome-wide association studies. Arthritis Rheumatol 68:2338–2344

López-Isac E, Acosta-Herrera M, Kerick M, Assassi S, Satpathy AT, Granja J, Mumbach MR, Beretta L, Simeón CP, Carreira P (2019) GWAS for systemic sclerosis identifies multiple risk loci and highlights fibrotic and vasculopathy pathways. Nat Commun 10:1–14

Lopez-Isac E, Bossini-Castillo L, Guerra SG, Assassi S, Zhou X, Simeón CP, Ortego-Centeno N, Castellvi I, Carreira P, Gorlova O (2014) Identification of IL12RB1 as a novel systemic sclerosis susceptibility locus. Arthritis Rheumatol (Hoboken, NJ) 66:3521

Lőrincz P, Tóth S, Benkő P, Lakatos Z, Boda A, Glatz G, Zobel M, Bisi S, Hegedűs K, Takáts S (2017) Rab2 promotes autophagic and endocytic lysosomal degradation. J Cell Biol 216:1937–1947

Lozano E, Dominguez-Villar M, Kuchroo V, Hafler DA (2012) The TIGIT/CD226 axis regulates human T cell function. J Immunol 188:3869–3875

Lu M-M, Ye Q-L, Feng C-C, Yang J, Zhang T, Li J, Leng R-X, Pan H-F, Yuan H, Ye D-Q (2012) Association of FAS gene polymorphisms with systemic lupus erythematosus: a case-control study and meta-analysis. Exp Ther Med 4:497–502

Lundholm M, Mayans S, Motta V, Löfgren-Burström A, Danska J, Holmberg D (2010) Variation in the CD3ζ (Cd247) gene correlates with altered T cell activation and is associated with autoimmune diabetes. J Immunol 184:5537–5544

Luo J, Treubert-Zimmermann U, Redies C (2004) Cadherins guide migrating Purkinje cells to specific parasagittal domains during cerebellar development. Mol Cell Neurosci 25:138–152

Luo J, Niu X, Liu H, Zhang M, Chen M, Deng S (2013) Up-regulation of transcription factor Blimp1 in systemic lupus erythematosus. Mol Immunol 56:574–582

Macias-Garcia A, Heizmann B, Sellars M, Marchal P, Dali H, Pasquali J-L, Muller S, Kastner P, Chan S (2016) Ikaros is a negative regulator of B1 cell development and function. J Biol Chem 291:9073–9086

Mandik-Nayak L, DuHadaway JB, Mulgrew J, Pigott E, Manley K, Sedano S, Prendergast GC, Laury-Kleintop LD (2017) RhoB blockade selectively inhibits autoantibody production in autoimmune models of rheumatoid arthritis and lupus. Dis Models Mech 10:1313–1322

Manetti M, Allanore Y, Saad M, Fatini C, Cohignac V, Guiducci S, Romano E, Airó P, Caramaschi P, Tinazzi I (2012) Evidence for caveolin-1 as a new susceptibility gene regulating tissue fibrosis in systemic sclerosis. Ann Rheum Dis 71:1034–1041

Manetti M, Allanore Y, Saad M, Fatini C, Cohignac V, Guiducci S, Romano E, Airó P, Caramaschi P, Riccieri V (2013) AB0242 Evidence for caveolin-1 (CAV1) as a new susceptibility gene regulating tissue fibrosis in systemic sclerosis. Ann Rheum Dis 71:651–651

Marangoni RG, Korman BD, Allanore Y, Dieude P, Armstrong LL, Rzhetskaya M, Hinchcliff M, Carns M, Podlusky S, Shah SJ (2015) A candidate gene study reveals association between a variant of the peroxisome proliferator-activated receptor gamma (PPAR-γ) gene and systemic sclerosis. Arthritis Res Ther 17:1–8

Marasini B, Casari S, Zeni S, Turri O, Biondi M (2001) Stromelysin promoter polymorphism is associated with systemic sclerosis. Rheumatology 40:475–476

Martin J-E, Broen JC, Carmona FD, Teruel M, Simeon CP, Vonk MC, van 't Slot R, Rodriguez-Rodriguez L, Vicente E, Fonollosa V (2012a) Identification of CSK as a systemic sclerosis genetic risk factor through genome wide association study follow-up. Hum Mol Genet 21:2825–2835

Martin J-E, Carmona FD, Broen JC, Simeon CP, Vonk MC, Carreira P, Ríos-Fernández R, Espinosa G, Vicente-Rabaneda E, Tolosa C (2012b) The autoimmune disease-associated IL2RA locus is involved in the clinical manifestations of systemic sclerosis. Genes Immun 13:191–196

Martin J-E, Assassi S, Diaz-Gallo L-M, Broen JC, Simeon CP, Castellvi I, Vicente-Rabaneda E, Fonollosa V, Ortego-Centeno N, González-Gay MA (2013) A systemic sclerosis and systemic lupus erythematosus pan-meta-GWAS reveals new shared susceptibility loci. Hum Mol Genet 22:4021–4029

Matsushita T, Hasegawa M, Hamaguchi Y, Takehara K, Sato S (2006) Longitudinal analysis of serum cytokine concentrations in systemic sclerosis: association of interleukin 12 elevation with spontaneous regression of skin sclerosis. J Rheumatol 33:275–284

Mattana TCC, Santos AS, Fukui RT, Mainardi-Novo DTO, Costa VS, Santos RF, Matioli SR, Rossi da Silva ME (2014) CD226 rs763361 is associated with the susceptibility to type 1 diabetes and greater frequency of GAD65 autoantibody in a Brazilian cohort. Mediators of inflammation

Mattuzzi S, Barbi S, Carletto A, Ravagnani V, Moore PS, Bambara LM, Scarpa A (2007) Association of polymorphisms in the IL1B and IL2 genes with susceptibility and severity of systemic sclerosis. J Rheumatol 34:997–1004

Matucci Cerinic M, Kahaleh M (2002) Beauty and the beast. The nitric oxide paradox in systemic sclerosis. Oxford University Press, City

Maul G, Jimenez S, Riggs E, Ziemnicka-Kotula D (1989) Determination of an epitope of the diffuse systemic sclerosis marker antigen DNA topoisomerase I: sequence similarity with retroviral p30gag protein suggests a possible cause for autoimmunity in systemic sclerosis. Proc Natl Acad Sci 86:8492–8496

Mayes MD (1998) Classification and epidemiology of scleroderma. Semin Cutan Med Surg 17(1):22–26

Mayes MD, Trojanowska M (2007) Genetic factors in systemic sclerosis. Arthritis Res Ther 9:1–7
Mayes MD, Bossini-Castillo L, Gorlova O, Martin JE, Zhou X, Chen WV, Assassi S, Ying J, Tan FK, Arnett FC (2014) Immunochip analysis identifies multiple susceptibility loci for systemic sclerosis. Am J Hum Genet 94:47–61
McGregor AR, Watson A, Yunis E, Pandey JP, Takehara K, Tidwell JT, Ruggieri A, Silver RM, LeRoy EC, Maricq HR (1988) Familial clustering of scleroderma spectrum disease. Am J Med 84:1023–1032
McKinney C, Fanciulli M, Merriman ME, Phipps-Green A, Alizadeh BZ, Koeleman BP, Dalbeth N, Gow PJ, Harrison AA, Highton J (2010) Association of variation in Fcγ receptor 3B gene copy number with rheumatoid arthritis in Caucasian samples. Ann Rheum Dis 69:1711–1716
McKinney C, Broen J, Vonk M, Beretta L, Hesselstrand R, Hunzelmann N, Riemekasten G, Scorza R, Simeon C, Fonollosa V (2012) Evidence that deletion at FCGR3B is a risk factor for systemic sclerosis. Genes Immun 13:458–460
Miraghazadeh B, Cook MC (2018) Nuclear factor-kappaB in autoimmunity: man and mouse. Front Immunol 9:613
Mitchell RA, Metz CN, Peng T, Bucala R (1999) Sustained mitogen-activated protein kinase (MAPK) and cytoplasmic phospholipase A2 activation by macrophage migration inhibitory factor (MIF): regulatory role in cell proliferation and glucocorticoid action. J Biol Chem 274:18100–18106
Mizushima N (2007) Autophagy: process and function. Genes Dev 21:2861–2873
Mogensen TH (2019) IRF and STAT transcription factors-from basic biology to roles in infection, protective immunity, and primary immunodeficiencies. Front Immunol 9:3047
Moncada S (1991) Nitric oxide: physiology, pathophysiology and pharmacology. Pharmacol Rev 43:109–142
Mulligan-Kehoe MJ, Drinane MC, Mollmark J, Casciola-Rosen L, Hummers LK, Hall A, Rosen A, Wigley FM, Simons M (2007) Antiangiogenic plasma activity in patients with systemic sclerosis. Arthritis Rheum Off J Am Coll Rheumatol 56:3448–3458
Nair RP, Duffin KC, Helms C, Ding J, Stuart PE, Goldgar D, Gudjonsson JE, Li Y, Tejasvi T, Feng B-J (2009) Genome-wide scan reveals association of psoriasis with IL-23 and NF-κB pathways. Nat Genet 41:199–204
Namjou B, Kothari PH, Kelly JA, Glenn SB, Ojwang JO, Adler A, Alarcón-Riquelme ME, Gallant CJ, Boackle SA, Criswell LA (2011) Evaluation of the TREX1 gene in a large multi-ancestral lupus cohort. Genes Immun 12:270–279
Nantel A, Mohammad-Ali K, Sherk J, Posner BI, Thomas DY (1998) Interaction of the Grb10 adapter protein with the Raf1 and MEK1 kinases. J Biol Chem 273:10475–10484
Negro R, Gobessi S, Longo PG, He Y, Zhang Z-Y, Laurenti L, Efremov DG (2012) Overexpression of the autoimmunity-associated phosphatase PTPN22 promotes survival of antigen-stimulated CLL cells by selectively activating AKT. Blood J Am Soc Hematol 119:6278–6287
Nihtyanova SI, Denton CP (2010) Autoantibodies as predictive tools in systemic sclerosis. Nat Rev Rheumatol 6:112
Nishikomori R, Usui T, Wu C-Y, Morinobu A, O'Shea JJ, Strober W (2002) Activated STAT4 has an essential role in Th1 differentiation and proliferation that is independent of its role in the maintenance of IL-12Rβ2 chain expression and signaling. J Immunol 169:4388–4398
O'Reilly S (2018) Toll like receptors in systemic sclerosis: an emerging target. Immunol Lett 195:2–8
Ogawa F, Shimizu K, Hara T, Muroi E, Hasegawa M, Takehara K, Sato S (2008) Serum levels of heat shock protein 70, a biomarker of cellular stress, are elevated in patients with systemic sclerosis: association with fibrosis and vascular damage. Clin Exp Rheumatol 26:659–662
Oh RS, Haak AJ, Smith KM, Ligresti G, Choi KM, Xie T, Wang S, Walters PR, Thompson MA, Freeman MR (2018) RNAi screening identifies a mechanosensitive ROCK-JAK2-STAT3 network central to myofibroblast activation. J Cell Sci 131:jcs209932
Ohtsuka T, Yamakage A, Yamazaki S (2002) The polymorphism of transforming growth factor-β1 gene in Japanese patients with systemic sclerosis. Br J Dermatol 147:458–463
Omori SA, Cato MH, Anzelon-Mills A, Puri KD, Shapiro-Shelef M, Calame K, Rickert RC (2006) Regulation of class-switch recombination and plasma cell differentiation by phosphatidylinositol 3-kinase signaling. Immunity 25:545–557
Ostojić P, Damjanov N (2006) Different clinical features in patients with limited and diffuse cutaneous systemic sclerosis. Clin Rheumatol 25:453–457
Park M-J, Moon S-J, Lee E-J, Jung K-A, Kim E-K, Kim D-S, Lee J-H, Kwok S-K, Min J-K, Park S-H (2018) IL-1-IL-17 signaling axis contributes to fibrosis and inflammation in two different murine models of systemic sclerosis. Front Immunol 9:1611
Parrish-Novak J, Dillon SR, Nelson A, Hammond A, Sprecher C, Gross JA, Johnston J, Madden K, Xu W, West J (2000) Interleukin 21 and its receptor are involved in NK cell expansion and regulation of lymphocyte function. Nature 408:57–63
Piskurich JF, Lin K-I, Lin Y, Wang Y, Ting JP-Y, Calame K (2000) BLIMP-1 mediates extinction of major histocompatibility class II transactivator expression in plasma cells. Nat Immunol 1:526–532
Pistoia V, Cocco C, Airoldi I (2009) Interleukin-12 receptor β2: from cytokine receptor to gatekeeper gene in human B-cell malignancies. J Clin Oncol 27:4809–4816
Powell B, Passmore E, Nesci A, Dunn S (1998) The Notch signalling pathway in hair growth. Mech Dev 78:189–192
Powell MD, Read KA, Sreekumar BK, Oestreich KJ (2019) Ikaros zinc finger transcription factors:

regulators of cytokine signaling pathways and CD4+ T helper cell differentiation. Front Immunol 10:1299

Powis SJ, Deverson EV, Coadweil WJ, Ciruela A, Huskisson NS, Smith H, Butcher GW, Howard JC (1992) Effect of polymorphism of an MHC-linked transporter on the peptides assembled in a class I molecule. Nature 357:211–215

Qian F, He M, Duan W, Mao L, Li Q, Yu Z, Zhou Z, Zhang Y (2015) Cross regulation between hypoxia-inducible transcription factor-1α (HIF-1α) and transforming growth factor (TGF)-ß1 mediates nickel oxide nanoparticles (NiONPs)-induced pulmonary fibrosis. Am J Transl Res 7:2364

Qian Y, Wang G, Xue F, Chen L, Wang Y, Tang L, Yang H (2017) Genetic association between TAP1 and TAP2 polymorphisms and ankylosing spondylitis: a systematic review and meta-analysis. Inflamm Res 66:653–661

Radstake TR, Gorlova O, Rueda B, Martin J-E, Alizadeh BZ, Palomino-Morales R, Coenen MJ, Vonk MC, Voskuyl AE, Schuerwegh AJ (2010) Genome-wide association study of systemic sclerosis identifies CD247 as a new susceptibility locus. Nat Genet 42:426–429

Rajabi F, Drake L, Senna M, Rezaei N (2018) Alopecia areata: a review of disease pathogenesis. Br J Dermatol

Randone SB, Guiducci S, Cerinic MM (2008) Systemic sclerosis and infections. Autoimmun Rev 8:36–40

Razani B, Zhang XL, Bitzer M, Von Gersdorff G, Böttinger EP, Lisanti MP (2001) Caveolin-1 regulates transforming growth factor (TGF)-β/SMAD signaling through an interaction with the TGF-β type I receptor. J Biol Chem 276:6727–6738

Reveille JD, Fischbach M, McNearney T, Friedman AW, Aguilar MB, Lisse J, Fritzler MJ, Ahn C, Arnett FC, Group GS (2001) Systemic sclerosis in 3 US ethnic groups: a comparison of clinical, sociodemographic, serologic, and immunogenetic determinants. In: Seminars in arthritis and rheumatism. Elsevier, pp 332–346

Rigat B, Hubert C, Alhenc-Gelas F, Cambien F, Corvol P, Soubrier F (1990) An insertion/deletion polymorphism in the angiotensin I-converting enzyme gene accounting for half the variance of serum enzyme levels. J Clin Investig 86:1343–1346

Roebuck KA (1999) Oxidant stress regulation of IL-8 and ICAM-1 gene expression: differential activation and binding of the transcription factors AP-1 and NF-kappaB. Int J Mol Med 4:223–253

Romagnani P, Maggi L, Mazzinghi B, Cosmi L, Lasagni L, Liotta F, Lazzeri E, Angeli R, Rotondi M, Filì L (2005) CXCR3-mediated opposite effects of CXCL10 and CXCL4 on TH1 or TH2 cytokine production. J Allergy Clin Immunol 116:1372–1379

Romero LI, Zhang D-N, Cooke JP, Ho H-KV, Avalos E, Herrera R, Herron GS (2000) Differential expression of nitric oxide by dermal microvascular endothelial cells from patients with scleroderma. Vasc Med 5:147–158

Rubio-Rivas M, Moreno R, Corbella X (2017) Occupational and environmental scleroderma. Systematic review and meta-analysis. Clin Rheumatol 36:569–582

Rueda B, Broen J, Simeon C, Hesselstrand R, Diaz B, Suarez H, Ortego-Centeno N, Riemekasten G, Fonollosa V, Vonk M (2009a) The STAT4 gene influences the genetic predisposition to systemic sclerosis phenotype. Hum Mol Genet 18:2071–2077

Rueda B, Simeon C, Hesselstrand R, Herrick A, Worthington J, Ortego-Centeno N, Riemekasten G, Fonollosa V, Vonk M, Van den Hoogen F (2009b) A large multicentre analysis of CTGF-945 promoter polymorphism does not confirm association with systemic sclerosis susceptibility or phenotype. Ann Rheum Dis 68:1618–1620

Rueda B, Gourh P, Broen J, Agarwal S, Simeon C, Ortego-Centeno N, Vonk M, Coenen M, Riemekasten G, Hunzelmann N (2010) BANK1 functional variants are associated with susceptibility to diffuse systemic sclerosis in Caucasians. Ann Rheum Dis 69:700–705

Saeedi M, Amoli M, Robati R, Sayahpour F, Namazi N, Toossi P (2013) Macrophage migration inhibitory factor gene polymorphism is not associated with pemphigus vulgaris in Iranian patients. J Eur Acad Dermatol Venereol 27:1127–1131

Salanueva IJ, Cerezo A, Guadamillas MC, Del Pozo MA (2007) Integrin regulation of caveolin function. J Cell Mol Med 11:969–980

Samuelson EM, Laird RM, Maue AC, Rochford R, Hayes SM (2012) Blk haploinsufficiency impairs the development, but enhances the functional responses, of MZ B cells. Immunol Cell Biol 90:620–629

Sasai M, Linehan MM, Iwasaki A (2010) Bifurcation of Toll-like receptor 9 signaling by adaptor protein 3. Science 329:1530–1534

Sato S, Hanakawa H, Hasegawa M, Nagaoka T, Hamaguchi Y, Nishijima C, Komatsu K, Hirata A, Takehara K (2000) Levels of interleukin 12, a cytokine of type 1 helper T cells, are elevated in sera from patients with systemic sclerosis. J Rheumatol 27:2838–2842

Sbaa E, Frérart F, Feron O (2005) The double regulation of endothelial nitric oxide synthase by caveolae and caveolin: a paradox solved through the study of angiogenesis. Trends Cardiovasc Med 15:157–162

Schachna L, Wigley FM, Morris S, Gelber AC, Rosen A, Casciola-Rosen L (2002) Recognition of granzyme B-generated autoantigen fragments in scleroderma patients with ischemic digital loss. Arthritis Rheum Off J Am Coll Rheumatol 46:1873–1884

Selvi E, Tripodi S, Catenaccio M, Lorenzini S, Chindamo D, Manganelli S, Romagnoli R, Ietta F, Paulesu L, Miracco C (2003) Expression of macrophage migration inhibitory factor in diffuse systemic sclerosis. Ann Rheum Dis 62:460–464

Servettaz A, Goulvestre C, Kavian N, Nicco C, Guilpain P, Chéreau C, Vuiblet V, Guillevin L, Mouthon L, Weill B (2009) Selective oxidation of DNA topoisomerase 1 induces systemic sclerosis in the mouse. J Immunol 182:5855–5864

Shah AA, Rosen A (2011) Cancer and systemic sclerosis: novel insights into pathogenesis and clinical implications. Curr Opin Rheumatol 23:530

Shi Y, Wu Q, Xuan W, Feng X, Wang F, Tsao BP, Zhang M, Tan W (2018) Transcription factor SOX5 promotes the migration and invasion of fibroblast-like synoviocytes in part by regulating MMP-9 expression in collagen-induced arthritis. Front Immunol 9:749

Shimoda K, Kato K, Aoki K, Matsuda T, Miyamoto A, Shibamori M, Yamashita M, Numata A, Takase K, Kobayashi S (2000) Tyk2 plays a restricted role in IFNα signaling, although it is required for IL-12-mediated T cell function. Immunity 13:561–571

Shiwen X, Stratton R, Nikitorowicz-Buniak J, Ahmed-Abdi B, Ponticos M, Denton C, Abraham D, Takahashi A, Suki B, Layne MD (2015) A role of myocardin related transcription factor-A (MRTF-A) in scleroderma related fibrosis. PLoS One 10: e0126015

Shu C, Du W, Mao X, Li Y, Zhu Q, Wang W, Wu N, Mao X, Jin H, Sun Q (2014) Possible single-nucleotide polymorphism loci associated with systemic sclerosis susceptibility: a genetic association study in a Chinese Han population. PLoS One 9: e113197

Sica A, Mantovani A (2012) Macrophage plasticity and polarization: in vivo veritas. J Clin Investig 122:787–795

Simpfendorfer KR, Armstead BE, Shih A, Li W, Curran M, Manjarrez-Orduño N, Lee AT, Diamond B, Gregersen PK (2015) Autoimmune disease-associated haplotypes of BLK exhibit lowered thresholds for B cell activation and expansion of Ig class-switched B cells. Arthritis Rheumatol 67:2866–2876

Sinici I, Kalyoncu U, Karahan S, Kiraz S, Atalar E (2010) Endothelial nitric oxide gene polymorphism and risk of systemic sclerosis: predisposition effect of T-786C promoter and protective effect of 27 bp repeats in Intron 4. Clin Exp Rheumatol 28:169

Skarmoutsou E, D'Amico F, Marchini M, Malaponte G, Scorza R, Mazzarino MC (2012) Association of TIMP-1+ 372 SNP with digital ulcer manifestation in female systemic sclerosis patients. Hum Immunol 73:950–953

Skarmoutsou et al., 2011Skarmoutsou E, d'AMIcO F, Marchini M, Stivala F, Malaponte G, Scorza R, Mazzarino MC (2011) Analysis of matrix metalloproteinase-9 gene polymorphism-1562 C/T in patients suffering from systemic sclerosis with and without ulcers. Int J Mol Med 27:873–877

Skhirtladze C, Distler O, Dees C, Akhmetshina A, Busch N, Venalis P, Zwerina J, Spriewald B, Pileckyte M, Schett G (2008) Src kinases in systemic sclerosis: central roles in fibroblast activation and in skin fibrosis. Arthritis Rheum 58:1475–1484

Song G, Lee Y (2017) Association between BLK polymorphisms and susceptibility to SLE. Zeitschrift Für Rheumatologie 76:176–182

Song YW, Lee EB, Whang DH, Kang SJ, Takeuchi F, Park MH (2005) Association of TAP1 and TAP2 gene polymorphisms with systemic sclerosis in Korean patients. Hum Immunol 66:810–817

Soroosh P, Ine S, Sugamura K, Ishii N (2006) OX40-OX40 ligand interaction through T cell-T cell contact contributes to CD4 T cell longevity. J Immunol 176:5975–5987

Spalinger MR, Kasper S, Gottier C, Lang S, Atrott K, Vavricka SR, Scharl S, Gutte PM, Grütter MG, Beer H-D (2016) NLRP3 tyrosine phosphorylation is controlled by protein tyrosine phosphatase PTPN22. J Clin Investig 126:1783–1800

Spalinger MR, Lang S, Gottier C, Dai X, Rawlings DJ, Chan AC, Rogler G, Scharl M (2017) PTPN22 regulates NLRP3-mediated IL1B secretion in an autophagy-dependent manner. Autophagy 13:1590–1601

Spalinger MR, Lang S, Vavricka SR, Fried M, Rogler G, Scharl M (2013) Protein tyrosine phosphatase non-receptor type 22 modulates NOD2-induced cytokine release and autophagy. PLoS One 8:e72384

Spalinger MR, Lang S, Weber A, Frei P, Fried M, Rogler G, Scharl M (2013) Loss of protein tyrosine phosphatase nonreceptor Type 22 regulates interferon-γ-induced signaling in human monocytes. Gastroenterology 144:978–988. e910

Stüber E, Strober W (1996) The T cell-B cell interaction via OX40-OX40L is necessary for the T cell-dependent humoral immune response. J Exp Med 183:979–989

Su L-C, Xu W-D, Huang A-F (2020) IRAK family in inflammatory autoimmune diseases. Autoimmunity Rev 19:102461

Susol E, Rands A, Herrick A, McHugh N, Barrett J, Ollier W, Worthington J (2000) Association of markers for TGFβ3, TGFβ2 and TIMP1 with systemic sclerosis. Rheumatology 39:1332–1336

Svegliati S, Amico D, Spadoni T, Fischetti C, Finke D, Moroncini G, Paolini C, Tonnini C, Grieco A, Rovinelli M (2017) Agonistic anti-PDGF receptor autoantibodies from patients with systemic sclerosis impact human pulmonary artery smooth muscle cells function in vitro. Front Immunol 8:75

Szilveszter KP, Németh T, Mócsai A (2019) Tyrosine kinases in autoimmune and inflammatory skin diseases. Front Immunol 10:1862

Tan F, Zhou X, Mayes M, Gourh P, Guo X, Marcum C, Jin L, Arnett F Jr (2006) Signatures of differentially regulated interferon gene expression and vasculotrophism in the peripheral blood cells of systemic sclerosis patients. Rheumatology 45:694–702

Tanida I (2011) Autophagosome formation and molecular mechanism of autophagy. Antioxid Redox Signal 14:2201–2214

Tao J-H, Zou Y-F, Feng X-L, Li J, Wang F, Pan F-M, Ye D-Q (2011) Meta-analysis of TYK2 gene polymorphisms association with susceptibility to autoimmune and inflammatory diseases. Mol Biol Rep 38:4663–4672

Taroni JN, Greene CS, Martyanov V, Wood TA, Christmann RB, Farber HW, Lafyatis RA, Denton CP,

Hinchcliff ME, Pioli PA (2017) A novel multi-network approach reveals tissue-specific cellular modulators of fibrosis in systemic sclerosis. Genome Med 9:1–24

Terao C, Kawaguchi T, Dieude P, Varga J, Kuwana M, Hudson M, Kawaguchi Y, Matucci-Cerinic M, Ohmura K, Riemekasten G (2017) Transethnic meta-analysis identifies GSDMA and PRDM1 as susceptibility genes to systemic sclerosis. Ann Rheum Dis 76:1150–1158

Teruel M, McKinney C, Balsa A, Pascual-Salcedo D, Rodriguez-Rodriguez L, Ortiz AM, Gómez-Vaquero C, González-Gay MA, Smith M, Witte T (2013) Association of CD247 polymorphisms with rheumatoid arthritis: a replication study and a meta-analysis. PLoS One 8:e68295

Texido G, Su I-h, Mecklenbräuker I, Saijo K, Malek SN, Desiderio S, Rajewsky K, Tarakhovsky A (2000) The B-cell-specific Src-family kinase Blk is dispensable for B-cell development and activation. Mol Cell Biol 20:1227–1233

Thannickal VJ, Lee DY, White ES, Cui Z, Larios JM, Chacon R, Horowitz JC, Day RM, Thomas PE (2003) Myofibroblast differentiation by transforming growth factor-1 Is dependent on cell adhesion and integrin signaling via focal adhesion kinase. J Biol Chem 278:12384–12389

Tian Y, Han C, Wei Z, Dong H, Shen X, Cui Y, Fu X, Tian Z, Wang S, Zhou J (2021) SOX-5 activates a novel RORγt enhancer to facilitate experimental autoimmune encephalomyelitis by promoting Th17 cell differentiation. Nat Commun 12:1–18

Touyz R, Schiffrin E (2004) Reactive oxygen species in vascular biology: implications in hypertension. Histochem Cell Biol 122:339–352

Trowsdale J, Hanson I, Mockridge I, Beck S, Townsendt A, Kelly A (1990) Sequences encoded in the class II region of the MHC related to the 'ABC' superfamily of transporters. Nature 348:741–744

Tsuchiya N, Kawasaki A, Hasegawa M, Fujimoto M, Takehara K, Kawaguchi Y, Kawamoto M, Hara M, Sato S (2009) Association of STAT4 polymorphism with systemic sclerosis in a Japanese population. Ann Rheum Dis 68:1375–1376

Tsuji-Yamada J, Nakazawa M, Takahashi K, Iijima K, Hattori S, Okuda K, Minami M, Ikezawa Z, Sasaki T (2001) Effect of IL-12 encoding plasmid administration on tight-skin mouse. Biochem Biophys Res Commun 280:707–712

Ueki M, Takeshita H, Fujihara J, Iida R, Yuasa I, Kato H, Panduro A, Nakajima T, Kominato Y, Yasuda T (2009) Caucasian-specific allele in non-synonymous single nucleotide polymorphisms of the gene encoding deoxyribonuclease I-like 3, potentially relevant to autoimmunity, produces an inactive enzyme. Clin Chim Acta 407:20–24

Ulanet DB, Flavahan NA, Casciola-Rosen L, Rosen A (2004) Selective cleavage of nucleolar autoantigen B23 by granzyme B in differentiated vascular smooth muscle cells: insights into the association of specific autoantibodies with distinct disease phenotypes. Arthritis Rheum Off J Am Coll Rheumatol 50:233–241

Ushio-Fukai M, Alexander RW (2004) Reactive oxygen species as mediators of angiogenesis signaling. Role of NAD (P) H oxidase. Mol Cell Biochem 264:85–97

van Bon L, Affandi AJ, Broen J, Christmann RB, Marijnissen RJ, Stawski L, Farina GA, Stifano G, Mathes AL, Cossu M (2014) Proteome-wide analysis and CXCL4 as a biomarker in systemic sclerosis. N Engl J Med 370:433–443

Van Den Hoogen F, Khanna D, Fransen J, Johnson SR, Baron M, Tyndall A, Matucci-Cerinic M, Naden RP, Medsger TA Jr, Carreira PE (2013) 2013 classification criteria for systemic sclerosis: an American College of Rheumatology/European League against rheumatism collaborative initiative. Arthritis Rheum 65:2737–2747

Varga J, Pasche B (2009) Transforming growth factor β as a therapeutic target in systemic sclerosis. Nat Rev Rheumatol 5:200–206

Verhoeven Y, Tilborghs S, Jacobs J, De Waele J, Quatannens D, Deben C, Prenen H, Pauwels P, Trinh XB, Wouters A (2020) The potential and controversy of targeting STAT family members in cancer. In: Seminars in cancer biology. Elsevier, pp 41–56

Vigone B, Santaniello A, Marchini M, Montanelli G, Caronni M, Severino A, Beretta L (2015) Role of class II human leucocyte antigens in the progression from early to definite systemic sclerosis. Rheumatology 54:707–711

Vittal R, Horowitz JC, Moore BB, Zhang H, Martinez FJ, Toews GB, Standiford TJ, Thannickal VJ (2005) Modulation of prosurvival signaling in fibroblasts by a protein kinase inhibitor protects against fibrotic tissue injury. Am J Pathol 166:367–375

Wallis DD, Tan FK, Kielty CM, Kimball MD, Arnett FC, Milewicz DM (2001) Abnormalities in fibrillin 1-containing microfibrils in dermal fibroblast cultures from patients with systemic sclerosis (scleroderma). Arthritis Rheum 44:1855–1864

Wang XM, Zhang Y, Kim HP, Zhou Z, Feghali-Bostwick CA, Liu F, Ifedigbo E, Xu X, Oury TD, Kaminski N (2006a) Caveolin-1: a critical regulator of lung fibrosis in idiopathic pulmonary fibrosis. J Exp Med 203:2895–2906

Wang Y, Fan PS, Kahaleh B (2006b) Association between enhanced type I collagen expression and epigenetic repression of the FLI1 gene in scleroderma fibroblasts. Arthritis Rheum Off J Am Coll Rheumatol 54:2271–2279

Wang Y, Shaked I, Stanford SM, Zhou W, Curtsinger JM, Mikulski Z, Shaheen ZR, Cheng G, Sawatzke K, Campbell AM (2013) The autoimmunity-associated gene PTPN22 potentiates toll-like receptor-driven, type 1 interferon-dependent immunity. Immunity 39:111–122

Wang J, Yi L, Guo X, He D, Li H, Guo G, Wang Y, Zou H, Gu Y, Tu W (2014) Lack of association of the

CD247 SNP rs2056626 with systemic sclerosis in Han Chinese. Open Rheumatol J 8:43

Wang W, Bhattacharyya S, Marangoni RG, Carns M, Dennis-Aren K, Yeldandi A, Wei J, Varga J (2020) The JAK/STAT pathway is activated in systemic sclerosis and is effectively targeted by tofacitinib. J Scleroderma Relat Disord 5:40–50

Warchoł T, Piotrowski P, Lianeri M, Cieślak D, Wudarski M, Hrycaj P, Łącki J, Jagodziński P (2009) The CD3Z 844 T> A polymorphism within the 3′-UTR of CD3Z confers increased risk of incidence of systemic lupus erythematosus. Tissue Antigens 74:68–72

Ward AM, Udnoon S, Watkins J, Walker AE, Darke C (1976) Immunological mechanisms in the pathogenesis of vinyl chloride disease. Br Med J 1:936–938

Wei J, Bhattacharyya S, Jain M, Varga J (2008) Regulation of matrix remodeling by peroxisome proliferatoractivated receptor-γ: a novel link between metabolism and fibrogenesis. Open Rheumatol J 2012; 6: 103–15. J Clin Endocrinol Metab 93:1433–1441

Wei P, Yang Y, Guo X, Hei N, Lai S, Assassi S, Liu M, Tan F, Zhou X (2016) Integrative studies of scleroderma-associated genetic and environmental factors with fibroblasts identify polymorphisms of TNFAIP3 in association with MMP expression. Arthritis Rheumatol (Hoboken, NJ) 68:749

Wei J, Ghosh AK, Sargent JL, Komura K, Wu M, Huang Q-Q, Jain M, Whitfield ML, Feghali-Bostwick C, Varga J (2010) PPARγ downregulation by TGFß in fibroblast and impaired expression and function in systemic sclerosis: a novel mechanism for progressive fibrogenesis. PLoS One 5:e13778

Wen Y, Cai W, Yang J, Fu X, Putha L, Xia Q, Windsor JA, Phillips AR, Tyndall JD, Du D (2021) Targeting macrophage migration inhibitory factor in acute pancreatitis and pancreatic cancer. Front Pharmacol 12:270

Wipff J, Allanore Y, Kahan A, Meyer O, Mouthon L, Guillevin L, Pierlot C, Glikmans E, Bardin T, Boileau C (2006) Lack of association between the protein tyrosine phosphatase non-receptor 22 (PTPN22)* 620W allele and systemic sclerosis in the French Caucasian population. Ann Rheum Dis 65:1230–1232

Wipff J, Gallier G, Dieude P, Avouac J, Tiev K, Hachulla E, Granel B, Diot E, Sibilia J, Mouthon L (2009) Angiotensin-converting enzyme gene does not contribute to genetic susceptibility to systemic sclerosis in European Caucasians. J Rheumatol 36:337–340

Wipff J, Dieude P, Avouac J, Tiev K, Hachulla E, Cracowski J-L, Diot E, Sibilia J, Mouthon L, Meyer O (2010) Association of metalloproteinase gene polymorphisms with systemic sclerosis in the European Caucasian population. J Rheumatol 37:599–602

Witkowska-Tobo[3]a et al., 2004 Witkowska-Tobo[3]a AM, Szczerkowska-Dobosz A, Nedoszytko B, Roszkiewicz J (2004) Polymorphism of the TAP1 gene in Polish patients with psoriasis vulgaris. J Appl Genet 45:391–393

Wu M, Assassi S (2013) The role of type 1 interferon in systemic sclerosis. Front Immunol 4:266

Wu SP, Leng L, Feng Z, Liu N, Zhao H, McDonald C, Lee A, Arnett FC, Gregersen PK, Mayes MD (2006) Macrophage migration inhibitory factor promoter polymorphisms and the clinical expression of scleroderma. Arthritis Rheum Off J Am Coll Rheumatol 54:3661–3669

Wu Y-Y, Georg I, Díaz-Barreiro A, Varela N, Lauwerys B, Kumar R, Bagavant H, Castillo-Martín M, El Salem F, Marañón C (2015) Concordance of increased B1 cell subset and lupus phenotypes in mice and humans is dependent on BLK expression levels. J Immunol 194:5692–5702

Xu J, Yang Y, Qiu G, Lal G, Yin N, Wu Z, Bromberg JS, Ding Y (2011) Stat4 is critical for the balance between Th17 cells and regulatory T cells in colitis. J Immunol 186:6597–6606

Xu Y, Wang W, Tian Y, Liu J, Yang R (2016) Polymorphisms in STAT 4 and IRF 5 increase the risk of systemic sclerosis: a meta-analysis. Int J Dermatol 55:408–416

Xu D, Mu R, Wei X (2019) The roles of IL-1 family cytokines in the pathogenesis of systemic sclerosis. Front Immunol 10:2025

Yamakage A, Kikuchi K, Smith EA, LeRoy EC, Trojanowska M (1992) Selective upregulation of platelet-derived growth factor alpha receptors by transforming growth factor beta in scleroderma fibroblasts. J Exp Med 175:1227–1234

Yazdani R, Ganjalikhani-Hakemi M, Esmaeili M, Abolhassani H, Vaeli S, Rezaei A, Sharifi Z, Azizi G, Rezaei N, Aghamohammadi A (2017) Impaired Akt phosphorylation in B-cells of patients with common variable immunodeficiency. Clin Immunol 175:124–132

Ye X, Zhou X-J, Zhang H (2018) Exploring the role of autophagy-related gene 5 (ATG5) yields important insights into autophagy in autoimmune/autoinflammatory diseases. Front Immunol 9:2334

Yousefi S, Perozzo R, Schmid I, Ziemiecki A, Schaffner T, Scapozza L, Brunner T, Simon H-U (2006) Calpain-mediated cleavage of Atg5 switches autophagy to apoptosis. Nat Cell Biol 8:1124–1132

Zakrzewska K, Arvia R, Torcia MG, Clemente AM, Tanturli M, Castronovo G, Sighinolfi G, Giuggioli D, Ferri C (2019) Effects of parvovirus B19 in vitro infection on monocytes from patients with systemic sclerosis: enhanced inflammatory pathways by caspase-1 activation and cytokine production. J Investig Dermatol 139:2125–2133. e2121

Zhang SL, Chabod J, Penfornis A, Reviron D, Tiberghien P, Wendling D, Toussirot E (2002) TAP1 and TAP2 gene polymorphism in rheumatoid arthritis in a population in eastern France. Eur J Immunogenet 29:241–249

Zhang X, Nie S, Si X, Luo Y, Tang W (2012) Association between the CTGF−945C/G polymorphism and systemic sclerosis: a meta-analysis. Gene 509:1–6

Zhang D-M, Cheng L-Q, Zhai Z-F, Feng L, Zhong B-Y, You Y, Zhang N, Song Z-Q, Yang X-C, Chen F-R

(2013a) Single-nucleotide polymorphism and haplotypes of TNIP1 associated with systemic lupus erythematosus in a Chinese Han population. J Rheumatol 40:1535–1544

Zhang Y, Choksi S, Chen K, Pobezinskaya Y, Linnoila I, Liu Z-G (2013b) ROS play a critical role in the differentiation of alternatively activated macrophages and the occurrence of tumor-associated macrophages. Cell Res 23:898–914

Zhang Q, Lenardo MJ, Baltimore D (2017) 30 years of NF-κB: a blossoming of relevance to human pathobiology. Cell 168:37–57

Zhang Y, Yang X, Qiu C, Liu F, Liu P, Liu Z (2018) Matrine suppresses AGE-induced HAEC injury by inhibiting ROS-mediated NRLP3 inflammasome activation. Eur J Pharmacol 822:207–211

Zhang X, Mei D, Zhang L, Wei W (2020) Src family protein kinase controls the fate of B cells in autoimmune diseases. Inflammation 1–11

Zhao W, Yue X, Liu K, Zheng J, Huang R, Zou J, Riemekasten G, Petersen F, Yu X (2017) The status of pulmonary fibrosis in systemic sclerosis is associated with IRF5, STAT4, IRAK1, and CTGF polymorphisms. Rheumatol Int 37:1303–1310

Zhou X, Lee JE, Arnett FC, Xiong M, Park MY, Yoo YK, Shin ES, Reveille JD, Mayes MD, Kim JH (2009) HLA–DPB1 and DPB2 are genetic loci for systemic sclerosis: a genome-wide association study in Koreans with replication in North Americans. Arthritis Rheum Off J Am Coll Rheumatol 60:3807–3814

Zhou X-j, Lu X-l, Lv J-c, Yang H-z, Qin L-x, Zhao M-h, Su Y, Li Z-g, Zhang H (2011) Genetic association of PRDM1-ATG5 intergenic region and autophagy with systemic lupus erythematosus in a Chinese population. Ann Rheum Dis 70:1330–1337

Zhou X, Li H, Guo S, Wang J, Shi C, Espitia M, Guo X, Wang Q, Liu M, Assassi S (2019) Associations of multiple NOTCH4 exonic variants with systemic sclerosis. J Rheumatol 46:184–189

Zilahi E, Tarr T, Papp G, Griger Z, Sipka S, Zeher M (2012) Increased microRNA-146a/b, TRAF6 gene and decreased IRAK1 gene expressions in the peripheral mononuclear cells of patients with Sjögren's syndrome. Immunol Lett 141:165–168

Zochling J, Newell F, Charlesworth JC, Leo P, Stankovich J, Cortes A, Zhou Y, Stevens W, Sahhar J, Roddy J (2014) An immunochip-based interrogation of scleroderma susceptibility variants identifies a novel association at DNASE1L3. Arthritis Res Ther 16:1–7

Zou Y, Wang F, Feng X, Tao J, Zhu J, Pan F, Su H (2011) Association of NFKB1-94ins/delATTG promoter polymorphism with susceptibility to autoimmune and inflammatory diseases: a meta-analysis. Tissue Antigens 77:9–17

The Immunogenetics of Vasculitis

Fotini B. Karassa, Eleftherios Pelechas, and Georgios Zouzos

Abstract

Vasculitides are a cluster of diseases defined by an immune attack targeting vessels of different sizes. While most types of vasculitis have an undetermined cause, progress has been achieved in the recent decade in elucidating the mechanisms that participate in the inflammatory damage of the blood vessel wall. Several studies have emphasized that genetic susceptibility is an important aspect of the pathogenesis of vasculitides. The most prominent genetic risk loci for vasculitides reside within the major histocompatibility complex region. This indicates that the immune system is a major contributor to the pathogenesis of this group of diseases. In this chapter, we provide an updated overview of the etiology and pathogenesis of these entities with an emphasis on the major insights gained from recent genetic studies in the highly studied types of vasculitides.

Keywords

Primary vasculitides · Pathogenesis · Genetic risk · GWAS · HLA associations

F. B. Karassa (✉) · E. Pelechas · G. Zouzos
Division of Rheumatology, Department of Medicine, School of Health Sciences, University of Ioannina, 45110 Ioannina, Greece
e-mail: fkarassa@uoi.gr

1 Introduction

Vasculitides represent a diverse group of diseases defined by inflammatory cell infiltration and necrosis of the vessel wall (Anwar and Karim 2017; Jennette et al. 2013). These disorders can cause an array of clinical symptoms, ranging from a mild self-limited cutaneous lesion to a life-threatening multisystem disease, based on the size, location, functional aspects, and intensity of the inflammatory process in the affected vessels (Gonzalez-Gay and Garcia-Porrua 2001). Despite their frequent onset with unspecified symptoms and signs, vasculitides usually evolve over several weeks to months with manifestations and clinical attributes reflecting organ- or tissue-specific involvement (Gonzalez-Gay and Garcia-Porrua 2001; Jennette et al. 2013). Though the cause of most types of vasculitis is still unclear, substantial advances have been made recently in understanding the mechanisms that contribute to the immune-mediated demolition of vessel walls (Hughes et al. 2013; Lyons et al. 2012; Millet et al. 2015; Sangaletti et al. 2012; Takeuchi et al. 2017; Terao et al. 2013). The pathogenic process may be considered primary (for instance when the etiology is unknown) or secondary (e.g., as a consequence of connective tissue disease or infection) (Jennette et al. 2013). Several studies highlight that genetic susceptibility is a fundamental aspect of the pathogenesis in most of the vasculitic

N. Rezaei and F. Rajabi (eds.), *The Immunogenetics of Dermatologic Diseases*, Advances in Experimental Medicine and Biology 1367,
https://doi.org/10.1007/978-3-030-92616-8_11

syndromes (Hughes et al. 2013; Lyons et al. 2012; Takeuchi et al. 2017; Terao et al. 2013). The advent of exome sequencing modalities and the analysis of high-throughput genotyping techniques constitute major advances in technology that enabled our understanding of the genetic substructure of systemic vasculitides over the recent decade.

In the current chapter, we provide an updated outline of the etiology and pathogenesis of the primary systemic vasculitides with a focus on the major insights gained from recent genetic studies such as genome-wide association studies (GWAS) that use single nucleotide polymorphism (SNP) genotyping, meta-analyses, fine-mapping, immunochip assays and studies performed across different forms of these disorders and/or populations of diverse ancestries. We emphasize pivotal genetic studies in the highly studied types of primary systemic vasculitides and discuss how they have improved our understanding of pathways to disease.

1.1 Search Strategy and Selection Criteria

The MEDLINE (via PubMed) was searched for original studies published until June 1, 2019, in the English language using the terms "vasculitis", or "Takayasu", or "giant cell arteritis", or "temporal arteritis", or "Kawasaki", or "antineutrophil cytoplasmic antibody-associated vasculitis", or "ANCA-associated vasculitis", or "microscopic polyangiitis", or "granulomatosis with polyangiitis", or "Wegener granulomatosis", or "eosinophilic granulomatosis with polyangiitis", or "Churg-Strauss", or Henoch-Schönlein purpura", or "IgA vasculitis", or "Behcet's", or "polyarteritis nodosa" in combination with the search terms "genetics", "pathogenesis", "genome-wide association studies", "genetic analysis", "meta-analysis". The most recent articles were mainly selected, yet highly referenced older publications were not excluded. The reference lists of the articles retrieved by the search strategy were also searched for additional eligible publications.

2 Classification: Epidemiology

The exact etiology of most types of vasculitides is not yet completely elucidated and furthermore, there is substantial heterogeneity and overlap across their clinical and pathologic manifestations; these have been significant obstacles to the development of a universally used classification system. A set of criteria for classifying all types of vasculitis established by the American College of Rheumatology in 1990 (Hunder et al. 1990) proved to have insufficient diagnostic accuracy and little value for the categorization of patients with cutaneous vasculitis. Currently, the most accepted system is the 2012 revised international Chapel Hill Consensus Conference (CHCC 2012) nomenclature (Jennette et al. 2013) with a subsequent dermatologic addendum that intended to systematize the names, definitions, and descriptions for cutaneous components of primary systemic vasculitides (Sunderkotter et al. 2018). Nevertheless, it ought to be emphasized that the CHCC 2012 created a nomenclature that was not intended to be used as a categorization or diagnostic criteria. It categorizes primary vasculitis by combining knowledge regarding etiopathogenesis, histopathology, epidemiology, and clinical signs and symptoms (Jennette et al. 2013). The first classification level adopted by the CHCC 2012 scheme was based on the primary type and size of the affected vessels, i.e., large-vessel, medium-vessel, and small-vessel vasculitis (Figs. 1 and 2). Large-vessel vasculitis attacks large arteries more frequently than medium-or small-vessel vasculitis, whereas medium-vessel vasculitis mostly involves medium-sized arteries and veins, and small-vessel vasculitis primarily attacks arterioles,

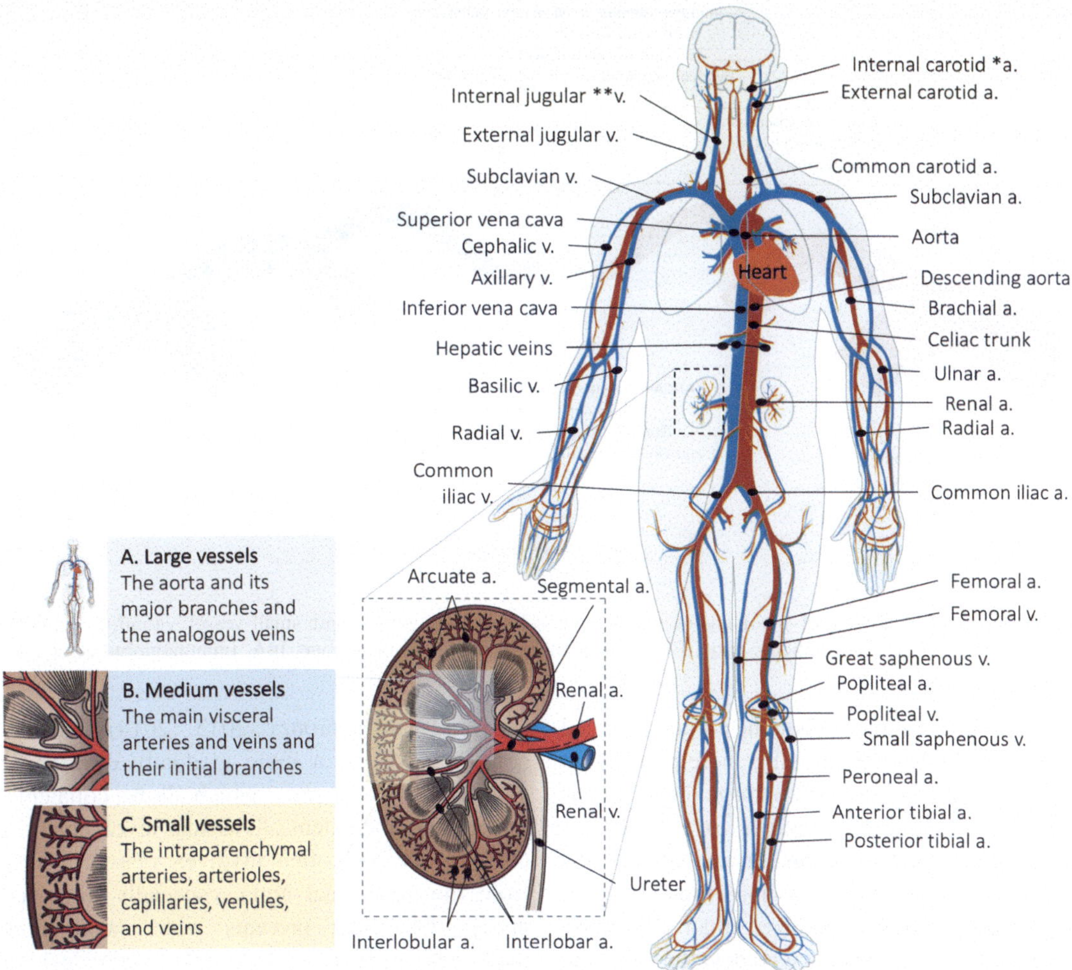

Fig. 1 Gross anatomy of the vessels (*a: artery, **v; vein)

capillaries, and postcapillary venules (Figs. 1 and 2), but the key point from the CHCC 2012 nomenclature (Table 1) is that vasculitis in all three main groups may eventually involve vessels with any diameter (Jennette et al. 2013).

While the vasculitides are considered relatively uncommon disorders, their incidence is not negligible, particularly in Western countries. About one in every 2.000 adults has some type of vasculitis whereas one in every 7.000 adults develops this disorder each year. The most common types of primary systemic vasculitides (Table 1), at least in the United States, are giant cell arteritis (GCA), granulomatosis with polyangiitis (GPA) which was formerly known as Wegener granulomatosis, and microscopic polyangiitis (MPA) (Gonzalez-Gay and Garcia-Porrua 2001).

3 Large-Vessel Vasculitis

3.1 General Aspects

Large-vessel vasculitis involves large arteries more frequently than the other forms of vasculitides (Table 1). These large arteries include the aorta and its first-level branches (Figs. 1 and 2). Due to the essential role of these blood vessels, this vasculitis variant is characterized by serious

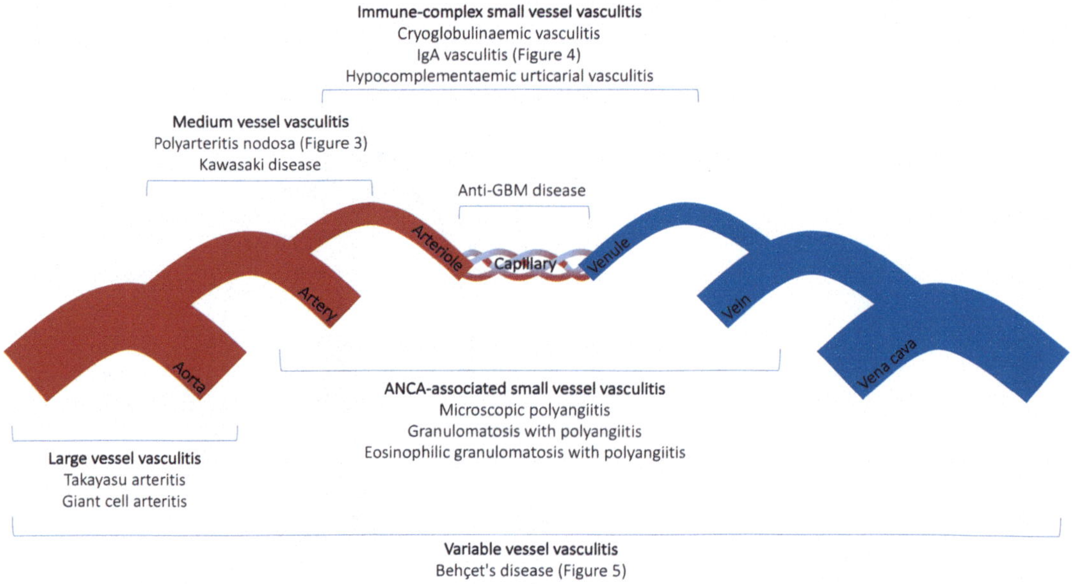

Fig. 2 Distribution of vessel involvement by large-vessel, medium-vessel, and small-vessel vasculitis (ANCA, antineutrophil cytoplasmic antibody; anti-GBM, anti-glomerular basement membrane; IgA, immunoglobulin A)

clinical manifestations. When the aorta is targeted by dysfunctional immunity, it is more probable to develop signs of vessel wall damage displaying as aneurysm formation, rupture, or dissection. Takayasu arteritis (TA) and giant cell arteritis (GCA) constitute the two major forms. TA usually affects women younger than 50 years whereas nearly all patients who develop GCA are elderly individuals (often above 50 years) (Harky et al. 2019; Jennette et al. 2013). Both entities are granulomatous arteritides predominantly affecting the large arteries. Yet, GCA has a preference for carotid and vertebral artery branches and generally affects the temporal artery. Even though there is no apparent aortic involvement at the onset, observational studies imply an increased incidence of aortic aneurysm in such individuals (Robson et al. 2015). GCA is often associated with polymyalgia rheumatica which is defined as a sense of stiffness and tenderness in the neck, shoulders, and hip. Headache, visual symptoms, constitutional symptoms, jaw claudication, and abnormally appearing temporal artery are the other typical manifestations of GCA (Weyand and Goronzy 2013, 2014). One of the most devastating complications is permanent visual loss (Weyand and Goronzy 2013, 2014). On the contrary, TA has a more gradually developing course of vessel stenosis which allows collaterals to form, yet the extent of vascular involvement is considerable and often involves vessels arising from the abdominal aorta, especially the renal artery. TA often presents with claudication, hypertension, fever of unknown origin, lack of pulse on the affected side, and presence of a bruit over the affected region (Harky et al. 2019). Large-vessel vasculitis rarely has cutaneous findings since there are no large arteries in the dermis or subcutaneous tissues (Jennette et al. 2013; Sunderkotter et al. 2018).

3.2 Pathogenesis

The two major variants of large-vessel vasculitis appear to have comparable pathogenesis given that their histopathologic features are indistinguishable. Because the media and intima are not vascularized, the major site of damage is assumed to be the vasa-vasorum located at the adventitia. The inflammatory process initiates in the adventitia and spreads to the other layers of

Table 1 The 2012 revised international Chapel Hill Consensus Conference (CHCC) Nomenclature of Vasculitides (Jennette et al. 2013) and the dermatologic addendum to the CHCC 2012 (Sunderkötter et al. 2018)

Large-vessel vasculitis
Takayasu arteritis
Giant cell Arteritis
Medium-vessel vasculitis
Polyarteritis nodosa
Kawasaki disease
Small-vessel vasculitis
Antineutrophil cytoplasmic antibody (ANCA)-associated vasculitis
Microscopic polyangiitis
Granulomatosis with polyangiitis (also known as Wegener granulomatosis)
Eosinophilic granulomatosis with polyangiitis (also known as Churg-Strauss syndrome)
Immune complex small-vessel vasculitis
Anti-glomerular basement membrane disease
Cryoglobulinemic vasculitis
IgA vasculitis (also known as Henoch-Schönlein purpura)
Hypocomplementemic urticarial vasculitis
Variable-vessel vasculitis
Behçet's disease
Cogan's syndrome
Single-organ vasculitis[a]
Cutaneous leukocytoclastic angiitis
Cutaneous arteritis
Primary central nervous system vasculitis
Isolated aortitis
Others
Vasculitis associated with systemic disease
Vasculitis associated with systemic lupus erythematosus
Vasculitis associated with rheumatoid arthritis
Vasculitis associated with sarcoidosis
Others
Vasculitis associated with probable etiology
Infection (e.g. hepatitis C virus, hepatitis B virus, syphilis)-associated vasculitis
Drug-associated immune complex or ANCA-associated vasculitis
Cancer-associated vasculitis
Others

[a]According to the nomenclature of cutaneous vasculitis (Sunderkötter et al. 2018) in the single-organ vasculitis category, 5 more forms (cutaneous IgM/IgG immune complex vasculitis, nodular cutaneous vasculitis, erythema elevatum et diutinum, recurrent macular vasculitis in hypergammaglobulinemia, normocomplementemic urticarial vasculitis) were added

the vessel wall (Weyand and Goronzy 2013, 2014; Weyand et al. 2019). Dendritic cells (DCs) are present at the border of the adventitia and the media. In large-vessel vasculitis, these cells recognize pathogen- or microorganism-associated molecular patterns via Toll-like receptors (TLRs) and become aberrantly activated (Harky et al. 2019; Robson et al. 2015; Weyand and Goronzy 2013, 2014; Weyand et al. 2019). However, the antigen(s) that trigger the pathogenic cascade remain elusive. The stimulation of DCs leads to loss of tissue tolerance and renders arteries susceptible to immune attack (Dejaco et al. 2017; Harky et al. 2019; Weyand and Goronzy 2013, 2014; Weyand et al. 2019). Vascular DCs in GCA increase in number, become trapped, and distribute throughout the layers of the vessel. Once activated, vascular DCs recruit CD4+ T-cells via variable expression of TLRs that can determine the extent of vessel wall penetration and the severity of the inflammatory response (Dejaco et al. 2017; Harky et al. 2019; Weyand and Goronzy 2013, 2014; Weyand et al. 2019). Specifically, TLR4 promotes transmural panarteritis with $CD4^+$ T-cells invading into the arterial wall, whereas TLR5 triggering mediates the building of a perivascular infiltrate in the adventitial space; hence, TA and GCA appear to induce the expression of particular TLRs (Deng et al. 2009; Pryshchep et al. 2008). Remarkably, DCs are a major factor in determining the pattern of vessel involvement in large-vessel vasculitis, since TLRs are found in a variety of combinations in different arteries. CCL20 is produced by activated vascular DCs and promotes the recruitment of CD4+ T-cells by binding to their CCR6 receptors (Deng et al. 2009; Pryshchep et al. 2008). Migration of $CD4^+$ T-cells and macrophages is enabled via the vasa-vasorum and these cells invade across the tissue space in an adventitial-to-intimal route. Usually, extremely activated macrophages are found in granulomas, with nearby T-cells whereas B-cells are largely lacking from the inflammation (Martinez-Taboada et al. 1996; Weyand and Goronzy 2013, 2014; Weyand et al. 2019). Additionally, in GCA, the DCs could downregulate PD-L1 (an immune-inhibitory ligand) and therefore accelerate T-cell recruitment and retention in the vessel wall (Zhang et al. 2017). In the peripheral blood of patients with GCA, the diminished expression of NOX2 on $CD8^+CCR7^+$ regulatory T-cells can interrupt their suppressive effect on $CD4^+$ T-cell responses (Wen et al. 2016). In addition, matrix metalloprotease (MMP)-9–producing monocytes degrade the basal lamina, which appears to be a crucial stage in the invasion process (Watanabe et al. 2018). T-cells are not able to penetrate through collagen IV-rich tissue unless they co-occur with monocytes that release proteinase. In GCA, monocyte-derived MMP-9 supports T-cells in the infiltrative process. The detection of considerably amplified expression of MMP-1,-3, and -9 in individuals with active illness supports the hypothesis that MMPs have a role in the etiology of TA (Mahajan et al. 2012). Another crucial event is the interaction among $CD4^+$ T-cells and microvascular endothelial cells (Wen et al. 2017). Adventitial microvessels in GCA-affected patients express Jagged-1, a NOTCH1 receptor ligand. NOTCH1(26) is expressed by circulating CD4 + T-cells, which receive stimulatory signals from Jagged-1 + endothelial cells, thus providing a milieu that supports the shifting of T-cell homeostasis toward inflammation. Activated $CD4^+$ T-cells and macrophages secrete cytokines and inflammatory mediators, resulting in further T-cell differentiation (Weyand and Goronzy 2013, 2014). Two major cytokine clusters have a major role in the pathogenesis of GCA, the interleukin-12 (IL-12)/interferon-γ (IFN-γ) axis (produced by type 1 helper T-cell (Th1)) and the IL-6/IL-17/IL-21 axis (produced by type 17 helper T-cell (Th17)). Nonetheless, there are distinctions in the pathophysiology of TA and GCA in terms of the subclasses of T-cell that they exhibit and the discrete cytokine milieu that they produce. In GCA, the IL-6/IL-17 cluster was found to be very much responsive to standard regimens of corticosteroids, but the IL-12/IFN-γ was resistant to standard therapy (Weyand and Goronzy 2013, 2014). The opposite finding was shown in TA, with only the Th1 lineage being highly susceptible to steroid-mediated immunosuppression (Saadoun et al. 2015). The ultimate stage of the pathological process of TA and GCA implicates remodeling of the vessels causing stenosis, obstruction, or aneurysm. In GCA, IFN-γ-stimulated macrophages release cytokines that expand the inflammation as well as proteolytic enzymes, such as MMPs, that act to degrade extracellular matrix components and also have an important role in the emergence and branching of vasa-vasorum (Dejaco et al. 2017; Harky et al. 2019). Apart from the activated macrophages, multinucleated giant cells, fibroblasts, and damaged vascular smooth-muscle cells similarly produce proangiogenic and growth-promoting factors resulting in neovascularization and lumen-obstructive intimal hyperplasia (Harky et al. 2019). On the other hand, stromal cells in the vessel wall and the matrix proteins, appear to strongly influence inflammatory events. Thus, the severity and course of the inflammatory response depend on the interactions among vascular and immune cells, thereby controlling the chronicity of vasculitis and remodeling of the arterial wall (Weyand and Goronzy 2013, 2014; Weyand et al. 2019).

3.2.1 Genetic Associations in Takayasu Arteritis

The genetic contribution to the pathogenesis of TA was largely unknown until relatively recently. A GWAS on Japanese patients, and more importantly, an immunochip study on Turkish and North American communities (Table 2) have allowed an improved characterization of the genetic constituent of TA (Saruhan-Direskeneli et al. 2013; Terao et al. 2013).

There are two classes of HLA molecules; class I (HLA-A, -B, and -C) that mainly expresses endogenous peptides, and class II (HLA-DR, -DP, and -DQ) that have restricted expression and processes exogenous peptides. HLAs facilitate the recognition of self from foreign antigens (McCluskey et al. 2017). The HLA region that encodes these molecules appears to be the most polymorphic section in the human genome and has been linked with >100 diseases, which are primarily autoimmune (Hosomichi et al. 2015).

Previous studies have demonstrated that the most consistent genetic predisposition for TA is within the major histocompatibility complex (MHC) class I genomic region (Table 2). Particularly, the *HLA-B*52:01* allele has been repeatedly linked to TA across different ethnicities including Asians, Turks, Mexicans, and North Americans, and subsequently confirmed at the genome-wide level of significance (Kimura et al. 1996; Sahin et al. 2012; Terao et al. 2013, 2014; Yoshida et al. 1993). A study using the immunochip genotyping platform including approximately 196 thousand genetic alleles also detected a linkage between TA and the extended HLA region. The data that was obtained by analyzing two groups of patients and healthy controls, each from diverse ethnicities, demonstrated the existence of two independent linkage signals within the HLA region in TA. The strongest association signal came from the *HLA–B/MHC class I polypeptide-related sequence A* (*MICA*) gene followed by another strong signal from the *HLA–DQB1/HLA–DRB1* gene (Saruhan-Direskeneli et al. 2013) (Table 2). The *HLA-B/MICA* region was also demonstrated to confer risk for TA in the Chinese Han population (Wen et al. 2018). Hence, there seem to be two independent loci in MHC-I (*HLA–B/MICA*) and II region (*HLA–DQB1/HLA–DRB1*) that confer genetic risk for TA.

The most important non-HLA susceptibility gene for TA identified up to this point is the *IL12B* (Table 2), which was shown to exceed the p-value of 10^{-6} in two subsequent studies (Saruhan-Direskeneli et al. 2013; Terao et al. 2013). It codes the P40 regulatory subunit of IL-12 and IL-23 cytokines and it could impact both disease susceptibility and progression in synergism with HLA-B*52:01. The genetic region encoding two surface proteins of the immunoglobulin family, Fc-gamma receptor IIA (FCGR2A) and Fc-gamma receptor IIIA (FCGR3A), was also associated with TA in an immunochip study (Saruhan-Direskeneli et al. 2013). A gene coding for a transcription factor

Table 2 Genetic susceptibility factors from genome-wide association studies[a], immunochip genotyping with or without imputed data for the highly studied types of vasculitides

Vasculitis	Locus or allele	SNP	Study method	Population(s)	No of cases/No of controls	Year of publication/References
Takayasu arteritis						
	IL12B	rs6871626	GWAS	Japanese	167/663	2013 (Brouwer et al. 1993)
	HLA-B	rs4947248	GWAS	Japanese	167/663	2013 (Brouwer et al. 1993)
	*HLA-B*52:01*	rs9263739	GWAS	Japanese	167/663	2013 (Brouwer et al. 1993)
	HLA-B/MICA	rs12524487	Immunochip genotyping/Imputed data	Turkish, European ancestry	411/1,036	2013 (Ge et al. 2013)
	HLA-DQB1/HLA-DRB1	rs113452171	Immunochip genotyping/Imputed data	Turkish, European ancestry	411/1,036	2013 (Ge et al. 2013)
	HLA-DQB1/HLA-DRB1	rs189754752	Immunochip genotyping/Imputed data	Turkish, European ancestry	411/1,036	2013 (Ge et al. 2013)
	FCGR2A/FCGR3A	rs10919543	Immunochip genotyping/Imputed data	Turkish, European ancestry	411/1,036	2013 (Ge et al. 2013)
	IL12B	rs56167332	Immunochip genotyping/Imputed data	Turkish, European ancestry	411/1,036	2013 (Ge et al. 2013)
	IL6	rs2069837	GWAS	Turkish, European ancestry	693/1,536	2015 (Harky et al. 2019)
	RPS9/LILRB3	rs11666543	GWAS	Turkish, European ancestry	693/1,536	2015 (Harky et al. 2019)
	21q22	rs2242944	GWAS	Turkish, European ancestry	693/1,536	2015 (Harky et al. 2019)
	21q22	rs2836878	GWAS	Turkish, European ancestry	693/1,536	2015 (Harky et al. 2019)

(continued)

Table 2 (continued)

Vasculitis	Locus or allele	SNP	Study method	Population(s)	No of cases/No of controls	Year of publication/References
	21q22	rs2836881	GWAS	Turkish, European ancestry	693/1,536	2015 (Harky et al. 2019)
	FCGR3A	rs2099684	GWAS	Japanese	633/5,928	2018 (He et al. 2013)
	DUSP22	rs17133698	GWAS	Japanese	633/5,928	2018 (He et al. 2013)
	PTK2B	rs2322599	GWAS	Japanese	633/5,928	2018 (He et al. 2013)
	KLHL33	rs1713450	GWAS	Japanese	633/5,928	2018 (He et al. 2013)
	LILR3A	rs103294	GWAS	Japanese	633/5,928	2018 (He et al. 2013)
	21q.22	rs4817988	GWAS	Japanese	633/5,928	2018 (He et al. 2013)
Giant cell arteritis						
	HLA-DRA/HLA-DRB1	rs9268905	Imputed GWAS	European ancestry	2,134/9,125	2017 (Henderson et al. 2013)
	HLA-DQA1/HLA-DQA2	rs9275592	Imputed GWAS	European ancestry	2,134/9,125	2017 (Henderson et al. 2013)
	PLG	rs4252134	Imputed GWAS	European ancestry	2,134/9,125	2017 (Henderson et al. 2013)
	P4HA2	rs128738	Imputed GWAS	European ancestry	2,134/9,125	2017 (Henderson et al. 2013)
	*DRB1*04*	–	Immunochip genotyping/Imputed data	European ancestry	1,651/15,306	2015 (Iwaki-Egawa and Watanabe 2006)
	*DQA1*03*	–	Immunochip genotyping/Imputed data	European ancestry	1,651/15,306	2015 (Iwaki-Egawa and Watanabe 2006)
	*DQA1*01*	–	Immunochip genotyping/Imputed data	European ancestry	1,651/15,306	2015 (Iwaki-Egawa and Watanabe 2006)
	*DQB1*03*	–	Immunochip genotyping/Imputed data	European ancestry	1,651/15,306	2015 (Iwaki-Egawa and Watanabe 2006)

(continued)

Table 2 (continued)

Vasculitis	Locus or allele	SNP	Study method	Population(s)	No of cases/No of controls	Year of publication/References
	*DQB1*05*	–	Immunochip genotyping/Imputed data	European ancestry	1,651/15,306	2015 (Iwaki-Egawa and Watanabe 2006)
	*DQB1*06*	–	Immunochip genotyping/Imputed data	European ancestry	1,651/15,306	2015 (Iwaki-Egawa and Watanabe 2006)
	*DRB1*14*	–	Immunochip genotyping/Imputed data	European ancestry	1,651/15,306	2015 (Iwaki-Egawa and Watanabe 2006)
	*DQA1*0301*	–	Immunochip genotyping/Imputed data	European ancestry	1,651/15,306	2015 (Iwaki-Egawa and Watanabe 2006)
	*DQB1*0302*	–	Immunochip genotyping/Imputed data	European ancestry	1,651/15,306	2015 (Iwaki-Egawa and Watanabe 2006)
	*DRB1*0404*	–	Immunochip genotyping/Imputed data	European ancestry	1,651/15,306	2015 (Iwaki-Egawa and Watanabe 2006)
	*DRB1*0401*	–	Immunochip genotyping/Imputed data	European ancestry	1,651/15,306	2015 (Iwaki-Egawa and Watanabe 2006)
	*DQA1*0101*	–	Immunochip genotyping/Imputed data	European ancestry	1,651/15,306	2015 (Iwaki-Egawa and Watanabe 2006)
	*DQA1*0102*	–	Immunochip genotyping/Imputed data	European ancestry	1,651/15,306	2015 (Iwaki-Egawa and Watanabe 2006)
	*DQB1*0503*	–	Immunochip genotyping/Imputed data	European ancestry	1,651/15,306	2015 (Iwaki-Egawa and Watanabe 2006)

(continued)

Table 2 (continued)

Vasculitis	Locus or allele	SNP	Study method	Population(s)	No of cases/No of controls	Year of publication/References
Kawasaki disease						
	NAALADL2	rs17531088	GWAS	Caucasian ethnicity	893/134	2009 (Lee et al. 2012)
	FCGR2A	rs1801274	GWAS	European, Taiwanese, Korean, Chinese	2,173/9,383	2011 (Lee et al. 2013)
	19q13	rs2233152	GWAS	European, Taiwanese, Korean, Chinese	2,173/9,383	2011 (Lee et al. 2013)
	ITPKC	rs28493229	GWAS	European, Taiwanese, Korean, Chinese	2,173/9,383	2011 (Lee et al. 2013)
	BLK	rs2736340	GWAS	Han Chinese	883/1,657	2012 (Little et al. 2009)
	CD40	rs2618476	GWAS	Han Chinese	883/1,657	2012 (Little et al. 2009)
	FAM167A-BLK	rs2254546	GWAS	Japanese	754/947	2012 (López-Mejías et al. 2017)
	CD40	rs4813003	GWAS	Japanese	754/947	2012 (López-Mejías et al. 2017)
	6p21.3	rs2857151	GWAS	Japanese	754/947	2012 (López-Mejías et al. 2017)
	COPB2	rs1873668	GWAS	Han Chinese	458/812	2011 (Mahajan et al. 2012)
	COPB2	rs4243399	GWAS	Han Chinese	458/812	2011 (Mahajan et al. 2012)
	COPB2	rs16849083	GWAS	Han Chinese	458/812	2011 (Mahajan et al. 2012)
	CASP3	rs72689236	Linkage and candidate gene	Japanese	920/1,409	2007 (Lyons et al. 2012), 2010 (Nakazawa et al. 2016)
	BLK	rs6993775	GWAS	Korean	915/4,553	2017 (McCluskey et al. 2017)
	6p21.3	rs9380242	GWAS	Korean	915/4,553	2017 (McCluskey et al. 2017)
	6p21.3	rs9378199	GWAS	Korean	915/4,553	2017 (McCluskey et al. 2017)
	6p21.3	rs9266669	GWAS	Korean	915/4,553	2017 (McCluskey et al. 2017)
	6p21.3	rs6938467	GWAS	Korean	915/4,553	2017 (McCluskey et al. 2017)

(continued)

Table 2 (continued)

Vasculitis	Locus or allele	SNP	Study method	Population(s)	No of cases/No of controls	Year of publication/References
ANCA-associated vasculitis						
	HLA-DP	rs3117242	GWAS	European	2,267 GPA and MPA/6,858	2012/(Anwar and Karim 2017)
	HLA-DP	rs3117242	GWAS	European	1,683 GPA/6,858	2012/(Anwar and Karim 2017)
	HLA-DP	rs3117242	GWAS	European	1,521 PR3(+)/ 6,858	2012/(Anwar and Karim 2017)
	HLA-DP	rs3117242	GWAS	European	1,521 PR3(+)/ 556 MPO(+)	2012/(Anwar and Karim 2017)
	HLA-DQ	rs5000634	GWAS	European	2,267 GPA and MPA/6,858	2012/(Anwar and Karim 2017)
	COL11A2	rs3130233	GWAS	European	2,267 GPA and MPA/6,858	2012/(Anwar and Karim 2017)
	COL11A2	rs3117016	GWAS	European	2,267 GPA and MPA/6,858	2012/(Anwar and Karim 2017)
	SERPINA1	rs7151526	GWAS	European	1,683 GPA/6,858	2012/(Anwar and Karim 2017)
	SERPINA1	rs7151526	GWAS	European	1,521 PR3(+)/ 6,858	2012/(Anwar and Karim 2017)
	HLA-DPB1	rs9277554	GWAS	European ancestry	750 GPA/1,820	2013 (Serrano et al. 2013)
	HLA-DPA1	rs9277341	GWAS	European ancestry	750 GPA/1,820	2013 (Serrano et al. 2013)
	HLA-DPB1	rs9277554	GWAS	European ancestry	578 C-ANCA(+)/ 1.820	2013 (Serrano et al. 2013)
	HLA-DPA1	rs9277341	GWAS	European ancestry	578 C-ANCA(+)/ 1.820	2013 (Serrano et al. 2013)
	HLA–DPB1	rs141530233	GWAS	Self-reported European ancestry	1,986 GPA and MPA/4,723	2017 (Shimizu et al. 2016)
	HLA–DPB1	rs1042169	GWAS	Self-reported European ancestry	1,986 GPA and MPA/4,723	2017 (Shimizu et al. 2016)
	HLA–DPA1	rs9277341	GWAS	Self-reported European ancestry	1,986 GPA and MPA/4,723	2017 (Shimizu et al. 2016)

(continued)

Table 2 (continued)

Vasculitis	Locus or allele	SNP	Study method	Population(s)	No of cases/No of controls	Year of publication/References
	HLA–DQA1	rs35242582	GWAS	Self-reported European ancestry	1,986 GPA and MPA/4,723	2017 (Shimizu et al. 2016)
	HLA–DQB1	rs1049072	GWAS	Self-reported European ancestry	1,986 GPA and MPA/4,723	2017 (Shimizu et al. 2016)
	PRTN3	rs62132293	GWAS	Self-reported European ancestry	1,986 GPA and MPA/4,723	2017 (Shimizu et al. 2016)
	SERPINA1	rs28929474	GWAS	Self-reported European ancestry	1,986 GPA and MPA/4,723	2017 (Shimizu et al. 2016)
IgA vasculitis (formerly Henoch-Schönlein purpura)						
	HLA-DQA1/HLA-DQB1	rs9275260	Imputed GWAS	European ancestry	308/1,018	2017/(Takahashi et al. 2014)
Behçet's disease						
	GIMAP4	rs1608157	GWAS	Korean, Japanese	742/1,072	2013 (Wen et al. 2016)
	HLA-B	rs4959053	GWAS	Japanese, Turkish, Korean	1,945/2,156	2010 (Wen et al. 2018)
	IL23R-IL12RB2	rs1495965	GWAS	Japanese, Turkish, Korean	1,945/2,156	2010 (Wen et al. 2018)
	IL10	rs1800871	GWAS	Japanese, Turkish, Korean	1,945/2,156	2010 (Wen et al. 2018)
	*HLA-B*51*	–	GWAS	Turkish, Middle Eastern, European, Asian	2,430/2,660	2010 (Wen et al. 2017)
	IL10	rs1518111	GWAS	Turkish, Middle Eastern, European, Asian	2,430/2,660	2010 (Wen et al. 2017)
	IL23R-IL12RB2	rs924080	GWAS	Turkish, Middle Eastern, European, Asian	2,430/2,660	2010 (Wen et al. 2017)
	6p21.33	–	GWAS	European, Middle Eastern, Turkish	336/5,843	2015 (Weyand and Goronzy 2013)
	IL12A	s17810546	GWAS	European, Middle Eastern, Turkish	336/5,843	2015 (Weyand and Goronzy 2013)
	*HLA-B*51*	rs1050502	Immunochip genotyping/Imputed data	Turkish, Iranian, Japanese	3,477/3,342	2017 (Burgner et al. 2009)

(continued)

Table 2 (continued)

Vasculitis	Locus or allele	SNP	Study method	Population(s)	No of cases/No of controls	Year of publication/References
	CEBPB–PTPN1	rs913678	Immunochip genotyping/Imputed data	Turkish, Iranian, Japanese	3,477/3,342	2017 (Burgner et al. 2009)
	IL10	rs1518110	Immunochip genotyping/Imputed data	Turkish, Iranian, Japanese	3,477/3,342	2017 (Burgner et al. 2009)
	CCR1	rs7616215	Immunochip genotyping/Imputed data	Turkish, Iranian, Japanese	3,477/3,342	2017 (Burgner et al. 2009)
	IL12A	rs17753641	Immunochip genotyping/Imputed data	Turkish, Iranian, Japanese	3,477/3,342	2017 (Burgner et al. 2009)
	IL1A–IL1B	rs3783550	Immunochip genotyping/Imputed data	Turkish, Iranian, Japanese	3,477/3,342	2017 (Burgner et al. 2009)
	IRF8	rs11117433	Immunochip genotyping/Imputed data	Turkish, Iranian, Japanese	3,477/3,342	2017 (Burgner et al. 2009)
	ADO–EGR2	rs7075773	Immunochip genotyping/Imputed data	Turkish, Iranian, Japanese	3,477/3,342	2017 (Burgner et al. 2009)
	LACC1	rs9316059	Immunochip genotyping/Imputed data	Turkish, Iranian, Japanese	3,477/3,342	2017 (Burgner et al. 2009)
	ERAP1	rs17482078	Immunochip genotyping/Imputed data	Turkish, Iranian, Japanese	3,477/3,342	2017 (Burgner et al. 2009)
	KLRC4	rs2617170	Immunochip genotyping/Imputed data	Turkish, Iranian, Japanese	3,477/3,342	2017 (Burgner et al. 2009)

(continued)

Table 2 (continued)

Vasculitis	Locus or allele	SNP	Study method	Population(s)	No of cases/No of controls	Year of publication/References
	RIPK2	rs2230801	Immunochip genotyping/Imputed data	Turkish, Iranian, Japanese	3,477/3,342	2017 (Burgner et al. 2009)
	FUT2	rs601338	Immunochip genotyping/Imputed data	Turkish, Iranian, Japanese	3,477/3,342	2017 (Burgner et al. 2009)
	FUT2	rs1047781	Immunochip genotyping/Imputed data	Turkish, Iranian, Japanese	3,477/3,342	2017 (Burgner et al. 2009)
	CCR1-CCR3	s7616215	Imputed GWAS	Turkish, Japanese	2,659/2,744	2013 (Weyand and Goronzy 2014)
	STAT4	rs7574070	Imputed GWAS	Turkish, Japanese	2,659/2,744	2013 (Weyand and Goronzy 2014)
	KLRC4	rs2617170	Imputed GWAS	Turkish, Japanese	2,659/2,744	2013 (Weyand and Goronzy 2014)
	KLRC4	rs1841958	Imputed GWAS	Turkish, Japanese	2,659/2,744	2013 (Weyand and Goronzy 2014)
	ERAP1	rs17482078	Imputed GWAS	Turkish, Japanese	2,659/2,744	2013 (Weyand and Goronzy 2014)
	STAT4	rs897200	GWAS	Han Chinese	703/1,657	2012 (Yazici et al. 2018)
	STAT4	rs7572482	GWAS	Han Chinese	703/1,657	2012 (Yazici et al. 2018)
	HLA–B	rs4959053	GWAS	Han Chinese	703/1,657	2012 (Yazici et al. 2018)
	HLA–B	rs9266406	GWAS	Han Chinese	703/1,657	2012 (Yazici et al. 2018)
	HLA–B	rs9266409	GWAS	Han Chinese	703/1,657	2012 (Yazici et al. 2018)

[a]At the genome-wide significance *P*-value of $<5 \times 10^{-8}$; *ANCA* antineutrophil cytoplasmic antibody; *C-ANCA* cytoplasmic ANCA; *GPA* granulomatosis with polyangiitis; *GWAS* genome-wide association studies; *HLA* human leukocyte antigen system; *MPA* microscopic polyangiitis; *MPO* myeloperoxidase *PR3* proteinase 3; *SNP* single-nucleotide polymorphism

own as the *MAX dimerization protein* (*MLX*), which is involved in the regulation of cell proliferation, and differentiation by forming heterodimers with Mad proteins has also been linked to TA susceptibility. The *proteasome assembly chaperone 1* (*PSMG1*) encoded protein that promotes the gathering of the 20S proteasome through forming a heterodimer with PSMG2 is another TA susceptibility gene (Saruhan-Direskeneli et al. 2013; Terao et al. 2013). A recent multiethnic GWAS study (Table 2), including two separate cohorts of North American and Turkish patients, demonstrated three novel genetic susceptibility loci for TA (Renauer et al. 2015); *IL-6*, *RSP/LILRB3* (*RPS9* stands for ribosomal protein S9 that encodes a segment of the ribosomal 40S subunit and *LILRB3* stands for *leukocyte immunoglobulin-like receptor B* that codes a peptide belonging to the subfamily B class of the leukocyte immunoglobulin-like receptors), and *PSMG1* that is the intergenic noncoding locus at 21q22 neighboring proteasome 26S subunit. The association of the genetic variants of *IL-6* and *RPS9/LILRB3* with a predisposition to TA indicates the role of central immunoregulatory pathways and could provide more insight into the pathogenesis of this large-vessel vasculitis. IL-6 regulates various phases of the immune response such as T-cells differentiation into Th17 cells and regulatory T-cells. The 19q13.4 containing the *RPS9/LILRB3* is a gene-rich locus that contains multiple genes belonging to the leukocyte immunoglobulin-like receptor superfamily. Members of this family are expressed by many mature immune cells and interact with class I HLA molecules. The third association signal (Table 2) comes from a locus at 21q22 (Renauer et al. 2015). This locus also appears to associate susceptibility to ankylosing spondylitis (AS) and ulcerative colitis (UC). A follow-up study of a previous GWAS on Japanese was able to find new significant loci (Terao et al. 2018) (Table 2) including protein tyrosine kinase 2 beta (*PTK2B* encoding a cytoplasmic protein tyrosine kinase), *LILRA3/LILRB2*, dual-specificity phosphatase 22 (*DUSP22* with phosphatase activity), and kelch like family member 33 (*KLHL33*). An additional susceptibility gene, unreported in non-European GWAS, was heat shock protein family A member 6 (*HSPA6)/FCGR3A*. It was also shown that a single variant capable of influencing the expression of *MHC Class I polypeptide-related sequence B* (*MICB*), a ligand for natural killer (NK) cell receptor (NKG2D), could account for the whole linkage within the *HLA-B* region. Prominent epistasis has also been reported between the *HLA-B*52* and *LILRA3*. Enhancer enrichment and pathway analysis along with the implication of both HLA and non-HLA regions in TA susceptibility indicated a substantial role for NK cells in disease pathogenesis (Terao et al. 2018).

3.2.2 Genetic Associations in Giant Cell Arteritis

In the only GWAS in GCA published very recently, 2,134 patients and 9,125 healthy controls from 10 independent cohorts with European ancestry were included (Carmona et al. 2017). This GWAS confirmed MHC-II as the most important susceptibility region (Carmona et al. 2017). Additionally, the plasminogen (*PLG*) and the prolyl 4-hydroxylase subunit alpha-2 (*P4HA2*) were recognized as GCA risk genes (Carmona et al. 2017) (Table 2). Notably, the association peaks were found to overlap with many regulatory molecules relevant to cells and tissues implicated in GCA pathogenesis. PLG and P4HA2 are implicated in vascular remodeling and angiogenesis (Miles and Parmer 2013; Moser et al. 1999; Myllyharju 2003), indicating their importance in the pathogenesis of this form of vasculitis. Previously reported genetic links of GCA that have been replicated by separate cohorts but yet have not reached genome-wide significance level include the *HLA-DRB1*04*, *IL10*, and vascular endothelial growth factor (*VEGF*) (Carmona et al. 2014; Gonzalez-Gay et al. 2003). A recently published, large-scale genetic analysis combing dense genotyping with the immunochip array on 1,651 participants with GCA and 15,306 controls from six European countries, also showed a significant contribution of the HLA class II region to the pathogenesis of the disease and identified few other potential susceptibility genes (Carmona et al. 2015). The *protein tyrosine phosphatase non-receptor type 22* (*PTPN22*) is one of these genes. A *PTPN22* variant with a gain-of-function mutation that has also been linked to several autoimmune diseases showed a strong GCA association (Carmona et al. 2015). *PTPN22* cis translated to a tyrosine phosphatase known as LYP, which has an important role in the T-cell receptor pathway, dendritic cell activation, and the humoral activity of B-cells (Zhang et al. 2011). Regardless of the debate over whether genome-wide significance thresholds are suitable for immunochip studies, the involvement of *PTPN22* appears to denote a risk factor for GCA (Carmona et al. 2015) and this variant was consistent across all of the four analyzed populations (Carmona et al. 2015; Serrano et al. 2013). Other assumed susceptibility genes outside the HLA region implicated in the large-scale genetic analysis using immunochip genotyping include the leucine-rich repeat-containing 32 (*LRRC32*) and *REL*, both of which code for proteins with important roles in T-cell function (Carmona et al. 2015). NOD-like receptor family pyrin domain containing 1 (*NLRP1*) and *IL17A* have also been linked to GCA at a nominal level of significance. However, in the replication phase, the association remained significant, revealing a critical function for the inflammasome and Th17 cells in the pathogenesis of the disease (Marquez et al. 2014; Serrano et al. 2013).

4 Medium-Vessel Vasculitis

4.1 General Aspects

Vasculitides that primarily affect medium-sized vessels, such as the visceral arteries and their first-degree branches, are known as medium-vessel vasculitis (Figs. 1 and 2). Although hypothetically any size artery may be affected, usually this vasculitis type spares the smallest blood vessels (Jennette et al. 2013). The most common forms are polyarteritis nodosa (PAN) and Kawasaki disease (KD) (Jennette et al. 2013).

PAN is characterized by inflammatory infiltration causing the necrosis of the vessel walls of medium-sized vessels or muscular arterioles. Although it is not associated with glomerulonephritis or lung involvement, the disease has a preference for certain tissue and organs, including the skin (Fig. 3), the kidneys, peripheral nerves, and the gastrointestinal (GI) tract primarily causing renovascular hypertension and renal infarctions (Stone 2002). Characterization and shaping of PAN have changed over time and it is still evolving. PAN has long been linked to

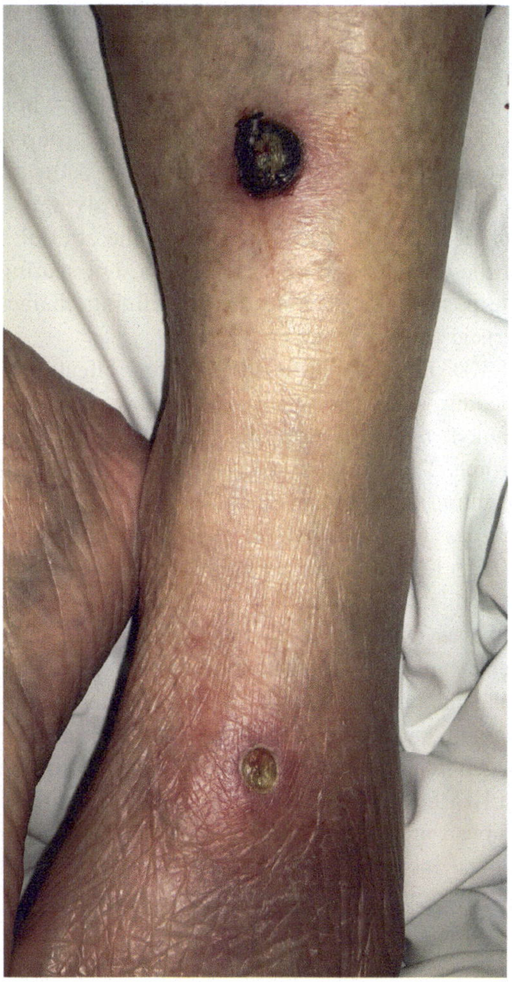

Fig. 3 Medium vessel vasculitis. Polyarteritis nodosa, ulcerated skin lesions

hepatitis B virus (HBV) infection (Guillevin et al. 2005; Stone 2002). Nevertheless, since the HBV vaccine became available, the proportion of HBV-related cases has decreased significantly. The CHCC 2012 terminology defines HBV-related PAN as a vasculitis "associated with a probable etiology" (Jennette et al. 2013); this description is reasonable, as we recognize the triggering factor for this type of PAN. Additionally, according to the CHCC 2012 definition (Jennette et al. 2013), PAN is not typified by the presence of the antineutrophil cytoplasmic antibodies (ANCAs) (Jennette et al. 2013), whereas mutations in specific genes or primary immunodeficiencies can lead to a necrotizing vasculopathy that strongly resembles this disease (Henderson et al. 2013; Navon Elkan et al. 2014; Ozen et al. 2001; Yalçinkaya et al. 2007; Zhou et al. 2014). Finally, a significant disease group is a cutaneous PAN, especially in the pediatric setting (Ozen et al. 2004). Arteritis involving the subcutaneous fat with extension to the arterioles at the dermo-subcutaneous junction, but sparing the postcapillary venules, is its defining characteristic (Sunderkotter et al. 2018).

KD is a vasculitis variant that affects the medium-sized and small vessels and is accompanied by mucocutaneous lymph node syndrome. The coronary vessels are often entangled resulting in aneurysm formation; aorta and large arteries may also be affected (Jennette et al. 2013). KD is among the most common types of systemic vasculitides that preferentially occur in children (Jennette et al. 2013). It typically presents with strawberry tongue and fissured lips, bilateral conjunctivitis, lymphadenopathy, swelling of hands and feet as well as a skin rash. Asian populations have a much higher incidence of KD than Western countries. Japan, Korea, and Taiwan are the three countries with the highest annual incidence of KD (Agarwal and Agrawal 2017).

4.2 Pathogenesis

The cause of classic PAN is still unknown. Patients with PAN do not have ANCAs, hence the etiology is not ANCA-driven (Jennette et al. 2013). However, innate and adaptive immune responses may be involved in the pathways leading to necrosis of the vessel wall. A recent study was able to demonstrate altered characteristics in regulatory T-cells in patients with PAN and also a dominance of Th1 cells over Th17 cells. Therefore, the authors proposed that defects in T-cells may be the underlying cause of the disease (Shimojima et al. 2017). In addition, the link between streptococcal infection and cutaneous PAN hints at the involvement of dendritic cells and the innate immune responses (Ozen et al. 2004). The pathological mechanisms involved in the HBV-related vasculitis, on the other hand, are distinct from that of classic disease and it is associated with the production and deposition of immune complexes (Guillevin et al. 2005; Stone 2002).

Although the pathogenesis of KD is yet unknown, it seems to be the result of genetic predisposition and infectious triggers, followed by a derailed inflammatory response (Agarwal and Agrawal 2017). The theory that an infectious trigger is implicated in the pathogenesis of the disease is mostly supported by results from epidemiological studies. Bacterial superantigens and viral infections have been linked with KD pathogenesis (Agarwal and Agrawal 2017). Yet, a dysregulated immune response is essential to the pathogenetic mechanisms in KD. T-cells have been the primary suspects with the involvement of inositol 1,4,5-triphosphate 3-kinase (ITPKC) as the most important mediator. ITPKC acts as an inhibitor for T-cells. Therefore, the loss of its regulatory effects is associated with an exaggerated T-cell activation and cytokines production (Agarwal and Agrawal 2017). IL-6, IL-20, IFN-γ, and tumor necrosis factor-α (TNF-α) are abundantly expressed in active KD and their levels drop after a successful intravenous immunoglobulin therapy (IVIg) (Wang et al. 2013). Recently, studies have also shown an imbalance between $CD4^+$ pro-inflammatory cells and regulatory T-cells (FOXP3+) in the acute stage of the disease. Activation of Th17 cells with upregulation of their cytokines and, at the same time, suppression of the differentiation of regulatory T-cells have been verified in children with KD (Jia et al. 2010). This imbalance between Th17 and regulatory T-cells shifts T-cell homeostasis toward inflammation (Jia et al. 2010; Ni et al. 2014). NKG2D is an activating ligand expressed by immune cells like NK cells and CD8+ cytotoxic T-cells; hence, its low levels in the acute stage of KD may be linked to dysregulated immune response (Ge et al. 2013). The crucial contribution of IL-1 in the development of KD has been confirmed through knockout mice models (Lee et al. 2015). Vascular endothelial cells incur histological changes consistent with both endothelial cell activation and damage. Through enhanced expression of adhesion molecules and chemokine release, IL-1 and TNF-α play a key role in enabling endothelial cell activation (Galeotti et al. 2010; Takahashi et al. 2014). TNF-α also promotes the activity of MMP-9 that leads to the destruction of elastin and the development of an aneurysm in the vessel wall (Agarwal and Agrawal 2017). The inducible nitric oxide (NO) synthase enzyme is found in vascular smooth muscle cells, myocardial cells, leukocytes, and other immune cells. It is upregulated throughout an inflammatory response and appears to increase NO production in KD patients. The excess production of NO may lead to vessel wall dilatation (Agarwal and Agrawal 2017; Song et al. 2015).

4.2.1 Genetic Associations in Kawasaki Disease

Multiple lines of evidence and the ethnic-preferential pattern suggest that genetic determinants contribute to KD's susceptibility and the potential outcome. The publication of a genome-wide linkage study (GWLS), eight subsequent GWA studies, and an extension study of a previous GWAS, in KD cohorts of different ancestries (Table 2) have provided a substantially more detailed understanding of its genetic basis (Burgner et al. 2009; Khor et al. 2011; Kim et al. 2011, 2017; Kuo et al. 2016; Lee et al. 2012; Onouchi et al. 2012, 2007; Shimizu et al. 2016; Tsai et al. 2011). These studies identified several biologically plausible loci associated with the occurrence of KD with great significance. The most relevant genetic variants that have been repeatedly associated with this vasculitis include the cluster domain 40 (*CD40*) that belongs to the TNF receptor family, the B lymphoid tyrosine kinase (*BLK*) that is implicated in B-cell receptor (BCR) signaling and B-cell development (Bewarder et al. 1996), and the *FCGR2A* (Chang et al. 2013; Khor et al. 2011; Kim et al. 2017; Lee et al. 2012; Nagelkerke et al. 2019; Onouchi et al. 2012). CD40 regulates the negative selection of autoreactive T-cells and the stimulation of B- and T-cells following antigen presentation, Interestingly, a recent study using bioinformatics analyses that integrated previous GWA studies with information on gene expression profiling, quantitative trait loci expression (eQTL), and epigenetic fine mapping, pointed out the significance of B-cells in the development of KD (Farh et al. 2015). Both decreased expression of messenger RNA from the common risk haplotype of *BLK* in B-cells (Simpfendorfer et al. 2015) and increased expression of a membrane-bound isoform of CD40 on these cells might lead to enhanced B-cell activity, and hence, the significance of SNPs of *BLK* and *CD40* genes is highlighted in KD pathogenesis (Field et al. 2015; Onouchi et al. 2012; Simpfendorfer et al. 2015). Other significant linkage loci included the inositol 1,4,5-triphosphate 3-kinase C (*ITPKC*) which adjusts T-cell activation, the caspase 3 (*CASP3*), a protease that plays a key role in apoptosis, and the nicotinamide nucleotide adenylyltransferase 2 (*NMNAT2*) which belongs to a family of enzymes that catalyze a crucial step in nicotinamide adenine dinucleotide biosynthetic (Burgner et al. 2009; Khoret al. 2011; Kim et al. 2011, 2017, 2007; Lee et al. 2012; Onouchi et al. 2012; Tsai et al. 2011) (Table 2). Subsequent studies, including meta-analyses, have established most of these associations across different ethnicities (Kuo et al. 2011, 2011; Onouchi et al. 2010; Xie et al. 2018; Yan et al. 2013). Potential links between several SNPs and the formation of coronary artery aneurysms (Kwon et al. 2019; Shimizu et al. 2016) as well as the responsiveness to IVIg (Kim et al. 2019) in KD patients have also been reported.

Suggestive association with KD was detected for N-acetylated alpha-linked acidic dipeptidase-like 2 (*NAALADL2*), a variant with unidentified function; yet, the result of transcriptome analyses demonstrated a decline in NAALADL2 mRNA expression in peripheral blood cells in the acute stage of KD in comparison to its expression in the quiescent stages (Burgner et al. 2009). This implies that this protein may play a role in immunological homeostasis. Other variants that demonstrate a suggestive linkage with KD included the Dab reelin signal transducer homolog 1(*DAB1*) that plays a role in the neuronal positioning in the brain but its function in immune response and vascular biology is unknown, the zinc finger homeobox 3 (*ZFHX3*) which is a transcriptional factor involved in the regulation of myogenic and neuronal differentiation, and the pellino E3 ubiquitin-protein ligase 1 (*PELI1*) that belongs to the TLR path (Kim et al. 2011; Tsai et al. 2011). Additional loci that have been pointed out as plausible candidates included the loci encoding for the heavy chain variable region of the immunoglobulin, the coatomer protein complex beta-2 subunit (*COPB2*) that is important for vesicular trafficking especially the Golgi budding and fusion and may play a role in regulating the T-cell receptor signal transduction and the endoplasmic reticulum aminopeptidase 1 (*ERAP1*) which is a ubiquitous metallopeptidase that trims the NH2-end residues from peptides and optimizes their length for fitting into MHC-I groove (Kim et al. 2011; Tsai et al. 2011).

The involvement of MHC in the pathogenesis of KD is still a debate because the positive results emanate from candidate gene studies with somewhat small sample sizes that have not been adequately confirmed in the following studies. The strongest association signals detected in the GWA study in KD Japanese patients were found in the MHC-II region at 6p21.3, according to earlier studies. This region harbors SNPs within the region between the *HLA-DQA2* and *HLA-DQB* genes (Onouchi et al. 2012) (Table 2). A recent GWAS with a replication study in a Korean population also demonstrated that the HLA region (*HLA-C, HLA-B, MICA*, and *HCP5*) was significantly associated with KD susceptibility (Kim et al. 2017). Unexpectedly, no association between this vasculitis form and the MHC region was demonstrated in the other GWA studies across different populations, in spite of the importance of the immune system in KD pathogenesis.

4.2.2 Genetics of PAN-Like Necrotizing Vasculitis

In 2014, two independent studies, using whole-exome sequencing, screened several familial cases of PAN-like necrotizing vasculitis for potential genetic defects (Navon Elkan et al. 2014; Zhou et al. 2014). Mutations of the cat eye syndrome chromosome region candidate 1 gene (*CECR1*) cause adenosine deaminase 2 (ADA2) deficiency (Navon Elkan et al. 2014; Zhou et al. 2014). ADA2 is an enzyme that catalyzes the degradation of adenosine to inosine, it is highly expressed in myeloid cells (Zavialov et al. 2010) and it is produced by activated monocytes, macrophages, and dendritic cells (Iwaki-Egawa and Watanabe 2006). ADA2 is a growth factor for leukocytes that allows them to have immunomodulatory functions (Caorsi et al. 2016). It is also essential for endothelial stability. Although endothelial cells do not express *CECR1*, the deficiency of ADA2 is associated with vascular endothelial damage and overexpression of endothelial activation markers. The deficiency of ADA2 (DADA2) results in vasculopathy associated with autoimmune characteristics and thus is regarded as a monogenic defect causing the same clinical phenotype as classic PAN (Navon Elkan et al. 2014; Zhou et al. 2014). Although the definite cause of vasculitis in DADA2 patients is unknown, brain biopsy samples from these individuals indicate endothelial activation (Zhou et al. 2014). These patients also have a distinct immunodeficiency of the B-cell compartment (Schepp et al. 2017). Additionally, monocytes from DADA2 individuals tend to transform into M1 macrophages (Caorsi et al. 2016). Consequently, ADA2 deficiency could damage the endothelial cells and vessel integrity and promote macrophage and monocyte polarization toward inflammatory phenotypes. The DADA2 is characterized by vascular characteristics that are similar to those seen in PAN. Due to the necrotizing vasculitis revealed in their histology, the cases described in the earliest publications regarding DADA2 were initially classified as PAN (Navon Elkan et al. 2014; Zhou et al. 2014). Since DADA2 is an autosomal recessive disorder, individuals with this disease usually have a positive PAN family history. Until now, there are more than 160 cases described with 61 disease-causing mutations with most of them being missense variants (Caorsi et al. 2016; Meyts and Aksentijevich 2018). However, the clinical spectrum of DADA2 extends beyond the features first described, and the variability of the disease, even among family members with similar mutations, is becoming more widely recognized (Caorsi et al. 2016; Meyts and Aksentijevich 2018).

5 Small-Vessel Vasculitis

5.1 ANCA-Associated Vasculitis: General Aspects

Following the initial association of ANCAs with glomerulonephritis in 1982 (Davies et al. 1982), ANCA-associated vasculitis was recognized as a disorder discrete from other forms of vasculitides (Jennette et al. 2013). Currently, it is described as a systemic vasculitis of small vessels that is characterized by the ANCA positivity (Jennette et al. 2013). Indirect immunofluorescence performed on neutrophils fixed with ethanol can visualize two major types of ANCAs based on their cellular location. Different cellular localization patterns of the two main types of ANCAs can be observed via the indirect immunofluorescence technique. Perinuclear ANCA (p-ANCA) is linked with staining at the periphery of the nucleus whereas cytoplasmic ANCA (c-ANCA) is accompanied by diffuse staining of the neutrophil cytoplasm. Myeloperoxidase (MPO, a lysosomal protein) and proteinase 3 (PR3, a serine proteinase) are the two primary proteins identified by these ANCAs, respectively. At present, the quantitative amount of ANCAs is measured via enzyme-linked immunosorbent assay (ELISA). According to the target antigen utilized, ANCAs demonstrated by ELISA are referred to as MPO-ANCA or PR3-ANCA (Hoffman 1998; Jennette et al. 2013).

ANCA-associated vasculitis encompasses microscopic polyangiitis (MPA), eosinophilic granulomatosis with polyangiitis (EGPA, also referred to as Churg-Strauss syndrome), and granulomatosis with polyangiitis (GPA, formerly known as Wegener granulomatosis), and (Table 1). The most prevalent cause of pulmonary-renal syndrome with glomerulonephritis and alveolar hemorrhage is MPA, which affects small arteries. MPO-ANCA positivity is found in the majority of MPA patients. Necrotizing vasculitis is the histological hallmark of MPA, whereas granulomatous inflammation is almost never present (Jennette et al. 2013). Granulomatous inflammation, on the other hand, is a feature of GPA with concurrent development of necrotizing small-vessel vasculitis (Jennette et al. 2013). It usually involves the respiratory tract. Classically, patients with GPA have high levels of PR3-ANCA in their serum. Crescentic glomerulonephritis and pauci-immune necrotizing glomerulonephritis can be present in both MPA and GPA (Jennette et al. 2013). EGPA is far less common and is histologically characterized by eosinophil-rich necrotizing vasculitis of small-to-medium-sized vessels associated with a granulomatous reaction. Adult-onset asthma, allergic rhinitis, and nasal polyposis often precede the overt symptoms of EGPA. Eosinophilia and infiltration of eosinophils in the affected tissues are its classic features. Approximately half of the patients diagnosed with EGPA have high levels of MPO-ANCA (Jennette et al. 2013). Epidemiological studies have indicated racial disparities in both ANCA specificity and presentations of ANCA-associated vasculitis (Furuta et al. 2014; Pearce et al. 2017). PR3-ANCAs and GPAs are more frequent in Western countries, while MPO-ANCA and MPA prevail in East Asia such as Japan (Furuta et al. 2014; Pearce et al. 2017).

5.2 Pathogenesis of ANCA-Associated Vasculitis

The pathogenesis of ANCA-associated vasculitis largely overlaps among MPA, GPA, and EGPA. Of these, MPA has been deemed the prototypic form since the mechanisms implicated in its pathophysiology are found in all varieties of ANCA-associated vasculitis. GPA and EGPA both have distinct features compared to MPA. Several animal models of ANCA-associated vasculitis are available. These models have revealed that ANCAs are not only a biomarker for this type of vasculitis but they also have pathogenic features (Brouwer et al. 1993; Little et al. 2009; Schreiber et al. 2006; Xiao et al. 2002). Through amplification of the complement activation loop, ANCAs promote endothelium damage by fully activating primed neutrophils. Specifically, inflammatory cytokines such as TNF and IL-1β along with the binding of C5a to its receptor on the surfaces of the cells appear to prime neutrophils (Jennette and Falk 2014; Nakazawa et al. 2019). Subsequently, the crystallizable fragment (Fc) region of ANCAs interacts with the Fc-gamma receptor on leukocytes, causing primed neutrophils to produce MPO and PR3 on to which corresponding ANCAs bind. This binding activates neutrophils causing aberrant cytokine production as well as the release of reactive oxygen species (ROS) and lytic enzymes, which cause damage to endothelial cells (Abdulahad and Kallenberg 2011; Flint et al. 2015). Interestingly, while ANCAs are aimed at self-antigens, the pathogenesis of tissue injury in ANCA-associated vasculitis is dissimilar to the pathways at work in other autoimmune diseases where tissue injury is primarily mediated by the immune complexes. The histological hallmark of ANCA-associated vasculitis is necrotizing glomerulonephritis lacking evident immune complex deposition (Jennette and Falk 2014; Nakazawa et al. 2019). Instead, substantial endothelial injury occurs as a result of ANCA-activated neutrophils and their inflammatory mediators, as well as the alternative complement pathway, given that patients with active disease have elevated serum levels of C3a and C5a (Xiao et al. 2007). Additionally, the ANCA-stimulated neutrophils also release neutrophil extracellular traps (NETs) (Sangaletti et al. 2012). While NETs are important components in innate immunity, disproportionate NET formation is detrimental to vascular endothelial cells. NETs are also implicated in the appearance of ANCAs themselves (Sangaletti et al. 2012). Low NET degradation activity has been recently found in patients with ANCA-associated vasculitis. These NETs are persistent and continued exposure to their contents causes MPO and PR3 tolerance to be disrupted (Kessenbrock et al. 2009; Millet et al. 2015; Nakazawa et al. 2019, 2016; Sangaletti et al. 2012). These autoantigens are subsequently presented to $CD4^+$ T-cells by DCs, causing further production of ANCAs (Kessenbrock et al. 2009; Nakazawa et al. 2019, 2016). Hence, the pathophysiology of ANCA-associated vasculitis appears to entail a vicious cycle of NET release and ANCA synthesis. Although innate immune system molecules play an important role in the pathogenesis of ANCA-associated vasculitis, dysregulation of T-cells and B-cells, as well as genetic susceptibility, are also crucial (Jennette and Falk 2014; Nakazawa et al. 2019).

5.2.1 Genetic Associations in ANCA-Associated Vasculitis

Three GWAS (Lyons et al. 2012; Merkel et al. 2017; Xie et al. 2013) and a meta-analysis (Rahmattulla et al. 2016) have been able to link susceptibility to ANCA-associated vasculitis with several genetic variants (Table 2). Among these, the *MHC II* genes harbored the peak associations. A GWAS conducted on European individuals confirmed that PR3-ANCA positive GPA is highly associated with variations in the *HLA-DP* gene (Table 2) and MPO-ANCA positive MPA appears to be related to *HLA-DQ* gene (Lyons et al. 2012). Remarkably, the HLA genomic signature had the strongest associated with ANCA specificity regardless of the clinical subtype. A GWAS study performed on a North American population was able to show that the locus containing *HLA-DP* harbored the most significant linkage with GPA (Xie et al. 2013). This study also recognized *HLA-DPB1*04* as a susceptibility allele for GPA. Instead, *HLA-DRB1*09:01* which is frequent in East Asia, yet uncommon in populations of European ancestry, shows a significant association with MPA in patients with Japanese ancestry (Kawasaki et al. 2016). These ethnic variations in the frequency of the MHC II polymorphisms may explain the epidemiological differences reported in ANCA-associated vasculitis; GPA with PR3-ANCA predominates in populations of European ancestry while MPA with MPO-ANCA is abundant in Asian populations. Another recent study that combined a GWAS, a replication study, and a meta-analysis of a population of self-reported European ancestry diagnosed with either GPA or MPA, confirmed the *HLA–DPB1* as a particularly significant risk factor (Merkel et al. 2017) (Table 2).

A recent meta-analysis including 62 articles published through 2014 investigating 140 genetic variants, identified 33 variants associated with ANCA-associated vasculitis (Rahmattulla et al. 2016). Outside the MHC region, *SERPINA1* encoding α1-antitrypsin which is a type of serine protease inhibitor (serpin), was described as the first GWAS hit for ANCA-associated vasculitis (Lyons et al. 2012; Merkel et al. 2017) (Table 2). A role has also been implied for α1-antitrypsin in negatively regulating PR3 protease activity and thus PR3-induced inflammatory responses (Duranton 2003). Other genes reported to confer risk for GPA and/or MPA include *PTPN22*, semaphorin-6A (*SEMA6A*), and proteinase 3 (*PRTN3*) coding PR3 (Lyons et al. 2012; Merkel et al. 2017; Rahmattulla et al. 2016; Xie et al. 2013). In white individuals with ANCA-associated vasculitis, the *PTPN22* gain-of-function variant is more frequent than in the general population. This SNP enhances the activity of PTPN22, a protein that decreases the production of the immunosuppressive IL-10 leading to a dysregulated immune response and autoimmunity (Cao et al. 2012). Also, direct causal effects of another SNP in *PTPN22* (Merkel et al. 2017) have been suggested by an earlier report linking the associated lymphoid protein tyrosine phosphatase (LYP) variant to several signaling pathways (Zhang et al. 2011). Similarly, an SNP located upstream of the *PRTN3* promoter is strongly associated with GPA or MPA (Merkel et al. 2017) (Table 2). The risk allele of this SNP was shown to increase *PRTN3* expression in neutrophils, an aberrancy frequently found in ANCA-associated vasculitis and linked to the pathogenic neutrophil activation (Ciavatta et al. 2010). In the combined analysis as well as the replication cohorts, an SNP in *SEMA6A* was recognized as a novel susceptibility locus for GPA, achieving a genome-wide level of significance (Xie et al. 2013). Although the function of semaphorins is uncertain, they appear to be involved in immune regulation.

5.3 Immune Complex Small-Vessel Vasculitis

5.3.1 General Aspects and Pathogenesis for IgA Vasculitis (Formerly Henoch-Schönlein Purpura)

IgA vasculitis is a form of systemic vasculitis characterized by infiltration of polymorphonuclear leukocytes and deposition of IgA1-predominant immune complexes (Jennette et al. 2013), in the vessel walls and glomerular mesangium (Gonzalez-Gay et al. 2018). IgA vasculitis usually affects the skin, resulting in symmetric erythematous petechiae or papules on the buttocks and lower extremities that progress to palpable purpura (Fig. 4). The disease also affects the GI tract, joints, and kidneys, often causing glomerulonephritis undifferentiated from

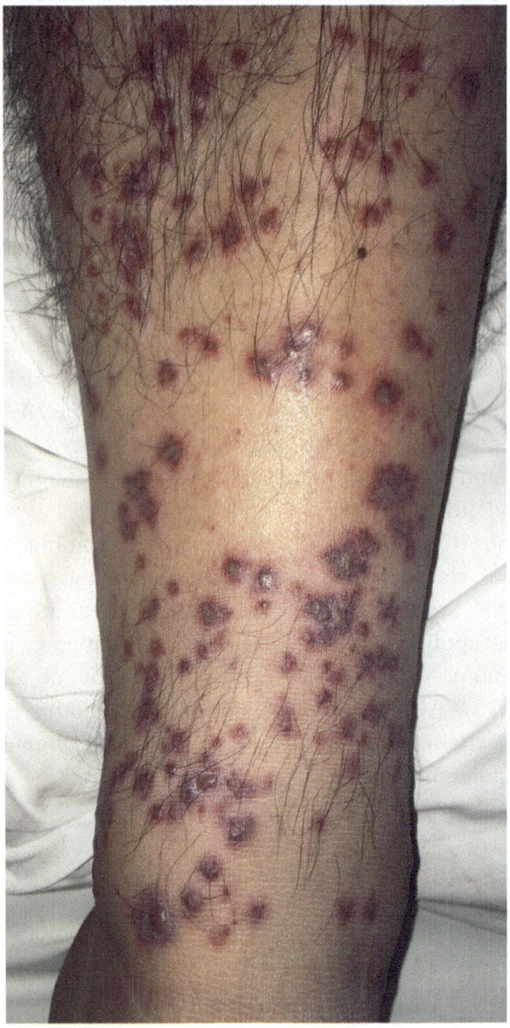

Fig. 4 Immune-complex small vessel vasculitis. IgA-vasculitis, palpable purpura

IgA nephropathy. Any portion of the GI tract could get involved, however, the small bowel is the most commonly affected due to mesenteric vasculitis (Gonzalez-Gay et al. 2018; Jennette et al. 2013). The CHCC 2012 consensus replaced the eponym "Henoch-Schönlein purpura" with IgA vasculitis (Table 1), based on convincing evidence demonstrating IgA deposition within the vessel walls as the pathologic hallmarks of the disease (Jennette et al. 2013). Patients diagnosed with systemic IgA vasculitis or renal limited IgA nephropathy exhibit altered glycosylation of the hinge region of the IgA1 molecule (Suzuki et al. 2009, 2011). These circulating abnormal glycosylated IgA1 may trigger the immune system to produce glycan-specific IgG antibodies that can form IgA1/anti-IgA1 IgG immune complexes that upon deposition in vessel walls induce inflammation (Suzuki et al. 2009, 2011). Isolated cutaneous IgA vasculitis is analogous to renal limited IgA nephropathy without systemic disease, yet patients with these forms may subsequently develop systemic IgA vasculitis (Gonzalez-Gay et al. 2018; Jennette et al. 2013).

5.3.2 Genetic Associations in IgA Vasculitis

Compared to other types of vasculitis, relatively few studies have investigated the genetic mechanisms involved in the pathogenesis of IgA vasculitis. The only GWAS published very recently, included patients of European ancestry and confirmed the association between IgA vasculitis and a linkage disequilibrium block located at the HLA class II region with a genome-wide level of significance (Table 2) (López-Mejías et al. 2017). While no specific SNPs were found to be linked to susceptibility to IgA vasculitis at the genome-wide level of significance, locations 13 and 11 of the *HLA-DRB1* were shown to be of possible importance for genetic predisposition (López-Mejías et al. 2017). In this regard, a subsequent meta-analysis was able to confirm the association with *HLA-DRB1*01* alleles and further elucidate the protective role of the *HLA-DRB1*07* allele (Amoli et al. 2001; He et al. 2013). A significant association of *HLA-B35* with renal involvement in IgA vasculitis has been reported, yet this association has not been replicated in a subsequent publication (He et al. 2013). Likewise, patients with IgA vasculitis who do not have the *469 K/E* variant of *ICAM-1* seem to develop less frequently severe gastrointestinal symptoms (Eleftheriou and Brogan 2009). However, further studies with the recruitment of larger numbers of patients as well as populations of diverse ancestries are required to properly demonstrate the genetic influence in the vulnerability to this type of vasculitis.

6 Variable-Vessel Vasculitis

6.1 General Aspects

It is a vasculitis that affects vessels of any size (large, small, and medium) and type (small capillaries, arteries, and veins). Behçet's disease (BD) and the Cogan's syndrome are the two forms included in the CHCC 2012 nomenclature (Table 1) and they are characterized as primary categories of vasculitis (Jennette et al. 2013). BD is more common in countries located across the ancient Silk Road; it is most prevalent in Turkey but also occurs frequently in Japan, Korea, China, Greece, and middle Eastern countries such as Iran and Saudi Arabia. The disease seldom develops elsewhere in the world. Striking clinical features include recurrent attacks of oral ulceration and/or genital aphthae (Fig. 5), skin lesions, uveitis, arthritis, gastrointestinal disease, and central nervous system involvement. BD vasculitis can involve both arteries and veins; small-vessel vasculitis, aneurysms, large-vessel events, and venous or arterial thrombosis may also develop (Gul 2015; Jennette et al. 2013; Leccese and Alpsoy 2019).

6.2 Pathogenesis

The pathogenesis of BD is still unknown; yet, the disorder appears to be at the intersection of autoimmune and autoinflammatory diseases. Systemic perivasculitis with early neutrophil infiltration and endothelial swelling is the most common pathologic lesion. Other less prevalent pathologic features are diffuse inflammation of all layers of large vessels resulting in pseudoaneurysms and vasculitis of vasa-vasorum within the adventitia (Gul 2015; Leccese and Alpsoy 2019). Separately from the activated neutrophils, there are more invading Th1, Th17, cytotoxic $CD8^+$, and $\gamma\delta$ + T-cells, implying a link between innate and adaptive autoreactive immune responses (Greco et al. 2018; Gul 2015; Leccese and Alpsoy 2019; Yazici et al. 2018). Due to the occurrence of episodes of inflammation without provocation and the lack of evidence of pathogenic high-titers of autoantibodies or antigen-specific T cells, increased neutrophil activity, and raised levels of IL-1b, some authors claim the disease should be classified as an autoinflammatory disease (Gul 2015). While environmental factors such as oral microbial flora have been linked to BD etiology, no infectious agent has been identified as the causative culprit. Instead, infectious pathogens or the microbiome appear to have a role in the progression of the disease by triggering dysregulation of the immune system in genetically predisposed individuals (Greco et al. 2018; Gul 2015; Leccese and Alpsoy 2019; Yazici et al. 2018).

6.2.1 Genetic Associations in Behçet's Disease

Despite a high sibling risk ratio (Gul and Ohno 2012) and a regional distribution of BD, the lack of consistency with anticipated Mendelian inheritance patterns suggests that multiple genetic and environmental factors contribute to disease pathogenesis (Greco et al. 2018; Gul 2015; Leccese and Alpsoy 2019; Yazici et al. 2018). BD represents the most-studied vasculitis to date (Table 2) in terms of genetic factors linked to disease susceptibility. In total, three GWAS in subjects of Turkish, Japanese, Korean, and Italian origin (Lee et al. 2013; Mizuki et al. 2010; Remmers et al. 2010), as well as a multicenter GWAS including Western Europeans, Middle Eastern, and Turkish individuals have been published (Kappen et al. 2015). Also, five different extension studies of the GWAS and a recent immunochip study have been conducted (Hughes et al. 2013; Kang et al. 2017; Kim et al. 2013; Kirino et al. 2013; Kirino et al. 2013; Takeuchi et al. 2017). The most prominent BD association signals come from the MHC-I region (Wallace 2014). Particularly, the *HLA-B*51* alleles (Table 2) have consistently been linked to BD across populations from different ethnicities and are considered the primary genetic

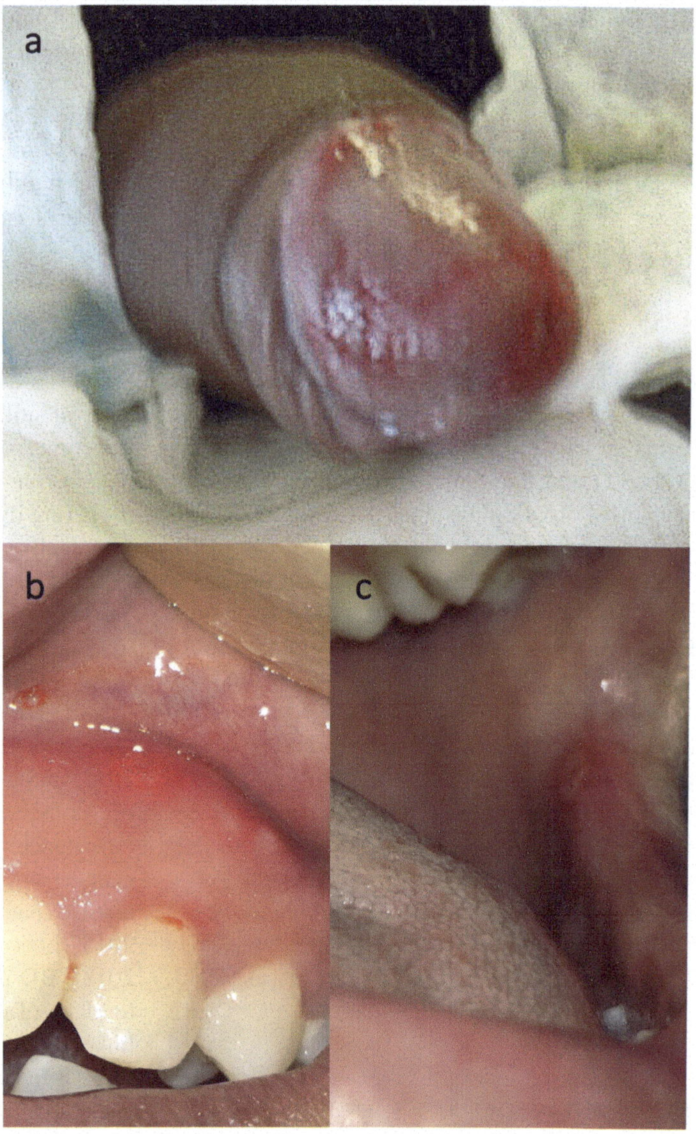

Fig. 5 Variable vessel vasculitis. Behcet's disease (**a** genital; **b** and **c**, oral ulcers)

susceptibility factor for BD (Menthon et al. 2009; Takeuchi et al. 2017). Nonetheless, a subsequent study that evaluated about eight thousand variants in the extended HLA locus and performed a meta-analysis on 24,834 variants extracted from two independent BD cohorts, was able to show that the robust association between *HLA-B*51* and BD might be better explained by an SNP in the *HLA-B/MICA* intergenic region (*rs116799036*) (Hughes et al. 2013). This study was also able to report some other independent disease susceptibility loci in the MHC region including the *HLA-Cw*16:02* allele, and the *rs12525170* and *rs114854070* SNPs (Hughes et al. 2013). In a subsequent study on Turkish subjects, the investigators analyzed both directly ascertained and imputed SNP genotypes in the HLA-B region together with data on amino acids and HLA types to better characterize the sources of BD risk allele within the MHC region (Ombrello et al. 2014). They also applied SNP mapping with stepwise, multivariate logistic regression and conditional analysis of the MHC region. They were not able to confirm the anticipated effect for *rs116799036* (Ombrello et al. 2014). Instead, they were able to identify the *HLA-B/MICA* region and the intragenic noncoding segment between *HLA-F* and *HLA-A* as independent areas associated with BD (Ombrello et al. 2014). In the *HLA-B/MICA* region, *HLA-B*51* was established as the strongest loci to confer risk for BD (Ombrello et al. 2014). The major advantage of this investigation was narrowing down the MHC associations of BD to amino acid levels. A model consisting of seven MHC-I amino acid residues was mapped that was able to explain all the detected independent associations (Ombrello et al. 2014). Notably, several of these amino acids had been previously demonstrated to modulate either antigen binding of the HLA molecule or the interactions between HLA-B molecules with CD8 + T-cells and NK cells, implying a role for cellular cytotoxicity in BD (Ombrello et al. 2014). Finally, the largest study thus far (Takeuchi et al. 2017), was able to confirm the strongest disease association for *HLA-B*51* among all markers within the MHC region, using the immunochip dense genotyping method in Turkish subjects and two additional populations (Iranian and Japanese subjects) in the replication phase (Table 2). Also, a huge meta-analysis of 78 studies established *HLA-B*51* as the major risk loci for developing BD (Menthon et al. 2009).

Using various techniques, multiple loci residing outside the MHC region have demonstrated associations with BD with a genome-wide level of significance. Two of these non-MHC association signals were identified in the *IL10* locus that encodes an immunoregulatory Th2 cytokine, and the IL-23 receptor/IL-12 receptor beta-2 (*IL23R/IL12RB2*) region which is important in the differentiation of Th1 and Th17 cells. These variants were the highest non-MHC linkages that were identified by two GWAS performed in Turkey and Japan, using deep exonic resequencing and immunochip genotyping, respectively (Kirino et al. 2013; Mizuki et al. 2010; Remmers et al. 2010; Takeuchi et al. 2017) (Table 2). More recently, association with *IL23R–IL12RB2* intergenic, rs1495965 SNP, was also confirmed in a Korean population (Kang et al. 2017). The same region *IL23R–IL12RB2* has also been implicated in disease susceptibility in two previously published GWAS (Mizuki et al. 2010; Remmers et al. 2010) (Table 2). Notably, a recent GWAS with subjects from Western European, Middle Eastern, and Turkish ancestry, established the involvement of a variant in the *IL12A* locus as the susceptibility factor (Kappen et al. 2015) (Table 2). A Korean GWAS was able to demonstrate a novel BD risk loci residing within the *guanosine-5'-triphosphatase IMAP family member 4* (*GIMAP4*) gene that is thought to be important in T-cell and B-cells development (Lee et al. 2013) (Table 2). Nevertheless, this finding was not replicated in European-based studies (Ortiz-Fernández et al. 2014).

The extraction and reanalysis of the data from the GWAS on Turkish and Japanese subjects according to imputed genotypes were able to reveal new BD associations signals at the loci encoding the ERAP1, the C–C motif chemokine receptor-1 (CCR1), the signal transducer and activator of transcription-4 (STAT4), and a cluster region consisting of several killer cell lectin-like receptor family members (*KLRK1*, *KLRC1-4*) (Kirino et al. 2013). A GWAS with a replication study in a Han Chinese population confirmed that *STAT4*, as well as the HLA–B region, are risk variants for BD (Hou et al. 2012). Another study in a Spanish population was able to confirm the association between *ERAP1* and BD and the epistasis between *HLA-B*51* and *ERAP1* (Conde-Jaldon et al. 2014). The disease associations of *CCR1*, *ERAP1*, and *KLRC4* loci have also been replicated in a recent publication using the immunochip array in Turkish subjects (Takeuchi et al. 2017) (Table 2). *ERAP1* gene encodes a metallopeptidase capable of processing the peptides to fit them into the MHC molecules.

In the most recent publication using immunochip genotyping, four new risk loci were identified (Takeuchi et al. 2017). In particular, the variants which displayed genome-wide significant associations with BD included the *IL1A–IL1B* region encoding the members of interleukin 1 cytokine family, the interferon regulatory factor family 8 region (*IRF8*; with DNA-binding transcription factor activity), the *CEBPB* (which codes for a transcription factor that has a basic leucine zipper domain)–*PTPN1* (encoding a protein which belongs to the protein tyrosine phosphatase family) loci, and finally the 2-aminoethanethiol dioxygenase (with cysteamine dioxygenase activity)-early growth response 2 (with DNA-binding transcription factor and ligase activity) (*ADO–EGR2*) loci (Takeuchi et al. 2017) (Table 2). The disease association of *IRF8, ADO–EGR2*, and *CEBPB–PTPN1* loci was confirmed by genotyping Iranian subjects while imputed data in Japanese further replicated *ADO–EGR2* and *IRF8* (Takeuchi et al. 2017). Furthermore, a meta-analysis demonstrated that *fucosyltransferase-2* (*FUT2*) genes were associated with susceptibility to BD in all three ethnic groups. The risk genotypes were the ones to be associated with non-secretor phenotypes (Table 2). This further confirmed the results of a previous meta-analysis on the GWA studies performed in Iran and Turkey (Takeuchi et al. 2017). *FUT2* encodes an enzyme responsible for the production of a precursor surface antigen, called the H antigen, that is an essential substrate for the last step in the ABO blood group antigen synthesis. Non-secretor individuals do not express active FUT2 enzymes, and therefore, they are not able to express the ABO antigens in bodily fluids and the GI mucosa (Ferrer-Admetlla et al. 2009). These findings provide evidence that non-secretory ABO genotypes, predominantly at mucus membranes, increase susceptibility to BD perhaps through altering the interaction between host and microbial agents (Takeuchi et al. 2017). Meta-analysis additionally identified the receptor-interacting serine/threonine kinase 2 (*RIPK2*) and the laccase domain containing 1 (*LACC1*) as newly identified BD susceptibility markers (Takeuchi et al. 2017). These variants are found in putative functional domains and have predictable consequences, either modifying protein configuration or the expression of adjacent genes. A previously reported disease association in a Han Chinese population for the TNFα-inducible protein 3 (*TNFAIP3*), a gene involved in the regulation of inflammatory response induced by cytokines (Li et al. 2013), was not confirmed in the immunochip study (Takeuchi et al. 2017) or a study on subjects of European ancestry (Ortiz-Fernandez et al. 2015). Despite these discrepancies, the overall findings from genetic studies suggest that hereditary factors play a role in the pathogenesis of BD through regulating the mucus barrier dynamics and the host's immune reaction to pathogens (Takeuchi et al. 2017). Interestingly, a genome-wide methylation study using pyrosequencing technology on a Han Chinese population was published very recently. This study revealed five differentially methylated CpG sites with substantial hypomethylation in the *RUNX2, FKBP5, FLJ43663*, and *NFIL3* genes. These findings imply that abnormal DNA methylation may have a role in the etiology of BD, regardless of previously recognized genetic variations (Yu et al. 2019). Yet, these results should be validated across populations of different ethnicities, and the mechanisms whereby altered methylation affects BD development that needs to be clarified.

7 Conclusions

Undoubtedly, we have considerably increased our understanding of the genetic basis of primary systemic vasculitides over the past decades. However, we have in turn discovered that we cannot deduce that associated SNPs affect the function of their nearest gene. Understanding how gene expression is regulated will be essential to unravel the role of vasculitis-associated genetic variants. Researchers have been able to pose probing questions about how disease-associated alleles affect the process of complex diseases owing to exponential breakthroughs in genetic engineering in recent years. Despite this, identifying the genetic component of primary vasculitides and dissecting these disorders remains a major challenge. Genome editing technology has the potential to give substantial empirical evidence of the processes through which these genetic components impact disease. Nevertheless, current insights and advances regarding the understanding of crucial pathways that play a role in the pathogenesis of these diseases are close to having an impact on the management of patients with different types of vasculitis through the development of novel drugs, the repositioning of existing therapies, and the implementation of a stratified treatment approach.

References

Abdulahad WHLP, Kallenberg CG (2011) T-helper cells as new players in ANCA-associated vasculitides. Arthritis Res Ther 13:236

Agarwal S, Agrawal DK (2017) Kawasaki disease: etiopathogenesis and novel treatment strategies. Expert Rev Clin Immunol 13:247–258

Amoli MM, Thomson W, Hajeer AH, Calvino MC, Garcia-Porrua C, Ollier WE, Gonzalez-Gay MA (2001) HLA-DRB1*01 association with Henoch-Schonlein purpura in patients from northwest Spain. J Rheumatol 28:1266–1270

Anwar S, Karim MY (2017) Update on systemic vasculitides. J Clin Pathol 70:476–482

Bewarder N, Weinrich V, Budde P, Hartmann D, Flaswinkel H, Reth M, Frey J (1996) In vivo and in vitro specificity of protein tyrosine kinases for immunoglobulin G receptor (FcgammaRII) phosphorylation. Mol Cell Biol 16:4735–4743

Brouwer E, Huitema MG, Klok PA, de Weerd H, Tervaert JW, Weening JJ, Kallenberg CG (1993) Antimyeloperoxidase-associated proliferative glomerulonephritis: an animal model. J Exp Med 177:905–914

Burgner D, Davila S, Breunis WB, Ng SB, Li Y, Bonnard C, Ling L, Wright VJ, Thalamuthu A, Odam M, Shimizu C, Burns JC, Levin M, Kuijpers TW, Hibberd ML, International Kawasaki Disease Genetics C (2009) A genome-wide association study identifies novel and functionally related susceptibility Loci for Kawasaki disease. PLoS Genet 5:e1000319

Cao Y, Yang J, Colby K, Hogan SL, Hu Y, Jennette CE, Berg EA, Zhang Y, Jennette JC, Falk RJ, Preston GA (2012) High basal activity of the PTPN22 gain-of-function variant blunts leukocyte responsiveness negatively affecting IL-10 production in ANCA vasculitis. PLoS One 7:e42783

Caorsi R, Penco F, Schena F, Gattorno M (2016) Monogenic polyarteritis: the lesson of ADA2 deficiency. Pediatr Rheumatol Online J 14:51

Carmona FD, Gonzalez-Gay MA, Martin J (2014) Genetic component of giant cell arteritis. Rheumatology (oxford) 53:6–18

Carmona FD, Mackie SL, Martin JE, Taylor JC, Vaglio A, Eyre S, Bossini-Castillo L, Castaneda S, Cid MC, Hernandez-Rodriguez J, Prieto-Gonzalez S, Solans R, Ramentol-Sintas M, Gonzalez-Escribano MF, Ortiz-Fernandez L, Morado IC, Narvaez J, Miranda-Filloy JA, Spanish GCAG, Beretta L, Lunardi C, Cimmino MA, Gianfreda D, Santilli D, Ramirez GA, Soriano A, Muratore F, Pazzola G, Addimanda O, Wijmenga C, Witte T, Schirmer JH, Moosig F, Schonau V, Franke A, Palm O, Molberg O, Diamantopoulos AP, Carette S, Cuthbertson D, Forbess LJ, Hoffman GS, Khalidi NA, Koening CL, Langford CA, McAlear CA, Moreland L, Monach PA, Pagnoux C, Seo P, Spiera R, Sreih AG, Warrington KJ, Ytterberg SR, Gregersen PK, Pease CT, Gough A, Green M, Hordon L, Jarrett S, Watts R, Levy S, Patel Y, Kamath S, Dasgupta B, Worthington J, Koeleman BP, de Bakker PI, Barrett JH, Salvarani C, Merkel PA, Gonzalez-Gay MA, Morgan AW, Martin J (2015) A large-scale genetic analysis reveals a strong contribution of the HLA class II region to giant cell arteritis susceptibility. Am J Hum Genet 96:565–580

Carmona FD, Vaglio A, Mackie SL, Hernandez-Rodriguez J, Monach PA, Castaneda S, Solans R, Morado IC, Narvaez J, Ramentol-Sintas M, Pease CT, Dasgupta B, Watts R, Khalidi N, Langford CA, Ytterberg S, Boiardi L, Beretta L, Govoni M, Emmi G, Bonatti F, Cimmino MA, Witte T, Neumann T, Holle J, Schonau V, Sailler L, Papo T, Haroche J, Mahr A, Mouthon L, Molberg O, Diamantopoulos AP, Voskuyl A, Brouwer E, Daikeler T, Berger CT, Molloy ES, O'Neill L, Blockmans D, Lie BA, McLaren P, Vyse TJ, Wijmenga C, Allanore Y, Koeleman BPC, Spanish CGAG, Consortium U, Vasculitis Clinical Research C, Barrett JH, Cid MC, Salvarani C, Merkel PA, Morgan AW, Gonzalez-Gay MA, Martin J (2017) A genome-wide association study identifies risk alleles in plasminogen and P4HA2 associated with giant cell arteritis. Am J Hum Genet 100:64–74

Chang CJ, Kuo HC, Chang JS, Lee JK, Tsai FJ, Khor CC, Chang LC, Chen SP, Ko TM, Liu YM, Chen YJ, Hong YM, Jang GY, Hibberd ML, Kuijpers T, Burgner D, Levin M, Burns JC, Davila S, International Kawasaki Disease Genetics C, Korean Kawasaki Disease Genetics C, Taiwan Kawasaki Disease Genetics C, Chen YT, Chen CH, Wu JY, Lee YC (2013) Replication and meta-analysis of GWAS identified susceptibility loci in Kawasaki disease confirm the importance of B lymphoid tyrosine kinase (BLK) in disease susceptibility. PLoS One 8:e72037

Ciavatta DJ, Yang J, Preston GA, Badhwar AK, Xiao H, Hewins P, Nester CM, Pendergraft WF 3rd, Magnuson TR, Jennette JC, Falk RJ (2010) Epigenetic basis for aberrant upregulation of autoantigen genes in humans with ANCA vasculitis. J Clin Invest 120:3209–3219

Conde-Jaldon M, Montes-Cano MA, Garcia-Lozano JR, Ortiz-Fernandez L, Ortego-Centeno N, Gonzalez-Leon R, Espinosa G, Grana-Gil G, Sanchez-Burson J, Gonzalez-Gay MA, Barnosi-Marin AC, Solans R, Fanlo P, Carballeira MR, Camps T, Castaneda S,

Martin J, Gonzalez-Escribano MF (2014) Epistatic interaction of ERAP1 and HLA-B in Behcet disease: a replication study in the Spanish population. PLoS One 9:e102100

Davies DJ, Moran JE, Niall JF, Ryan GB (1982) Segmental necrotising glomerulonephritis with antineutrophil antibody: possible arbovirus aetiology? Br Med J (clin Res Ed) 285:606

de Menthon M, Lavalley MP, Maldini C, Guillevin L, Mahr A (2009) HLA-B51/B5 and the risk of Behcet's disease: a systematic review and meta-analysis of case-control genetic association studies. Arthritis Rheum 61:1287–1296

Dejaco C, Brouwer E, Mason JC, Buttgereit F, Matteson EL, Dasgupta B (2017) Giant cell arteritis and polymyalgia rheumatica: current challenges and opportunities. Nat Rev Rheumatol 13:578–592

Deng J, Ma-Krupa W, Gewirtz AT, Younge BR, Goronzy JJ, Weyand CM (2009) Toll-like receptors 4 and 5 induce distinct types of vasculitis. Circ Res 104:488–495

Duranton JBJ (2003) Inhibition of proteinase 3 by [alpha] 1-antitrypsin in vitro predicts very fast inhibition in vivo. Am J Respir Cell Mol Biol 29:57–61

Eleftheriou D, Brogan PA (2009) Vasculitis in children. Best Pract Res Clin Rheumatol 23:309–323

Farh KK, Marson A, Zhu J, Kleinewietfeld M, Housley WJ, Beik S, Shoresh N, Whitton H, Ryan RJ, Shishkin AA, Hatan M, Carrasco-Alfonso MJ, Mayer D, Luckey CJ, Patsopoulos NA, De Jager PL, Kuchroo VK, Epstein CB, Daly MJ, Hafler DA, Bernstein BE (2015) Genetic and epigenetic fine mapping of causal autoimmune disease variants. Nature 518:337–343

Ferrer-Admetlla A, Sikora M, Laayouni H, Esteve A, Roubinet F, Blancher A, Calafell F, Bertranpetit J, Casals F (2009) A natural history of FUT2 polymorphism in humans. Mol Biol Evol 26:1993–2003

Field JSF, Schibeci S; Australia and New Zealand MS Genetics Consortium (ANZgene), Johnson L, Gresle M, Laverick L, Parnell G, Stewart G, McKay F, Kilpatrick T, Butzkueven H, Booth D (2015) The MS risk allele of CD40 is associated with reduced cell-membrane bound expression in antigen presenting cells: implications for gene function. PLoS One 10

Flint SM, McKinney EF, Smith KG (2015) Emerging concepts in the pathogenesis of antineutrophil cytoplasmic antibody-associated vasculitis. Curr Opin Rheumatol 27:197–203

Furuta SCA, Hamano Y, Fujimoto S, Nagafuchi H, Makino H, Matsuo S, Ozaki S, Endo T, Muso E, Ito C, Kusano E, Yamagata M, Ikeda K, Kashiwakuma D, Iwamoto I, Westman K, Jayne D (2014) Comparison of phenotype and outcome in microscopic polyangiitis between Europe and Japan. J Rheumatol 41:325–333

Galeotti C, Bayry J, Kone-Paut I, Kaveri SV (2010) Kawasaki disease: aetiopathogenesis and therapeutic utility of intravenous immunoglobulin. Autoimmun Rev 9:441–448

Ge X, Li CR, Yang J, Wang GB (2013) Aberrantly decreased levels of NKG2D expression in children with kawasaki disease. Scand J Immunol 77:389–397

Gonzalez-Gay MA, Amoli MM, Garcia-Porrua C, Ollier WE (2003) Genetic markers of disease susceptibility and severity in giant cell arteritis and polymyalgia rheumatica. Semin Arthritis Rheum 33:38–48

Gonzalez-Gay MA, Garcia-Porrua C (2001) Epidemiology of the vasculitides. Rheum Dis Clin North Am 27:729–749

Gonzalez-Gay MA, Lopez-Mejias R, Pina T, Blanco R, Castaneda S (2018) IgA vasculitis: genetics and clinical and therapeutic management. Curr Rheumatol Rep 20:24

Greco ADVA, Ralli M, Ciofalo A, Mancini P, Attanasio G, de Vincentiis M, Lambiase A (2018) Behçet's disease: new insights into pathophysiology, clinical features and treatment options. Autoimmun Rev 17:567–575

Guillevin L, Mahr A, Callard P, Godmer P, Pagnoux C, Leray E, Cohen P, French Vasculitis Study G (2005) Hepatitis B virus-associated polyarteritis nodosa: clinical characteristics, outcome, and impact of treatment in 115 patients. Medicine (Baltimore) 84:313–322

Gul A (2015) Pathogenesis of Behcet's disease: autoinflammatory features and beyond. Semin Immunopathol 37:413–418

Gul A, Ohno S (2012) HLA-B*51 and Behcet disease. Ocul Immunol Inflamm 20:37–43

Harky A, Fok M, Balmforth D, Bashir M (2019) Pathogenesis of large vessel vasculitis: implications for disease classification and future therapies. Vasc Med 24:79–88

He X, Yu C, Zhao P, Ding Y, Liang X, Zhao Y, Yue X, Wu Y, Yin W (2013) The genetics of Henoch-Schonlein purpura: a systematic review and meta-analysis. Rheumatol Int 33:1387–1395

Henderson LA, Frugoni F, Hopkins G, de Boer H, Pai SY, Lee YN, Walter JE, Hazen MM, Notarangelo LD (2013) Expanding the spectrum of recombination-activating gene 1 deficiency: a family with early-onset autoimmunity. J Allergy Clin Immunol 132(969–971):e961-962

Hoffman GSSU (1998) Antineutrophil cytoplasmic antibodies. Arthritis Rheum 41:1521–1533

Hosomichi K, Shiina T, Tajima A, Inoue I (2015) The impact of next-generation sequencing technologies on HLA research. J Hum Genet 60:665–673

Hou S, Yang Z, Du L, Jiang Z, Shu Q, Chen Y, Li F, Zhou Q, Ohno S, Chen R, Kijlstra A, Rosenbaum JT, Yang P (2012) Identification of a susceptibility locus in STAT4 for Behcet's disease in Han Chinese in a genome-wide association study. Arthritis Rheum 64:4104–4113

Hughes T, Coit P, Adler A, Yilmaz V, Aksu K, Duzgun N, Keser G, Cefle A, Yazici A, Ergen A, Alpsoy E, Salvarani C, Casali B, Kotter I, Gutierrez-Achury J, Wijmenga C, Direskeneli H, Saruhan-Direskeneli G,

Sawalha AH (2013) Identification of multiple independent susceptibility loci in the HLA region in Behcet's disease. Nat Genet 45:319–324

Hunder GG, Arend WP, Bloch DA, Calabrese LH, Fauci AS, Fries JF, Leavitt RY, Lie JT, Lightfoot RW Jr, Masi AT et al (1990) The American College of Rheumatology 1990 criteria for the classification of vasculitis. Introduction. Arthritis Rheum 33:1065–1067

Iwaki-Egawa SYT, Watanabe Y (2006) Human plasma adenosine deaminase 2 is secreted by activated monocytes. Biol Chem 387:319–321

Jennette JC, Falk R, Bacon P, Basu N, Cid M, Ferrario F, Flores-Suarez L, Gross W, Guillevin L, Hagen E (2013) 2012 revised international chapel hill consensus conference nomenclature of vasculitides

Jennette JC, Falk RJ (2014) Pathogenesis of antineutrophil cytoplasmic autoantibody-mediated disease. Nat Rev Rheumatol 10:463–473

Jennette JCFR, Bacon PA, Basu N, Cid MC, Ferrario F, Flores-Suarez LF, Gross WL, Guillevin L, Hagen EC, Hoffman GS, Jayne DR, Kallenberg CG, Lamprecht P, Langford CA, Luqmani RA, Mahr AD, Matteson EL, Merkel PA, Ozen S, Pusey CD, Rasmussen N, Rees AJ, Scott DG, Specks U, Stone JH, Takahashi K, Watts RA (2013) 2012 revised International Chapel Hill consensus conference nomenclature of vasculitides. Arthritis Rheum 65:1–11

Jia S, Li C, Wang G, Yang J, Zu Y (2010) The T helper type 17/regulatory T cell imbalance in patients with acute Kawasaki disease. Clin Exp Immunol 162:131–137

Kang EH, Kim S, Park MY, Choi JY, Choi IA, Kim MJ, Ha YJ, Lee EY, Lee YJ, Lee EB, Kang C, Song YW (2017) Behcet's disease risk association fine-mapped on the IL23R-IL12RB2 intergenic region in Koreans. Arthritis Res Ther 19:227

Kappen JH M-GC, van Hagen PM, Stolk L, Estrada K, Rivadeneira F, Uitterlinden AG, Stanford MR, Ben-Chetrit E, Wallace GR, Soylu M, van Laar JA (2015) Genome-wide association study in an admixed case series reveals IL12A as a new candidate in Behçet disease. PLoS One 10

Kawasaki A, Hasebe N, Hidaka M, Hirano F, Sada KE, Kobayashi S, Yamada H, Furukawa H, Yamagata K, Sumida T, Miyasaka N, Tohma S, Ozaki S, Matsuo S, Hashimoto H, Makino H, Arimura Y, Harigai M, Tsuchiya N (2016) Protective role of HLA-DRB1*13:02 against microscopic polyangiitis and MPO-ANCA-positive vasculitides in a Japanese population: a case-control study. PLoS One 11:e0154393

Kessenbrock K, Krumbholz M, Schonermarck U, Back W, Gross WL, Werb Z, Grone HJ, Brinkmann V, Jenne DE (2009) Netting neutrophils in autoimmune small-vessel vasculitis. Nat Med 15:623–625

Khor CC DS, Breunis WB, Lee YC, Shimizu C, Wright VJ, Yeung RS, Tan DE, Sim KS, Wang JJ, Wong TY, Pang J, Mitchell P, Cimaz R, Dahdah N, Cheung YF, Huang GY, Yang W, Park IS, Lee JK, Wu JY, Levin M, Burns JC, Burgner D, Kuijpers TW, Hibberd ML, Hong Kong–Shanghai Kawasaki Disease Genetics Consortium, Korean Kawasaki Disease Genetics Consortium, Taiwan Kawasaki Disease Genetics Consortium, International Kawasaki Disease Genetics Consortium, US Kawasaki Disease Genetics Consortium, Blue Mountains Eye Study (2011) Genome-wide association study identifies FCGR2A as a susceptibility locus for Kawasaki disease. Nat Genet 43:1241–1246

Kim JJ HY, Sohn S, Jang GY, Ha KS, Yun SW, Han MK, Lee KY, Song MS, Lee HD, Kim DS, Lee JE, Shin ES, Jang JH, Lee YS, Kim SY, Lee JY, Han BG, Wu JY, Kim KJ, Park YM, Seo EJ, Park IS, Lee JK, Korean Kawasaki Disease Genetics Consortium (2011) A genome-wide association analysis reveals 1p31 and 2p13.3 as susceptibility loci for Kawasaki disease. Hum Genet 129:487–495

Kim JJYS, Yu JJ, Yoon KL, Lee KY, Kil HR, Kim GB, Han MK, Song MS, Lee HD, Ha KS, Sohn S, Johnson TA, Takahashi A, Kubo M, Tsunoda T, Ito K, Onouchi Y, Hong YM, Jang GY, Lee JK, Korean Kawasaki Disease Genetics Consortium (2017) A genome-wide association analysis identifies NMNAT2 and HCP5 as susceptibility loci for Kawasaki disease. J Hum Genet 62:1023–1029

Kim JJ, Yun SW, Yu JJ, Yoon KL, Lee KY, Kil HR, Kim GB, Han MK, Song MS, Lee HD, Ha KS, Sohn S, Ebata R, Hamada H, Suzuki H, Ito K, Onouchi Y, Hong YM, Jang GY, Lee JK, and the Korean Kawasaki Disease Genetics C (2019) Identification of SAMD9L as a susceptibility locus for intravenous immunoglobulin resistance in Kawasaki disease by genome-wide association analysis. Pharmacogenomics J

Kim SJ, Lee S, Park C, Seo JS, Kim JI, Yu HG (2013) Targeted resequencing of candidate genes reveals novel variants associated with severe Behcet's uveitis. Exp Mol Med 45:e49

Kimura A, Kitamura H, Date Y, Numano F (1996) Comprehensive analysis of HLA genes in Takayasu arteritis in Japan. Int J Cardiol 54(Suppl):S61-69

Kirino YBG, Ishigatsubo Y, Mizuki N, Tugal-Tutkun I, Seyahi E, Ozyazgan Y, Sacli FS, Erer B, Inoko H, Emrence Z, Cakar A, Abaci N, Ustek D, Satorius C, Ueda A, Takeno M, Kim Y, Wood GM, Ombrello MJ, Meguro A, Gül A, Remmers EF, Kastner DL (2013) Genome-wide association analysis identifies new susceptibility loci for Behçet's disease and epistasis between HLA-B*51 and ERAP1. Nat Genet 45:202–207

Kirino Y, Zhou Q, Ishigatsubo Y, Mizuki N, Tugal-Tutkun I, Seyahi E, Ozyazgan Y, Ugurlu S, Erer B, Abaci N, Ustek D, Meguro A, Ueda A, Takeno M, Inoko H, Ombrello MJ, Satorius CL, Maskeri B, Mullikin JC, Sun HW, Gutierrez-Cruz G, Kim Y, Wilson AF, Kastner DL, Gul A, Remmers EF (2013) Targeted resequencing implicates the familial Mediterranean fever gene MEFV and the toll-like receptor 4 gene TLR4 in Behcet disease. Proc Natl Acad Sci U S A 110:8134–8139

Kuo HC, Li SC, Guo MM, Huang YH, Yu HR, Huang FC, Jiao F, Kuo HC, Andrade J, Chan WC (2016) Genome-wide association study identifies novel susceptibility genes associated with coronary artery aneurysm formation in Kawasaki disease. PLoS One 11:e0154943

Kuo HC, Yang KD, Juo SH, Liang CD, Chen WC, Wang YS, Lee CH, Hsi E, Yu HR, Woon PY, Lin IC, Huang CF, Hwang DY, Lee CP, Lin LY, Chang WP, Chang WC (2011) ITPKC single nucleotide polymorphism associated with the Kawasaki disease in a Taiwanese population. PLoS One 6:e17370

Kuo HC, Yu HR, Juo SH, Yang KD, Wang YS, Liang CD, Chen WC, Chang WP, Huang CF, Lee CP, Lin LY, Liu YC, Guo YC, Chiu CC, Chang WC (2011) CASP3 gene single-nucleotide polymorphism (rs72689236) and Kawasaki disease in Taiwanese children. J Hum Genet 56:161–165

Kwon YCKJ, Yu JJ, Yun SW, Yoon KL, Lee KY, Kil HR, Kim GB, Han MK, Song MS, Lee HD, Ha KS, Sohn S, Hong YM, Jang GY, Lee JK, Korean Kawasaki Disease Genetics Consortium (2019) Identification of the TIFAB gene as a susceptibility locus for coronary artery aneurysm in patients with Kawasaki disease. Pediatr Cardiol 40:483–488

Leccese P, Alpsoy E (2019) Behcet's disease: an overview of etiopathogenesis. Front Immunol 10:1067

Lee YWD, Dagvadorj J, Shimada K, Chen S, Huang G et al (2015) IL-1 signaling is critically required in stromal cells in Kawasaki disease vasculitis mouse model: role of both IL-1α and IL-1β. Arterioscler Thromb Vasc Biol 35:2605–2616

Lee YCKH, Chang JS, Chang LY, Huang LM, Chen MR, Liang CD, Chi H, Huang FY, Lee ML, Huang YC, Hwang B, Chiu NC, Hwang KP, Lee PC, Chang LC, Liu YM, Chen YJ, Chen CH, Taiwan Pediatric ID, Alliance CYT, Tsai FJ, Wu JY (2012) Two new susceptibility loci for Kawasaki disease identified through genome-wide association analysis. Nat Genet 44:522–525

Lee YJHY, Wallace GR, Choi YS, Park JA, Choi JY, Song R, Kang YM, Kang SW, Baek HJ, Kitaichi N, Meguro A, Mizuki N, Namba K, Ishida S, Kim J, Niemczyk E, Lee EY, Song YW, Ohno S, Lee EB (2013) Genome-wide association study identifies GIMAP as a novel susceptibility locus for Behcet's disease. Ann Rheum Dis 72:1510–1516

Li H, Liu Q, Hou S, Du L, Zhou Q, Zhou Y, Kijlstra A, Li Z, Yang P (2013) TNFAIP3 gene polymorphisms confer risk for Behcet's disease in a Chinese Han population. Hum Genet 132:293–300

Little MA, Smyth L, Salama AD, Mukherjee S, Smith J, Haskard D, Nourshargh S, Cook HT, Pusey CD (2009) Experimental autoimmune vasculitis: an animal model of anti-neutrophil cytoplasmic autoantibody-associated systemic vasculitis. Am J Pathol 174:1212–1220

López-Mejías RCF, Castañeda S, Genre F, Remuzgo-Martínez S, Sevilla-Perez B, Ortego-Centeno N, Llorca J, Ubilla B, Mijares V, Pina T, Miranda-Filloy JA, Navas Parejo A, de Argila D, Aragües M, Rubio E, Luque ML, Blanco-Madrigal JM, Galíndez-Aguirregoikoa E, Jayne D, Blanco R, Martín J, González-Gay MA (2017) A genome-wide association study suggests the HLA Class II region as the major susceptibility locus for IgA vasculitis. Sci Rep 7:5088

Lyons PART, Trivedi S, Holle JU, Watts RA, Jayne DR, Baslund B, Brenchley P, Bruchfeld A, Chaudhry AN, Cohen Tervaert JW, Deloukas P, Feighery C, Gross WL, Guillevin L, Gunnarsson I, Harper L, Hrušková Z, Little MA, Martorana D, Neumann T, Ohlsson S, Padmanabhan S, Pusey CD, Salama AD, Sanders JS, Savage CO, Segelmark M, Stegeman CA, Tesař V, Vaglio A, Wieczorek S, Wilde B, Zwerina J, Rees AJ, Clayton DG, Smith KG (2012) Genetically distinct subsets within ANCA-associated vasculitis. N Engl J Med 367:214–223

Mahajan N, Dhawan V, Mahmood S, Malik S, Jain S (2012) Extracellular matrix remodeling in Takayasu's arteritis: role of matrix metalloproteinases and adventitial inflammation. Arch Med Res 43:406–410

Marquez A, Hernandez-Rodriguez J, Cid MC, Solans R, Castaneda S, Fernandez-Contreras ME, Ramentol M, Morado IC, Narvaez J, Gomez-Vaquero C, Martinez-Taboada VM, Ortego-Centeno N, Sopena B, Monfort J, Garcia-Villanueva MJ, Caminal-Montero L, de Miguel E, Blanco R, Spanish GCAC, Palm O, Molberg O, Latus J, Braun N, Moosig F, Witte T, Beretta L, Santaniello A, Pazzola G, Boiardi L, Salvarani C, Gonzalez-Gay MA, Martin J (2014) Influence of the IL17A locus in giant cell arteritis susceptibility. Ann Rheum Dis 73:1742–1745

Martinez-Taboada V, Brack A, Hunder GG, Goronzy JJ, Weyand CM (1996) The inflammatory infiltrate in giant cell arteritis selects against B lymphocytes. J Rheumatol 23:1011–1014

McCluskey J, Kanaan C, Diviney M (2017) Nomenclature and serology of HLA class I and class II alleles. Curr Protoc Immunol 118:A 1S 1–A 1S 6

Merkel PA, Xie G, Monach PA, Ji X, Ciavatta DJ, Byun J, Pinder BD, Zhao A, Zhang J, Tadesse Y, Qian D, Weirauch M, Nair R, Tsoi A, Pagnoux C, Carette S, Chung S, Cuthbertson D, Davis JC Jr, Dellaripa PF, Forbess L, Gewurz-Singer O, Hoffman GS, Khalidi N, Koening C, Langford CA, Mahr AD, McAlear C, Moreland L, Seo EP, Specks U, Spiera RF, Sreih A, St Clair EW, Stone JH, Ytterberg SR, Elder JT, Qu J, Ochi T, Hirano N, Edberg JC, Falk RJ, Amos CI, Siminovitch KA, Vasculitis Clinical Research C (2017) Identification of functional and expression polymorphisms associated with risk for antineutrophil cytoplasmic autoantibody-associated vasculitis. Arthritis Rheumatol 69:1054–106

Meyts I, Aksentijevich I (2018) Deficiency of adenosine deaminase 2 (DADA2): updates on the phenotype, genetics, pathogenesis, and treatment. J Clin Immunol 38:569–578

Miles LA, Parmer RJ (2013) Plasminogen receptors: the first quarter century. Semin Thromb Hemost 39:329–337

Millet A, Martin KR, Bonnefoy F, Saas P, Mocek J, Alkan M, Terrier B, Kerstein A, Tamassia N, Satyanarayanan SK, Ariel A, Ribeil JA, Guillevin L, Cassatella MA, Mueller A, Thieblemont N, Lamprecht P, Mouthon L, Perruche S, Witko-Sarsat V (2015) Proteinase 3 on apoptotic cells disrupts immune silencing in autoimmune vasculitis. J Clin Invest 125:4107–4121

Mizuki NMA, Ota M, Ohno S, Shiota T, Kawagoe T, Ito N, Kera J, Okada E, Yatsu K, Song YW, Lee EB, Kitaichi N, Namba K, Horie Y, Takeno M, Sugita S, Mochizuki M, Bahram S, Ishigatsubo Y, Inoko H (2010) Genome-wide association studies identify IL23R-IL12RB2 and IL10 as Behçet's disease susceptibility loci. Nat Genet 42:703–706

Moser TL, Stack MS, Asplin I, Enghild JJ, Hojrup P, Everitt L, Hubchak S, Schnaper HW, Pizzo SV (1999) Angiostatin binds ATP synthase on the surface of human endothelial cells. Proc Natl Acad Sci U S A 96:2811–2816

Myllyharju J (2003) Prolyl 4-hydroxylases, the key enzymes of collagen biosynthesis. Matrix Biol 22:15–24

Nagelkerke SQ TC, Breunis WB, Tanck MWT, Geissler J, Png E, Hoang LT, van der Heijden J, Naim ANM, Yeung RSM, Levin ML, Wright VJ, Burgner DP, Ponsonby AL, Ellis JA, Cimaz R, Shimizu C, Burns JC, Fijnvandraat K, van der Schoot CE, van den Berg TK, de Boer M, Davila S, Hibberd ML, Kuijpers TW, International Kawasaki Disease Genetics Consortium. (2019) Extensive ethnic variation and linkage disequilibrium at the FCGR2/3 locus: different genetic associations revealed in Kawasaki disease. Front Immunol 10

Nakazawa DMS, Tomaru U, Ishizu A (2019) Pathogenesis and therapeutic interventions for ANCA-associated vasculitis. Nat Rev Rheumatol 15:91–101

Nakazawa DSH, Kusunoki Y, Miyoshi A, Nishio S, Tomaru U, Atsumi T, Ishizu A (2016) The responses of macrophages in interaction with neutrophils that undergo NETosis. J Autoimmun 67:19–28

Navon Elkan P, Pierce SB, Segel R, Walsh T, Barash J, Padeh S, Zlotogorski A, Berkun Y, Press JJ, Mukamel M, Voth I, Hashkes PJ, Harel L, Hoffer V, Ling E, Yalcinkaya F, Kasapcopur O, Lee MK, Klevit RE, Renbaum P, Weinberg-Shukron A, Sener EF, Schormair B, Zeligson S, Marek-Yagel D, Strom TM, Shohat M, Singer A, Rubinow A, Pras E, Winkelmann J, Tekin M, Anikster Y, King MC, Levy-Lahad E (2014) Mutant adenosine deaminase 2 in a polyarteritis nodosa vasculopathy. N Engl J Med 370:921–931

Ni CRLQ, Xia Y, Wang GB, Yang J, FF L (2014) Regulatory T cell microRNA expression changes in children with acute Kawasaki disease. Clin Exp Immunol 178:384–393

Ombrello MJ, Kirino Y, de Bakker PI, Gul A, Kastner DL, Remmers EF (2014) Behcet disease-associated MHC class I residues implicate antigen binding and regulation of cell-mediated cytotoxicity. Proc Natl Acad Sci USA 111:8867–8872

Onouchi Y, Ozaki K, Buns JC, Shimizu C, Hamada H, Honda T, Terai M, Honda A, Takeuchi T, Shibuta S, Suenaga T, Suzuki H, Higashi K, Yasukawa K, Suzuki Y, Sasago K, Kemmotsu Y, Takatsuki S, Saji T, Yoshikawa T, Nagai T, Hamamoto K, Kishi F, Ouchi K, Sato Y, Newburger JW, Baker AL, Shulman ST, Rowley AH, Yashiro M, Nakamura Y, Wakui K, Fukushima Y, Fujino A, Tsunoda T, Kawasaki T, Hata A, Nakamura Y, Tanaka T (2010) Common variants in CASP3 confer susceptibility to Kawasaki disease. Hum Mol Genet 19:2898–2906

Onouchi Y, Ozaki K, Burns JC, Shimizu C, Terai M, Hamada H, Honda T, Suzuki H, Suenaga T, Takeuchi T, Yoshikawa N, Suzuki Y, Yasukawa K, Ebata R, Higashi K, Saji T, Kemmotsu Y, Takatsuki S, Ouchi K, Kishi F, Yoshikawa T, Nagai T, Hamamoto K, Sato Y, Honda A, Kobayashi H, Sato J, Shibuta S, Miyawaki M, Oishi K, Yamaga H, Aoyagi N, Iwahashi S, Miyashita R, Murata Y, Sasago K, Takahashi A, Kamatani N, Kubo M, Tsunoda T, Hata A, Nakamura Y, Tanaka T, Japan Kawasaki Disease Genome C, Consortium USKDG (2012) A genome-wide association study identifies three new risk loci for Kawasaki disease. Nat Genet 44:517–521

Onouchi YTM, Takahashi A, Tsunoda T, Yashiro M, Nakamura Y, Yanagawa H, Wakui K, Fukushima Y, Kawasaki T, Nakamura Y, Hata A (2007) A genome-wide linkage analysis of Kawasaki disease: evidence for linkage to chromosome 12. J Hum Genet 52:179–190

Ortiz-Fernández LC-JM, García-Lozano JR, Montes-Cano MA, Ortego-Centeno N, Castillo-Palma MJ, Espinosa G, Graña-Gil G, Sánchez-Bursón J, González-Gay MA, Barnosi-Marín AC, Solans R, Fanlo P, Rodríguez Carballeira M, Camps T, Castañeda S, Martín J, González-Escribano MF (2014) GIMAP and Behçet disease: no association in the European population. Ann Rheum Dis 73:1433–1434

Ortiz-Fernandez L, Garcia-Lozano JR, Montes-Cano MA, Conde-Jaldon M, Ortego-Centeno N, Garcia-Hernandez FJ, Espinosa G, Grana-Gil G, Sanchez-Burson J, Julia MR, Blanco R, Barnosi-Marin AC, Solans R, Fanlo P, Rodriguez Carballeira M, Camps T, Castaneda S, Martin J, Gonzalez-Escribano MF (2015) Lack of association of TNFAIP3 and JAK1 with Behcet's disease in the European population. Clin Exp Rheumatol 33:S36-39

Ozen S, Anton J, Arisoy N, Bakkaloglu A, Besbas N, Brogan P, Garcia-Consuegra J, Dolezalova P, Dressler F, Duzova A, Ferriani VP, Hilario MO, Ibanez-Rubio M, Kasapcopur O, Kuis W, Lehman TJ, Nemcova D, Nielsen S, Oliveira SK, Schikler K, Sztajnbok F, Terreri MT, Zulian F, Woo P (2004)

Juvenile polyarteritis: results of a multicenter survey of 110 children. J Pediatr 145:517–522
Ozen S, Ben-Chetrit E, Bakkaloglu A, Gur H, Tinaztepe K, Calguneri M, Turgan C, Turkmen A, Akpolat I, Danaci M, Besbas N, Akpolat T (2001) Polyarteritis nodosa in patients with Familial Mediterranean Fever (FMF): a concomitant disease or a feature of FMF? Semin Arthritis Rheum 30:281–287
Pearce FACA, Merkel PA, Luqmani RA, Watts RA (2017) Global ethnic and geographic differences in the clinical presentations of antineutrophil cytoplasm antibody-associated vasculitis. Rheumatology (oxford) 56:1962–1969
Pryshchep O, Ma-Krupa W, Younge BR, Goronzy JJ, Weyand CM (2008) Vessel-specific Toll-like receptor profiles in human medium and large arteries. Circulation 118:1276–1284
Rahmattulla C, Mooyaart AL, van Hooven D, Schoones JW, Bruijn JA, Dekkers OM, European Vasculitis Genetics C, Bajema IM (2016) Genetic variants in ANCA-associated vasculitis: a meta-analysis. Ann Rheum Dis 75:1687–1692
Remmers EF, Cosan F, Kirino Y, Ombrello MJ, Abaci N, Satorius C, Le JM, Yang B, Korman BD, Cakiris A, Aglar O, Emrence Z, Azakli H, Ustek D, Tugal-Tutkun I, Akman-Demir G, Chen W, Amos CI, Dizon MB, Kose AA, Azizlerli G, Erer B, Brand OJ, Kaklamani VG, Kaklamanis P, Ben-Chetrit E, Stanford M, Fortune F, Ghabra M, Ollier WE, Cho YH, Bang D, O'Shea J, Wallace GR, Gadina M, Kastner DL, Gul A (2010) Genome-wide association study identifies variants in the MHC class I, IL10, and IL23R-IL12RB2 regions associated with Behcet's disease. Nat Genet 42:698–702
Renauer PA, Saruhan-Direskeneli G, Coit P, Adler A, Aksu K, Keser G, Alibaz-Oner F, Aydin SZ, Kamali S, Inanc M, Carette S, Cuthbertson D, Hoffman GS, Akar S, Onen F, Akkoc N, Khalidi NA, Koening C, Karadag O, Kiraz S, Langford CA, Maksimowicz-McKinnon K, McAlear CA, Ozbalkan Z, Ates A, Karaaslan Y, Duzgun N, Monach PA, Ozer HT, Erken E, Ozturk MA, Yazici A, Cefle A, Onat AM, Kisacik B, Pagnoux C, Kasifoglu T, Seyahi E, Fresko I, Seo P, Sreih AG, Warrington KJ, Ytterberg SR, Cobankara V, Cunninghame-Graham DS, Vyse TJ, Pamuk ON, Tunc SE, Dalkilic E, Bicakcigil M, Yentur SP, Wren JD, Merkel PA, Direskeneli H, Sawalha AH (2015) Identification of susceptibility loci in IL6, RPS9/LILRB3, and an intergenic locus on chromosome 21q22 in Takayasu arteritis in a genome-wide association study. Arthritis Rheumatol 67:1361–1368
Robson JC, Kiran A, Maskell J, Hutchings A, Arden N, Dasgupta B, Hamilton W, Emin A, Culliford D, Luqmani RA (2015) The relative risk of aortic aneurysm in patients with giant cell arteritis compared with the general population of the UK. Ann Rheum Dis 74:129–135
Saadoun D, Garrido M, Comarmond C, Desbois AC, Domont F, Savey L, Terrier B, Geri G, Rosenzwajg M, Klatzmann D, Fourret P, Cluzel P, Chiche L, Gaudric J, Koskas F, Cacoub P (2015) Th1 and Th17 cytokines drive inflammation in Takayasu arteritis. Arthritis Rheumatol 67:1353–1360
Sahin Z BM, Aksu K, Kamali S, Akar S, Onen F, Karadag O, Ozbalkan Z, Ates A, Ozer HT, Yilmaz V, Seyahi E, Ozturk MA, Cefle A, Cobankara V, Onat AM, Tunc E, Düzgün N, Aydin SZ, Yilmaz N, Fresko İ, Karaaslan Y, Kiraz S, Akkoc N, Inanc M, Keser G, Uyar FA, Direskeneli H, Saruhan-Direskeneli G, Turkish Takayasu Study Group (2012) Takayasu's arteritis is associated with HLA-B*52, but not with HLA-B*51, in Turkey. Arthritis Res Ther 14
Sangaletti S, Tripodo C, Chiodoni C, Guarnotta C, Cappetti B, Casalini P, Piconese S, Parenza M, Guiducci C, Vitali C, Colombo MP (2012) Neutrophil extracellular traps mediate transfer of cytoplasmic neutrophil antigens to myeloid dendritic cells toward ANCA induction and associated autoimmunity. Blood 120:3007–3018
Saruhan-Direskeneli G, Hughes T, Aksu K, Keser G, Coit P, Aydin SZ, Alibaz-Oner F, Kamali S, Inanc M, Carette S, Hoffman GS, Akar S, Onen F, Akkoc N, Khalidi NA, Koening C, Karadag O, Kiraz S, Langford CA, McAlear CA, Ozbalkan Z, Ates A, Karaaslan Y, Maksimowicz-McKinnon K, Monach PA, Ozer HT, Seyahi E, Fresko I, Cefle A, Seo P, Warrington KJ, Ozturk MA, Ytterberg SR, Cobankara V, Onat AM, Guthridge JM, James JA, Tunc E, Duzgun N, Bicakcigil M, Yentur SP, Merkel PA, Direskeneli H, Sawalha AH (2013) Identification of multiple genetic susceptibility loci in Takayasu arteritis. Am J Hum Genet 93:298–305
Schepp J, Proietti M, Frede N, Buchta M, Hubscher K, Rojas Restrepo J, Goldacker S, Warnatz K, Pachlopnik Schmid J, Duppenthaler A, Lougaris V, Uriarte I, Kelly S, Hershfield M, Grimbacher B (2017) Screening of 181 patients With antibody deficiency for deficiency of adenosine deaminase 2 sheds new light on the disease in adulthood. Arthritis Rheumatol 69:1689–1700
Schreiber A, Xiao H, Falk RJ, Jennette JC (2006) Bone marrow-derived cells are sufficient and necessary targets to mediate glomerulonephritis and vasculitis induced by anti-myeloperoxidase antibodies. J Am Soc Nephrol 17:3355–3364
Serrano A, Carmona FD, Castaneda S, Solans R, Hernandez-Rodriguez J, Cid MC, Prieto-Gonzalez S, Miranda-Filloy JA, Rodriguez-Rodriguez L, Morado IC, Gomez-Vaquero C, Blanco R, Sopena B, Ortego-Centeno N, Unzurrunzaga A, Mari-Alfonso B, Sanchez-Martin J, Garcia-Villanueva MJ, Hidalgo-Conde A, Pazzola G, Boiardi L, Salvarani C, Gonzalez-Gay MA, Martin J (2013) Evidence of association of the NLRP1 gene with giant cell arteritis. Ann Rheum Dis 72:628–630
Serrano AMA, Mackie SL, Carmona FD, Solans R, Miranda-Filloy JA, Hernández-Rodríguez J, Cid MC, Castañeda S, Morado IC, Narváez J, Blanco R,

Sopeña B, García-Villanueva MJ, Monfort J, Ortego-Centeno N, Unzurrunzaga A, Marí-Alfonso B, Sánchez Martín J, de Miguel E, Magro C, Raya E, UK GCA Consortium; Spanish GCA Consortium, Braun N, Latus J, Molberg O, Lie BA, Moosig F, Witte T, Morgan AW, González-Gay MA, Martín J (2013) Identification of the PTPN22 functional variant R620W as susceptibility genetic factor for giant cell arteritis. Ann Rheum Dis 72:1882–1886

Shimizu CEH, Wright VJ, Kim J, Alphonse MP, Perry JC, Cimaz R, Burgner D, Dahdah N, Hoang LT, Khor CC, Salgado A, Tremoulet AH, Davila S, Kuijpers TW, Hibberd ML, Johnson TA, Takahashi A, Tsunoda T, Kubo M, Tanaka T, Onouchi Y, Yeung RS, Coin LJ, Levin M, Burns JC, International Kawasaki Disease Genetics Consortium (2016) Genetic variation in the SLC8A1 calcium signaling pathway is associated with susceptibility to Kawasaki disease and coronary artery abnormalities. Circ Cardiovasc Genet 9:559–568

Shimojima Y, Ishii W, Kishida D, Fukushima K, Ikeda SI (2017) Imbalanced expression of dysfunctional regulatory T cells and T-helper cells relates to immunopathogenesis in polyarteritis nodosa. Mod Rheumatol 27:102–109

Simpfendorfer KR, Armstead BE, Shih A, Li W, Curran M, Manjarrez-Orduno N, Lee AT, Diamond B, Gregersen PK (2015) Autoimmune disease-associated haplotypes of BLK exhibit lowered thresholds for B cell activation and expansion of Ig class-switched B cells. Arthritis Rheumatol 67:2866–2876

Song RLG, Li X, Xu W, Liu J, Jin H (2015) Elevated inducible nitric oxide levels and decreased hydrogen sulfide levels can predict the risk of coronary artery ectasia in Kawasaki disease. Pediatr Cardiol 37:322–329

Stone JH (2002) Polyarteritis nodosa. JAMA 288:1632–1639

Sunderkötter CH, Zelger B, Chen KR, Requena L, Piette W, Carlson JA, Dutz J, Lamprecht P, Mahr A, Aberer E (2018) Nomenclature of cutaneous vasculitis: dermatologic addendum to the 2012 revised international Chapel Hill consensus conference nomenclature of vasculitides. Arthritis Rheumatol 70:171–184

Sunderkotter CH, Zelger B, Chen KR, Requena L, Piette W, Carlson JA, Dutz J, Lamprecht P, Mahr A, Aberer E, Werth VP, Wetter DA, Kawana S, Luqmani R, Frances C, Jorizzo J, Watts JR, Metze D, Caproni M, Alpsoy E, Callen JP, Fiorentino D, Merkel PA, Falk RJ, Jennette JC (2018) Nomenclature of cutaneous vasculitis: dermatologic addendum to the 2012 revised international Chapel Hill consensus conference nomenclature of vasculitides. Arthritis Rheumatol 70:171–184

Suzuki HFR, Zhang Z, Brown R, Hall S, Julian BA, Chatham WW, Suzuki Y, Wyatt RJ, Moldoveanu Z, Lee JY, Robinson J, Tomana M, Tomino Y, Mestecky J, Novak J (2009) Aberrantly glycosylated IgA1 in IgA nephropathy patients is recognized by IgG antibodies with restricted heterogeneity. J Clin Invest 119:1668–1677

Suzuki HKK, Novak J, Moldoveanu Z, Herr AB, Renfrow MB, Wyatt RJ, Scolari F, Mestecky J, Gharavi AG, Julian BA (2011) The pathophysiology of IgA nephropathy. J Am Soc Nephrol 22:1795–1803

Takahashi K, Oharaseki T, Yokouchi Y (2014) Update on etio and immunopathogenesis of Kawasaki disease. Curr Opin Rheumatol 26:31–36

Takeuchi M, Mizuki N, Meguro A, Ombrello MJ, Kirino Y, Satorius C, Le J, Blake M, Erer B, Kawagoe T, Ustek D, Tugal-Tutkun I, Seyahi E, Ozyazgan Y, Sousa I, Davatchi F, Francisco V, Shahram F, Abdollahi BS, Nadji A, Shafiee NM, Ghaderibarmi F, Ohno S, Ueda A, Ishigatsubo Y, Gadina M, Oliveira SA, Gul A, Kastner DL, Remmers EF (2017) Dense genotyping of immune-related loci implicates host responses to microbial exposure in Behcet's disease susceptibility. Nat Genet 49:438–443

Terao C, Yoshifuji H, Kimura A, Matsumura T, Ohmura K, Takahashi M, Shimizu M, Kawaguchi T, Chen Z, Naruse TK, Sato-Otsubo A, Ebana Y, Maejima Y, Kinoshita H, Murakami K, Kawabata D, Wada Y, Narita I, Tazaki J, Kawaguchi Y, Yamanaka H, Yurugi K, Miura Y, Maekawa T, Ogawa S, Komuro I, Nagai R, Yamada R, Tabara Y, Isobe M, Mimori T, Matsuda F (2013) Two susceptibility loci to Takayasu arteritis reveal a synergistic role of the IL12B and HLA-B regions in a Japanese population. Am J Hum Genet 93:289–297

Terao C, Yoshifuji H, Matsumura T, Naruse TK, Ishii T, Nakaoka Y, Kirino Y, Matsuo K, Origuchi T, Shimizu M, Maejima Y, Amiya E, Tamura N, Kawaguchi T, Takahashi M, Setoh K, Ohmura K, Watanabe R, Horita T, Atsumi T, Matsukura M, Miyata T, Kochi Y, Suda T, Tanemoto K, Meguro A, Okada Y, Ogimoto A, Yamamoto M, Takahashi H, Nakayamada S, Saito K, Kuwana M, Mizuki N, Tabara Y, Ueda A, Komuro I, Kimura A, Isobe M, Mimori T, Matsuda F (2018) Genetic determinants and an epistasis of LILRA3 and HLA-B*52 in Takayasu arteritis. Proc Natl Acad Sci USA 115:13045–13050

Terao C, Yoshifuji H, Mimori T (2014) Recent advances in Takayasu arteritis. Int J Rheum Dis 17:238–247

Tsai FJ, Lee YC, Chang JS, Huang LM, Huang FY, Chiu NC, Chen MR, Chi H, Lee YJ, Chang LC, Liu YM, Wang HH, Chen CH, Chen YT, Wu JY (2011) Identification of novel susceptibility Loci for kawasaki disease in a Han chinese population by a genome-wide association study. PLoS One 6:e16853.

Wallace G (2014) HLA-B*51 the primary risk in Behçet disease. Proc Natl Acad Sci USA 111:8706–8707

Wang Y, Wang W, Gong F, Fu S, Zhang Q, Hu J, Qi Y, Xie C, Zhang Y (2013) Evaluation of intravenous immunoglobulin resistance and coronary artery lesions in relation to Th1/Th2 cytokine profiles in patients with Kawasaki disease. Arthritis Rheum 65:805–814

Watanabe R, Maeda T, Zhang H, Berry GJ, Zeisbrich M, Brockett R, Greenstein AE, Tian L, Goronzy JJ,

Weyand CM (2018) MMP (Matrix Metalloprotease)-9-producing monocytes enable T cells to invade the vessel wall and cause vasculitis. Circ Res 123:700–715

Wen XCS, Li J, Li Y, Li L, Wu Z, Yuan H, Tian X, Zhang F, Li Y (2018) Association between genetic variants in the human leukocyte antigen-B/MICA and Takayasu arteritis in Chinese Han population. Int J Rheum Dis 21:271–277

Wen Z, Shen Y, Berry G, Shahram F, Li Y, Watanabe R, Liao YJ, Goronzy JJ, Weyand CM (2017) The microvascular niche instructs T cells in large vessel vasculitis via the VEGF-Jagged1-Notch pathway. Sci Transl Med 9

Wen Z, Shimojima Y, Shirai T, Li Y, Ju J, Yang Z, Tian L, Goronzy JJ, Weyand CM (2016) NADPH oxidase deficiency underlies dysfunction of aged CD8 + Tregs. J Clin Invest 126:1953–1967

Weyand CM, Goronzy JJ (2013) Immune mechanisms in medium and large-vessel vasculitis. Nat Rev Rheumatol 9:731–740

Weyand CM, Goronzy JJ (2014) Clinical practice. Giant-cell arteritis and polymyalgia rheumatica. N Engl J Med 371:50–57

Weyand CM, Watanabe R, Zhang H, Akiyama M, Berry GJ, Goronzy JJ (2019) Cytokines, growth factors and proteases in medium and large vessel vasculitis. Clin Immunol 206:33–41

Xiao H, Heeringa P, Hu P, Liu Z, Zhao M, Aratani Y, Maeda N, Falk RJ, Jennette JC (2002) Antineutrophil cytoplasmic autoantibodies specific for myeloperoxidase cause glomerulonephritis and vasculitis in mice. J Clin Invest 110:955–963

Xiao H, Schreiber A, Heeringa P, Falk RJ, Jennette JC (2007) Alternative complement pathway in the pathogenesis of disease mediated by anti-neutrophil cytoplasmic autoantibodies. Am J Pathol 170:52–64

Xie G, Roshandel D, Sherva R, Monach PA, Lu EY, Kung T, Carrington K, Zhang SS, Pulit SL, Ripke S, Carette S, Dellaripa PF, Edberg JC, Hoffman GS, Khalidi N, Langford CA, Mahr AD, St Clair EW, Seo P, Specks U, Spiera RF, Stone JH, Ytterberg SR, Raychaudhuri S, de Bakker PI, Farrer LA, Amos CI, Merkel PA, Siminovitch KA (2013) Association of granulomatosis with polyangiitis (Wegener's) with HLA-DPB1*04 and SEMA6A gene variants: evidence from genome-wide analysis. Arthritis Rheum 65:2457–2468

Xie X, Shi X, Liu M (2018) The roles of genetic factors in Kawasaki disease: a systematic review and meta-analysis of genetic association studies. Pediatr Cardiol 39:207–225

Yalçinkaya FOZ, Kasapçopur O, Oztürk A, Akar N, Bakkaloğlu A, Arisoy N, Ekim M, Ozen S (2007) J Pediatr 151:675–678

Yan Y, Ma Y, Liu Y, Hu H, Shen Y, Zhang S, Ma Y, Tao D, Wu Q, Peng Q, Yang Y (2013) Combined analysis of genome-wide-linked susceptibility loci to Kawasaki disease in Han Chinese. Hum Genet 132:669–680

Yazici HSE, Hatemi G, Yazici Y (2018) Behçet syndrome: a contemporary view. Nat Rev Rheumatol 14:119

Yoshida M, Kimura A, Katsuragi K, Numano F, Sasazuki T (1993) DNA typing of HLA-B gene in Takayasu's arteritis. Tissue Antigens 42:87–90

Yu H, Du L, Yi S, Wang Q, Zhu Y, Qiu Y, Jiang Y, Li M, Wang D, Wang Q, Yuan G, Cao Q, Kijlstra A, Yang P (2019) Epigenome-wide association study identifies Behcet's disease-associated methylation loci in Han Chinese. Rheumatology (oxford) 58:1574–1584

Zavialov AVGE, Glaichenhaus N, Franco R, Zavialov AV, Lauvau G (2010) Human adenosine deaminase 2 induces differentiation of monocytes into macrophages and stimulates proliferation of T helper cells and macrophages. J Leukoc Biol 88:279–290

Zhang H, Watanabe R, Berry GJ, Vaglio A, Liao YJ, Warrington KJ, Goronzy JJ, Weyand CM (2017) Immunoinhibitory checkpoint deficiency in medium and large vessel vasculitis. Proc Natl Acad Sci USA 114:E970–E979

Zhang J, Zahir N, Jiang Q, Miliotis H, Heyraud S, Meng X, Dong B, Xie G, Qiu F, Hao Z, McCulloch CA, Keystone EC, Peterson AC, Siminovitch KA (2011) The autoimmune disease-associated PTPN22 variant promotes calpain-mediated Lyp/Pep degradation associated with lymphocyte and dendritic cell hyperresponsiveness. Nat Genet 43:902–907

Zhou Q, Yang D, Ombrello AK, Zavialov AV, Toro C, Zavialov AV, Stone DL, Chae JJ, Rosenzweig SD, Bishop K, Barron KS, Kuehn HS, Hoffmann P, Negro A, Tsai WL, Cowen EW, Pei W, Milner JD, Silvin C, Heller T, Chin DT, Patronas NJ, Barber JS, Lee CC, Wood GM, Ling A, Kelly SJ, Kleiner DE, Mullikin JC, Ganson NJ, Kong HH, Hambleton S, Candotti F, Quezado MM, Calvo KR, Alao H, Barham BK, Jones A, Meschia JF, Worrall BB, Kasner SE, Rich SS, Goldbach-Mansky R, Abinun M, Chalom E, Gotte AC, Punaro M, Pascual V, Verbsky JW, Torgerson TR, Singer NG, Gershon TR, Ozen S, Karadag O, Fleisher TA, Remmers EF, Burgess SM, Moir SL, Gadina M, Sood R, Hershfield MS, Boehm M, Kastner DL, Aksentijevich I (2014) Early-onset stroke and vasculopathy associated with mutations in ADA2. N Engl J Med 370:911–920

The Immunogenetics of Behcet's Disease

Mustafa Anıl Yılmaz and Ümit Türsen

Abstract

Behcet's disease (BD) is an autoimmune disorder that affects the blood vessels and thus could entangle virtually every organ of the body. Oral ulceration, genital aphthous lesions, and ocular inflammation are the main manifestations of the disease that tend to have a chronic, relapsing–remitting course. The disease comes from an association between environmental and genetic backgrounds. The clustering of cases in families and the high rate of co-occurrence of the disease in siblings were the initial findings that proposed a genetic basis for BD. Later on, multiple case–control studies and genome-wide association studies were able to clarify particular genes included in the etiopathogenesis of BD. The major gene polymorphisms include HLA and HLA-related genes, interleukins, and other genes involved in inflammation and transcription activation. Herein we have summarized the susceptibility genes that are associated with BD. Investigations on the genetics of BD could potentially clarify the disease pathogenesis and provide insights for the development of better treatments.

Keywords

Behcet's disease · Immunogenetics · Single nucleotide polymorphism · Pathogenesis · GWAS

1 Introduction

Behcet's disease (BD) is a multi-systemic, immune-mediated disorder, marked by chronic, relapsing–remitting oral exulcerations, genital aphthous lesions, and eye lesions (Fig. 1) (Behcet 1937). It is more prevalent in the middle east, the Mediterranean region, and eastern Asia. Turkey has one of the highest prevalence of BD in the world with 110–420 cases in every 100,000 residents (Azizlerli et al. 2003). Although the etiology of BD is unknown, it is proposed to be related to exogen etiologic factors, ranging from contagious microorganisms to environmental pollution as opposed to a setting of genetic sensitivity (Taheri et al. 2015). Familial studies have been able to provide some evidence for the involvement of genetics in the pathogenesis of BD. Gül. et al. Was the first to quantify this association by showing a recurrence risk of 11.4–52.5 in siblings of those affected in different populations within Turkey (Gül et al. 2000). Among several candidate genes suspected to cause BD, *HLA-B51* has the most significant association with the disease occurrence (Demirseren et al. 2014). It has been reported that

M. A. Yılmaz · Ü. Türsen (✉)
Department of Dermatology, Mersin University, Mersin, Turkey
e-mail: utursen@mersin.edu.tr

N. Rezaei and F. Rajabi (eds.), *The Immunogenetics of Dermatologic Diseases*, Advances in Experimental Medicine and Biology 1367,
https://doi.org/10.1007/978-3-030-92616-8_12

carriers of *HLA-B51* are almost 5 times more likely to start Behçet syndrome compared to non-carriers (O.R 5.8) (Menthon et al. 2009). This allele accounts for about 19% of the heritability of BD among siblings highlighting the importance of other non-MHC genes (Gül et al. 2001). In addition, genome-wide association studies (GWAS) have linked Behçet disease to polymorphisms in genes encoding cytokines, activator factors, and chemokines (Puccetti et al. 2018). The major gene polymorphisms linked with BD consist of HLAs (*HLA-B* and *HLA-A*), HLA related genes (*CIITA, ERAP1*, and *MICA*), interleukins (*IL33, IL10, IL12A, IL12RB2*, and *IL23R*), pattern recognition receptors and transcription factors (*MEFV, STAT4, IRF8, TNFAIP3, REL, TLR4, NOD1, NOD2, KLRC4, NCOA5*, and *FOXP3*), chemokine and chempkine receptors (*CCR1* and *CCR3*), and several other unclassified genes (*FUT2, ADO-EGR2, UBAC2, SUMO4, JPKL-CNTN5*, and *CEBPB-PTPN1*) (Deng et al. 2018; Talei et al. 2019) (Fig. 2).

2 HLA and HLA-Related Genes

The HLA-B51 is a split-antigens of the greater HLA-B5 serotype (Sugisaki et al. 2005). Even in high-risk populations, the *HLA-B51* gene has a significantly higher prevalence (50–72%) in individuals with BD compared to healthy controls (10–15%) (Maldini et al. 2012). Male patients with BD are more likely to harbor the HLA-B51 allele than females (Maldini et al. 2012). As mentioned earlier *HLA-B51* is the most powerful genetic predictor of BD accounting for about 20% of the heritability of the disease in various reports from different ethnic backgrounds (Deng et al. 2018). The HLA-B*51 belongs to the class I major histocompatibility complex (MHC) and thus binds and presents 8–11 amino acid long peptides to CD8+ T-cells (Sakaguchi and Takiguchi 1997). The spontaneous activation of HLA-B51-positive neutrophils promotes a T-helper 1 (Th1) dominant immune reaction that leads to perivascular tissue injury (Eksioglu-Demiralp et al. 2001; Takeno et al. 1995). HLA-

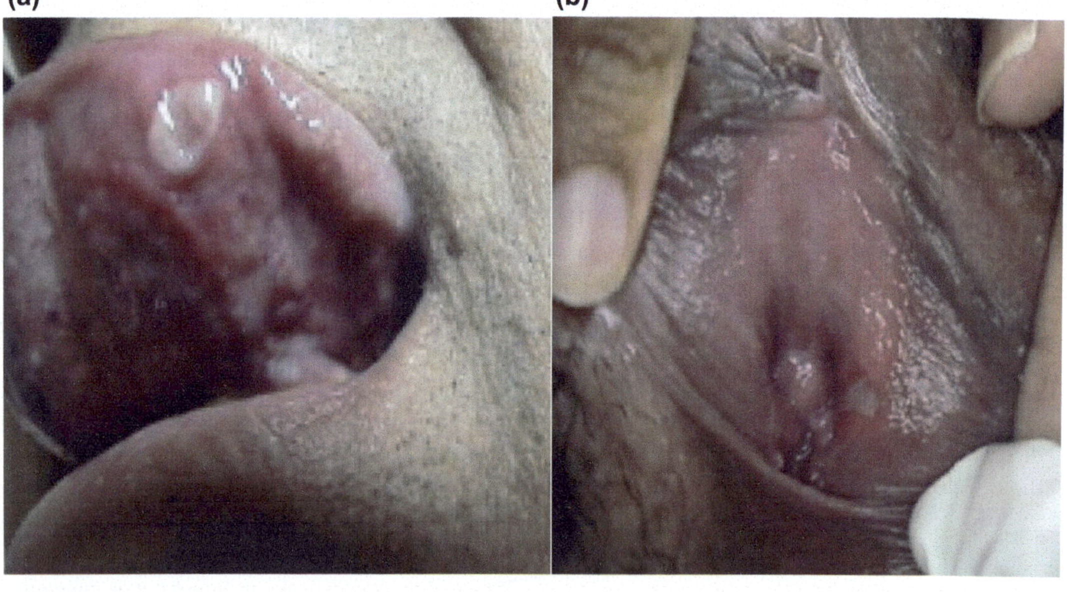

Fig. 1 Clinical findings in Behcet's disease. **a** Oral aphthous lesions. **b** Genital ulcers

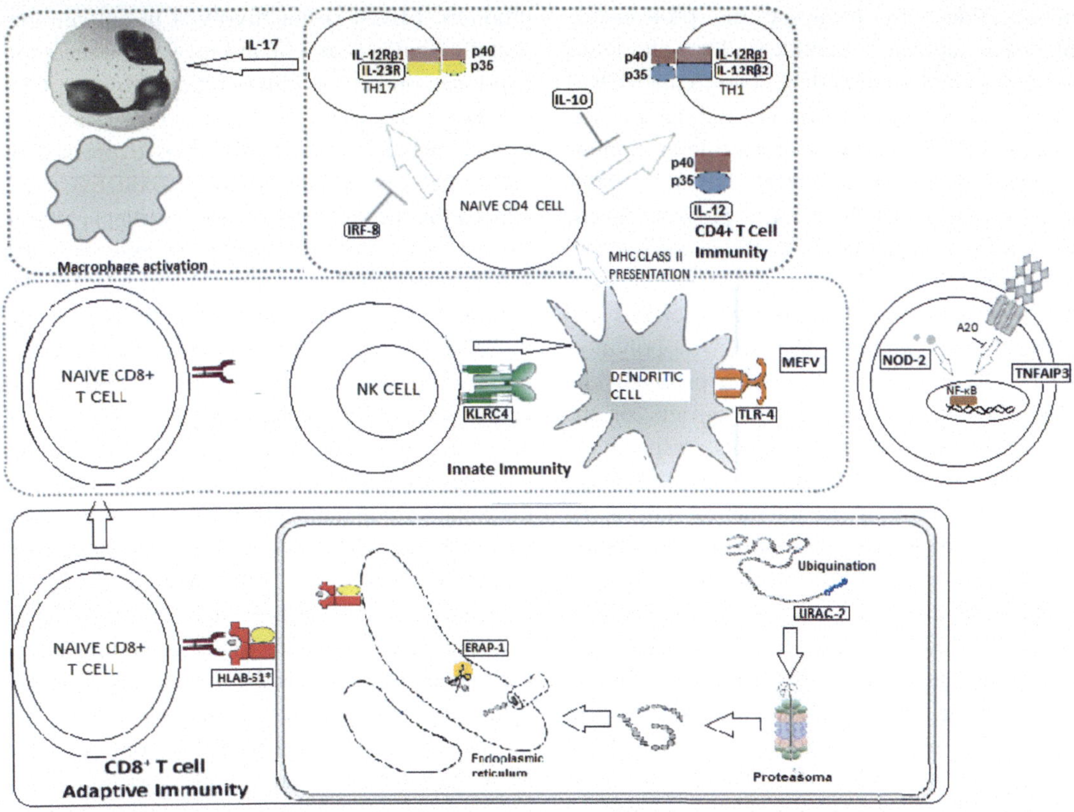

Fig. 2 The immunopathogenesis of Behcet's disease

B51 can interfere with T-cell responses as apparent from the difference in the dominant gamma-delta T-cells type in patients with and without this HLA. Both Vd1 (CD5-/dull, CD28-, and CD57+) and Vd2 (CD5+, CD28+, and CD57-) gamma-delta T-cells have a significantly higher in vivo activity in individuals with active BD disease whereas only Vd1 gamma-delta T-cells show an over proportional activity in HLAB51 positive patients (Yasuoka et al. 2008). The Vd1 cells are a subset of memory T-cells that can mature independent of the thymus.

The HLA-B51A positivity also possesses some prognostic value as it has been shown that carriers of this allele have a higher risk of genital ulcers and ocular complications (Maldini et al. 2012). *HLA-A*26* is another allele found to be linked with BD in Taiwanese, Greek, Japanese, South Korean, Saudi Arabian, Turk patients (Al-Okaily et al. 2016; Chung et al. 1990; Kamiishi et al. 2008; Mizuki et al. 1997; Nakamura et al. 2019; Ombrello et al. 2014). Prognostic value has been attributed to *HLA-A*26* with Japanese and South Korean BD carriers of this allele having a higher risk of eye involvement (Hughes et al. 2013; Kang et al. 2011, 2013). The *HLA-A02, HLA-A24, HLA-A26, HLA-A31, HLA-B27, HLA-B57* confer susceptibility to BD and *HLA-A03, HLA-B15, HLA-B35, HLA-B49, HLA-B58* confer protection from developing BD in different populations (Al-Okaily et al. 2016; Giza et al. 2018; Kaburaki et al. 2010; Meguro et al. 2010; Mizuki et al. 1997; Montes-Cano et al. 2013; Ortiz-Fernández et al. 2016; Takeuchi et al. 2015).

The endoplasmic reticulum aminopeptidase-1 (ERAP1)

The *ERAP1* gene is located at 5q15 (Amirzargar et al. 2010). It encodes a protein that serves as an aminopeptidase by trimming the proteasome-processed antigenic peptides. The shortened antigenic peptides could then bond to the MHC-I groove and be expressed on the cellular surface. Thus the ERAP1 has an essential role in immune responses (Rock et al. 2004). Several studies have suggested that the *ERAP1* polymorphisms might have interactions with disease-associated HLA alleles. These gene–gene interactions have been reported in diseases such as psoriasis and ankylosing spondylitis. The *ERAP1* polymorphisms affect the susceptibility to psoriasis and ankylosing spondylitis only in carriers of the *HLA-C*06* and *HLA-B*27* alleles, respectively (Burton et al. 2007; Evans et al. 2011; Strange et al. 2010). This epistatic interaction reflects the role of peptide loading and antigen presentation in the pathogenesis of autoimmune disease (Cortes et al. 2015; Kirino et al. 2013). The BD-associated low activity *ERAP1* variant (p. Arg725Gln) generates longer length peptides, an increase in the sub-peptidome with p2 Pro peptides, and a peptide-pool (peptidome) with an overall lower affinity for HLA-B*51. This achieves understandable proof for the outcome of disease-associated *ERAP1* allotypes on altering the peptide repertoire in individuals carrying HLA-B*51. An ERAP-BD association has been shown in a Chinese cohort and further confirmed in the analysis of the Turkish and Spanish cohorts (Zhang et al. 2015). Iranian cohorts have linked another *ERAP1* variant, rs30187 T allele homozygotes (Arg528Lys), to BD susceptibility. This variant also acts through epistatic interactions with the *HLA-B*51* (Conde-Jaldón et al. 2014; Kirino et al. 2013; Mahmoudi et al. 2018). Kirino et al. (Ortiz-Fernández et al. 2016) revealed that in the Turkish population, the p. Arg725Gln (rs17482078) polymorphism of the *ERAP1* gene, had a higher association with BD in *HLA-B*51* positive individuals compared to those negative for *HLA-B*51* (odds ratio 3.78 versus 1.48, respectively).

MICA

The *MHC-I chain-related gene A* (*MICA*) gene located at the 46 kb centromeric region of *HLA-B*, carries six exons. Unlike HLA class I gene products, MICA is not involved in antigen presentation but acts as a ligand for several receptors expressed on natural killer cells (NK cells), CD8 + T cells, and γδT cells bearing NKG2D receptors (Groh et al. 1998). MICA is expressed on cell surfaces in response to major oxidative stress and facilitates cell destruction by innate immunity. A polymorphism located in exon 5 of the *MICA* gene has at least five alleles, A4, A5, A6, A9, and A5.1, reflecting the number of the (GCT/AGC) repeats (Mizuki et al. 1997). *MICA* has another 102 alleles that result from single nucleotide polymorphisms (SNP) in exons 2, 3, and 4. Susceptibility to BD has been linked to the presence of the *MICA*009* and **019* alleles in the Spanish population (Muñoz-Saá et al. 2006) and with the *MICA-A6* allele in Japanese individuals (Mizuki et al. 1997; Wei et al. 2016). A Korean study showed that the association between *MICA-A6* and BD was significant in individuals negative for *HLA-B51* and thus confirmed the independence of this association from the linkage disequilibrium (LD) present in the MHC region (Park et al. 2002). A meta-analysis published in 2016 also confirmed this association with a pooled OR of 2.34, despite the heterogeneity among different ethnic groups (Zhang et al. 2016).

3 Interleukin Gens

IL-10

The *interleukin-10* (*IL-10*) gene, located 1q21-32, has five exons and four introns. This interleukin plays a key regulatory role in inflammatory responses and is produced by T helper-2 cells (Th2), regulatory T cells (Treg), and to a lesser extent monocyte. IL-10 inhibits antigen presentation by lowering the expression of HLA molecules on cellular surfaces and reduces Th1 activity by reducing the expression of co-stimulatory molecules (Ozbey et al. 2009). A GWA study reported numerous BD-associated variants including the rs1800872, the rs1518111, the rs1554286, and the rs1800871 within the *IL-10* gene in Chinese, Turkish, Japanese, Korean, and Iranian populations (Afkari et al. 2018; Hu et al. 2015; Mizuki et al. 2010; Remmers et al. 2010; Wallace et al. 2007).

IL-12

IL-12 is a pro-inflammatory cytokine that promotes Th1 differentiation and function (Teng et al. 2015). IL-12 is made up of two particles, a 35 kD chain encoded by the *p35* (*IL-12A*) gene and a 40 kD chain coded by the *p40* (*IL-12B*) gene (Hall et al. 2000). IL-12 attaches to its heterodimeric receptor that is also made up of two particles, IL-12Rβ1 and IL-12Rβ2 (coded by *IL-12RB1* and *IL-12RB2* genes respectively) (Watford et al. 2004). The *IL-12A* rs1780546 variant has been linked to BD in both Turkish and European populations (Kappen et al. 2015).

IL-23R and IL-12RB2

The IL-23 is another dimeric pro-inflammatory cytokine with two subunits, p19 and p40 (Goff et al. 2010). Unlike IL-12 that promotes the differentiation of Th1 cells and the secretion interferon- γ (IFNγ), IL-23 is involved in the Th17 differentiation especially when transforming growth factor β (TGF-β) and IL-6 are present in the milieu. IL-23 also stimulates antigen presentation by dendritic cells (Bettelli et al. 2006; Langrish et al. 2005).

The β1 subunit of the IL-12 receptor (IL-12Rβ1) is present in both IL-12 and IL-23 signaling complexes, IL-12Rβ1/IL-12Rβ2 and IL-12Rβ1/IL-23R, respectively (Presky et al. 1996). STAT molecules only bind to the intracellular sections of IL-12Rβ2 and IL-23R and have no interactions with IL-12Rβ1. As a result, authors have shown it to be the only signal-relaying component of the IL-12 and IL-23 receptors (Collison and Vignali 2008). A GWAS identified *IL- 23R* SNP rs17375018 to be linked with BD in Turkish patients (Yalçin et al. 2014). In addition, multiple SNPs within the *IL-23R* and *IL-12RB2* genes including the rs11209032, rs1495965, 10,489,629, rs924080, rs17375018, rs7517847, and rs1966176 were linked to BD in the Turkish (Remmers et al. 2010), Japanese (Mizuki et al. 2010), Chinese (Han) (Qin et al. 2016; Yu et al. 2017), Iranian (Xavier et al. 2012), Western Algerian (Khaib Dit Naib et al. 2013), and Korean patients (Kang et al. 2017).

IL-33

IL-33 is a member of the IL-1 superfamily and is involved in both innate and adaptive immune responses (Liew et al. 2010). IL-33 stimulates the production of both IL-2 via dendritic cells and IL-4, IL-5, IL-6, and IL-13 via Th2 cells. It can also stimulate CD8+ T lymphocytes and contribute to the expansion of serum stimulation-2 positive (ST2+) Treg cells. The presence of the ST2 receptor on the surfaces of NK cells, mast cells, and basophils makes them reactive to IL-33 (Çerçi et al. 2017). The *IL-33* rs1342326 T/G SNP which affects gene expression has been shown to confer susceptibility to BD in Iranian patients (Talei et al. 2019).

4 Other Immune-Related Genes

Mediterranean fever (*MEFV*)

The *MEVF* gene encodes a protein of 781 amino acid protein known as pyrin responsible for the induction of Familial Mediterranean Fever (FMF). Pyrin is primarily expressed in the myeloid cells and promotes the excessive production of IL-1β (Centola et al. 2000). Multiple studies confirmed the association of *MEFV* mutations, M694V and M680I, with BD (pooled OR: 2.60 and pooled OR: 1.74) (Esmaeili et al. 2011; Kirino et al. 2013; Tasliyurt et al. 2013; Wu et al. 2015).

IRF8

IRF8, a member of the IRF family21 proteins attaches to the IFN-stimulated response element (ISRE) and controls the translation of genes induced by type I IFNs (IFNα and IFNβ) (Lee et al. 2006; Tsujimura et al. 2003; Zhao et al. 2006). It is the main modulator of numerous features of dendritic cell development, differentiation, and function (Gabriele and Ozato 2007) and an important transcriptional inhibitor for the differentiation of Th17 cells (Ouyang et al. 2011). The rs17445836 and rs11642873 SNPs of the *IRF8* gene have been linked to susceptibility to BD in a Chinese report. The risk variants of these SNPs seem to affect *IRF8* gene expression and thus the subsequent cytokine production (Jiang et al. 2016). The *IRF8* rs11117433, rs142105922, and rs7203487 were also linked to susceptibility to BD in the patients with Turkish, Iranian, and Japanese ancestry (Takeuchi et al. 2017).

TNFAIP3

TNFα induced protein 3 (TNF/AIP3), also called A20, is a 790 amino acid peptide encoded by the *TNFAIP3* gene. A20 is a ubiquitinating enzyme that is capable of inhibiting the NF-κB pathway. The absence of A20 promotes IL1β production (Oda and Kastner 2017).

Loss-of-function mutations of the *TNFAIP3* gene cause a monogenic disease known as haploinsufficiency of A20 (HA20) which was formerly categorized as a clinical subtype of BD. Recent studies have classified HA20 as an NF-kB-mediated autoinflammatory disease. HA20 differs from classical BD in the age of onset (occurring in early childhood instead of adulthood), the prominence of gastrointestinal involvement, and the presence of recurrent fevers (Aeschlimann et al. 2018; Berteau et al. 2018).

The rs9494885, rs7753873, and rs10499194 SNPs of the *TNFAIP3* gene have been associated with BD in the Han Chinese patients (Li et al. 2012), but not in the European individuals (Ortiz-Fernández et al. 2015).

REL

The *REL* gene located at 2p16.1 codes a member of the NF-κB family known as c-Rel (Chen et al. 2011). The c-Rel is responsible for regulating the transcription of genes involved in antigen presentation, CD40 signaling, and T-cell development. Its expression is confined to mature hematopoietic cells (Lamhamedi-Cherradi et al. 2003).

The GG genotype of the *REL* rs842647 SNP and the G allele of the rs842647 SNP were founded to confer risk to BD, with the latter also conferring susceptibility to cutaneous complication (Chen et al. 2016).

5 Toll-Like Receptors

Toll-like receptors (TLRs) are non-specific innate immune receptors that have a crucial role in the protection against external antigens. They are defined by their capability to reply to attacked microorganisms urgently by recognizing special microbial patterns, including flagellin, lipopolysaccharides (LPS), nucleic acids derived from virus and bacteria, and zymosan of fungi (Takeuchi et al. 2002).

The *TLR4* gene has been linked to BD in multiple studies from Japan, Korea, China, and Turkey patients. However, studies on Italian and Tunisian patients failed to replicate these findings (Ben Dhifallah et al. 2009; Boiardi et al. 2009; Fang et al. 2013; Horie et al. 2009; Meguro et al. 2007).

Nucleotide-binding and oligomerization domain-containing proteins (NOD)

The NOD1 and NOD2 are two intracellular pattern recognition receptors belonging to the nucleotide-binding oligomerization (NOD)-like receptor (NLR) family (Chamaillard et al. 2003).

NOD1 recognizes epitopes unique to peptidoglycans originated from bacteria (mostly Gram-negative and some forms of Gram-positive). NOD2 responds to muramyl dipeptide (MDP) which is also a type of bacterial peptidoglycan (Girardin 2003). These proteins are encoded by the *NOD1/ CARD4* and *NOD2/CARD15* genes, mapping on chromosome 7p14.3 and 16q12.1 respectively (Kawai and Akira 2009). NOD2 variants have been linked to BD (Ahmad et al. 2005; Burillo-Sanz et al. 2017).

Lately, *NOD1* was also shown as a BD-linked gene, in which the less frequent G allele of *NOD1* rs2075818 was remarkably diminished in Chinese patients with BD (Li et al. 2016).

CCR1-CCR3

C–C chemokine receptor type 1 (*CCR1*) and *CCR3* code for G protein-coupled chemokine receptors. They show a crucial contribution in the aggregation and stimulation of inflammatory cells (Marzio et al. 2005; Penido et al. 2001;

Saeki and Naya 2003). The rs7616215 SNP within the *CCR1-CCR3* locus was first reported to be linked with BD in a GWAS conducted in Turkey (Remmers et al. 2010). A later study of the Chinese patients showed a powerful linkage between BD and rs13084057, rs13092160, and rs13075270 SNPs within the *CCR1-CCR3* region (Hou et al. 2012). The *CCR1* association was also confirmed in studies from Turkey, Japan, and Iran (Penido et al. 2001; Sousa et al. 2015).

KLRC4

NKG2F protein encoded by the *Killer Cell Lectin Like Receptor C4 (KLRC4)* gene codes for a protein that is a member of the NKG2 family (Yabe et al. 1993). The NKG2 family members bind to homologous MHC class I molecules expressed by stressed cells and act a crucial role in the modulation of NK cell tasks against tumoral cells and virus-infected cells (Sun 2010).

A suggestive linkage between SNPs within the *KLRC1-4* genes and BD was found in a GWAS conducted in Turkey and Japan (Kaburaki et al. 2009; Kirino et al. 2013) and was later verified by an Iranian cohort (Sousa et al. 2015).

Signal transducer and activator of transcription factor 4 (STAT4)

The *STAT4* gene codes a transcription factor expressed in dendritic cells, macrophages, and lymphocytes. STAT4 is essential to the functions of the innate and adaptive immune cells. It mediates the proliferation and differentiation of both Th1 and Th17 cells (Mathur et al. 2007).

The *STAT4* gene variants and BD were first found to be linked by a study on Han Chinese patients (Hou et al. 2012). Later on, the same findings were replicated in Korean, Turkish, Iranian cohorts (Kaburaki et al. 2009) (Sousa et al. 2015).

NCOA5

The *nuclear receptor coactivator-5* (*NCOA5*) gene is located at 20q13.1 and encodes a coregulator that interacts with the estrogen receptor 1 and 2 (ESR1 and ESR2) and nuclear receptor subfamily 1 group D member 2 (NR1D2) (Böser et al. 2013). The rs2903908 SNP of the *NCOA5* gene was linked with BD in the Turkish studies with the CT genotype conferring risk for the development of genital ulcers and uveitis in patients with BD (Rustemoglu et al. 2017).

FOXP3

Forkhead box P3 (FOXP3) is a transcription factor with a key role in the development and maintenance of Treg cells (Ziegler 2006). Treg cells were originally founded as a group of CD4 + T cells harboring the CD25 (also known as IL-2 receptor α chain) and CD45 that were also able to protect the mouse from developing autoimmune diseases (Noval Rivas and Chatila 2016). Tregs produce immune-regulatory cytokines and are required for fine-tuning the immune system.

The rs3761548 (3279 C/A) SNP of the *FOXP3* gene is linked to susceptibility to BD in Iranian patients from the North-Western region (Hosseini et al. 2015).

6 Genes with Miscellaneous Functions

FUT2

FUT2 codes the fucosyltransferase 2 that mediates in the formation of the precursor of the ABO-histo-blood group antigens, the H antigen in bodily fluids, and on the mucosa of the gastrointestinal tract (Ferrer-Admetlla et al. 2009).

Several *FUT2* SNPs including rs601338, rs632111, rs602662, rs492602, rs281377, and rs681343 have been linked to BD susceptibility in studies from both Iran and Turkey (Xavier et al. 2015).

UBAC2

UBAC2 codes a ubiquitination-related structural domain involved in proteasomal degradation. The SNP rs9513584 of the *UBAC2* gene was found to confer susceptibility to BD by a study on patients with Turkish ancestry (Fei et al. 2009). Later on, several other SNPs including the rs3825427, rs7999348, rs9517723, rs9517668, and rs9517701 of this gene were linked to BD susceptibility in Chinese, Italian, and Japanese studies (Hou et al. 2012; Jiang et al. 2016; Sawalha et al. 2011; Yamazoe et al. 2017).

SUMO4

Small ubiquitin-like modifier 4 (*SUMO4*) gene at the long arm of the 6th chromosome maintains the negative regulation of NF-kB-dependent transcription of the *IL12B* gene and the activation of heat shock transcriptional factors (Mabb and Miyamoto 2007). The linkage between Behcet's diseases and the *SUMO4* SNPs, rs237024, and rs237026, was first found by a study conducted in China. This association was independent of the status of the *HLA-B51* allele and was replicated by subsequent Tunisian and Korean studies (Hou et al. 2008; Kamoun et al. 2010; Park et al. 2011). Some of these variants were also conferred risk for disease severity and cutaneous involvement in the setting of BD (Kamoun et al. 2010; Park et al. 2011).

7 Conclusion

Although the exact pathogenesis of BD is not fully understood, both environmental agents and a genetic predisposition are vital for the onset of BD. The GWA studies have revolutionized our understanding of the pathogenesis of autoimmune diseases including BD by making data gathering on the genetics of disease easier and feasible. Although BD was initially described as an MHC-related inflammatory disease, other genes mediating both innate and adaptive immune responses have also been linked to the disease. Some discrepancy exists in the reported genetic association of BD in different study cohorts which might indicate the ethnic-specific pathogenesis of BD.

Immunogenetic studies are expected to decode clinical-genetic association, clarify pathogenesis, and provide insights for the better development of treatments capable of inducing long-lasting remissions in BD.

References

Aeschlimann FA, Batu ED, Canna SW, Go E, Gül A, Hoffmann P, Leavis HL, Ozen S, Schwartz DM, Stone DL, van Royen-Kerkof A, Kastner DL, Aksentijevich I, Laxer RM (2018) A20 haploinsufficiency (HA20): clinical phenotypes and disease course of patients with a newly recognised NF-kB-mediated autoinflammatory disease. Ann Rheum Dis 77:728–735

Afkari B, Babaloo Z, Dolati S, Khabazi A, Jadidi-Niaragh F, Talei M, Shanehbandi D, Mahmoudi S, Hazhirkarzar B, Sakhinia E (2018) Molecular analysis of interleukin-10 gene polymorphisms in patients with Behçet's disease. Immunol Lett 194:56–61

Ahmad T, Zhang L, Gogus F, Verity D, Wallace G, Madanat W, Fayyad F, James T, Neville M, Kanawati C, Fortune F, Celik A, Stanford M, Jewell DP, Marshall SE (2005) CARD15polymorphisms in Behçet's disease. Scand J Rheumatol 34:233–237

Al-Okaily F, Al-Rashidi S, Al-Balawi M, Mustafa M, Arfin M, Al-Asmari A (2016) Genetic Association of HLA-A*26, -A*31, and -B*51 with Behcet's Disease in Saudi Patients. Clin Med Insights Arthritis Musculoskelet Disord 9:167–173

Amirzargar A, Shahram F, Nikoopour E, Rezaei N, Saeedfar K, Ziaei N, Davatchi F (2010) Proinflammatory cytokine gene polymorphisms in Behçet's disease. Eur Cytokine Netw 21:292–296

Azizlerli G, Köse AA, Sarica R, Gül A, Tutkun IT, Kulaç M, Tunç R, Urgancioğlu M, Dişçi R (2003) Prevalence of Behçet's disease in Istanbul, Turkey. Int J Dermatol 42:803–806

Behcet H (1937) Uber rezidivierende, aphthose, durchein Virus verusachte Gaschwure am Mund, am Auge und an den Genitalien. Dermat Wochsch 105:1152–1157

Ben Dhifallah I, Lachheb J, Houman H, Hamzaoui K (2009) Toll-like-receptor gene polymorphisms in a Tunisian population with Behçet's disease. Clin Exp Rheumatol 27:S58-62

Berteau F, Rouviere B, Delluc A, Nau A, Le Berre R, Sarrabay G, Touitou I, de Moreuil C (2018) Autosomic dominant familial Behçet disease and haploinsufficiency A20: a review of the literature. Autoimmun Rev 17:809–815

Bettelli E, Carrier Y, Gao W, Korn T, Strom TB, Oukka M, Weiner HL, Kuchroo VK (2006) Reciprocal developmental pathways for the generation of pathogenic effector TH 17 and regulatory T cells. Nature 441:235–238

Boiardi L, Atzeni F, Casali B, Farnetti E, Nicoli D, Pipitone N, Catanoso MG, Olivieri I, Cantini F, Salvi F, La Corte R, Triolo G, Filippini D, Paolazzi G, Salvarani C (2009) Toll-like receptor 4 (TLR4) gene polymorphisms in Italian patients with Behçet's disease. Clin Exp Rheumatol 27:S43-47

Böser A, Drexler Hannes CA, Reuter H, Schmitz H, Wu G, Schöler Hans R, Gentile L, Bartscherer K (2013) SILAC proteomics of planarians identifies Ncoa5 as a conserved component of pluripotent stem cells. Cell Rep 5:1142–1155

Burillo-Sanz S, Montes-Cano M-A, García-Lozano J-R, Ortiz-Fernández L, Ortego-Centeno N, García-Hernández F-J, Espinosa G, Graña-Gil G, Sánchez-Bursón J, Rosa Juliá M, Solans R, Blanco R, Barnosi-Marín A-C, Gómez De la Torre R, Fanlo P, Rodríguez-Carballeira M, Rodríguez-Rodríguez L, Camps T, Castañeda S, Alegre-Sancho J-J, Martín J, González-Escribano MF (2017) Mutational profile of rare variants in inflammasome-related genes in Behçet disease: a next generation sequencing approach. Sci Rep 7:8453–8453

Burton P, Clayton D, Cardon L, Craddock N, Deloukas P, Duncanson A, Kwiatkowski D, McCarthy M, Ouwehand W, Samani N (2007) Wellcome trust case control consortium Australo-Anglo-American Spondylitis Consortium (TASC) biologics in RA Genetics and Genomics Study Syndicate (BRAGGS) Steering Committee Breast Cancer Susceptibility Collaboration (UK): Association scan of 14,500 nonsynonymous SNPs in four diseases identifies autoimmunity variants. Nat Genet 39:1329–1337

Centola M, Wood G, Frucht DM, Galon J, Aringer M, Farrell C, Kingma DW, Horwitz ME, Mansfield E, Holland SM (2000) The gene for familial Mediterranean fever, MEFV, is expressed in early leukocyte development and is regulated in response to inflammatory mediators. Blood J Am Soc Hematol 95:3223–3231

Çerçi P, Altıner S, İnal A, Köse K, Keskin G, Ölmez Ü (2017) Investigating the role of IL-33 in the pathogenesis of Behçet's disease. Acta Clin Belg 72:434–438

Chamaillard M, Hashimoto M, Horie Y, Masumoto J, Qiu S, Saab L, Ogura Y, Kawasaki A, Fukase K, Kusumoto S, Valvano MA, Foster SJ, Mak TW, Nuñez G, Inohara N (2003) An essential role for NOD1 in host recognition of bacterial peptidoglycan containing diaminopimelic acid. Nat Immunol 4:702–707

Chen F, Xu L, Zhao T, Xiao X, Pan Y, Hou S (2016) Genetic Variation in the REL gene increases risk of Behcet's disease in a Chinese Han population but that of PRKCQ does not. PLoS ONE 11:e0147350–e0147350

Chen G, Hardy K, Pagler E, Ma L, Lee S, Gerondakis S, Daley S, Shannon MF (2011) The NF-κB transcription factor c-Rel is required for Th17 effector cell development in experimental autoimmune encephalomyelitis. J Immunol 187:4483–4491

Chung YM, Yeh TS, Sheu MM, Chen MS, Wen MS, Tsai HY, Liao HR (1990) Behcet's disease with ocular involvement in Taiwan: a joint survey of six major ophthalmological departments. J Formos Med Assoc 89:413–417

Collison LW, Vignali DA (2008) Interleukin-35: odd one out or part of the family? Immunol Rev 226:248–262

Conde-Jaldón M, Montes-Cano MA, García-Lozano JR, Ortiz-Fernández L, Ortego-Centeno N, González-León R, Espinosa G, Graña-Gil G, Sánchez-Bursón J, González-Gay MA, Barnosi-Marín AC, Solans R, Fanlo P, Carballeira MR, Camps T, Castañeda S, Martín J, González-Escribano MF (2014) Epistatic interaction of ERAP1 and HLA-B in Behçet disease: a replication study in the Spanish population. PLoS One 9:e102100

Cortes A, Pulit SL, Leo PJ, Pointon JJ, Robinson PC, Weisman MH, Ward M, Gensler LS, Zhou X, Garchon H-J (2015) Major histocompatibility complex associations of ankylosing spondylitis are complex and involve further epistasis with ERAP1. Nat Commun 6:1–8

de Menthon M, Lavalley MP, Maldini C, Guillevin L, Mahr A (2009) HLA–B51/B5 and the risk of Behçet's disease: a systematic review and meta-analysis of case–control genetic association studies. Arthritis Care Res 61:1287–1296

Demirseren DD, Ceylan GG, Akoglu G, Emre S, Erten S, Arman A, Metin A (2014) HLA-B51 subtypes in Turkish patients with Behçet's disease and their correlation with clinical manifestations. Genet Mol Res 13:4788–4796

Deng Y, Zhu W, Zhou X (2018) Immune regulatory genes are major genetic factors to Behcet disease: systematic review. Open Rheumatol J 12:123

Deng Y, Zhu W, Zhou X (2018) Immune regulatory genes are major genetic factors to Behcet disease: systematic review. Open Rheumatol J 12:70–85

Di Marzio P, Dai WW, Franchin G, Chan AY, Symons M, Sherry B (2005) Role of Rho family GTPases in CCR1- and CCR5-induced actin reorganization in macrophages. Biochem Biophys Res Commun 331:909–916

Eksioglu-Demiralp E, Direskeneli H, Kibaroglu A, Yavuz S, Ergun T, Akoglu T (2001) Neutrophil activation in Behçet's disease. Clin Exp Rheumatol 19: S-19

Esmaeili M, Bonyadi M, Khabbazi A, Ebrahimi AA, Sharif SK, Hajialilo M, Kolahi S, Dastgiri S (2011) Common MEFV mutations in Iranian Azeri Turkish patients with Behçet's disease. Scand J Rheumatol 40:383–386

Evans DM, Spencer CC, Pointon JJ, Su Z, Harvey D, Kochan G, Oppermann U, Dilthey A, Pirinen M, Stone MA (2011) Interaction between ERAP1 and HLA-B27 in ankylosing spondylitis implicates peptide handling in the mechanism for HLA-B27 in disease susceptibility. Nat Genet 43:761–767

Fang J, Hu R, Hou S, Ye Z, Xiang Q, Qi J, Zhou Y, Kijlstra A, Yang P (2013) Association ofTLR2Gene polymorphisms with ocular Behçet's disease in a Chinese Han population. Invest Opthalmol vis Sci 54:8384

Fei Y, Webb R, Cobb BL, Direskeneli H, Saruhan-Direskeneli G, Sawalha AH (2009) Identification of novel genetic susceptibility loci for Behçet's disease using a genome-wide association study. Arthritis Res Ther 11:R66

Ferrer-Admetlla A, Sikora M, Laayouni H, Esteve A, Roubinet F, Blancher A, Calafell F, Bertranpetit J, Casals F (2009) A natural history of FUT2 polymorphism in humans. Mol Biol Evol 26:1993–2003

Gabriele L, Ozato K (2007) The role of the interferon regulatory factor (IRF) family in dendritic cell development and function. Cytokine Growth Factor Rev 18:503–510

Girardin SE (2003) Nod1 detects a unique muropeptide from gram-negative bacterial peptidoglycan. Science 300:1584–1587

Giza M, Koftori D, Chen L, Bowness P (2018) Is Behçet's disease a "class 1-opathy"? The role of HLA-B*51 in the pathogenesis of Behçet's disease. Clin Exp Immunol 191:11–18

Groh V, Steinle A, Bauer S, Spies T (1998) Recognition of stress-induced MHC molecules by intestinal epithelial γδ T cells. Science 279:1737–1740

Gül A, Hajeer AH, Worthington J, Barrett JH, Ollier WE, Silman AJ (2001) Evidence for linkage of the HLA–B locus in Behçet's disease, obtained using the transmission disequilibrium test. Arthritis Rheum off J Am College Rheumatol 44:239–241

Gül A, Inanç M, Öcal L, Aral O, Koniçe M (2000) Familial aggregation of Behcet's disease in Turkey. Ann Rheum Dis 59:622–625

Hall M, McGlinn E, Coakley G, Fisher S, Boki K, Middleton D, Kaklamani E, Moutsopoulos H, Loughran T, Ollier W (2000) Genetic polymorphism of IL-12 p40 gene in immune-mediated disease. Genes Immun 1:219–224

Horie Y, Meguro A, Ota M, Kitaichi N, Katsuyama Y, Takemoto Y, Namba K, Yoshida K, Song YW, Park KS, Lee EB, Inoko H, Mizuki N, Ohno S (2009) Association of TLR4 polymorphisms with Behcet's disease in a Korean population. Rheumatology 48:638–642

Hosseini A, Shanehbandi D, Estiar MA, Gholizadeh S, Khabbazi A, Khodadadi H, Sakhinia E, Babaloo Z (2015) A single nucleotide polymorphism in the FOXP3 gene associated with Behçet's disease in an Iranian population. Clin Lab 61:1897–1903

Hou S, Xiao X, Li F, Jiang Z, Kijlstra A, Yang P (2012) Two-stage association study in Chinese Han identifies two independent associations in CCR1/CCR3 locus as candidate for Behçet's disease susceptibility. Hum Genet 131:1841–1850

Hou S, Yang P, Du L, Zhou H, Lin X, Liu X, Kijlstra A (2008) SUMO4 gene polymorphisms in Chinese Han patients with Behcet's disease. Clin Immunol 129:170–175

Hou S, Yang Z, Du L, Jiang Z, Shu Q, Chen Y, Li F, Zhou Q, Ohno S, Chen R, Kijlstra A, Rosenbaum JT, Yang P (2012) Identification of a susceptibility locus inSTAT4for Behçet's disease in Han Chinese in a genome-wide association study. Arthritis Rheum 64:4104–4113

Hu J, Hou S, Zhu X, Fang J, Zhou Y, Liu Y, Bai L, Kijlstra A, Yang P (2015) Interleukin-10 gene polymorphisms are associated with Behcet's disease but not with Vogt-Koyanagi-Harada syndrome in the Chinese Han population. Mol vis 21:589–603

Hughes T, Coit P, Adler A, Yilmaz V, Aksu K, Düzgün N, Keser G, Cefle A, Yazici A, Ergen A, Alpsoy E, Salvarani C, Casali B, Kötter I, Gutierrez-Achury J, Wijmenga C, Direskeneli H, Saruhan-Direskeneli G, Sawalha AH (2013) Identification of multiple independent susceptibility loci in the HLA region in Behçet's disease. Nat Genet 45:319–324

Jiang Y, Wang H, Yu H, Li L, Xu D, Hou S, Kijlstra A, Yang P (2016) Two Genetic Variations in the IRF8 region are associated with Behçet's disease in Han Chinese. Sci Rep 6:19651–19651

Kaburaki T, Araki F, Takamoto M, Okinaga K, Yoshida A, Numaga J, Fujino Y, Kawashima H (2009) Best-corrected visual acuity and frequency of ocular attacks during the initial 10 years in patients with Behçet's disease. Graefes Arch Clin Exp Ophthalmol 248:709–714

Kaburaki T, Takamoto M, Numaga J, Kawashima H, Araie M, Ohnogi Y, Harihara S, Kuwata S, Takeuchi F (2010) Genetic association of HLA-A*2601 with ocular Behçet's disease in Japanese patients. Clin Exp Rheumatol 28:S39-44

Kamiishi T, Itoh Y, Meguro A, Nishida T, Sasaki S, Nanba K, Ohno S, Inoko H, Mizuki N (2008) Four-digit allele genotyping of HLA-A and HLA-B genes in Japanese patients with Behçet's disease (BD) by a PCR-SSOP-luminex method and stratification analysis according to each major symptom of BD. Nippon Ganka Gakkai Zasshi 112:451–458

Kamoun M, Ben Dhifallah I, Karray E, Zakraoui L, Hamzaoui K (2010) Association of small ubiquitin-like modifier 4 (SUMO4) polymorphisms in a Tunisian population with Behçet's disease. Clin Exp Rheumatol 28:S45-49

Kang EH, Kim JY, Takeuchi F, Kim JW, Shin K, Lee EY, Lee YJ, Lee EB, Park MH, Song YW (2011) Associations between the HLA-A polymorphism and the clinical manifestations of Behcet's disease. Arthritis Res Ther 13:R49

Kang EH, Kim S, Park MY, Choi JY, Choi IA, Kim MJ, Ha YJ, Lee EY, Lee YJ, Lee EB, Kang C, Song YW (2017) Behçet's disease risk association fine-mapped on the IL23R-IL12RB2 intergenic region in Koreans. Arthritis Res Ther 19:227

Kang EH, Park JW, Park C, Yu HG, Lee EB, Park MH, Song YW (2013) Genetic and non-genetic factors affecting the visual outcome of ocular Behcet's disease. Hum Immunol 74:1363–1367

Kappen JH, Medina-Gomez C, van Hagen PM, Stolk L, Estrada K, Rivadeneira F, Uitterlinden AG, Stanford MR, Ben-Chetrit E, Wallace GR, Soylu M, van Laar JA (2015) Genome-wide association study in an admixed case series reveals IL12A as a new candidate in Behçet disease. PLoS One 10:e0119085

Kawai T, Akira S (2009) The roles of TLRs, RLRs and NLRs in pathogen recognition. Int Immunol 21:317–337
Khaib Dit Naib O, Aribi M, Idder A, Chiali A, Sairi H, Touitou I, Lefranc G, Barat-Houari M (2013) Association analysis of IL10, TNF-α, and IL23R-IL12RB2 SNPs with Behçet's disease risk in Western Algeria. Front Immunol 4:342
Kirino Y, Bertsias G, Ishigatsubo Y, Mizuki N, Tugal-Tutkun I, Seyahi E, Ozyazgan Y, Sacli FS, Erer B, Inoko H, Emrence Z, Cakar A, Abaci N, Ustek D, Satorius C, Ueda A, Takeno M, Kim Y, Wood GM, Ombrello MJ, Meguro A, Gül A, Remmers EF, Kastner DL (2013) Genome-wide association analysis identifies new susceptibility loci for Behçet's disease and epistasis between HLA-B*51 and ERAP1. Nat Genet 45:202–207
Kirino Y, Zhou Q, Ishigatsubo Y, Mizuki N, Tugal-Tutkun I, Seyahi E, Özyazgan Y, Ugurlu S, Erer B, Abaci N, Ustek D, Meguro A, Ueda A, Takeno M, Inoko H, Ombrello MJ, Satorius CL, Maskeri B, Mullikin JC, Sun HW, Gutierrez-Cruz G, Kim Y, Wilson AF, Kastner DL, Gül A, Remmers EF (2013) Targeted resequencing implicates the familial Mediterranean fever gene MEFV and the toll-like receptor 4 gene TLR4 in Behçet disease. Proc Natl Acad Sci U S A 110:8134–8139
Lamhamedi-Cherradi S-E, Zheng S, Hilliard BA, Xu L, Sun J, Alsheadat S, Liou H-C, Chen YH (2003) Transcriptional regulation of type I diabetes by NF-κ B. J Immunol 171:4886–4892
Langrish CL, Chen Y, Blumenschein WM, Mattson J, Basham B, Sedgwick JD, McClanahan T, Kastelein RA, Cua DJ (2005) IL-23 drives a pathogenic T cell population that induces autoimmune inflammation. J Exp Med 201:233–240
Le Goff B, Blanchard F, Berthelot J-M, Heymann D, Maugars Y (2010) Role for interleukin-6 in structural joint damage and systemic bone loss in rheumatoid arthritis. Joint Bone Spine 77:201–205
Lee CH, Melchers M, Wang H, Torrey TA, Slota R, Qi C-F, Kim JY, Lugar P, Kong HJ, Farrington L (2006) Regulation of the germinal center gene program by interferon (IFN) regulatory factor 8/IFN consensus sequence-binding protein. J Exp Med 203:63–72
Li H, Liu Q, Hou S, Du L, Zhou Q, Zhou Y, Kijlstra A, Li Z, Yang P (2012) TNFAIP3 gene polymorphisms confer risk for Behcet's disease in a Chinese Han population. Hum Genet 132:293–300
Li L, Yu H, Jiang Y, Deng B, Bai L, Kijlstra A, Yang P (2016) Corrigendum: genetic variations of NLR family genes in Behcet's disease. Sci Rep 6:26423–26423
Liew FY, Pitman NI, McInnes IB (2010) Disease-associated functions of IL-33: the new kid in the IL-1 family. Nat Rev Immunol 10:103–110
Mabb AM, Miyamoto S (2007) SUMO and NF-κB ties. Cell Mol Life Sci 64:1979–1996
Mahmoudi M, Ashraf-Ganjouei A, Javinani A, Shahram F, Meguro A, Mizuki N, Ahmadzadeh N, Jafarinejad-Farsangi S, Mostafaei S, Kavosi H, Faezi ST, Akhlaghi M, Davatchi F (2018) Epistatic interaction of ERAP1 and HLA-B*51 in Iranian patients with Behçet's disease. Sci Rep 8:17612
Maldini C, Lavalley MP, Cheminant M, de Menthon M, Mahr A (2012) Relationships of HLA-B51 or B5 genotype with Behcet's disease clinical characteristics: systematic review and meta-analyses of observational studies. Rheumatology (oxford) 51:887–900
Mathur AN, Chang H-C, Zisoulis DG, Stritesky GL, Yu Q, O'Malley JT, Kapur R, Levy DE, Kansas GS, Kaplan MH (2007) Stat3 and Stat4 direct development of IL-17-secreting Th cells. J Immunol 178:4901–4907
Meguro A, Inoko H, Ota M, Katsuyama Y, Oka A, Okada E, Yamakawa R, Yuasa T, Fujioka T, Ohno S, Bahram S, Mizuki N (2010) Genetics of Behçet disease inside and outside the MHC. Ann Rheum Dis 69:747–754
Meguro A, Ota M, Katsuyama Y, Oka A, Ohno S, Inoko H, Mizuki N (2007) Association of the toll-like receptor 4 gene polymorphisms with Behcet's disease. Ann Rheum Dis 67:725–727
Mizuki N, Inoko H, Ohno S (1997) Molecular genetics (HLA) of Behçet's disease. Yonsei Med J 38:333–349
Mizuki N, Meguro A, Ota M, Ohno S, Shiota T, Kawagoe T, Ito N, Kera J, Okada E, Yatsu K (2010) Genome-wide association studies identify IL23R-IL12RB2 and IL10 as Behcet's disease susceptibility loci. Nat Genet 42:703–706
Mizuki N, Ohno S, Ando H, Chen L, Palimeris GD, Stavropoulos-Ghiokas E, Ishihara M, Goto K, Nakamura S, Shindo Y, Isobe K, Ito N, Inoko H (1997) A strong association between HLA-B*5101 and Behçet's disease in Greek patients. Tissue Antigens 50:57–60
Mizuki N, Ota M, Kimura M, Ohno S, Ando H, Katsuyama Y, Yamazaki M, Watanabe K, Goto K, Nakamura S, Bahram S, Inoko H (1997) Triplet repeat polymorphism in the transmembrane region of the MICA gene: a strong association of six GCT repetitions with Behçet disease. Proc Natl Acad Sci USA 94:1298–1303
Montes-Cano MA, Conde-Jaldón M, García-Lozano JR, Ortiz-Fernández L, Ortego-Centeno N, Castillo-Palma MJ, Espinosa G, Graña-Gil G, González-Gay MA, Barnosi-Marín AC, Solans R, Fanlo P, Camps T, Castañeda S, Sánchez-Bursón J, Núñez-Roldán A, Martín J, González-Escribano MF (2013) HLA and non-HLA genes in Behçet's disease: a multicentric study in the Spanish population. Arthritis Res Ther 15: R145
Muñoz-Saá I, Cambra A, Pallarés L, Espinosa G, Juan A, Pujalte F, Matamoros N, Milà J, Julià MR (2006) Allelic diversity and affinity variants of MICA are imbalanced in Spanish patients with Behçet's disease. Scand J Immunol 64:77–82
Nakamura J, Meguro A, Ishii G, Mihara T, Takeuchi M, Mizuki Y, Yuda K, Yamane T, Kawagoe T, Ota M, Mizuki N (2019) The association analysis between HLA-A*26 and Behçet's disease. Sci Rep 9:4426

Noval Rivas M, Chatila TA (2016) Regulatory T cells in allergic diseases. J Allergy Clin Immunol 138:639–652

Oda H, Kastner DL (2017) Genomics, biology, and human illness: advances in the monogenic autoinflammatory diseases. Rheum Dis Clin North Am 43:327–345

Ombrello MJ, Kirino Y, de Bakker PI, Gül A, Kastner DL, Remmers EF (2014) Behcet disease-associated MHC class I residues implicate antigen binding and regulation of cell-mediated cytotoxicity. Proc Natl Acad Sci 111:8867–8872

Ortiz-Fernández L, Carmona FD, Montes-Cano MA, García-Lozano JR, Conde-Jaldón M, Ortego-Centeno N, Castillo MJ, Espinosa G, Graña-Gil G, Sánchez-Bursón J, Juliá MR, Solans R, Blanco R, Barnosi-Marín AC, Gómez de la Torre R, Fanlo P, Rodríguez-Carballeira M, Rodríguez-Rodríguez L, Camps T, Castañeda S, Alegre-Sancho JJ, Martín J, González-Escribano MF (2016) Genetic analysis with the immunochip platform in Behçet disease. Identification of residues associated in the HLA class I region and new susceptibility loci. PLoS One 11:e0161305

Ortiz-Fernández L, García-Lozano JR, Montes-Cano MA, Conde-Jaldón M, Ortego-Centeno N, García-Hernández FJ, Espinosa G, Graña-Gil G, Sánchez-Bursón J, Juliá MR, Blanco R, Barnosi-Marín AC, Solans R, Fanlo P, Rodríguez Carballeira M, Camps T, Castañeda S, Martín J, González-Escribano MF (2015) Lack of association of TNFAIP3 and JAK1 with Behçet's disease in the European population. Clin Exp Rheumatol 33:S36-39

Ouyang X, Zhang R, Yang J, Li Q, Qin L, Zhu C, Liu J, Ning H, Shin MS, Gupta M (2011) Transcription factor IRF8 directs a silencing programme for TH 17 cell differentiation. Nat Commun 2:1–12

Ozbey U, Tug E, Namli M (2009) Interleukin-10 gene promoter polymorphism in patients with schizophrenia in a region of East Turkey. World J Biol Psychiatry 10:461–468

Park G, Kim H-S, Choe J-Y, Kim S-K (2011) SUMO4 C438T polymorphism is associated with papulopustular skin lesion in Korean patients with Behçet's disease. Rheumatol Int 32:3031–3037

Park SH, Park KS, Seo YI, Min DJ, Kim WU, Kim TG, Cho CS, Mok JW, Park KS, Kim HY (2002) Association of MICA polymorphism with HLA-B51 and disease severity in Korean patients with Behcet's disease. J Korean Med Sci 17:366–370

Penido C, Castro-Faria-Neto HC, Vieira-de-Abreu A, Figueiredo RT, Pelled A, Martins MA, Jose PJ, Williams TJ, PcT B (2001) LPS induces Eosinophil migration via CCR3 signaling through a mechanism independent of RANTES and eotaxin. Am J Respir Cell Mol Biol 25:707–716

Presky DH, Yang H, Minetti LJ, Chua AO, Nabavi N, Wu C-Y, Gately MK, Gubler U (1996) A functional interleukin 12 receptor complex is composed of two β-type cytokine receptor subunits. Proc Natl Acad Sci 93:14002–14007

Puccetti A, Fiore PF, Pelosi A, Tinazzi E, Patuzzo G, Argentino G, Moretta F, Lunardi C, Dolcino M (2018) Gene expression profiling in Behcet's disease indicates an autoimmune component in the pathogenesis of the disease and opens new avenues for targeted therapy. J Immunol Res 2018:4246965

Qin X, Xu J, Wu Z, Sun F, Chen H, Zheng W, Li S, Li P, Chen S, Shen M, Zhang W, You X, Wu Q, Zhang F, Li YZ (2016) Association study of rs924080 and rs11209032 polymorphisms of IL23R-IL12RB2 in a Northern Chinese Han population with Behcet's disease. Hum Immunol 77:1284–1290

Remmers EF, Cosan F, Kirino Y, Ombrello MJ, Abaci N, Satorius C, Le JM, Yang B, Korman BD, Cakiris A, Aglar O, Emrence Z, Azakli H, Ustek D, Tugal-Tutkun I, Akman-Demir G, Chen W, Amos CI, Dizon MB, Kose AA, Azizlerli G, Erer B, Brand OJ, Kaklamani VG, Kaklamanis P, Ben-Chetrit E, Stanford M, Fortune F, Ghabra M, Ollier WE, Cho YH, Bang D, O'Shea J, Wallace GR, Gadina M, Kastner DL, Gül A (2010) Genome-wide association study identifies variants in the MHC class I, IL10, and IL23R-IL12RB2 regions associated with Behçet's disease. Nat Genet 42:698–702

Rock KL, York IA, Goldberg AL (2004) Post-proteasomal antigen processing for major histocompatibility complex class I presentation. Nat Immunol 5:670–677

Rustemoglu A, Erkol Inal E, Inanir A, Ekinci D, Gul U, Yigit S, Ates O, Karakus N (2017) Clinical significance of NCOA5 gene rs2903908 polymorphism in Behçet's disease. Excli j 16:609–617

Saeki T, Naya A (2003) CCR1 chemokine receptor antagonist. Curr Pharm Des 9:1201–1208

Sakaguchi T, Takiguchi M (1997) Peptide binding motif for HLA class I and autoimmune disease. Nihon Rinsho 55:1397–1402

Sawalha AH, Hughes T, Nadig A, Yılmaz V, Aksu K, Keser G, Cefle A, Yazıcı A, Ergen A, Alarcón-Riquelme ME, Salvarani C, Casali B, Direskeneli H, Saruhan-Direskeneli G (2011) A putative functional variant within the UBAC2 gene is associated with increased risk of Behçet's disease. Arthritis Rheum 63:3607–3612

Sousa I, Shahram F, Francisco D, Davatchi F, Abdollahi BS, Ghaderibarmi F, Nadji A, Mojarad Shafiee N, Xavier JM, Oliveira SA (2015) Brief report: association ofCCR1, KLRC4, IL12A-AS1, STAT4, andERAP1With Behçet's disease in Iranians. Arthritis Rheumatol 67:2742–2748

Strange A, Capon F, Spencer C, Knight J, Weale M, Allen M, Barton A, Band G, Bellenguez C, Bergboer J (2010) Genetic Analysis of Psoriasis Consortium & the Wellcome Trust Case Control Consortium 2 A genome-wide association study identifies new psoriasis susceptibility loci and an interaction between HLA-C and ERAP1. Nat Genet 42:985–990

Sugisaki K, Saito R, Takagi T, Shio K, Shioya Y, Fukaya E, Iwadate H, Sekine H, Orikasa H, Kobayashi H, Watanabe H, Sato Y (2005) HLA-B52-positive vasculo-Behçet disease: usefulness of magnetic resonance angiography, ultrasound study, and computed tomographic angiography for the early evaluation of multiarterial lesions. Mod Rheumatol 15:56–61

Sun (2010) Up-regulation of NKG2F receptor, a functionally unknown killer receptor, of human natural killer cells by interleukin-2 and interleukin-15. Oncol Rep 24

Taheri S, Borlu M, Evereklioglu C, Ozdemir SY, Ozkul Y (2015) mRNA expression level of interleukin genes in the determining phases of Behçet's disease. Ann Dermatol 27:291–297

Takeno M, Kariyone A, Yamashita N, Takiguchi M, Mizushima Y, Kaneoka H, Sakane T (1995) Excessive function of peripheral blood neutrophils from patients with Behçet's disease and from HLA-B51 transgenic mice. Arthritis Rheum 38:426–433

Takeuchi M, Kastner DL, Remmers EF (2015) The immunogenetics of Behçet's disease: a comprehensive review. J Autoimmun 64:137–148

Takeuchi M, Mizuki N, Meguro A, Ombrello MJ, Kirino Y, Satorius C, Le J, Blake M, Erer B, Kawagoe T, Ustek D, Tugal-Tutkun I, Seyahi E, Ozyazgan Y, Sousa I, Davatchi F, Francisco V, Shahram F, Abdollahi BS, Nadji A, Shafiee NM, Ghaderibarmi F, Ohno S, Ueda A, Ishigatsubo Y, Gadina M, Oliveira SA, Gül A, Kastner DL, Remmers EF (2017) Dense genotyping of immune-related loci implicates host responses to microbial exposure in Behçet's disease susceptibility. Nat Genet 49:438–443

Takeuchi O, Sato S, Horiuchi T, Hoshino K, Takeda K, Dong Z, Modlin RL, Akira S (2002) Cutting edge: role of toll-like receptor 1 in mediating immune response to microbial lipoproteins. J Immunol 169:10–14

Talei M, Abdi A, Shanebandi D, Jadidi-Niaragh F, Khabazi A, Babaie F, Alipour S, Afkari B, Sakhinia E, Babaloo Z (2019) Interleukin-33 gene expression and rs1342326 polymorphism in Behçet's disease. Immunol Lett 212:120–124

Tasliyurt T, Yigit S, Rustemoglu A, Gul U, Ates O (2013) Common MEFV gene mutations in Turkish patients with Behcet's disease. Gene 530:100–103

Teng MW, Bowman EP, McElwee JJ, Smyth MJ, Casanova J-L, Cooper AM, Cua DJ (2015) IL-12 and IL-23 cytokines: from discovery to targeted therapies for immune-mediated inflammatory diseases. Nat Med 21:719–729

Tsujimura H, Tamura T, Ozato K (2003) Cutting edge: IFN consensus sequence binding protein/IFN regulatory factor 8 drives the development of type I IFN-producing plasmacytoid dendritic cells. J Immunol 170:1131–1135

Wallace GR, Kondeatis E, Vaughan RW, Verity DH, Chen Y, Fortune F, Madanat W, Kanawati CA, Graham EM, Stanford MR (2007) IL-10 genotype analysis in patients with Behçet's disease. Hum Immunol 68:122–127

Watford WT, Hissong BD, Bream JH, Kanno Y, Muul L, O'Shea JJ (2004) Signaling by IL-12 and IL-23 and the immunoregulatory roles of STAT4. Immunol Rev 202:139–156

Wei F, Zhang YU, Li W (2016) A meta-analysis of the association between Behçet's disease and MICA-A6. Biomed Rep 4:741–745

Wu Z, Zhang S, Li J, Chen S, Li P, Sun F, Wen X, Zheng W, Zhang F, Li Y (2015) Association between MEFV mutations M694V and M680I and Behçet's disease: a meta-analysis. PLoS One 10:e0132704

Xavier JM, Shahram F, Davatchi F, Rosa A, Crespo J, Abdollahi BS, Nadji A, Jesus G, Barcelos F, Patto JV, Shafiee NM, Ghaderibarim F, Oliveira SA (2012) Association study of IL10 and IL23R-IL12RB2 in Iranian patients with Behçet's disease. Arthritis Rheum 64:2761–2772

Xavier JM, Shahram F, Sousa I, Davatchi F, Matos M, Abdollahi BS, Sobral J, Nadji A, Oliveira M, Ghaderibarim F, Shafiee NM, Oliveira SA (2015) FUT2: filling the gap between genes and environment in Behçet's disease? Ann Rheum Dis 74:618–624

Yabe T, McSherry C, Bach F, Fisch P, Schall R, Sondel P, Houchins J (1993) A multigene family on human chromosome 12 encodes natural killer-cell lectins. Immunogenetics 37

Yalçin B, Atakan N, Dogan S (2014) Association of interleukin-23 receptor gene polymorphism with Behçet disease. Clin Exp Dermatol 39:881–887

Yamazoe K, Meguro A, Takeuchi M, Shibuya E, Ohno S, Mizuki N (2017) Comprehensive analysis of the association between UBAC2 polymorphisms and Behçet's disease in a Japanese population. Sci Rep 7:742–742

Yasuoka H, Yamaguchi Y, Mizuki N, Nishida T, Kawakami Y, Kuwana M (2008) Preferential activation of circulating CD8+ and gammadelta T cells in patients with active Behçet's disease and HLA-B51. Clin Exp Rheumatol 26:S59-63

Yu H, Zheng M, Zhang L, Li H, Zhu Y, Cheng L, Li L, Deng B, Kijlstra A, Yang P (2017) Identification of susceptibility SNPs in IL10 and IL23R-IL12RB2 for Behçet's disease in Han Chinese. J Allergy Clin Immunol 139:621–627

Zhang J, Liao D, Yang L, Hou S (2016) Association between functional MICA-TM and Behcet's disease: a systematic review and meta-analysis. Sci Rep 6:21033

Zhang L, Yu H, Zheng M, Li H, Liu Y, Kijlstra A, Yang P (2015) Association of ERAP1 gene polymorphisms with Behçet's disease in Han Chinese. Invest Ophthalmol vis Sci 56:6029–6035

Zhao J, Kong HJ, Li H, Huang B, Yang M, Zhu C, Bogunovic M, Zheng F, Mayer L, Ozato K (2006) IRF-8/interferon (IFN) consensus sequence-binding protein is involved in Toll-like receptor (TLR) signaling and contributes to the cross-talk between TLR and IFN-γ signaling pathways. J Biol Chem 281:10073–10080

Ziegler SF (2006) FOXP3: of mice and men. Annu Rev Immunol 24:209–226

The Immunogenetics of Granulomatous Diseases

Gizem Filazi Kök and Ümit Türsen

Abstract

Non-infectious granulomatous skin diseases are a wide category of well-defined reactive inflammatory conditions that share main similarities. While cutaneous sarcoidosis is the prototype of non-infectious (sterile) granulomatous dermatitides, there are several other entities in this group including granuloma annulare and necrobiosis lipoidica. Non-infectious granulomatous diseases are caused by complex associations between genetic situations and environmental triggers resulting in a variety of cutaneous and systemic manifestations. The genetic backgrounds of these diseases are the main topic of this manuscript.

Keywords

Non-infectious · Granulomatous · Skin · Diseases · Dermatology

G. F. Kök · Ü. Türsen (✉)
Department of Dermatology, Mersin University, Mersin, Turkey
e-mail: utursen@mersin.edu.tr

1 Introduction

The term non-infectious granulomatous skin disease is designated to a collection of reactive inflammatory lesions with prominent infiltration of histiocytes forming granulomas. While cutaneous sarcoidosis is the prototype of non-infectious (sterile) granulomatous dermatitides, several other entities are also present in this group including granuloma annulare (GA), necrobiosis lipoidica (NL), the more recently described actinic granuloma also known as "annulare elastolytic giant cell granuloma" or "AEGCG", cutaneous Crohn's disease, and foreign body granulomas. Two rheumatoid arthritis-associated skin conditions were coined "interstitial granulomatous dermatitis" by Dubey and Merry (2007) and "palisaded neutrophilic and granulomatous dermatitis" by Chu et al. (1994) also belong to this category of diseases (Hawryluk et al. 2010).

The diverse clinical manifestations of granulomatous diseases make their diagnosis hard and the overlapping histological features between the different entities in this group of diseases make it relatively difficult to distinguish one from another and increases the chance of misdiagnosis (Hawryluk et al. 2010; Kamil et al. 2015; Schmitt and Volz 2019). Moreover, counseling these patients regarding the prognosis of their diseases is also challenging because of the possible systemic co-morbidities that they may subsequently encounter.

N. Rezaei and F. Rajabi (eds.), *The Immunogenetics of Dermatologic Diseases*, Advances in Experimental Medicine and Biology 1367,
https://doi.org/10.1007/978-3-030-92616-8_13

Non-infectious granulomatous disorders come from a complex association between genetic settings and environmental triggers. Infectious agents, altered self-peptides, and organic/inorganic material have all been suggested to act as the triggering antigens. Regardless of the initiative events, the immunopathogenesis of all granulomatous diseases follows a few similar steps in the cascade of events (Ali et al. 2010; Iannuzzi et al. 2007). The inciting antigen is presented by dendritic cells and processed to the immune system accompanied by a major histocompatibility complex (MHC)molecule. The peptide-MHC complex is recognized by the αβ type of the T-cell receptors (TCR) on CD4 +helper T-cell. This interaction polarizes the differentiation of naive T-cells toward interferon-γ (IFN-γ) and interleukin-2 (IL-2) producing T-helper-1 (Th-1) cells and triggers antigen-presenting cells (APCs) to release tumor necrosis factor (TNF)-alpha, IL-12, IL-15, and IL-18 along with macrophage inflammatory protein-1 (MIP1), monocyte chemotactic protein-1 (MCP1), and granulocyte–macrophage colony-stimulating factor (GMCSF) (Ali et al. 2010). This cytokine milieu promotes the differentiation of macrophages into less phagocytic epithelioid cells which can then fuse to form multinucleated giant cells. Although the predominant response in granulomatous diseases is Th1 mediated, other immune pathways are also involved. The pathogens can directly stimulate innate immunity via toll-like receptors (TLRs). Furthermore, the involvement of Th17 and B-cell-induced hypergammaglobulinemia has also been documented (Fontenot and King 2018).

As the above-mentioned immune-mediated responses are chief to the etiopathogenesis of granulomatous diseases, the genes encoding the elements of this immune reaction can also play a major role. Polymorphisms in genes encoding antigen processing proteins, MHCs, immune receptors, and cytokines can alter the pathogenic process and ultimately determine the status of disease susceptibility or the clinic manifestation way of the disease. These genetic factors were originally discovered through case–control genetic association studies on candidate genes. Thereafter, observational non-candidate-driven methods such as genome-wide association studies (GWAS) were employed.

The focal point of this chapter is mostly about the contribution of genetic polymorphism to the pathogenesis of granulomatous diseases. The clinical application of these immunogenetic studies is in the acceleration of drug discovery.

2 Sarcoidosis

Sarcoidosis is a multisystem disease defined by the presence of a specific type of non-infectious granuloma known as sarcoidal granuloma in different tissues and organs. The usually affected systems are the pulmonary system, lymph nodes, and skin (Dai et al. 2019; Haimovic et al. 2012; Luisetti et al. 2000; Schmitt and Volz 2019). The skin is affected in approximately 25% of the cases (Heath et al. 2012). The most frequent cutaneous manifestation of sarcoidosis is erythema nodosum that typically confers a favorable prognosis. Other manifestations include lupus pernio, papules, plaques, and subcutaneous lesions all of which are related to a more chronic disease course (Dai et al. 2019). Owing to the diverse clinical manifestations of cutaneous sarcoidosis it has been called one of the "great imitators" (Fig. 1).

On histopathological examination, cutaneous sarcoidosis demonstrates multiple dermal collections of epithelioid and multinucleated giant

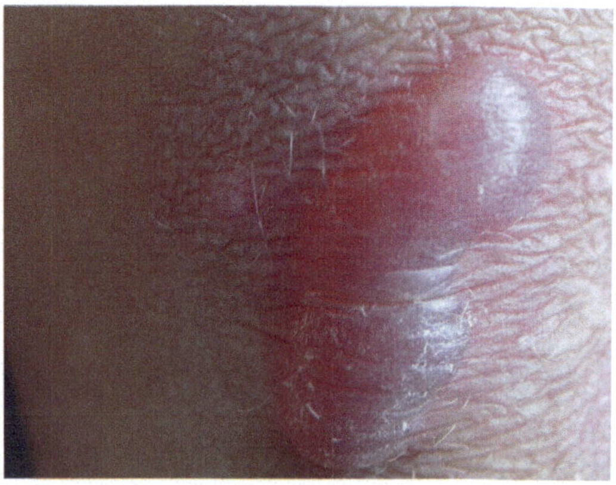

Fig. 1 Scar sarcoidosis on the right knee

cells devoid of lymphocytes. These nodular aggregations are encased by fibrotic tissue but lack central caseation (Ali et al. 2010).

2.1 The Pathogenesis of Sarcoidosis

Similar to all other granulomatous diseases, sarcoidosis results from a Th1 mediated immune response with IFN-γ and TNF-α acting as the dominant cytokines. Several agents have been suggested to act as inciting antigens responsible for the oligoclonal $\alpha\beta$ T-cell expansion including zirconium, talc, mycobacterium (specifically the catalase-peroxidase protein, mKatG), viruses, and Propionibacterium acne (Chen and Moller 2014; Eishi 2013; Song et al. 2005). Some have proposed autoimmunity as a trigger of T-cell activation with vimentin as a possible autoantigen (Starshinova et al. 2019; Wahlström et al. 2007). Serum amyloid-A (SAA) is another possible initiating factor identified in recent years. SSA is capable of activating APCs via TLR-2 and thus inducing the expression of TNF-α, IL-18, and IL-10 (Vadasz and Toubi 2017). Misfolded/fragmented SSA collections in the sarcoidal granuloma can also contribute to disease chronicity by traping circulating antigens that can constantly stimulate the immune system (Patterson and Chen 2018).

2.2 The Immunogenetics of Sarcoidosis

Genetic backgrounds are noted to participate in the progress of sarcoidosis based on two main observations: epidemiological studies identifying ethnicity as the main risk factor and frequent reports of familial clustering (up to six times more frequent in the siblings of those affected with the condition) (Rybicki et al. 2001; Sverrild et al. 2008). The genetic component of sarcoidosis is also supported by twin studies reporting a higher prevalence of the disease in monozygotic twins compared to dizygotic twins. A nationwide twin cohort was able to show an 80-fold increase in the prevalence of sarcoidosis in monozygotic twins compared to only a 7-folds increase for dizygotic twins (both compared to the general population) (Sverrild et al. 2008). Based on these observations, multiple association investigations have been done to clarify the initiative genes.

2.2.1 HLA Candidate Genes

The main focus of genetic studies on sarcoidosis has been on the MHC genes. These membrane-attached molecules play a major role in immune recognition of self and foreign antigens and show significant diversity among human beings. Although six genes and two pseudogenes encode the proteins belonging to the MHC class I group, the three most polymorphic ones, *HLA-A*, *HLA-B*, and *HLA-C* are considered the classic MHC-I genes which are co-dominantly expressed are on almost all nucleated cells (Neefjes et al. 2011). The MHC-II genes encompass five major groups from which *HLA-DP*, *HLA-DQ*, and *HLA-DR* are the most polymorphous ones expressed by antigen-presenting cells (Neefjes et al. 2011). In contrast to most autoimmune disorders, the association between HLAs and sarcoidosis is still controversial with the impact of HLA alleles varying significantly depending upon disease subtype and racial group. There is, on the other hand, a common agreement that some HLA might be linked to specific subtypes of sarcoidosis (Fischer et al. 2012; Luisetti et al. 2000; Smith et al. 2008).

Histological evaluation of pulmonary lesions of sarcoidosis demonstrates infiltration of CD4 +T-cells resulting from an oligoclonal expansion probably triggered by a specific antigen (Forman et al. 1994). The same scenario could hold for cutaneous sarcoidosis with the presentation of specific unknown antigens via HLA molecules to T-cell receptors (TCRs) triggering the subsequent immune activation and its pathological consequences. Since HLA molecules seem to play a significant role in the pathogenesis of immune response in sarcoidosis, investigators have taken a great interest in these molecules. In fact, the exploration of the association between HLA polymorphisms and sarcoidosis began in the early 1970s (Iannuzzi and Rybicki 2007; Müller-Quernheim et al. 2008; Yanardag et al. 2017).

The *HLA-B7* and *HLA-B8* form MHC-I and the *HLA-DRB1* from MHC-II are the most commonly reported genetic association of sarcoidosis in the literature. The polymorphisms of the *HLA-DRB1* gene are linked to both susceptibility and prognosis of sarcoidosis (Iannuzzi and Rybicki 2007; Ishihara et al. 1994; Rossman et al. 2003). Several studies have demonstrated an association between the *HLADRB1*01* and *DRB1*04* variants and reduced risk of sarcoidosis while reporting an increased risk of the disease in carriers of the *DRB1*11*, *DRB1*12*, *DRB1*14*, *DRB1*15*, and *DRB1*03* alleles (Fischer et al. 2012; Grutters et al. 2003b). Another study found several alleles including *DRB1*0402, HLA-DRB1*1101*, *DRB1*1201, and DRB1*1501* to confer risk for sarcoidosis (Rossman et al. 2003). In this study, the risk of developing extrapulmonary involvement was higher in the carriers of the *DRB1*1101* allele with a history of insecticide exposure. The *DRB1*1101* allele also conferred risk for the development of pulmonary-restricted sarcoidosis in those who had been subjected to molds and must odors. This evidence further supports the notion that interactions between specific genetic backgrounds and environmental factors could provoke the development of sarcoidosis (Moller et al. 2017). The HLA associations of sarcoidosis are listed in Table 1.

Regarding the clinical phenotypes, the *HLA-B8/DR3* haplotype has been linked to the Löfgren syndrome (designated to the constellation of the following presentations: bilateral hilar lymphadenopathy, ankle joint arthritis, and erythema nodosum) (Fischer et al. 2012).

2.2.2 Non-HLA Candidate Genes

Aside from HLAs, other immune-related genes such as those involved in the recruitment and activation of immune cells (T-cells and macrophages), antigen processing, and repair mechanisms may also influence the pathogenesis of sarcoidosis. Some of these non-HLA candidate genes are showed in Table 2 and more detailedly discussed in the following sections.

Angiotensin-converting enzyme (ACE)

The ACE is a zinc-metallopeptidase that inactivates bradykinin and converts angiotensin I to II. Its main target organ is the vessel wall where it promotes constriction. In normal circumstances, the serum level of ACE is determined by genetic polymorphisms. In particular, an insertion (I)/ deletion (D) polymorphisms of a 287 bp sequence in the 16th intron is the main factor determining the production rate of this enzyme (Rigat et al. 1990). Since ACE is produced by epithelioid cells (developed from monocytes and macrophages) in sarcoidal granulomas its serum levels may also increase in sarcoidosis. The ACE level in these settings is thought to reflect the overall body granuloma burden (Gilbert et al. 1993). Though ACE shows a significant part in the etiopathogenesis of sarcoidosis, an association between *ACE* polymorphisms and disease susceptibility or severity is a matter of debate (Maliarik et al. 1998; Sharma and Smith 1997).

Multiple studies have been conducted in different ethnicities. Some have shown increased susceptibility to sarcoidosis in individuals carrying the D allele (normally accompanied by higher ACE levels), while others were unable to detect such a correlation (McGrath et al. 2001; Schürmann et al. 2001). Three major meta-analyses have also led to inconclusive results. The first one conducted in 2007 on 12 case–control studies demonstrated no association between the genetic variants of the *ACE* and sarcoidosis (Medica et al. 2007). The second one enrolled 17 studies and revealed a notable association between sarcoidosis and *ACE* genotypes in the subgroup analysis of different ethnicities which followed the dominant mode of inheritance (DD and DI vs. II) in East Asians and the recessive mode of inheritance (DD vs. DI and II) in Europeans (Song et al. 2014). The third study analyzed data from 20 case–control studies and was able to indicate an important relation only for the recessive model in all ethnicities (both Caucasian and Asian) (Zhu et al. 2015). Nevertheless, these associations do not appear in GWAS studies.

Table 1 The HLA associations of sarcoidosis

	Allele	Association	References
MHC class I	*HLA-A3, HLA-B7*	Confers risk for sarcoidosis. Associated with prolonged disease course	Grunewald et al. (2004), McIntyre et al. (1977)
	HLA-A1, HLA-B8	Confers risk for sarcoidosis. Associated with arthritis and with a favorable prognosis	Gardner et al. (1984), Grunewald et al. (2004)
MHC class II	*HLA-DQB1*0201*	Protects against sarcoidosis, mild disease in several populations, Lofgren's syndrome	Iannuzzi et al. (2003), Sato et al. (2002)
	*HLA-DQB1*0602*	Confers risk. Associated with progressive disease in several groups	Iannuzzi et al. (2003), Voorter et al. (2005)
	*HLA-DRB1*0301*	Confers risk. Acute onset, good prognosis, Lofgren's syndrome. Also in strong LD with HLA-DQB1*201	Berlin et al. (1997), Gardner et al. (1984), Hedfors and Lindström (1983)
	*HLA-DRB1*04*	Confers protection against sarcoidosis in several populations. Associated with ocular sarcoidosis and Heerfordt's syndrome	Martinetti et al. (1995)
	*HLA-DRB1*01*	Confers protection against sarcoidosis in several populations	Grunewald et al. (2010), Sato et al. (2010)
	*HLADRB1*1101*	Confers risk for sarcoidosis in Caucasians and African Americans. Associated with progressive stage II/III on chest X-ray. Associated with exposure to insecticides, molds, and must	Rossman et al. (2003, 2008)
	*HLADRB1*12*	Confers risk for sarcoidosis	Sato et al. (2010)
	*HLADRB1*14*	Confers risk for sarcoidosis	Berlin et al. (1997), Grunewald et al. (2010)
	*HLADRB1*15*	Confers risk for sarcoidosis. Associates with prolonged disease course. In strong LD with DQB1*0602	Rossman et al. (2003), Sato et al. (2002)
	*HLA-DRB1*0803*	Confers risk. For sarcoidosis. Associated with ocular sarcoidosis a Japanese study	Sato et al. (2010)
	*DRB3*0101*	Confers risk to progressive disease in Caucasians	Bogunia-Kubik et al. (2001)
	*DRB3*1501*	Lofgren's syndrome	Rossman et al. (2003), Voorter et al. (2005)

Chemokine Receptors

The chemoattractant and their receptors have a significant role in the pathogenesis of sarcoidosis since they facilitate immune cell trafficking and recruitment (Boring et al. 1997; Li et al. 2017). From all these chemokines a single nucleotide polymorphism (SNP), corresponding to the substitution of isoleucine instead of valine at position 64, on the *CC-chemokine receptor 2 (CCR2)* gene has been shown to confer protection from sarcoidosis in Japanese patients (Hizawa et al. 1999). A haplotype of eight–single nucleotide polymorphisms at this gene has also been linked to Löfgren's syndrome in individuals with Dutch ancestry (Spagnolo et al. 2003). However, a large-scale German study was unable to confirm these associations (Valentonyte et al. 2005a).

Though the CC-chemokine receptor 5 (CCR5) has a major role in the recruitment and activation of immune cells, no firm association with susceptibility to sarcoidosis has been detected for the gene encoding this protein.

Table 2 Non-HLA genes associated with sarcoidosis

Candidate gene	Location	Comment	References
Angiotensin-converting enzyme (ACE)	17q23	Increased risk for DD genotypes in association studies and metanalysis of association studies but not GWAS	Song et al. (2015)
Butyrophilin-Like 2 (BTNL-2)	6p21.32	Associated with sarcoidosis in Caucasian patients in both GWAS and association studies	Schurmann et al. (2001), Valentonyte et al. (2005b)
CC chemokine receptor 2 (CCR2)	3p21.3	Mixed results from association studies. Confers protection from sarcoidosis in a Japanese study and Linked to Löfgren's syndrome in Germans	Hizawa et al. (1999), Spagnolo et al. (2003)
CC chemokine receptor 5 (CCR5)	3p21.3	Mixed results from association studies. Female-restricted association with Löfgren's syndrome	Fischer et al. (2008)
Complement receptor 1 (CR1)	1q32	Confers risk for sarcoidosis in association studies	Zorzetto et al. (2002)
Cystic fibrosis transmembrane regulator (CFTR)	7q31.2	Mixed results. Confers risk for sarcoidosis in association studies	Bombieri et al. (2000)
CCDC88B	11q13.1	Susceptibility to sarcoidosis in GWAS	Fischer et al. (2012)
Chemokine (C–C motif) ligand 5 (CCL5)	17q.12	Confers risk for organ involvement (≥ 3 organs) in an association study	Takada et al. (2001)
CD14	5q31.1	Susceptibility to sarcoidosis with milder symptoms	Fridlender et al. (2010)
Chromosome 10 open reading frame 67 (C10ORF67)	10p12.31	A protein-coding gene that confers susceptibility to both sarcoidosis and Crohn's disease in a GWAS	Franke et al. (2008)
Cyclooxygenase-2 (COX2)	1q25.2-q25.3	Confers susceptibility to sarcoidosis. Associated with a greater risk factor for pulmonary fibrosis. Identified through associations studies	Hill et al. (2006; Lopez-Campos et al. 2009)
GREM1	15q13-q15	Confers risk factor for pulmonary fibrosis in sarcoidosis	Heron et al. (2011)
Heat shock protein 70 1 like (HSPA1L)	6p21.3	Confers risk for sarcoidosis in association studies	Bogunia-Kubik et al. (2006)
Inhibitor kβ-α	14q13	Confers risk for sarcoidosis in association studies	Abdallah et al. (2003)
Interleukin-1α	2q14	Confers risk for sarcoidosis in association studies	Hutyrova et al. (2002)
IL7R	5p13	Confers susceptibility to sarcoidosis and Löfgren's syndrome in an association study	Heron et al. (2009a)
IL23R	1p31.3	Confers susceptibility to chronic sarcoidosis and sarcoid uveitis both in GWAS and association studies	Fischer et al. (2011), Kim et al. (2011)
IFN-γ	9p22	Confers susceptibility to sarcoidosis in an association study	Akahoshi et al. (2004)
Integrin, alpha E (ITGAE)	17p13.3–13.2	Confers susceptibility to sarcoidosis in an association study	Heron et al. (2009b)

(continued)

Table 2 (continued)

Candidate gene	Location	Comment	References
Matrix metalloproteinase (MMP9)	20q11.2-q13.1	Confers susceptibility to sarcoidosis in an association study	Piotrowski et al. (2011)
Mannose receptor C-type 1 (MRC1)	10p12.33	Confers susceptibility to sarcoidosis in an association study	Hattori et al. (2010)
MyD88	3p22	Confers susceptibility to sarcoidosis in an association study	Daniil et al. (2013)
Neurogenic locus notch homolog 4 (NOTCH4)	6p21.3	Confers susceptibility to sarcoidosis in GWAS	Adrianto et al. (2012)
Osteosarcoma amplified 9 *(OS9)*	12q13.3-q14.1	The protein plays a central role in protein degradation and aToll-like receptor-induced myeloid cell activation. Confers susceptibility to sarcoidosis in GWAS	Hofmann et al. (2013)
RAB23	6p11	Member of the RAS oncogene family. Confers susceptibility to sarcoidosis. Identified through GWAS	Adrianto et al. (2012), Hofmann et al. (2011, 2013)
TGF-β1	19q13.1	Associated with severe sarcoidosis. Case–control association study	Jonth et al. (2007)
TGF-β2	1q41	Associated with acute/self-limiting disease. Case–control association study	Pabst et al. (2011)
TGF-β3	14q24	Associated with increased risk of pulmonary fibrosis. Case–control association study	Kruit et al. (2006)
Toll-like receptors (TLR10-TLR1-TLR6)	4p14	Confers protection from chronic sarcoidosis	Veltkamp et al. (2012)
TLR9	9q33.1	Confers risk for chronic sarcoidosis. Case–control association study	Pabst et al. (2013)
TLR4	9q32	Confers risk for chronic sarcoidosis. Case–control association study	Pabst et al. (2006)
TNF-α	6p21.3	Confers risk for Löfgren's syndrome and erythema nodosum. Identified through association studies	Labunski et al. (2001), McDougal et al. (2009), Medica et al. (2007), Seitzer et al. (1997), Grutters et al. (2002)
Vascular endothelial growth factor A (VEGFA)	6p12	Associated with protection from sarcoidosis and susceptibility to acute disease. Identified through association studies	Morohashi et al. (2003), Pabst et al. (2010), Seyhan et al. (2008)
Vascular endothelial growth factor receptor 1 (VEGFR1)	13q12	Confers risk for sarcoidosis. Identified through association studies	Pabst et al. (2010)
VEGFR2	4q11-q12	Associated with acute and chronic disease courses. Identified through association studies	Pabst et al. (2010)
Vitamin D receptor	12q12-14	Increased risk of sarcoidosis confirmed through association studies	Niimi et al. (1999)

Moreover, the gene expression profiling of peripheral blood mononuclear cells demonstrated lower expression of the *chemokine (C-X3-C motif) receptor 1* in patients with sarcoidosis (Zhou et al. 2012). The same study also conducted a GWAS and was able to show a significant association between SNPs of the *CX3CR* gene and sarcoidosis susceptibility and severity (Zhou et al. 2012).

The cluster of differentiation (CD) surface molecules

The two TCR/MHC-I co-stimulatory B7 molecules, the CD80 and CD86, on the surface of antigen-presenting cells interact with CD28 and CD152 expressed on T-cells and relay activating signals to T-cells. Studies have been able to demonstrate higher levels of these two molecules (CD80 and CD86) along with elevated levels *CD40* and *CD30L* on the surface of alveolar macrophages of patients with sarcoidosis compared to healthy control subjects (Grutters 2005). This inspired scientists to explore the association between genetic polymorphisms of the genes encoding these proteins with sarcoidosis. A study conducted on 146 Japanese patients failed to show an association between the sarcoidosis susceptibility and the promoter and exon 3 polymorphisms of the *CD80* gene and the exon 8 variants of the *CD86* genes. These variants were not linked to sarcoidosis severity or phenotypes either (Handa et al. 2005).

The CD27 which regulates B-cell activation and immunoglobulin synthesis through its interaction with CD70 and the CD3γ which is a TCR complex subunit responsible for activation of both cytotoxic and helper T-cells are two key signature genes downregulated in the peripheral blood samples of sarcoidosis patients compared to normal individuals (Koth et al. 2011). However, the genes encoding these two proteins do not appear in genetic association studies.

Complements

Zorzetto et al. have been the only team to indicate an association between the *complement receptor 1* (*CR1*) polymorphisms and susceptibility to sarcoidosis (Zorzetto et al. 2002). Individuals harboring the GG genotype of the *CR1* 507C > G polymorphism were at greater risk for developing sarcoidosis. Though the presence of the GG genotype was a significant predictor of sarcoidosis in female patients, no correlations with clinical factors were demonstrable.

Cystic Fibrosis Transmembrane Conductance Regulator (CFTR)

The *CFTR* gene is known for its role in the pathogenesis of cystic fibrosis (CF). The R75Q variant of this gene appears to be more frequent in patients with atypical mild CF (Hughes et al. 2001). Bombieri and colleagues reported an association between this same variant and susceptibility to sarcoidosis (Bombieri et al. 2000). However, in a follow-up study utilizing the whole CF gene mutation screening panels, these findings were not replicated for sarcoidosis (Kishore and Petrek 2013).

Heat Shock Protein

Antibodies to 70 kDa HSPs (HSP70) have been detected in sarcoidosis (Smet and Ramadan 2001). To furthermore clarify their contribution to the pathogenesis of sarcoidosis the *HSPA1L* gene encoding for an HSP70 and located within the MHC class III region was evaluated (Bogunia-Kubik et al. 2006). The *HSP70*+2437 C allele was noted to be linked to susceptibility to sarcoidosis and Löfgren's syndrome in patients with Polish ancestry. These findings were not replicated for patients with Japanese ancestry (Ishihara et al. 1995).

Inhibitor KB-α

The nuclear factor kappa B (NF-κB) is an inducible transcription factor that mediates most signaling pathways in the alveolar macrophages and CD4+T-cells and is thus involved in the pathogenesis of sarcoidosis. The inhibitor kappa B-alpha (IκB) controls the activity of the NF-κB by halting its entrance to the nucleus (Conron et al. 2001). Abdallah and colleagues hypothesized that genetic variations of the *IκB-α* gene, especially those within the promoter region, might show a role in the etiopathogenesis of sarcoidosis by influencing the expression of *IκB-α* and subsequently affecting the intensity of the inflammation. From the three studied SNPs, the −297 T allele was indicated to be related to sensitivity to sarcoidosis (Abdallah et al. 2003).

Interleukins

IL-1 superfamily contains 11 cytokines that have structural and functional similarities and except IL-18 and IL-33 are all encoded by a gene cluster on the second chromosome (2q12-14). The two main members, IL-1α and IL-1β, are strong proinflammatory cytokines that bind to the IL-1 receptor (IL-1R) and act through activation of the MyD88 adaptor. The functions of these two cytokines are regulated by the natural antagonist of the IL-1R (IL-1Ra) which competes with them over binding sites (Veerdonk and Netea 2013)

The role of this cytokine superfamily in the pathogenesis of sarcoidosis has been vastly investigated. IL-1β which is mainly produced by macrophages is thought to have a role in maintaining T-cell alveolitis and granuloma formation. The bronchoalveolar lavage drained from patients suffering from pulmonary sarcoidosis demonstrates higher levels of IL-1β activity (Hunninghake 1984). It has been concluded that the IL-1Ra/IL-1β ratio in alveolar macrophage culture supernatants of individuals with sarcoidosis could predict disease chronicity (Mikuniya et al. 2000). Genetic polymorphisms in the IL-1α gene have also shown an association with sarcoidosis susceptibility. The—889 C allele on the 5′–flanking region of *the IL-1α* gene is twice as common in sarcoidosis patients from Czechia compared with healthy controls (Hutyrova et al. 2002). Investigations of genetic polymorphisms on *IL-1β* and *IL-1 receptor antagonist* (*IL-1RA*) have failed to show a relationship with sarcoidosis (Grutters et al. 2003a; Hutyrova et al. 2002; Niimi et al. 2000; Pandey JP, Frederick M, Group AR 2002).

As another member of the IL-1 superfamily, IL-18 is suspected in the etiopathogenesis of sarcoidosis by stimulating the production of IFN-γ (Shigehara et al. 2001). There have been contradictory results about the association between *IL-18* 607 (A/C) SNP and susceptibility to sarcoidosis in Japanese (Zhou et al. 2005) and Caucasian patients (Janssen et al. 2004).

Recently, two SNPs, one on the *IL-23 receptor* gene (rs11209026, Arg381Gln) and the other near *the IL-12B* gene (rs4921492) were found to confer risk for sarcoidosis. These SNPs are thought to influence the expression of the respective genes (Fischer et al. 2015). IL-12 and IL-23 are involved in the Th1 and Th17 mediated immunity which are well-known contributors to the development of granulomas and sarcoidosis (Berge et al. 2012). Moreover, the genetic polymorphisms on these two loci also confer risk for psoriasis and Crohn's disease (Berge et al. 2012). Since drugs targeting IL-12/IL-23 such as Ustekinumab are already available, confirmation of this association would be of clinical value (Judson et al. 2014).

TNF-α

TNF-α is a prominent proinflammatory cytokine with several effects that make it relevant to the pathogenesis of sarcoidosis: it upregulates the production and release of other proinflammatory cytokines such as IL-1; it attracts neutrophils; it enhances the phagocytic ability of macrophages, and it promotes the activity of T-cell. Although a study on familial cases of sarcoidosis in African-American subjects failed to demonstrate a link between sarcoidosis and TNF-α levels (Rybicki et al. 2004), multiple other reports have documented elevated levels of TNF-α production in macrophages isolated from the alveolar lavages of patients with active sarcoidosis (Zheng et al. 1995). Studies have also demonstrated a dramatic drop in TNF levels after successful treatment or spontaneous resolution of sarcoidosis (Müller-Quernheim et al. 1992; Ziegenhagen et al. 2002). Furthermore, using TNF-α inhibitors in the treatment of patients with sarcoidosis is associated with promising results (Doty et al. 2005; Pritchard and Nadarajah 2004). Proceeding on the tract of the mentioned evidence, multiple studies have investigated the contribution of *TNFα* genetic polymorphisms to sarcoidosis susceptibility and severity. The *TNF* gene locus is located within the MHC III domain of the 6th chromosome and contains multiple functional variants. One particular polymorphism located at position −308 (rs1800629) of the promoter segment has been linked to variations in TNFα production in normal and pathological states. The uncommon allele of this SNP, *TNFA2* (adenine instead of guanine at position-308) is linked to higher levels of *TNFα* translation. This variant was indicated to be connected with Löfgren syndrome or sarcoidosis-related erythema nodosum in multiple ethnicities (Labunski et al. 2001; Seitzer et al. 1997). The association was not apparent in patients with non-Löfgren sarcoidosis and therefore predicted a more favorable disease outcome (Grutters et al. 2002; Swider et al. 1999). Moreover, a meta-analysis consisting of seven cohorts investigating *−308/TNF-α* polymorphism, confirmed the association and showed that the dominant model had the highest Odds ratio for predicting sarcoidosis (Medica et al. 2007).

Another uncommon allele (T) at position −857 within the promoter region of the *TNF-α* was also shown to increase the susceptibility to sarcoidosis (Grutters et al. 2002). Sharma et al. have demonstrated that the *TNF-A1031* and -A863 polymorphisms also increase the risk of developing sarcoidosis in Asian Indians (Sharma et al. 2008).

Whether these TNFα associations are of functional relevance or due to the linkage disequilibrium (LD) in the MHC segment remains to be elucidated.

The butyrophilin-like 2 (BTNL2) gene

BTNL2 belongs to the immunoglobulin superfamily, is a coinhibitory molecule closely related to CD80 and CD86. BTNL2 impedes T-cell activity and cytokine production (Arnett et al. 2007; Valentonyte et al. 2005b). This protein is encoded by a gene located on 6p21.3 (within the MHC region). The links between sarcoidosis and genetic polymorphisms of the *BTNL-2* were discovered by a German familial genome-wide linkage study consisting of 63 families with sarcoidosis (Schurmann et al. 2001). Further investigations revealed the association to be due to the rs2076530 A allele. This allele triggers a functional change in the coded protein by disrupting the transmembrane helix and the C-terminal immunoglobulin C domain (Valentonyte et al. 2005b).

Although there is strong linkage disequilibrium (LD) between *BTNL2* and HLA alleles, some have argued that the associations between *BTNL2* variants and sarcoidosis might be independent of this LD (Rybicki BA, Walewski JL, Maliarik MJ, Kian H, Iannuzzi MC, Group AR 2005).

Although multiple studies in different ethnicities have marked the association between the rs2076530 and susceptibility to sarcoidosis, in a recent GWAS the strongest association signal was found on another SNP within the promoter region precisely at the transcription factor binding site (rs5007259) which remained significant even after conditioning for HLA- alleles and the rs2076530 variant (Fischer et al. 2015).

The annexin A11 (ANXA11) gene

ANXA11 gene is located at 10q22.3 and encodes a type of calcium-dependent, phospholipid-binding protein. It is involved in apoptosis, cell division, exocytosis, and vesicular trafficking (Gerke and Moss 2002). The link between the polymorphisms of the *ANXA11* gene and sarcoidosis was revealed by GWA studies (Hofmann et al. 2008; Levin et al. 2013; Mrazek et al. 2011). The rs1049550 showed the strongest association with sarcoidosis with the C allele protecting against the disease in Caucasians and African Americans (Hofmann et al. 2008; Levin et al. 2013). Also, the uncommon A allele of rs61860052 conferred protection from sarcoidosis in African Americans (Levin et al. 2013). The exact consequence of these polymorphisms and the role of ANXA11 in the etiopathogenesis of sarcoidosis is not understandable. It has been proposed that the dysregulation of apoptosis resulting from AXNA11 variants could increase the survival of inflammatory cells and slow down the resolution of inflammatory granulomas (Hofmann et al. 2008).

Ras-related protein Rab-23

This protein is involved in signal transduction, cellular transportation of proteins, and autophagosome formation required for antibacterial effects (Smith et al. 2007; Zheng et al. 2017). It is encoded by the

Rab-23 gene located on chromosome 6p12.1. The T allele of the rs1040461 is associated with sarcoidosis susceptibility in general and sarcoidosis associated with uveitis in particular (Davoudi et al. 2018; Hofmann et al. 2011). This relationship might be due to the ineffective clearing of bacterial pathogens that have been involved in the etiopathogenesis of sarcoidosis as triggering antigens (Davoudi et al. 2018).

Neurogenic locus notch homolog protein 4 (NOTCH4)

The association between the *NOTCH4* gene and sarcoidosis was revealed through GWAS studies indicating a higher prevalence of the rs715299 G allele in patients with sarcoidosis (Adrianto et al. 2012). The NOTCH is involved in regulating the T-cell activity (Maillard et al. 2003) and has also been linked to multiple autoimmune diseases (Duvefelt et al. 2004; Gorlova et al. 2011).

The 11q13.1 region

A recent GWAS in individuals from European ancestry identified the 11q13.1 chromosome region to be associated with sarcoidosis susceptibility (Fischer et al. 2012). Several genes and SNPs reside within this region but the rs479777 followed by the rs671976 had the strongest association signals with sarcoidosis. Both SNPs are cis-eQTLs for the expression of the *coiled-coil domain containing 88 (CCDC88B)* gene with the C allele of the rs479777 and the G alleles of the rs671976 positively correlating with the expression level of the *CCDC88B* gene (independent of the tissue or cell being investigated). This gene encodes a protein implicated in protection against the endoplasmic reticulum (ER)-related cellular stress response (Matsushita et al. 2011).

Besides the CCDC88B gene, three other promising candidate genes have also been suggested as the risk gene in the 11q13.1 region based on the data extracted from fine-mapping studies and expression profile investigations. All three genes are located within the risk region and their expression is under the influence of the mentioned SNPs. The candidate genes include the *potassium channel subfamily K member 4* (*KCNK4*) which regulates airway mechanosensing (Lembrechts et al. 2011), the *phospholipase C β 3* (*PLCB3*) which may have an act in T-cell chemotaxis and macrophage sensitivity to apoptosis (Bach et al. 2007; Wang et al. 2008), and the *peroxiredoxin 5* (*PRDX5*) which is an antioxidant that protects cells against nitro-oxidative stress (Knoops et al. 2011). Dysregulation of *PRDX5* may be joined in the etiopathogenesis of sarcoidosis and granuloma formation by affecting the phagocytic function of macrophages through the impairment of the respiratory burst. All three genes had higher expression in the bronchoalveolar lavage of individuals with sarcoidosis (Fischer et al. 2012).

3 Granuloma Annulare

Granuloma annulare (GA) is classified as a type of non-infectious granulomatous skin condition with polymorphous clinical features. Although the prototype lesions of GA are small coalescing papules that form a ringlike structure, other variants including generalized, subcutaneous, macular, patch, and perforating lesions have also been described (Piette and Rosenbach 2016a; Rubin and Rosenbach 2019). GA is more common in women, with a women-to-men ratio of 2:1, and it commonly occurs before the age of thirty. Though subcutaneous GA prons appear more frequently in children, generalized GA is often reported in elderly patients (Davids et al. 1993; Wang and Khachemoune 2018). Histologically, GA exhibits granulomatous inflammation with either interstitial or palisading configuration of lymphocytes and histiocytes accompanied by mucin deposition (Rubin and Rosenbach 2019). Although the etiology of GA is unknown, there is a very well-recognized link between the disorders and systemic associations such as diabetes mellitus, hyperlipidemia, thyroid disease, malignancies, and human immunodeficiency virus (HIV) (Piette and Rosenbach 2016b; Rubin and Rosenbach 2019). Moreover, some studies have suggested trauma, bites, infections, and vaccines as inciting agents (Barron et al. 1997; Baykal et al. 2002; Piette and Rosenbach 2016b). Primarily, the disease was thought to result from an insult to the blood vessels (vasculopathy/ vasculitis) based on the evidence showing thickened blood vessel walls in GA lesions. Since deposits of fibrinogen, immunoglobulin, and complement were found within these vessels it was supposed that the mechanism underlying the vasculitis was a type III immune complex reaction (Dahl et al. 1977; Friedman-Birnbaum and Ludatscher 1986). However, further studies were unable to replicate these findings (Bergman et al. 1993) and an alternative hypothesis of the involvement of cell-mediated immunity was proposed. This theory was supported by the evidence showing the presence of activated macrophages, helper T-cells, CD3+T-cells, and fibroblasts in the GA lesions (Buechner et al. 1983; Fayyazi et al. 2000). Nevertheless, neutrophil migration was also indicated to be damaged in GA patients. This could result in the recruitment of macrophages instead of neutrophils for pathogen clearing which may promote the formation of granulomas (Gange et al. 1979; Piette and Rosenbach 2016b).

Hence a presumed scenario for GA pathogenesis could start with an as yet unknown stimulus that triggers a delayed-type hypersensitivity reaction with sequestration of macrophages and histiocytes which release matrix metalloproteinases and secondarily damage the connective tissues and vessel walls (Fayyazi et al. 2000). The T-cell-mediated immune reaction can also trigger collagen synthesis via fibroblast-activating chemokines (Kallioinen et al. 1992; Mempel et al. 2002).

3.1 The Immunogenetics of GA

Due to the low prevalence of the disease, there is a substantial paucity of data regarding the immunogenetics of GA. The contribution of genetics, however, has been suggested by the presence of familial cases of GA and reports on the co-occurrence of the disease in identical twins. A relatively small study has been able to document a link between generalized GA and *HLA-Bw35* allele (Friedman-Birnbaum et al. 1978; Friedman and Winkelmann 1987). The same HLA also confers susceptibility to autoimmune thyroid disease which is known to be associated with GA (Vázquez-López et al. 2003). A case report on the successful treatment of GA with adalimumab (TNFα inhibitor) provides another clue to the importance of genetic factors in the pathogenesis of GA. This case describes a 67-year-old female with generalized disseminated GA who experienced marked improvement after 3 months on 40 mg of adalimumab weekly. Her identical twin sister who developed similar lesions also responded favorably to adalimumab. Further evaluations showed that the patients harbored the *HLA-AH8.1* known to be linked to high levels of TNFα release from peripheral blood mononuclear cells (Knoell 2009). Thus so far only two genetic loci have been identified to presumably confer risks for GA.

4 Necrobiosis Lipoidica

Necrobiosis lipoidica (NL) is a rare idiopathic granulomatous disease characterized by the degeneration of collagen fibers. Clinically, NL lesions appear as expanding annular plaques that are red-brown at the edges and yellow at the center. The central area often demonstrates some degree of atrophy and telangiectasia. Ulceration occurs in roughly one-third of the cases and long-standing lesions are at increased for squamous cell carcinomas. NL is more frequent in women with a women-to-men ratio of almost 3:1. There is a debatable association between NL and systemic associations such as type 1 and 2 diabetes mellitus, thyroiditis, and celiac disease. The incidence of NL in diabetic patients is estimated to be about 0.3–1.2%. Meanwhile, the prevalence of diabetes in patients with NL is about 65%. NL precedes the onset of diabetes in about 14%, appears simultaneously in approximately 24%, and develops after the diagnosis of diabetes in 62% of the patients (Piette and Rosenbach 2016b). The prevalence of thyroiditis in individuals with NL is reported to be about 15% (Erfurt-Berge et al. 2012). Other reported associated conditions such as hyperlipidemia, inflammatory bowel disease (Crohn's disease or ulcerative colitis), rheumatoid arthritis (RA), and sarcoidosis are relatively rare and limited to case reports (Wanat and Rosenbach 2018).

Histologically lesions of NL are composed of layers of interstitial granulomatous inflammation and homogenized necrobiotic collagen depositions forming a sandwich-like appearance. The inflammation extends deep into the dermis and contains plasma cells (Alegre and Winkelmann 1988).

Numerous hypotheses have been proposed regarding the etiopathogenesis of NL. One popular theory emphasizes diabetic microangiopathy as the initial event (Reid et al. 2013) holding the lower oxygen tensions of the NL lesions, the higher rate of retinopathy in diabetic patients with NL, and the increased expression of glucose transporter-1 receptor on NL fibroblasts as supportive evidence (Boateng et al. 1993; Muller and Winkelmann 1966; Reid et al. 2013). The deposition of glycoproteins in vessel walls could compromise blood supply which could then result in collagen degeneration and recruitment of inflammation. Other vascular etiologies such as venous insufficiency and immune complex depositions have also been suggested (Nakajima et al. 2009). Moreover, the increased plasma fibronectin and α_2-macroglobulin in individuals with NL could influence the blood viscosity and promote inflammation (Koh et al. 1984; Majewski et al. 1981). However, the higher blood flow in Doppler studies of NL vessels contradicts these blood supply-related theories (Ngo et al. 2008). It has been concluded that abnormalities in collagen synthesis and metabolism can also cause NL. Studies have been able to demonstrate lower levels of collagen synthesis accompanied by defective cross-linking of the fibers in NL lesions (Oikarinen et al. 1987). Moreover, antibodies against different types of collagen have been shown in the sera of individuals with NL (Evans et al. 1988). Impaired neutrophil migration and increases TNFα concentration have also been detected in NL lesions but the significance of these results remains unknown (Wanat and Rosenbach 2018).

4.1 The Immunogenetics of NL

Familial cases of NL are very scarce. Although most of these reports are in individuals with diabetes (Seviour and Elkeles 1985; Shimanovich et al. 2008) some are not and can provide an opportunity to demonstrate the genetic background of the disorder(Ho et al. 1992; Roche-Gamón et al. 2007). On the other hand, to date, such a report has not been performed and the genetic background of the NL remains unclear.

5 Conclusion

In conclusion, non-infectious granulomatous skin diseases are associated with a complex interplay between genetic background and environmental factors. Although sarcoidosis as the prototype of these reactions has been extensively investigated, other diseases in this category remain elusive.

References

Abdallah A, Sato H, Grutters J, Veeraraghavan S, Lympany P, Ruven H, van den Bosch J, Wells A, Du Bois R, Welsh K (2003) Inhibitor kappa B-alpha (IκB-α) promoter polymorphisms in UK and Dutch sarcoidosis. Genes Immun 4:450–454

Adrianto I, Lin CP, Hale JJ, Levin AM, Datta I, Parker R, Adler A, Kelly JA, Kaufman KM, Lessard CJ (2012) Genome-wide association study of African and European Americans implicates multiple shared and ethnic specific loci in sarcoidosis susceptibility. PloS One 7

Akahoshi M, Ishihara M, Remus N, Uno K, Miyake K, Hirota T, Nakashima K, Matsuda A, Kanda M, Enomoto T (2004) Association between IFNA genotype and the risk of sarcoidosis. Hum Genet 114:503–509

Alegre V, Winkelmann R (1988) A new histopathologic feature of necrobiosis lipoidica diabeticorum: lymphoid nodules. J Cutan Pathol 15:75–77

Ali M, Atwan A, Gonzalez M (2010) Cutaneous sarcoidosis: updates in the pathogenesis. J Eur Acad Dermatol Venereol 24:747–755

Arnett HA, Escobar SS, Gonzalez-Suarez E, Budelsky AL, Steffen LA, Boiani N, Zhang M, Siu G, Brewer AW, Viney JL (2007) BTNL2, a butyrophilin/B7-like molecule, is a negative costimulatory molecule modulated in intestinal inflammation. J Immunol 178:1523–1533

Bach TL, Chen Q-M, Kerr WT, Wang Y, Lian L, Choi JK, Wu D, Kazanietz MG, Koretzky GA, Zigmond S (2007) Phospholipase Cβ is critical for T cell chemotaxis. J Immunol 179:2223–2227

Barron D, Cootauco M, Cohen BA (1997) Granuloma annulare. A clinical review. Lippincotts Prim Care Pract 1:33–39

Baykal C, Özkaya-Bayazit E, Kaymaz R (2002) Granuloma annulare possibly triggered by antitetanus vaccination. J Eur Acad Dermatol Venereol 16:516–518

Bergman R, Pam Z, Lichtig C, Reiter I, Friedman-Birnbaum R (1993) Localized granuloma annulare. Histopathological and direct immunofluorescence study of early lesions, and the adjacent normal-looking skin of actively spreading lesions. Am J Dermatopathol 15:544–548

Berlin M, Fogdell-Hahn A, Olerup O, Eklund A, Grunewald J (1997) HLA-DR predicts the prognosis in Scandinavian patients with pulmonary sarcoidosis. Am J Respir Crit Care Med 156:1601–1605

Boateng B, Hiller D, Albrecht H, Hornstein O (1993) Cutaneous microcirculation in pretibial necrobiosis lipoidica. Comparative laser Doppler flowmetry and oxygen partial pressure determinations in patients and healthy probands. Der Hautarzt; Zeitschrift fur Dermatologie. Venerologie, Und Verwandte Gebiete 44:581–586

Bogunia-Kubik K, Koscinska K, Suchnicki K, Lange A (2006) HSP70-hom gene single nucleotide (+ 2763 G/A and+ 2437 C/T) polymorphisms in sarcoidosis. Int J Immunogenet 33:135–140

Bogunia-Kubik K, Tomeczko J, Suchnicki K, Lange A (2001) HLA-DRB1* 03, DRB1* 11 or DRB1* 12 and their respective DRB3 specificities in clinical variants of sarcoidosis. Tissue Antigens 57:87–90

Bombieri C, Luisetti M, Belpinati F, Zuliani E, Beretta A, Baccheschi J, Casali L, Pignatti PF (2000) Increased frequency of CFTR gene mutations in sarcoidosis: a case/control association study. Eur J Hum Genet 8:717–720

Boring L, Gosling J, Chensue SW, Kunkel SL, Farese RV, Broxmeyer HE, Charo IF (1997) Impaired monocyte migration and reduced type 1 (Th1) cytokine responses in CC chemokine receptor 2 knockout mice. J Clin Investig 100:2552–2561

Buechner S, Winkelmann R, Banks PM (1983) Identification of T-cell subpopulations in granuloma annulare. Arch Dermatol 119:125–128

Chen ES, Moller DR (2014) Etiologic role of infectious agents. In: (eds) Seminars in respiratory and critical care medicine. Thieme Medical Publishers, pp 285–295

Chu P, Connolly MK, LeBoit PE (1994) The histopathologic spectrum of palisaded neutrophilic and granulomatous dermatitis in patients with collagen vascular disease. Arch Dermatol 130:1278–1283

Conron M, Bondeson J, Pantelidis P, Beynon HL, Feldmann M, duBois RM, Foxwell BM (2001) Alveolar macrophages and T cells from sarcoid, but not normal lung, are permissive to adenovirus infection and allow analysis of NF-κ B–dependent signaling pathways. Am J Respir Cell Mol Biol 25:141–149

Dahl MV, Ullman S, Goltz RW (1977) Vasculitis in granuloma annulare: histopathology and direct immunofluorescence. Arch Dermatol 113:463–467

Dai C, Shih S, Ansari A, Kwak Y, Sami N (2019) Biologic therapy in the treatment of cutaneous sarcoidosis: a literature review. Am J Clin Dermatol 20:409–422

Daniil Z, Mollaki V, Malli F, Koutsokera A, Antoniou K, Rodopoulou P, Gourgoulianis K, Zintzaras E, Vassilopoulos G (2013) Polymorphisms and haplotypes in MyD88 are associated with the development of sarcoidosis: a candidate-gene association study. Mol Biol Rep 40:4281–4286

Davids JR, Kolman BH, Billman GF, Krous HF (1993) Subcutaneous granuloma annulare: recognition and treatment. J Pediatr Orthop 13:582–586

Davoudi S, Chang VS, Navarro-Gomez D, Stanwyck LK, Sevgi DD, Papavasileiou E, Ren A, Uchiyama E, Sullivan L, Lobo A-M (2018) Association of genetic variants in RAB23 and ANXA11 with uveitis in sarcoidosis. Mol Vis 24:59

de Smet MD, Ramadan A (2001) Circulating antibodies to inducible heat shock protein 70 in patients with uveitis. Ocul Immunol Inflamm 9:85–92

Doty JD, Mazur JE, Judson MA (2005) Treatment of sarcoidosis with infliximab. Chest 127:1064–1071

Dubey S, Merry P (2007) Interstitial granulomatous dermatitis (Ackerman's syndrome) in SLE presenting with the 'rope sign.' Rheumatology 46:80

Duvefelt K, Anderson M, Fogdell-Hahn A, Hillert J (2004) A NOTCH4 association with multiple sclerosis is secondary to HLA-DR* 1501. Tissue Antigens 63:13–20

Eishi Y (2013) Etiologic link between sarcoidosis and Propionibacterium acnes. Respir Investig 51:56–68

Erfurt-Berge C, Seitz A-T, Rehse C, Wollina U, Schwede K, Renner R (2012) Update on clinical and laboratory features in necrobiosis lipoidica: a retrospective multicentre study of 52 patients. Eur J Dermatol 22:770–775

Evans C, Pereira R, Yuen C, Holden C (1988) Anti-collagen antibodies in granuloma annulare and necrobiosis lipoidica. Clin Exp Dermatol 13:252–254

Fayyazi A, Schweyer S, Eichmeyer B, Herms J, Hemmerlein B, Radzun H, Berger H (2000) Expression of IFNγ, coexpression of TNFα and matrix metalloproteinases and apoptosis of T lymphocytes and macrophages in granuloma annulare. Arch Dermatol Res 292:384–390

Fischer A, Ellinghaus D, Nutsua M, Hofmann S, Montgomery CG, Iannuzzi MC, Rybicki BA, Petrek M, Mrazek F, Pabst S (2015) Identification of immune-relevant factors conferring sarcoidosis genetic risk. Am J Respir Crit Care Med 192:727–736

Fischer A, Nothnagel M, Franke A, Jacobs G, Saadati HR, Gaede KI, Rosenstiel P, Schürmann M, Müller-Quernheim J, Schreiber S (2011) Association of inflammatory bowel disease risk loci with sarcoidosis, and its acute and chronic subphenotypes. Eur Respir J 37:610–616

Fischer A, Schmid B, Ellinghaus D, Nothnagel M, Gaede KI, Schürmann M, Lipinski S, Rosenstiel P, Zissel G, Höhne K (2012) A novel sarcoidosis risk locus for Europeans on chromosome 11q13. 1. Am J Respir Crit Care Med 186:877–885

Fischer A, Valentonyte R, Nebel A, Nothnagel M, Müller-Quernheim J, Schürmann M, Schreiber S (2008) Female-specific association of CC chemokine receptor 5 gene polymorphisms with Löfgren's syndrome. J Mol Med 86:553–561

Fontenot A, King T (2018) Pathology and pathogenesis of sarcoidosis. U: UpToDate, Post TW ur. UpToDate [Internet]. UpToDate, Waltham, MA

Forman JD, Klein JT, Silver RF, Liu MC, Greenlee BM, Moller DR (1994) Selective activation and accumulation of oligoclonal V beta-specific T cells in active pulmonary sarcoidosis. J Clin Investig 94:1533–1542

Franke A, Fischer A, Nothnagel M, Becker C, Grabe N, Till A, Lu T, Müller-Quernheim J, Wittig M, Hermann A (2008) Genome-wide association analysis in sarcoidosis and Crohn's disease unravels a common susceptibility locus on 10p12. 2. Gastroenterology 135:1207–1215

Fridlender ZG, Schwartz A, Kohan M, Amir G, Glazer M, Berkman N (2010) Association between CD14 gene polymorphisms and disease phenotype in sarcoidosis. Respir Med 104:1336–1343

Friedman-Birnbaum R, Ludatscher RM (1986) Comparative ultrastructural study of generalized and localized granuloma annulare. Am J Dermatopathol 8:302–308

Friedman-Birnbaum R, Haim S, Gideone O, Barzilai A (1978) Histocompatibility antigens in granuloma annulare: comparative study of the generalized and localized types. Br J Dermatol 98:425–428

Friedman SJ, Winkelmann R (1987) Familial granuloma annulare. Report of two cases and review of the literature. J Am Acad Dermatol 16:600–605

Gange R, Black MM, Carrington P (1979) Defective neutrophil migration in granuloma annulare, necrobiosis lipoidica, and sarcoidosis. Arch Dermatol 115:32–35

Gardner J, Kennedy HG, Hamblin A, Jones E (1984) HLA associations in sarcoidosis: a study of two ethnic groups. Thorax 39:19–22

Gerke V, Moss SE (2002) Annexins: from structure to function. Physiol Rev 82:331–371

Gilbert S, Steinbrech DS, Landas SK, Hunninghake GW (1993) Amounts of angiotensin-converting enzyme mRNA reflect the burden of granulomas in granulomatous lung disease. Am Rev Respir Dis 148: 483–486

Gorlova O, Martin J-E, Rueda B, Koeleman BP, Ying J, Teruel M, Diaz-Gallo L-M, Broen JC, Vonk MC, Simeon CP (2011) Identification of novel genetic markers associated with clinical phenotypes of systemic sclerosis through a genome-wide association strategy. PLoS Genet 7

Grunewald J, Brynedal B, Darlington P, Nisell M, Cederlund K, Hillert J, Eklund A (2010) Different HLA-DRB1 allele distributions in distinct clinical subgroups of sarcoidosis patients. Respir Res 11:25

Grunewald J, Eklund A, Olerup O (2004) Human leukocyte antigen class I alleles and the disease course in sarcoidosis patients. Am J Respir Crit Care Med 169:696–702

Grutters J (2005) Genetics of sarcoidosis: Role of co-stimulatory genes? Respiration 72:227–228

Grutters J, Sato H, Pantelidis P, Ruven H, McGrath D, Wells A, Van den Bosch J, Welsh K, Du Bois R (2003a) Analysis of IL6 and IL1A gene polymorphisms in UK and Dutch patients with sarcoidosis. Sarcoidosis Vasculitis Diff Lung Dis Offic J Wasog 20:20–27

Grutters JC, Sato H, Pantelidis P, Lagan AL, McGrath DS, Lammers J-WJ, van den Bosch JM, Wells AU, du Bois RM, Welsh KI (2002) Increased frequency of the uncommon tumor necrosis factor−857T allele in British and Dutch patients with sarcoidosis. Am J Respir Crit Care Med 165:1119–1124

Grutters JC, Sato H, Welsh KI, du Bois RM (2003b) The importance of sarcoidosis genotype to lung phenotype. Am J Respir Cell Mol Biol 29:S59

Haimovic A, Sanchez M, Judson MA, Prystowsky S (2012) Sarcoidosis: a comprehensive review and update for the dermatologist: part I. Cutaneous disease. J Am Acad Dermatol 66:699. e691–699. e618

Handa T, Nagai S, Ito I, Tabuena R, Shigematsu M, Hamada K, Kitaichi M, Izumi T, Aoyama T, Toguchida J (2005) Polymorphisms of B7 (CD80 and CD86) genes do not affect disease susceptibility to sarcoidosis. Respiration 72:243–248

Hattori T, Konno S, Takahashi A, Isada A, Shimizu K, Shimizu K, Taniguchi N, Gao P, Yamaguchi E, Hizawa N (2010) Genetic variants in mannose receptor gene (MRC1) confer susceptibility to increased risk of sarcoidosis. BMC Med Genet 11:151

Hawryluk EB, Izikson L, English JC (2010) Non-infectious granulomatous diseases of the skin and their associated systemic diseases. Am J Clin Dermatol 11:171–181

Heath CR, David J, Taylor SC (2012) Sarcoidosis: are there differences in your skin of color patients? J Am Acad Dermatol 66:121. e121–121. e114

Hedfors E, Lindström F (1983) HLA-B8/DR3 in sarcoidosis: correlation to acute onset disease with arthritis. Tissue Antigens 22:200–203

Heron M, Grutters J, Van Moorsel C, Ruven H, Huizinga T, Van Der Helm-van MA, Claessen A, Van Den Bosch J (2009a) Variation in IL7R predisposes to sarcoid inflammation. Genes Immun 10: 647–653

Heron M, Grutters JC, Van Moorsel CH, Ruven HJ, Kazemier KM, Claessen AM, Van den Bosch JM (2009b) Effect of variation in ITGAE on risk of sarcoidosis, CD103 expression, and chest radiography. Clin Immunol 133:117–125

Heron M, Van Moorsel C, Grutters J, Huizinga T, van der Helm-van MA, Nagtegaal M, Ruven H, van den Bosch J (2011) Genetic variation in GREM1 is a risk factor for fibrosis in pulmonary sarcoidosis. Tissue Antigens 77:112–117

Hill MR, Papafili A, Booth H, Lawson P, Hubner M, Beynon H, Read C, Lindahl G, Marshall RP, McAnulty RJ (2006) Functional prostaglandin-endoperoxide synthase 2 polymorphism predicts poor outcome in sarcoidosis. Am J Respir Crit Care Med 174:915–922

Hizawa N, Yamaguchi E, Furuya K, Jinushi E, ITO A, Kawakami Y (1999) The role of the CC chemokine receptor 2 gene polymorphism V64I (CCR2-64I) in sarcoidosis in a Japanese population. Am J Respir Crit Care Med 159:2021–2023

Ho KKL, O'loughlin S, Powell F (1992) Familial non-diabetic necrobiosis lipoidica. Australas J Dermatol 33:31–34

Hofmann S, Fischer A, Nothnagel M, Jacobs G, Schmid B, Wittig M, Franke A, Gaede KI, Schürmann M, Petrek M (2013) Genome-wide association analysis reveals 12q13. 3–q14. 1 as new risk locus for sarcoidosis. Eur Respir J 41:888–900

Hofmann S, Fischer A, Till A, Müller-Quernheim J, Häsler R, Franke A, Gäde K, Schaarschmidt H, Rosenstiel P, Nebel A (2011) A genome-wide association study reveals evidence of association with sarcoidosis at 6p12. 1. Eur Respir J 38:1127–1135

Hofmann S, Franke A, Fischer A, Jacobs G, Nothnagel M, Gaede KI, Schürmann M, Müller-Quernheim J, Krawczak M, Rosenstiel P (2008) Genome-wide association study identifies ANXA11 as a new susceptibility locus for sarcoidosis. Nat Genet 40:1103

Hughes D, Dörk T, Stuhrmann M, Graham C (2001) Mutation and haplotype analysis of the CFTR gene in atypically mild cystic fibrosis patients from Northern Ireland. J Med Genet 38:136–139

Hunninghake G (1984) Release of interleukin-1 by alveolar macrophages of patients with active pulmonary sarcoidosis. Am Rev Respir Dis 129:569–572

Hutyrova B, Pantelidis P, Drabek J, Zurkova M, Kolek V, Lenhart K, Welsh KI, du Bois RM, Petrek M (2002) Interleukin-1 gene cluster polymorphisms in sarcoidosis and idiopathic pulmonary fibrosis. Am J Respir Crit Care Med 165:148–151

Iannuzzi MC, Maliarik MJ, Poisson LM, Rybicki BA (2003) Sarcoidosis susceptibility and resistance HLA-DQB1 alleles in African Americans. Am J Respir Crit Care Med 167:1225–1231

Iannuzzi MC, Rybicki BA (2007) Genetics of sarcoidosis: candidate genes and genome scans. Proc Am Thorac Soc 4:108–116

Iannuzzi MC, Rybicki BA, Teirstein AS (2007) Medical progress. Sarcoidosis. N Eng J Med 357:2153–2165

Ishihara M, Ohno S, Ishida T, Ando H, Naruse T, Nose Y, Inoko H (1994) Molecular genetic studies of HLA class II alleles in sarcoidosis. Tissue Antigens 43:238–241

Ishihara M, Ohno S, Ishida T, Mizuki N, Ando H, Naruse T, Ishihara H, Inoko H (1995) Genetic polymorphisms of the TNFB and HSP70 genes located in the human major histocompatibility complex in sarcoidosis. Tissue Antigens 46:59–62

Janssen R, Grutters J, Ruven H, Zanen P, Sato H, Welsh K, Du Bois R, Van Den Bosch J (2004) No association between interleukin-18 gene polymorphisms and haplotypes in Dutch sarcoidosis patients. Tissue Antigens 63:578–583

Jonth AC, Silveira L, Fingerlin TE, Sato H, Luby JC, Welsh KI, Rose CS, Newman LS, Du Bois RM, Maier LA (2007) TGF-β1 variants in chronic beryllium disease and sarcoidosis. J Immunol 179:4255–4262

Judson MA, Baughman RP, Costabel U, Drent M, Gibson KF, Raghu G, Shigemitsu H, Barney JB, Culver DA, Hamzeh NY (2014) Safety and efficacy of ustekinumab or golimumab in patients with chronic sarcoidosis. Eur Respir J 44:1296–1307

Kallioinen M, Sandberg M, Kinnunen T, Oikarinen A (1992) Collagen synthesis in granuloma annulare. J Invest Dermatol 98

Kamil ZS, Chen T, Ghazarian D (2015) Non-infectious granulomatous conditions of the skin: a clinicopathological approach to diagnosis. J Clin Pathol 68:982–991

Kim HS, Choi D, Lim LL, Allada G, Smith JR, Austin CR, Doyle TM, Goodwin KA, Rosenbaum JT, Martin TM (2011) Association of interleukin 23 receptor gene with sarcoidosis. Dis Markers 31:17–24

Kishore A, Petrek M (2013) Immunogenetics of sarcoidosis. J Int Trends Immun 1:43–53

Knoell KA (2009) Efficacy of adalimumab in the treatment of generalized granuloma annulare in monozygotic twins carrying the 8.1 ancestral haplotype. Arch Dermatol 145:610–611

Knoops B, Goemaere J, Van der Eecken V, Declercq J-P (2011) Peroxiredoxin 5: structure, mechanism, and function of the mammalian atypical 2-Cys peroxiredoxin. Antioxid Redox Signal 15:817–829

Koh M, Majewski B, Barter S, Rhodes E (1984) Increased plasma fibronectin in diabetes mellitus, necrobiosis lipoidica and widespread granuloma annulare. Clin Exp Dermatol 9:293–297

Koth LL, Solberg OD, Peng JC, Bhakta NR, Nguyen CP, Woodruff PG (2011) Sarcoidosis blood transcriptome reflects lung inflammation and overlaps with tuberculosis. Am J Respir Crit Care Med 184:1153–1163

Kruit A, Grutters JC, Ruven HJ, van Moorsel CH, Weiskirchen R, Mengsteab S, van den Bosch JM (2006) Transforming growth factor-β gene polymorphisms in sarcoidosis patients with and without fibrosis. Chest 129:1584–1591

Labunski S, Posern G, Ludwig S, Kundt G, Brocker E-B, Kunz M (2001) Tumour necrosis factor-a promoter polymorphism in erythema nodosum. Acta Derm Venereol 81:18–21

Lembrechts R, Pintelon I, Schnorbusch K, Timmermans J-P, Adriaensen D, Brouns I (2011) Expression of mechanogated two-pore domain potassium channels in mouse lungs: special reference to mechanosensory airway receptors. Histochem Cell Biol 136:371

Levin A, Iannuzzi M, Montgomery C, Trudeau S, Datta I, McKeigue P, Fischer A, Nebel A, Rybicki B (2013) Association of ANXA11 genetic variation with sarcoidosis in African Americans and European Americans. Genes Immun 14:13–18

Li H, Zhao X, Wang J, Zong M, Yang H (2017) Bioinformatics analysis of gene expression profile data to screen key genes involved in pulmonary sarcoidosis. Gene 596:98–104

Lopez-Campos JL, Rodriguez-Rodriguez D, Rodriguez-Becerra E, Michavila IA, Guerra JF, Hernandez FJG, Casanova A, de Córdoba Gamero JF, Romero-Ortiz A, Arellano-Orden E (2009) Cyclooxygenase-2 polymorphisms confer susceptibility to sarcoidosis but are not related to prognosis. Respir Med 103:427–433

Luisetti M, Beretta A, Casali L (2000) Genetic aspects in sarcoidosis. Eur Respir J 16:768–780

Maillard I, Adler SH, Pear WS (2003) Notch and the immune system. Immunity 19:781–791

Majewski B, Barter S, Rhodes E (1981) Serum α2 globulin levels in granuloma annulare and necrobiosis lipoidica. Br J Dermatol 105:557–562

Maliarik MJ, Rybicki BA, Malvitz E, Sheffer RG, Major M, Popovich J Jr, Iannuzzi MC (1998) Angiotensin-converting enzyme gene polymorphism and risk of sarcoidosis. Am J Respir Crit Care Med 158:1566–1570

Martinetti M, Tinelli C, Kolek V, Cuccia M, Salvaneschi L, Pasturenzi L, Semenzato G, Cipriani A, Bartova A, Luisetti M (1995) " The sarcoidosis map": a joint survey of clinical and immunogenetic findings in two European countries. Am J Respir Crit Care Med 152:557–564

Matsushita E, Asai N, Enomoto A, Kawamoto Y, Kato T, Mii S, Maeda K, Shibata R, Hattori S, Hagikura M (2011) Protective role of Gipie, a Girdin family protein, in endoplasmic reticulum stress responses in endothelial cells. Mol Biol Cell 22:736–747

McDougal KE, Fallin MD, Moller DR, Song Z, Cutler DJ, Steiner LL, Cutting GR (2009) Variation in the lymphotoxin-α/tumor necrosis factor locus modifies risk of erythema nodosum in sarcoidosis. J Investig Dermatol 129:1921–1926

McGrath DS, Foley PJ, Petrek M, Izakovicova-Holla L, Dolek V, Veeraraghavan S, Lympany PA, Pantelidis P, Vasku A, Wells AU (2001) Ace gene I/D polymorphism and sarcoidosis pulmonary disease severity. Am J Respir Crit Care Med 164:197–201

McIntyre J, McKee K, Loadholt C, Mercurio S, Lin I (1977) Increased HLA-B7 antigen frequency in South Carolina blacks in association with sarcoidosis. In: (eds) Transplantation proceedings, pp 173–176

Medica I, Kastrin A, Maver A, Peterlin B (2007) Role of genetic polymorphisms in ACE and TNF-α gene in sarcoidosis: a meta-analysis. J Hum Genet 52:836–847

Mempel M, Musette P, Flageul B, Schnopp C, Remling R, Gachelin G, Kourilsky P, Ring J, Abeck D (2002) T-cell receptor repertoire and cytokine pattern in granuloma annulare: defining a particular type of cutaneous granulomatous inflammation. J Investig Dermatol 118:957–966

Mikuniya T, Nagai S, Takeuchi M, Mio T, Hoshino Y, Miki H, Shigematsu M, Hamada K, Izumi T (2000) Significance of the interleukin-1 receptor antagonist/interleukin-1β ratio as a prognostic factor in patients with pulmonary sarcoidosis. Respiration 67:389–396

Moller DR, Rybicki BA, Hamzeh NY, Montgomery CG, Chen ES, Drake W, Fontenot AP (2017) Genetic, immunologic, and environmental basis of sarcoidosis. Ann Am Thorac Soc 14:S429–S436

Morohashi K, Takada T, Omori K, Suzuki E, Gejyo F (2003) Vascular endothelial growth factor gene polymorphisms in Japanese patients with sarcoidosis. Chest 123:1520–1526

Mrazek F, Stahelova A, Kriegova E, Fillerova R, Zurkova M, Kolek V, Petrek M (2011) Functional variant ANXA11 R230C: true marker of protection and candidate disease modifier in sarcoidosis. Genes Immun 12:490–494

Müller-Quernheim J, Pfeifer S, Männel DN, Strausz J, Ferlinz R (1992) Lung-restricted activation of the alveolar macrophage/monocyte system in pulmonary sarcoidosis. Am Rev Respir Dis 145:187–192

Müller-Quernheim J, Schürmann M, Hofmann S, Gaede KI, Fischer A, Prasse A, Zissel G, Schreiber S (2008) Genetics of sarcoidosis. Clin Chest Med 29:391–414

Muller SA, Winkelmann R (1966) Necrobiosis lipoidica diabeticorum: histopathologic study of 98 cases. Arch Dermatol 94:1–10

Nakajima T, Tanemura A, Inui S, Katayama I (2009) Venous insufficiency in patients with necrobiosis lipoidica. J Dermatol 36:166–169

Neefjes J, Jongsma ML, Paul P, Bakke O (2011) Towards a systems understanding of MHC class I and MHC class II antigen presentation. Nat Rev Immunol 11:823–836

Ngo B, Wigington G, Hayes K, Huerter C, Hillman B, Adler M, Rendell M (2008) Skin blood flow in necrobiosis lipoidica diabeticorum. Int J Dermatol 47:354–358

Niimi T, Sato S, Tomita H, Yamada Y, Akita K, Maeda H, Kawaguchi H, Sugiura Y, Ueda R (2000) Lack of association with interleukin 1 receptor antagonist and interleukin-1 β gene polymorphisms in sarcoidosis patients. Respir Med 94:1038–1042

Niimi T, Tomita H, Sato S, Kawaguchi H, Akita K, Maeda H, Sugiura Y, Ueda R (1999) Vitamin D receptor gene polymorphism in patients with sarcoidosis. Am J Respir Crit Care Med 160:1107–1109

Oikarinen A, Mörtenhumer M, Kallioninen M, Savolainen ER (1987) Necrobiosis lipoidica: ultrastructural and biochemical demonstration of a collagen defect. J Investig Dermatol 88:227–232

Pabst S, Baumgarten G, Stremmel A, Lennarz M, Knüfermann P, Gillissen A, Vetter H, Grohe C (2006) Toll-like receptor (TLR) 4 polymorphisms

are associated with a chronic course of sarcoidosis. Clin Exp Immunol 143:420–426
Pabst S, Bradler O, Gillissen A, Nickenig G, Skowasch D, Grohe C (2013) Toll-like receptor-9 polymorphisms in sarcoidosis and chronic obstructive pulmonary disease. In: (eds) Respiratory regulation-the molecular approach. Springer, pp 239–245
Pabst S, Fränken T, Schönau J, Stier S, Nickenig G, Meyer R, Skowasch D, Grohé C (2011) Transforming growth factor-β gene polymorphisms in different phenotypes of sarcoidosis. Eur Respir J 38:169–175
Pabst S, Karpushova A, Diaz-Lacava A, Herms S, Walier M, Zimmer S, Cichon S, Nickenig G, Nöthen MM, Wienker TF (2010) VEGF gene haplotypes are associated with sarcoidosis. Chest 137:156–163
Pandey JP, Frederick M, Group AR (2002) TNF-α, IL1-β, and immunoglobulin (GM and KM) gene polymorphisms in sarcoidosis. Hum Immun 63:485–491
Patterson KC, Chen ES (2018) The pathogenesis of pulmonary sarcoidosis and implications for treatment. Chest 153:1432–1442
Piette EW, Rosenbach M (2016a) Granuloma annulare: clinical and histologic variants, epidemiology, and genetics. J Am Acad Dermatol 75:457–465
Piette EW, Rosenbach M (2016b) Granuloma annulare: pathogenesis, disease associations and triggers, and therapeutic options. J Am Acad Dermatol 75:467–479
Piotrowski WJ, Górski P, Pietras T, Fendler W, Szemraj J (2011) The selected genetic polymorphisms of metalloproteinases MMP2, 7, 9 and MMP inhibitor TIMP2 in sarcoidosis. Med Sci Mon Int Med J Exp Clin Res 17:CR598
Pritchard C, Nadarajah K (2004) Tumour necrosis factor α inhibitor treatment for sarcoidosis refractory to conventional treatments: a report of five patients. Ann Rheum Dis 63:318–320
Reid SD, Ladizinski B, Lee K, Baibergenova A, Alavi A (2013) Update on necrobiosis lipoidica: a review of etiology, diagnosis, and treatment options. J Am Acad Dermatol 69:783–791
Rigat B, Hubert C, Alhenc-Gelas F, Cambien F, Corvol P, Soubrier F (1990) An insertion/deletion polymorphism in the angiotensin I-converting enzyme gene accounting for half the variance of serum enzyme levels. J Clin Investig 86:1343–1346
Roche-Gamón E, Vilata-Corell JJ, Velasco-Pastor M (2007) Familial necrobiosis lipoidica not associated with diabetes. Dermatol Online J 13
Rossman MD, Thompson B, Frederick M, Iannuzzi MC, Rybicki BA, Pander J, Newman LS, Rose C, Magira E, Monos D (2008) HLA and environmental interactions in sarcoidosis. Sarcoidosis Vasculitis Diff Lung Dis Offic J WASOG 25:125–132
Rossman MD, Thompson B, Frederick M, Maliarik M, Iannuzzi MC, Rybicki BA, Pandey JP, Newman LS, Magira E, Beznik-Cizman B (2003) HLA-DRB1* 1101: a significant risk factor for sarcoidosis in blacks and whites. Am J Hum Genet 73:720–735
Rubin CB, Rosenbach M (2019) Granuloma annulare: a retrospective series of 133 patients. Cutis 103:102–106
Rybicki B, Maliarik M, Poisson L, Iannuzzi M (2004) Sarcoidosis and granuloma genes: a family-based study in African-Americans. Eur Respir J 24:251–257
Rybicki BA, Iannuzzi MC, Frederick MM, Thompson BW, Rossman MD, Bresnitz EA, Terrin ML, Moller DR, Barnard J, Baughman RP (2001) Familial aggregation of sarcoidosis: a case–control etiologic study of sarcoidosis (ACCESS). Am J Respir Crit Care Med 164:2085–2091
Rybicki BA, Walewski JL, Maliarik MJ, Kian H, Iannuzzi MC, Group AR (2005) The BTNL2 gene and sarcoidosis susceptibility in African Americans and Whites. Am J Hum Genet 77:491–499
Sato H, Grutters JC, Pantelidis P, Mizzon AN, Ahmad T, van Houte A-J, Lammers J-WJ, van den Bosch JM, Welsh KI, du Bois RM (2002) HLA-DQB1* 0201: a marker for good prognosis in British and Dutch patients with sarcoidosis. Am J Respir Cell Mol Biol 27:406–412
Sato H, Woodhead FA, Ahmad T, Grutters JC, Spagnolo P, van den Bosch JM, Maier LA, Newman LS, Nagai S, Izumi T (2010) Sarcoidosis HLA class II genotyping distinguishes differences of clinical phenotype across ethnic groups. Hum Mol Genet 19:4100–4111
Schmitt A, Volz A (2019) Non-infectious granulomatous dermatoses. Journal der Deutschen Dermatologischen Gesellschaft [J Ger Soc Dermatol JDDG] 17:518–533
Schurmann M, Reichel P, Muller-Myhsok B, Schlaak M, Muller-Quernheim J, Schwinger E (2001) Results from a genome-wide search for predisposing genes in sarcoidosis. Am J Respirat Crit Care Med 164:840–846
Schürmann M, Reichel P, Müller-Myhsok B, Dieringer T, Wurm K, Schlaak M, Müller-Quernheim J, Schwinger E (2001) Angiotensin-converting enzyme (ACE) gene polymorphisms and familial occurrence of sarcoidosis. J Intern Med 249:77–83
Seitzer U, Swider C, Stüber F, Suchnicki K, Lange A, Richter E, Zabel P, Müller-Quernheim J, Flad H-D, Gerdes J (1997) Tumour necrosis factor alpha promoter gene polymorphism in sarcoidosis. Cytokine 9:787–790
Seviour P, Elkeles R (1985) Necrobiosis lipoidica in two diabetic sisters. Clin Exp Dermatol 10:159–161
Seyhan E, Cetinkaya E, Altin S, Gunluoglu M, Demir A, Koksal V, Issever H (2008) Vascular endothelial growth factor gene polymorphisms in Turkish patients with sarcoidosis. Tissue Antigens 72:162–165
Sharma P, Smith I (1997) Clinical value of ACE genotyping in diagnosis of sarcoidosis. Lancet 349:1602–1603
Sharma S, Ghosh B, Sharma S (2008) Association of TNF polymorphisms with sarcoidosis, its prognosis and tumour necrosis factor (TNF)-α levels in Asian Indians. Clin Exp Immunol 151:251–259

Shigehara K, Shijubo N, Ohmichi M, Takahashi R, Kon S-i, Okamura H, Kurimoto M, Hiraga Y, Tatsuno T, Abe S (2001) IL-12 and IL-18 are increased and stimulate IFN-γ production in sarcoid lungs. J Immunol 166:642–649

Shimanovich I, Erdmann H, Grabbe J, Zillikens D, Rose C (2008) Necrobiosis lipoidica in monozygotic twins. Arch Dermatol 144:119–120

Smith AC, Heo WD, Braun V, Jiang X, Macrae C, Casanova JE, Scidmore MA, Grinstein S, Meyer T, Brumell JH (2007) A network of Rab GTPases controls phagosome maturation and is modulated by Salmonella enterica serovar Typhimurium. J Cell Biol 176:263–268

Smith G, Brownell I, Sanchez M, Prystowsky S (2008) Advances in the genetics of sarcoidosis. Clin Genet 73:401–412

Song GG, Kim J-H, Lee YH (2014) Associations between TNF-α− 308 a/G and lymphotoxin-α+ 252 a/G polymorphisms and susceptibility to sarcoidosis: a meta-analysis. Mol Biol Rep 41:259–267

Song GG, Kim J-H, Lee YH (2015) Associations between the angiotensin-converting enzyme insertion/deletion polymorphism and susceptibility to sarcoidosis: a meta-analysis. J Renin-Angiotensin-Aldosterone Syst 16:219–226

Song Z, Marzilli L, Greenlee BM, Chen ES, Silver RF, Askin FB, Teirstein AS, Zhang Y, Cotter RJ, Moller DR (2005) Mycobacterial catalase–peroxidase is a tissue antigen and target of the adaptive immune response in systemic sarcoidosis. J Exp Med 201: 755–767

Spagnolo P, Renzoni EA, Wells AU, Sato H, Grutters JC, Sestini P, Abdallah A, Gramiccioni E, Ruven HJ, du Bois RM (2003) CC chemokine receptor 2 and sarcoidosis: association with Lofgren's syndrome. Am J Respir Crit Care Med 168:1162–1166

Starshinova AA, Malkova AM, Basantsova NY, Zinchenko YS, Kudryavtsev IV, Ershov GA, Soprun LA, Mayevskaya VA, Churilov LP, Yablonskiy PK (2019) Sarcoidosis as an autoimmune disease. Front Immun 10

Sverrild A, Backer V, Kyvik KO, Kaprio J, Milman N, Svendsen CB, Thomsen SF (2008) Heredity in sarcoidosis: a registry-based twin study. Thorax 63:894–896

Swider C, Schnittger L, Bogunia-Kubik K, Gerdes J, Flod H, Lange A, Seitzer U (1999) TNF- and HLA-DR genotyping as potential prognostic markers in pulmonary sarcoidosis. Eur Cytokine Netw 10: 143–146

Takada T, Suzuki E, Ishida T, Moriyama H, Ooi H, Hasegawa T, Tsukuda H, Gejyo F (2001) Polymorphism in RANTES chemokine promoter affects extent of sarcoidosis in a Japanese population. Tissue Antigens 58:293–298

ten Berge B, Paats MS, Bergen IM, van den Blink B, Hoogsteden HC, Lambrecht BN, Hendriks RW, KleinJan A (2012) Increased IL-17A expression in granulomas and in circulating memory T cells in sarcoidosis. Rheumatology 51:37–46

Vadasz Z, Toubi E (2017) FoxP3 expression in macrophages, cancer, and B cells—is it real? Clin Rev Allergy Immunol 52:364–372

Valentonyte R, Hampe J, Croucher PJ, Müller-Quernheim J, Schwinger E, Schreiber S, Schürmann M (2005a) Study of CC chemokine receptor 2 alleles in sarcoidosis, with emphasis on family-based analysis. Am J Respir Crit Care Med 171:1136–1141

Valentonyte R, Hampe J, Huse K, Rosenstiel P, Albrecht M, Stenzel A, Nagy M, Gaede KI, Franke A, Haesler R (2005b) Sarcoidosis is associated with a truncating splice site mutation in BTNL2. Nat Genet 37:357–364

Vázquez-López F, Pereiro M Jr, Haces JM, López MG, Sánchez TS, Coto TF, Oliva NP, Toribio J (2003) Localized granuloma annulare and autoimmune thyroiditis in adult women: a case-control study. J Am Acad Dermatol 48:517–520

Veerdonk FVD, Netea M (2013) New insights in the immunobiology of IL-1 family members. Front Immunol 4:167

Veltkamp M, van Moorsel CH, Rijkers GT, Ruven HJ, Grutters J (2012) Genetic variation in the Toll-like receptor gene cluster (TLR10-TLR1-TLR6) influences disease course in sarcoidosis. Tissue Antigens 79: 25–32

Voorter CE, Drent M, van den Berg-Loonen EM (2005) Severe pulmonary sarcoidosis is strongly associated with the haplotype HLA-DQB1* 0602–DRB1* 150101. Hum Immunol 66:826–835

Wahlström J, Dengjel J, Persson B, Duyar H, Rammensee H-G, Stevanović S, Eklund A, Weissert R, Grunewald J (2007) Identification of HLA-DR–bound peptides presented by human bronchoalveolar lavage cells in sarcoidosis. J Clin Investig 117:3576–3582

Wanat K, Rosenbach M (2018) Necrobiosis lipoidica. UpToDate. Waltham (MA): UpToDate. Accessed May 29

Wang J, Khachemoune A (2018) Granuloma annulare: a focused review of therapeutic options. Am J Clin Dermatol 19:333–344

Wang Z, Liu B, Wang P, Dong X, Fernandez-Hernando C, Li Z, Hla T, Li Z, Claffey K, Smith JD (2008) Phospholipase C β3 deficiency leads to macrophage hypersensitivity to apoptotic induction and reduction of atherosclerosis in mice. J Clin Investig 118: 195–204

Yanardag H, Tetikkurt C, Bilir M, Yılmaz E (2017) Association of HLA antigens with the clinical course of sarcoidosis and familial disease. Monaldi Arch Chest Dis 87

Zheng L-Q, Chi S-M, Li C-X (2017) Rab23's genetic structure, function and related diseases: a review. Bioscience Rep 37

Zheng L, Teschler H, Guzman J, Hübner K, Striz I, Costabel U (1995) Alveolar macrophage TNF-alpha release and BAL cell phenotypes in sarcoidosis. Am J Respir Crit Care Med 152:1061–1066

Zhou T, Zhang W, Sweiss NJ, Chen ES, Moller DR, Knox KS, Ma S-F, Wade MS, Noth I, Machado RF (2012) Peripheral blood gene expression as a novel genomic biomarker in complicated sarcoidosis. PloS One 7

Zhou Y, Yamaguchi E, Hizawa N, Nishimura M (2005) Roles of functional polymorphisms in the interleukin-18 gene promoter in sarcoidosis. Sarcoidosis Vasculitis Diff Lung Dis Offic J WASOG 22:105–113

Zhu R, Bi L, Kong H, Tilley S, Wang H, Xie W (2015) Meta-analytical association between angiotensin-converting enzyme gene polymorphisms and sarcoidosis risk. Genet Mol Res 14:3590–3600

Ziegenhagen MW, Rothe ME, Zissel G, Müller-Quernheim J (2002) Exaggerated TNF alpha release of alveolar macrophages in corticosteroid resistant sarcoidosis. Sarcoidosis Vasculitis Diff Lung Dis Offic J WASOG 19:185–190

Zorzetto M, Bombieri C, Ferrarotti I, Medaglia S, Agostini C, Tinelli C, Malerba G, Carrabino N, Beretta A, Casali L (2002) Complement receptor 1 gene polymorphisms in sarcoidosis. Am J Respir Cell Mol Biol 27:17–23

The Immunogenetics of Photodermatoses

Chaw-Ning Lee, Tzu-Ying Chen, and Tak-Wah Wong

Abstract

Photodermatosis is an abnormal skin inflammatory reaction to light. The major classifications of photodermatoses are idiopathic photodermatoses, photodermatoses due to exogenous or endogenous agents, photo-exacerbated dermatoses, and photosensitive genodermatoses. In this chapter, we focus on idiopathic photodermatoses and drug-related photodermatoses and emphasize on the epidemiology and immunogenetic backgrounds. Idiopathic photodermatoses, a spectrum of diseases with abnormal responses to ultraviolet radiation (UVR), include polymorphous light eruption, actinic prurigo, hydroa vacciniforme, chronic actinic dermatitis, and solar urticaria. Young people are more susceptible to most idiopathic photodermatoses except for chronic actinic dermatitis. Interestingly, idiopathic photodermatoses exhibit different characteristics between Caucasians and Asians. For example, the average age of Asian actinic prurigo patients is older than that of Caucasians in which genetic backgrounds or Fitzpatrick skin type might play a role. Drug-induced photodermatoses can be classified into phototoxic and photoallergic drug reactions. Certain drug-induced photodermatoses may mimic other dermatoses. For instance, drug-induced lupus erythematosus (LE) should be considered if an old man is diagnosed with LE but had a poor response to standard treatments.

Keywords

Actinic prurigo · Chronic actinic dermatitis · Hydroa vacciniforme · Photodermatoses · Polymorphous light eruption · Solar urticaria

1 Introduction

Photodermatoses are skin disorders that are precipitated by sunlight exposure. They can be classified into four major categories according to etiology: idiopathic photodermatoses, photodermatoses due to exogenous or endogenous agents, genetic photodermatoses, and photo-exacerbated dermatoses. Genetic photodermatoses are beyond the scope of this book and photo-exacerbated dermatoses will be discussed as individual

C.-N. Lee · T.-Y. Chen · T.-W. Wong (✉)
Department of Dermatology, National Cheng Kung University Hospital, College of Medicine, Tainan, Taiwan
e-mail: twwong@mail.ncku.edu.tw

T.-W. Wong
Department of Biochemistry & Molecular Biology, College of Medicine, Tainan, Taiwan

T.-W. Wong
Center of Applied Nanomedicine, National Cheng Kung University, Tainan, Taiwan

N. Rezaei and F. Rajabi (eds.), *The Immunogenetics of Dermatologic Diseases*, Advances in Experimental Medicine and Biology 1367,
https://doi.org/10.1007/978-3-030-92616-8_14

dermatoses in other chapters. The other categories will be reviewed in this and the following chapter.

2 Idiopathic Photodermatoses

The precise pathogenesis and etiology of idiopathic photodermatoses remain unclear. The idiopathic photodermatoses include polymorphous light eruption (PMLE), actinic prurigo (AP), hydroa vacciniforme (HV), chronic actinic dermatitis (CAD), and solar urticaria (SU). They are differentiated based on their distinct demographics, clinical features, and disease course (Fig. 1).

2.1 Polymorphous Light Eruption

Polymorphic light eruption (PMLE) occurs preferentially in young female adults. Although a recent report has claimed that PMLE is more common in individuals with skin of color, the disease is classically considered to be more common in Caucasians or people with Fitzpatrick skin type I (Gutierrez et al. 2018). PMLE patients develop itchy symmetric skin lesions at sun-exposed areas during spring or summer that appear within hours after exposure to ultraviolet A (UVA). The cutaneous signs are usually polymorphous and can include papules, plaques, vesicles, bullae, insect bite (strophulus)-like lesions, and erythema multiforme-like targets. However, in a single patient, the lesions are quite monomorphous and tend to recur in the same place (Fig. 2) (Dover and Hawk 1988; Jansen and Karvonen 1984).

PMLE is a delayed-type hypersensitivity (DTH) response to unknown light-induced photoantigens (Gruber-Wackernagel et al. 2014; Norris et al. 1991, 1989a). The presence of a DTH response is supported by the expression of endothelial leukocyte adhesion molecule-1, intercellular adhesion molecule-1 (ICAM-1), and vascular cell adhesion molecule-1 in PMLE lesions (Norris et al. 1991). It has been hypothesized that in genetically predisposed subjects, light (UVA more than UVB) triggers a reaction in the skin that leads to the formation of a photoantigen that induces a strong immune response in PMLE patients. In a healthy person, the immune response is abrogated by UV radiation-induced immune suppression (Gruber-Wackernagel et al. 2014). The $CD11b^{+}$ macrophage-like cells play an important role in the induction of immune suppression and tolerance after UVB irradiation by producing Interleukin (IL)-10 (Gruber-Wackernagel et al. 2014; Hammerberg et al. 1996). In PMLE skin, there is an extensive CD4+ T lymphocyte infiltration for up to 72 h after UVB irradiation in early lesions that are followed by CD8+ T cell infiltrations (Norris et al. 1992). Epidermal Langerhans cells (LC), dermal macrophages, plasmacytoid dendritic cells, and T regulatory cells are also increased in the papillary dermis in PMLE lesions (Rossi et al. 2018). Kölgen et al. showed that UVB irradiation failed to deplete CD1a + epidermal LCs and augment CD11b+ cells in PMLE (Kolgen et al. 1999). Neutrophils also

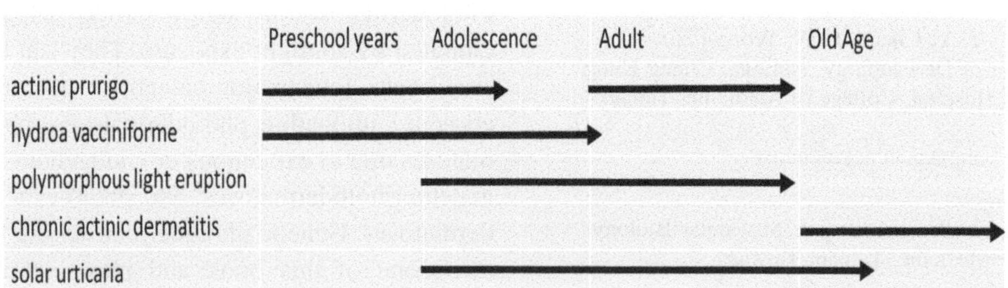

Fig. 1 The age of onset of idiopathic photodermatoses in a lifetime

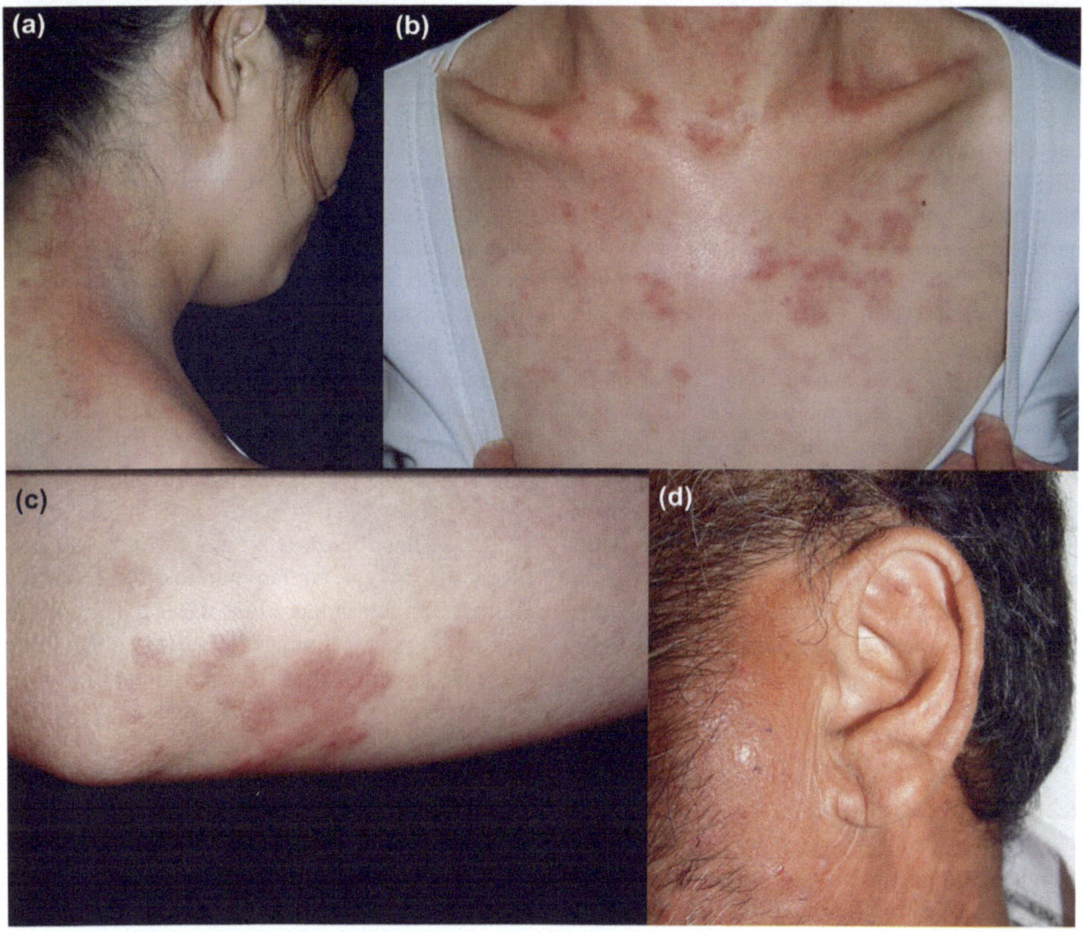

Fig. 2 Clinical pictures of polymorphic light eruption. **a** PMLE lesions presented as plaques; **b** papules; **c** insect bite-like, and **d** papulovesicles

migrate into normal human skin after UV exposure (Gruber-Wackernagel et al. 2014) but this does not occur in PMLE skin (Wolf et al. 2009). Whereas a T_H2 response is favored in normal skin after UV light, a T_H1 response is favored in patients with PMLE (Kolgen et al. 2004).

PMLE has a higher prevalence among twins and family members that suggests a genetic predisposition for the disease (Guarrera et al. 1993; Millard et al. 2000). Although not conclusive, a few candidate genes have shown associations with PMLE including *glutathione S-transferases (GST)* genes (*GSTM1, GSTT1 and GSTP1*), *IL-10*, *Fc fragment of IgG receptor (FCGR2A)*, *selectin-E* (*SELE*), *intercellular adhesion molecule-1* (*ICAM1*), *IL1A*, *IL1B*, *IL-1 receptor antagonist (IL1RN)*, and *tumor necrosis factor* (*TNF*)*-alpha* (Millard et al. 2008, 2001; Zirbs et al. 2013). Lembo et al. used genome-wide expression analysis to identify possible candidate genes and found 14 genes with lower expression and 2 genes with higher expression in patients with PMLE than in controls (Lembo et al. 2017). Among them, six genes, including *C1S* and *SCARB1* are related to apoptotic cell clearance. Reduced expression of these genes might impair normal apoptosis, lessen UV-induced immunosuppression and finally resulted in an active response to photoantigens after irradiation in PMLE susceptible skin (Lembo et al. 2017).

Moreover, some studies have hypothesized that UV-induced damage to microbial communities might lead to PMLE (Patra et al. 2016; Patra and Wolf 2016). Patra et al. reported increased expression of psoriasin, ribonuclease 7 (RNase7), HBD-2, and cathelicidin (LL-37) and decreased HBD-3 in PMLE skin (Lembo and Raimondo 2018; Patra et al. 2016, 2018). Vitamin D may have an antimicrobial effect in the skin and PMLE patients were found to have lower vitamin D levels (Patra and Wolf 2016). In fact, twice-daily administration of topical vitamin D_3 analog, calcipotriol, for more than 2 weeks before heavy sun exposure can alleviate symptoms in PMLE patients (Felton et al. 2013). Kim et al. revealed that calcipotriol suppressed some antimicrobial peptides (AMPs), which were stimulated by UVB in keratinocytes (Kim et al. 2009).

2.2 Actinic Prurigo

Actinic prurigo (AP) occurs preferentially in female Caucasian children. Although most of the patients with AP may spontaneously improve by adolescence, some features of the disease may persist into adulthood (Crouch et al. 2002). In contrary to Caucasians, AP mostly develops in adults in their 40 s and has male predominance in Asians (Chen et al. 2016c). About 20% of AP patients have a positive family history (McGregor et al. 2000). AP is reported to have a strong link to the human leukocyte antigen with *(HLA)-DRB1*0407 (DR4)* (60–80%) being the most prevalent subtype especially in Mexicans (Ross et al. 2008; Vega Memije et al. 2017), followed by *HLA DRB1*0401* (Ross et al. 2008). In Singapore, there is a closer association with *HLA-DRB1*0301* in affected patients (Chen et al. 2016b). AP patients develop intensely pruritic papules or nodules at sun-exposed (mainly the UVA wavelength) areas including lower lip and eyes during spring or summer season. These lesions are usually eczematous, excoriated or crusted, with additional scarring or post-inflammatory pigmentation after repeated scratching. Some patients may have conjunctivitis (Fig. 3).

AP is a DTH reaction and the immunogenic features are similar to PMLE. Some patients may primarily present with features of PMLE and later develop AP or vice versa which suggests a relationship between these two diseases (Grabczynska et al. 1999).

DTH has 4 major subtypes: type IVa with the dominance of T_H1, IFN-γ, IL-1, and IL-2; type IVb with the dominance of T_H2, eosinophils, IL-5, IL-4, and IL-13; type IVc with CD8+ T-cells, perforin, granzyme B, and Fas Ligand as major players; and type IVd with CD4+ T-cells, CD8 + T-cells, neutrophil, IL8, and GM-CSF all participating in the inflammation (Czarnobilska et al. 2007). AP induces both DTH T_H1 and T_H2 reactions (Vega Memije et al. 2017). One study was able to demonstrate dense nodular or diffuse inflammation in the dermis in skin samples of 20 Mexican AP patients (Arrese et al. 2001). B lymphocytes were identified in the central part of the follicle and T lymphocytes were identified in the periphery of lymphoid follicles (Arrese et al. 2001). TNF-alpha appeared mainly in the suprabasal keratinocytes. Another study was able to show elevated serum IgE levels in patients with AP (Cuevas-Gonzalez et al. 2016a). The presence of eosinophils and mast cells in AP tissue suggested a type IVb hypersensitivity reaction (Martinez-Luna et al. 2015). Cuevas-Gonzalez et al. found a higher expression of p53, Bcl-2 and caspase 3 in AP skin that suggested apoptotic pathways to be the last step in the immune response in AP patients after UV irradiation (Cuevas-Gonzalez et al. 2016b).

2.3 Hydroa Vacciniforme

Hydroa vacciniforme (HV) is a rare, chronic, scarring photodermatosis that occurs in children aged 1 to 15 years with spontaneous remission in puberty or young adulthood (Gupta et al. 2000). HV is commonly associated with Epstein–Barr virus (EBV) infection in endemic areas (Chen

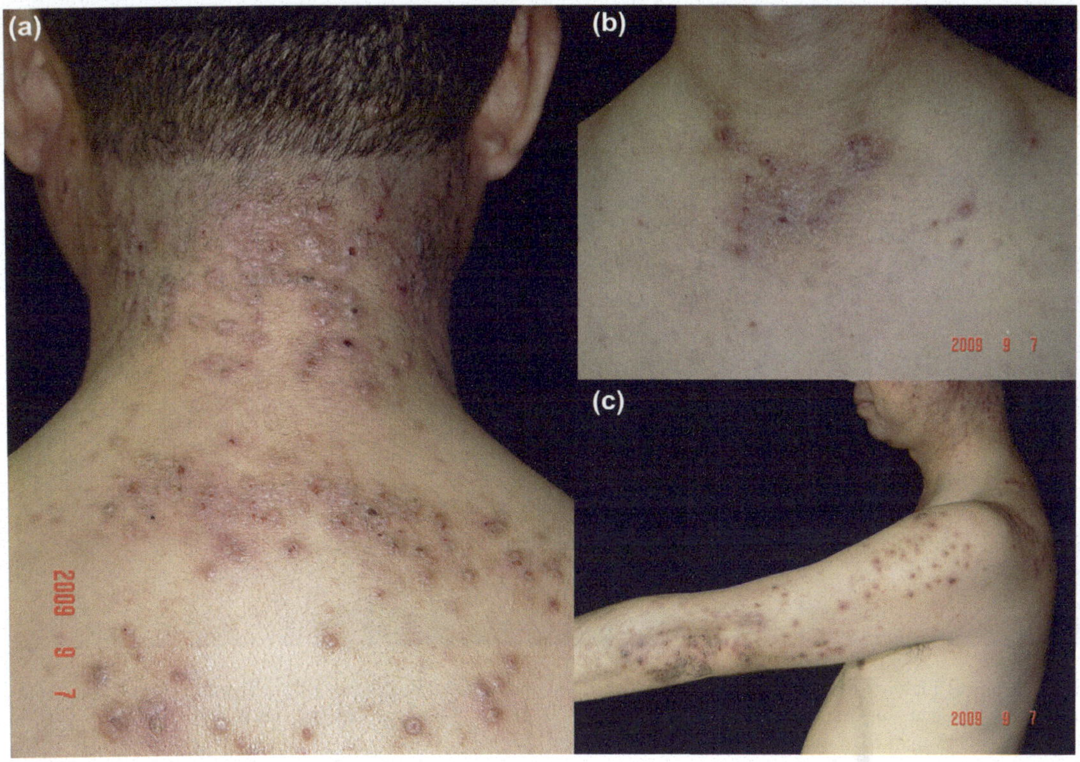

Fig. 3 Clinical pictures of adult-onset actinic prurigo. Papules, erosions and crustic ulcers are distributed on the sun-exposed skin (**a**, **b**, and **c**)

et al. 2016a). Within 30 min to 2 h after UV exposure, multiple eruptive pruritic erythematous macules develop mainly over bilateral cheeks, lower lip, and dorsal hands. These lesions are usually associated with pruritus or a burning sensation. They eventually evolve into symmetric hemorrhagic papulovesicular lesions and crusted blisters (Fig. 4) that heal with characteristic varioliform scars (Fig. 5). HV is sometimes associated with chronic EBV infection but it should be differentiated from hydroa vacciniforme-like lymphoma (HVLL) (Fig. 6). HVLL is a T-cell lymphoproliferative disorder that is believed to be caused by chronic EBV infection. However, the skin lesions in HVLL are prone to necrosis and ulcerations in both sun-exposed and covered skin and they are accompanied by systemic symptoms such as fever, anemia, hepatosplenomegaly, and wasting (Iwatsuki et al. 2006). The pathogenesis of HV is unknown. It has been reported that in 17% of cases, HV may evolve to HVLL (Chen et al. 2016a). Several genetic immunodeficiencies or gene mutations including *GATA2 deficiency, SH2D1, BIRC4, ITK, MAGT1*, and *CD27* mutations are associated with severe EBV disease and EBV-associated cancers but precise genetic studies regarding HV as missing (Cohen 2015; Cohen et al. 2016; Dropulic and Cohen 2011).

2.4 Chronic Actinic Dermatitis

Chronic actinic dermatitis (CAD) is a rare chronic disease that presents with eczematous or lichenified itchy patches or plaques in sun-exposed skin. In Caucasians, it usually occurs in elderly men (Fig. 7) but in darker skin type, it occurs more frequently in females and its onset is earlier (Gutierrez et al. 2018). The precise pathogenesis of CAD is unknown but it is quite similar to DTH reaction of allergic contact

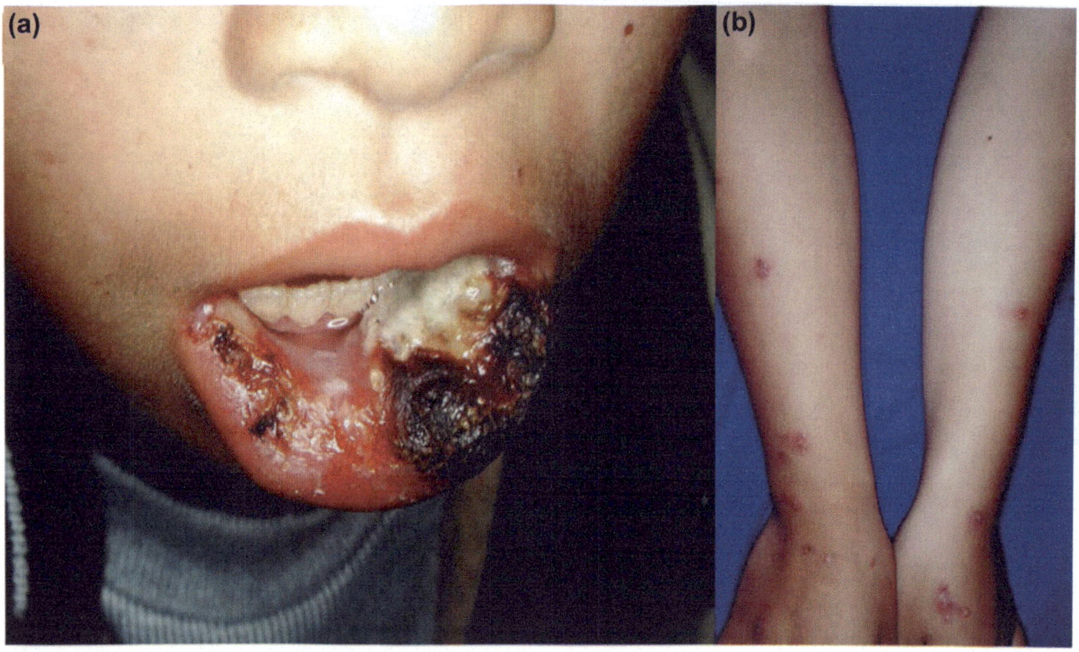

Fig. 4 Clinical pictures of hydroa vacciniforme on the face, lower lip and upper extremities in a 10-year-old child. Noted the marked necrosis of his lower lip and many papulovesicles on both forearms and dorsal hands after sunlight exposure (**a** and **b**)

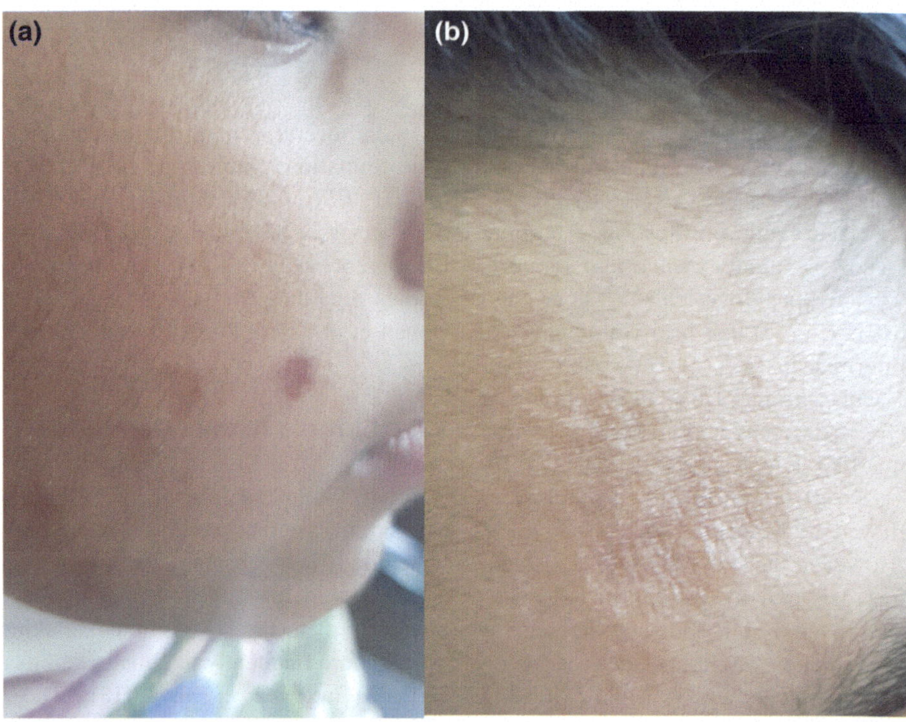

Fig. 5 Skin lesions in hydroa vacciniforme patients are healed with varioliform scars (**a** and **b**)

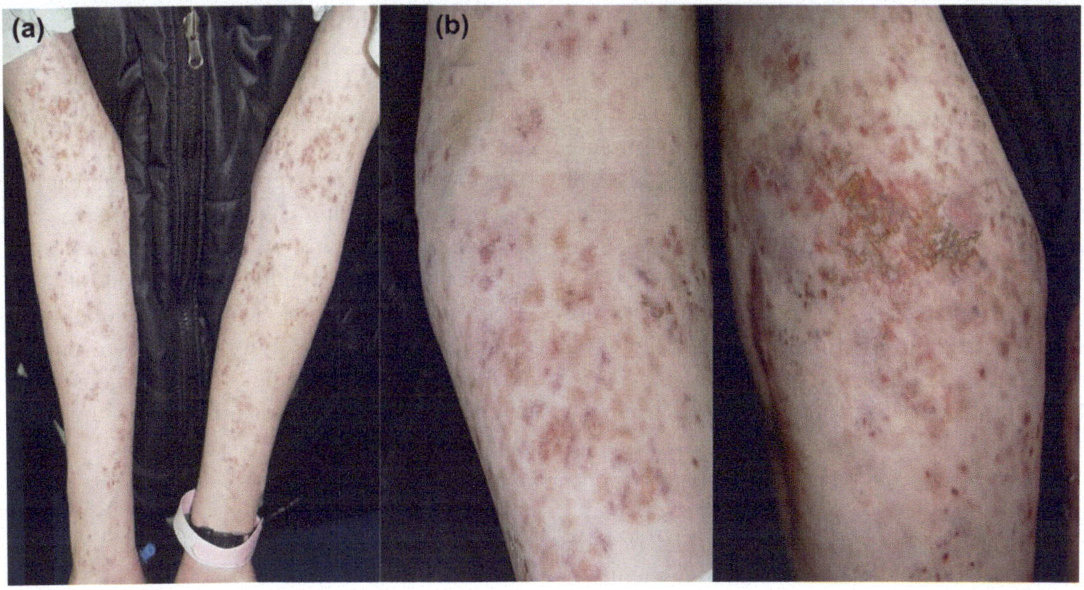

Fig. 6 Clinical pictures of a hydroa vacciniforme-like lymphoma patient with crustic papuloveiscles on his arms and thighs (**a** and **b**)

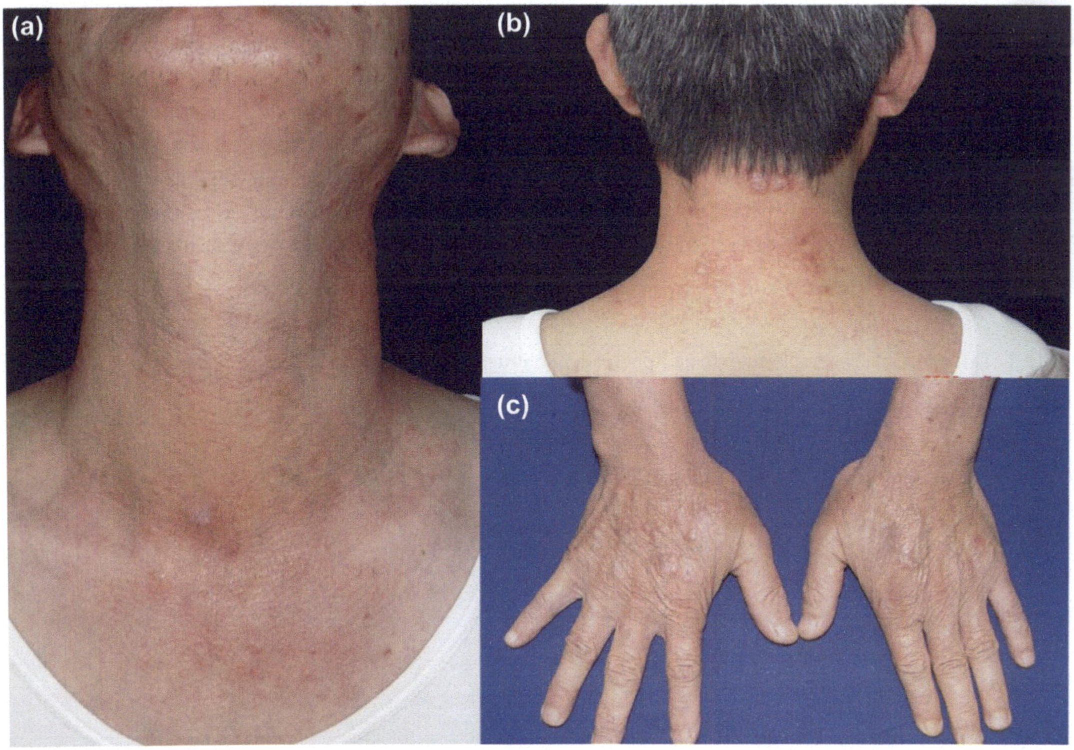

Fig. 7 Clinical pictures of chronic actinic dermatitis with lichenoid papules and plaques on the neck, upper chest, and dorsal hands (**a**, **b**, and **c**)

dermatitis in which $CD8^+$ cytotoxic suppressor T cells are predominant in the dermis of lesional skin (Hamada et al. 2017; Norris et al. 1989b).

The DTH response presumably results from cumulative UV irradiation especially in summer (Pas et al. 2004). In Asians, CAD is reported to be related to air pollution and other allergens such as sunscreens and plants (Kim and Kim 2018; Sharma and Verma 2012; Tan et al. 2011). Lei et al. reported the differences in mRNAs and long noncoding RNAs (lncRNAs) between CAD patients and normal controls (Lei et al. 2017). The presence of inflammatory and immune response-related genes such as TNFAIP3 among the differentially expressed genes (DEGs) suggested that they may play an important role in the pathogenesis of CAD (Lei et al. 2017). In their study, 4401 mRNAs (including 2310 upregulated and 2091 downregulated genes) and 243 lncRNAs (198 annotated and 45 novel lncRNAs) with differential expression levels were obtained between CAD samples and normal controls.

Moreover, in CAD, the expression of extracellular matrix-related genes is altered with an elevated *matrix metallopeptidase (MMP)-1* resulting in degeneration of elastin fibers, and deposition of elastin and fibrillin-1 (Liu et al. 2008). Other studies have failed in demonstrating an association between CAD and the *filaggrin* gene although its role in the pathogenesis of DTH and atopic dermatitis has been confirmed (Harkins et al. 2015).

2.5 Solar Urticaria

Solar urticaria (SU) is a variant of urticaria. After 5–10 min of exposure to UV or visible light (Komarow et al. 2015), pruritic and erythematous wheals develop over light-exposed areas and they resolve within hours. Angioedema and anaphylaxis are rare but have been reported. Unlike the other idiopathic photodermatoses, SU is an immediate type I (immunoglobulin E-mediated) hypersensitivity response against cutaneous or circulating photoallergens. The precise genetic associations of SU have not been studied but a detailed discussion on the immunogenetics of urticaria, in general, is discussed in a separate chapter.

3 Drug-Related Photodermatoses

3.1 Phototoxic and Photoallergic Reactions

Drug-induced photodermatoses can be classified into phototoxic and photoallergic reactions (Table 1). Phototoxicity can occur in any patient whenever the threshold concentration of the compound has been reached while photoallergy is a cell-mediated immune response induced by a small amount of chemical or drug in a previously sensitized patient. However, some phototoxic agents induce idiosyncratic reactions that affect

Table 1 Differences between phototoxic and photoallergic drugs induced reactions

Disease	Phototoxicity	Photoallergy
Incidence	High	Low
Onset after exposure to sunlight	Within hours	24–72 h
Mechanism	Non-immunological, dose-dependent	Immune-mediated
Light dose	Dependent	Independent
Distribution	Sun-exposed area only	May extend to non-sun exposed skin
Clinical presentation	Sunburn-like reaction (Khandpur et al. 2017)	Eczematous change

only a few specific patients. UVA is the major wavelength that elicits drug-induced photodermatoses. UVB and visible light can also induce photodermatoses.

Aminolevulinic acid (ALA), methyl aminolevulinate (MAL), and porfimer sodium used as photosensitizers in photodynamic therapy are examples of drugs that lead to phototoxic reactions activated by visible light. A possible explanation is that the offending drugs are activated by sunlight leading to the generation of reactive oxygen species (ROS) that cause tissue damage (Khandpur et al. 2017). Irradiation could also induce the binding of photosensitizer to cellular DNA (photoadducts) which results in DNA destructions (Khandpur et al. 2017). The common systemic phototoxic drugs are tetracyclines (especially doxycycline), quinolones, griseofulvin, voriconazole, retinoids, sulfonamides/trimethoprim, hydrochlorothiazide, phenothiazines amiodarone, nonsteroidal anti-inflammatory drugs (NSAIDs), taxane, vemurafenib (Dummer et al. 2012), methotrexate, psoralens, ALA, MAL, and porfimer sodium (Trakatelli et al. 2009). Some of the most common topical phototoxic drugs are coal tar, ketoprofen, and furocoumarins (Monteiro et al. 2016). Long-term use of voriconazole may induce severe phototoxic skin reactions and subsequently result in squamous cell carcinoma or melanoma in the up-coming years (Miller et al. 2010; Vohringer et al. 2011). The pediatric population is at a higher risk. Photoprotection should be warranted in children under voriconazole treatment. Su et al. reported the increased risk of cutaneous squamous cell carcinoma with an adjusted hazard ratio of 1.17 among patients treated with photosensitizing antihypertensive drugs (Su et al. 2018).

Photoallergy is DTH response induced by sunlight (usually UVA). The offending drug covalently binds to an endogenous protein to form a photoallergen (haptenization) (Khandpur et al. 2017). The subsequent immune-related cytokines and chemokines then cause inflammation and eczematous reactions identical to allergic contact dermatitis. Photoallergic reactions occur more frequently in the administration of topical agents compared to that of systemic drugs (Gonzalez and Gonzalez 1996; Khandpur et al. 2017). The common topical photoallergic agents are ingredients in sunscreens (e.g., benzophenones, cinnamates, dibenzoyl methanes), fragrances (such as musk ambrette, sandalwood oil), phenothiazines (promethazine, chlorpromazine), NSAIDs, bithionol, chlorhexidine, hexachlorophene, and fenticlor. Systemic photoallergic drugs include quinine, quinidine, griseofulvin, quinolones, sulfonamides, and NSAIDs (especially diclofenac and ketoprofen) (Kutlubay et al. 2014; Trakatelli et al. 2009).

The clinical manifestations vary from mild erythema to severe blisters. In some instances, the photoallergic reactions may even cause lupus erythematosus and pseudoporphyria (Table 2).

3.2 Genes Related to Drug-Induced Photodermatoses

Phototoxic drug reactions are found more commonly in Caucasians while photoallergic reactions occur equally between different races (Nakamura et al. 2014). There is a genetic predisposition to drug-induced lupus erythematosus and drug-induced subacute cutaneous lupus erythematosus. The former has increased expression of HLA DR-4 and the latter has increased expression of HLA-B8 and HLA DR3 (Ho and Chauhan 2018). Nakamura et al. revealed a higher incidence of drug-induced phototoxicity in Caucasians compared to African-Americans (15.9% vs. 0.7%) (Nakamura et al. 2014). This can be explained by the different amounts of melanin in colored skin and white skin. Melanin can form stable complexes with certain drugs in the epidermis (Wrzesniok et al. 2005). Few genetic polymorphisms have been suggested to be associated with susceptibility to developing phototoxic reactions. The *ATP-binding cassette (ABC) transporter ABCG2* gene is one of these genes. This transporter maintains a role in

Table 2 Drug-induced photodermatoses

Diseases	Drug	Duration/mechanism/ref
Drug-induced lupus erythematosus (DILE)	Hydralazine, procainamide, isoniazid, minocycline, diltiazem and TNF antagonist (Ho and Chauhan 2018)	Usually months to two years
Drug-induced subacute cutaneous lupus erythematosus (DISCLE)	Terbinafine, TNF antagonist, anti-epileptics, proton pump inhibitor (PPI), NSAIDs (especially naproxen), calcium channel blockers (CaCB), and ACE inhibitors, nab-paclitaxel (Gonzalez and Gonzalez 1996; Ho and Chauhan 2018)	PPI: 3 days to 5 months (Aggarwal 2016)
Pseudoporphyria	Voriconazole, NSAIDs of the propionic acid family, naproxen, nalidixic acid, tetracyclines, sulfonylureas, furosemide, bumetanide, dapsone, pyridoxine, benoxaprofen, tiaprofenic acid, amiodarone, erythropoietin, and etretinate family	Skin lesions similar to porphyria cutanea tarda but the symptoms usually continue for months after the drug has been discontinued
Erythema multiforme	Paclitaxel	
Onycholysis	Taxane, tetracyclines, psoralens, NSAIDs, fluoroquinolones	Nail plate absorbs and focuses UV energy on the nail bed (Kutlubay et al. 2014)
Photo recall phenomenon	Taxane	
Blue-gray hyperpigmentation	Amiodarone, chlorpromazine, tricyclic antidepressants, or diltiazem, minocycline	Drug metabolite–melanin complex (Kutlubay et al. 2014)

porphyrin hemostasis and can be inhibited by various drugs such as novobiocin and imatinib. Certain polymorphisms in this gene can alter the functions of ABCG2 transporter leading to the accumulation of porphyrin and increased sensitivity to light. This becomes clinically relevant when a susceptibility SNP is accompanied by an inhibitory drug (Tamura et al. 2007). The *glutathione S-transferase (GST)* genes are another group associated with photosensitivity. They are one of the main agents responsible for the detoxifying reactive oxygen species that result from UV exposure. Individuals with a homozygous deletion of *GST theta-1 (GSTT1)* are more sensitive toward UVB. *GST mu-1 (GSTM1)* deletion does not singlehandedly effect UVB sensitivity but its effects become apparent in individuals that are homozygous null for *GSTT1*. Conversely, individuals with functional *GSTM1* alleles are more susceptible to Hypericum (St. John's wort) induced phototoxicity (Kerb et al. 2002). GST polymorphisms are also associated with sensitivity to psoralen-ultraviolet A (PUVA). In GSTM1, the null allele confers risk for developing PUVA-related phototoxicity (Ibbotson et al. 2012). Hypothetically, polymorphisms in genes encoding drug-metabolizing enzymes, transporters, and binding proteins can all be involved in susceptibility to drug-induced phototoxicity.

References

Aggarwal N (2016) Drug-induced subacute cutaneous lupus erythematosus associated with proton pump inhibitors. Drugs Real World Outcomes 3:145–154

Arrese JE, Dominguez-Soto L, Hojyo-Tomoka MT, Vega-Memije E, Cortes-Franco R, Guevara E, Pierard GE (2001) Effectors of inflammation in actinic prurigo. J Am Acad Dermatol 44:957–961

Chen CC, Chang KC, Medeiros LJ, Lee JY (2016a) Hydroa vacciniforme and hydroa vacciniforme-like T-cell lymphoma: an uncommon event for transformation. J Cutan Pathol 43:1102–1111

Chen Q, Shen M, Heng YK, Theng TSC, Tey HL, Ren EC, Chong WS (2016b) Actinic prurigo in

Singaporean Chinese: a positive association with HLA-DRB1*03:01. Photochem Photobiol 92:355–359

Chen YA, Yang CC, Ting SW, Lee JY, Chen W (2016c) Adult-onset actinic prurigo: report of 19 patients from Taiwan. J Eur Acad Dermatol Venereol 30:e140–e142

Cohen JI (2015) primary immunodeficiencies associated with EBV disease. Curr Top Microbiol Immunol 390:241–265

Cohen JI, Dropulic L, Hsu AP, Zerbe CS, Krogmann T, Dowdell K, Hornung RL, Lovell J, Hardy N, Hickstein D, Cowen EW, Calvo KR, Pittaluga S, Holland SM (2016) Association of GATA2 deficiency with severe primary Epstein-Barr Virus (EBV) infection and EBV-associated cancers. Clin Infect Dis 63:41–47

Crouch R, Foley P, Baker C (2002) Actinic prurigo: a retrospective analysis of 21 cases referred to an Australian photobiology clinic. Australas J Dermatol 43:128–132

Cuevas-Gonzalez JC, Lievanos-Estrada Z, Vega-Memije ME, Hojyo-Tomoka MT, Dominguez-Soto L (2016a) Correlation of serum IgE levels and clinical manifestations in patients with actinic prurigo. An Bras Dermatol 91:23–26

Cuevas-Gonzalez JC, Vega-Memije ME, Garcia-Vazquez FJ, Rodriguez-Lobato E, Farfan-Morales JE (2016b) Apoptosis and apoptotic pathway in actinic prurigo by immunohistochemistry. Med Oral Patol Oral Cir Bucal 21:e53-58

Czarnobilska E, Obtułowicz K, Wsołek K (2007) Type IV of hypersensitivity and its subtypes. Przegl Lek 64:506–508

Dover JS, Hawk JL (1988) Polymorphic light eruption sine eruption. Br J Dermatol 118:73–76

Dropulic LK, Cohen JI (2011) Severe viral infections and primary immunodeficiencies. Clin Infect Dis 53:897–909

Dummer R, Rinderknecht J, Goldinger SM (2012) Ultraviolet A and photosensitivity during vemurafenib therapy. N Engl J Med 366:480–481

Felton S, Navid F, Schwarz A, Schwarz T, Glaser R, Rhodes LE (2013) Ultraviolet radiation-induced upregulation of antimicrobial proteins in health and disease. Photochem Photobiol Sci 12:29–36

Gonzalez E, Gonzalez S (1996) Drug photosensitivity, idiopathic photodermatoses, and sunscreens. J Am Acad Dermatol 35:871–885; quiz 886–877

Grabczynska SA, McGregor JM, Kondeatis E, Vaughan RW, Hawk JL (1999) Actinic prurigo and polymorphic light eruption: common pathogenesis and the importance of HLA-DR4/DRB1*0407. Br J Dermatol 140:232–236

Gruber-Wackernagel A, Byrne SN, Wolf P (2014) Polymorphous light eruption: clinic aspects and pathogenesis. Dermatol Clin 32:315–334, viii

Guarrera M, Micalizzi C, Rebora A (1993) Heterogeneity of polymorphous light eruption: a study of 105 patients. Arch Dermatol 129:1060–1061

Gupta G, Man I, Kemmett D (2000) Hydroa vacciniforme: a clinical and follow-up study of 17 cases. J Am Acad Dermatol 42:208–213

Gutierrez D, Gaulding JV, Motta Beltran AF, Lim HW, Pritchett EN (2018) Photodermatoses in skin of colour. J Eur Acad Dermatol Venereol 32:1879–1886

Hamada T, Aoyama Y, Shirafuji Y, Iwatsuki K (2017) Phenotypic analysis of circulating T-cell subset and its association with burden of skin disease in patients with chronic actinic dermatitis: a hematologic and clinicopathologic study of 20 subjects. Int J Dermatol 56:540–546

Hammerberg C, Duraiswamy N, Cooper KD (1996) Reversal of immunosuppression inducible through ultraviolet-exposed skin by in vivo anti-CD11b treatment. J Immunol 157:5254–5261

Harkins CP, Waters A, Kerr A, Campbell L, McLean WI, Brown SJ, Ibbotson SH (2015) Loss-of-function mutations in the gene encoding filaggrin are not strongly associated with chronic actinic dermatitis. J Investig Dermatol 135:1919–1921

Ho CH, Chauhan K (2018) Lupus erythematosus, drug-induced. In: (eds) StatPearls, Treasure Island (FL)

Ibbotson S, Dawe R, Dinkova-Kostova A, Weidlich S, Farr P, Ferguson J, Wolf C, Smith G (2012) Glutathione S-transferase genotype is associated with sensitivity to psoralen–ultraviolet A photochemotherapy. Br J Dermatol 166:380–388

Iwatsuki K, Satoh M, Yamamoto T, Oono T, Morizane S, Ohtsuka M, Xu ZG, Suzuki D, Tsuji K (2006) Pathogenic link between hydroa vacciniforme and Epstein-Barr virus-associated hematologic disorders. Arch Dermatol 142:587–595

Jansen CT, Karvonen J (1984) Polymorphous light eruption. a seven-year follow-up evaluation of 114 patients. Arch Dermatol 120:862–865

Kerb R, Brockmöller J, Schlagenhaufer R, Sprenger R, Roots I, Brinkmann U (2002) Influence of GSTT1 and GSTM1 genotypes on sunburn sensitivity. Am J Pharmacogenomics 2:147–154

Khandpur S, Porter RM, Boulton SJ, Anstey A (2017) Drug-induced photosensitivity: new insights into pathomechanisms and clinical variation through basic and applied science. Br J Dermatol 176:902–909

Kim BJ, Rho YK, Lee HI, Jeong MS, Li K, Seo SJ, Kim MN, Hong CK (2009) The effect of calcipotriol on the expression of human beta defensin-2 and LL-37 in cultured human keratinocytes. Clin Dev Immunol 2009:645898

Kim HJ, Kim KH (2018) Increased incidence of chronic actinic dermatitis in relation to climate changes and air pollution during the past 15 years in Korea. Photodermatol Photoimmunol Photomed 34:387–392

Kolgen W, van Meurs M, Jongsma M, van Weelden H, Bruijnzeel-Koomen CA, Knol EF, van Vloten WA, Laman J, de Gruijl FR (2004) Differential expression of cytokines in UV-B-exposed skin of patients with polymorphous light eruption: correlation with Langerhans cell migration and immunosuppression. Arch Dermatol 140:295–302

Kolgen W, Van Weelden H, Den Hengst S, Guikers KL, Kiekens RC, Knol EF, Bruijnzeel-Koomen CA, Van Vloten WA, de Gruijl FR (1999) CD11b+ cells and ultraviolet-B-resistant CD1a+ cells in skin of patients with polymorphous light eruption. J Invest Dermatol 113:4–10

Komarow HD, Eisch AR, Young M, Nelson C, Metcalfe DD (2015) Solar Urticaria. J Allergy Clin Immunol Pract 3:789–790

Kutlubay Z, Sevim A, Engin B, Tuzun Y (2014) Photodermatoses, including phototoxic and photoallergic reactions (internal and external). Clin Dermatol 32:73–79

Lei D, Lv L, Yang L, Wu W, Liu Y, Tu Y, Xu D, Jin Y, Nong X, He L (2017) Genome-wide analysis of mRNA and long noncoding RNA profiles in chronic actinic dermatitis. Biomed Res Int 2017:7479523

Lembo S, Hawk JLM, Murphy GM, Kaneko K, Young AR, McGregor JM, Walker SL, Palmer RA (2017) Aberrant gene expression with deficient apoptotic keratinocyte clearance may predispose to polymorphic light eruption. Br J Dermatol 177:1450–1453

Lembo S, Raimondo A (2018) Polymorphic light Eruption: what's new in pathogenesis and management. Front Med (lausanne) 5:252

Liu P, Tan S, Wang Q, Zhang P (2008) Expressions of fibrillin-1, elastin and matrix metalloproteinase-1 and-9 in chronic actinic dermatitis in elderly patients. Nan fang yi ke da xue xue bao. J South Med Univ 28:1354–1357

Martinez-Luna E, Bologna-Molina R, Mosqueda-Taylor A, Cuevas-Gonzalez JC, Rodriguez-Lobato E, Martinez-Velasco MA, Vega-Memije ME (2015) Inmunohistochemical detection of mastocytes in tissue from patients with actinic prurigo. J Clin Exp Dent 7: e656-659

McGregor JM, Grabczynska S, Vaughan R, Hawk JL, Lewis CM (2000) Genetic modeling of abnormal photosensitivity in families with polymorphic light eruption and actinic prurigo. J Invest Dermatol 115:471–476

Millard TP, Bataille V, Snieder H, Spector TD, McGregor JM (2000) The heritability of polymorphic light eruption. J Invest Dermatol 115:467–470

Millard TP, Fryer AA, McGregor JM (2008) A protective effect of glutathione-S-transferase GSTP1*Val(105) against polymorphic light eruption. J Invest Dermatol 128:1901–1905

Millard TP, Kondeatis E, Cox A, Wilson AG, Grabczynska SA, Carey BS, Lewis CM, Khamashta MA, Duff GW, Hughes GR, Hawk JL, Vaughan RW, McGregor JM (2001) A candidate gene analysis of three related photosensitivity disorders: cutaneous lupus erythematosus, polymorphic light eruption and actinic prurigo. Br J Dermatol 145:229–236

Miller DD, Cowen EW, Nguyen JC, McCalmont TH, Fox LP (2010) Melanoma associated with long-term voriconazole therapy: a new manifestation of chronic photosensitivity. Arch Dermatol 146:300–304

Monteiro AF, Rato M, Martins C (2016) Drug-induced photosensitivity: photoallergic and phototoxic reactions. Clin Dermatol 34:571–581

Nakamura M, Henderson M, Jacobsen G, Lim HW (2014) Comparison of photodermatoses in African-Americans and Caucasians: a follow-up study. Photodermatol Photoimmunol Photomed 30:231–236

Norris P, Poston RN, Thomas DS, Thornhill M, Hawk J, Haskard DO (1991) The expression of endothelial leukocyte adhesion molecule-1 (ELAM-1), intercellular adhesion molecule-1 (ICAM-1), and vascular cell adhesion molecule-1 (VCAM-1) in experimental cutaneous inflammation: a comparison of ultraviolet B erythema and delayed hypersensitivity. J Invest Dermatol 96:763–770

Norris PG, Barker JN, Allen MH, Leiferman KM, MacDonald DM, Haskard DO, Hawk JL (1992) Adhesion molecule expression in polymorphic light eruption. J Invest Dermatol 99:504–508

Norris PG, Morris J, McGibbon DM, Chu AC, Hawk JL (1989a) Polymorphic light eruption: an immunopathological study of evolving lesions. Br J Dermatol 120:173–183

Norris PG, Morris J, Smith NP, Chu AC, Hawk JL (1989b) Chronic actinic dermatitis: an immunohistologic and photobiologic study. J Am Acad Dermatol 21:966–971

Patra V, Byrne SN, Wolf P (2016) The skin microbiome: is It affected by UV-induced immune suppression? Front Microbiol 7:1235

Patra V, Mayer G, Gruber-Wackernagel A, Horn M, Lembo S, Wolf P (2018) Unique profile of antimicrobial peptide expression in polymorphic light eruption lesions compared to healthy skin, atopic dermatitis, and psoriasis. Photodermatol Photoimmunol Photomed 34:137–144

Patra V, Wolf P (2016) Microbial elements as the initial triggers in the pathogenesis of polymorphic light eruption? Exp Dermatol 25:999–1001

Ross G, Foley P, Baker C (2008) Actinic prurigo. Photodermatol Photoimmunol Photomed 24:272–275

Rossi MT, Arisi M, Lonardi S, Lorenzi L, Ungari M, Serana F, Fusano M, Moggio E, Calzavara-Pinton PG, Venturini M (2018) Cutaneous infiltration of plasmacytoid dendritic cells and T regulatory cells in skin lesions of polymorphic light eruption. J Eur Acad Dermatol Venereol 32:985–991

Sharma VK, Verma P (2012) Parthenium dermatitis in India: past, present and future. Indian J Dermatol Venereol Leprol 78:560

Su KA, Habel LA, Achacoso NS, Friedman GD, Asgari MM (2018) Photosensitizing antihypertensive drug use and risk of cutaneous squamous cell carcinoma. Br J Dermatol 179:1088–1094

Tamura A, Onishi Y, An R, Koshiba S, Wakabayashi K, Hoshijima K, Priebe W, Yoshida T, Kometani S, Matsubara T (2007) In vitro evaluation of photosensitivity risk related to genetic polymorphisms of human ABC transporter ABCG2 and inhibition by drugs. Drug Metab Pharmacokinet 22:428–440

Tan AW, Lim KS, Theng C, Chong WS (2011) Chronic actinic dermatitis in Asian skin: a Singaporean experience. Photodermatol Photoimmunol Photomed 27:172–175

Trakatelli M, Charalampidis S, Novakovic LB, Patsatsi A, Kalabalikis D, Sotiriadis D (2009) Photodermatoses with onset in the elderly. Br J Dermatol 161(Suppl 3):69–77

van de Pas CB, Kelly DA, Seed PT, Young AR, Hawk JL, Walker SL (2004) Ultraviolet-radiation-induced erythema and suppression of contact hypersensitivity responses in patients with polymorphic light eruption. J Invest Dermatol 122:295–299

Vega Memije ME, Cuevas Gonzalez JC, Hojyo-Tomoka MT, Rodriguez Lobato E (2017) Actinic prurigo as a hypersensitivity reaction type 4. Int J Dermatol 56: e135–e136

Vohringer S, Schrum J, Ott H, Hoger PH (2011) Severe phototoxicity associated with long-term voriconazole treatment. J Dtsch Dermatol Ges 9:274–276

Wolf P, Byrne SN, Gruber-Wackernagel A (2009) New insights into the mechanisms of polymorphic light eruption: resistance to ultraviolet radiation-induced immune suppression as an aetiological factor. Exp Dermatol 18:350–356

Wrzesniok D, Surazynski A, Karna E, Buszman E, Palka J (2005) Melanin counter act puromycin-induced inhibition of collagen and DNA biosynthesis in human skin fibroblasts. Life Sci 77:528–538

Zirbs M, Purner C, Buters JT, Effner R, Weidinger S, Ring J, Eberlein B (2013) GSTM1, GSTT1 and GSTP1 gene polymorphism in polymorphous light eruption. J Eur Acad Dermatol Venereol 27:157–162

The Immunogenetics of Melanoma

Farzaneh Darbeheshti

Abstract

Melanoma is a relatively common and deadly type of skin cancer that originates from melanocytes. Cutaneous malignant melanoma results from the interplay between genetic susceptibility and environmental factors. Though the majority of melanoma cases are sporadic, several high and low penetrance mutations have been identified as underlying factors of heritable melanoma. Genetic variations in immune system components are among the most studied factors in melanoma heritability. They are involved in several aspects of the pathogenesis of the tumor including predisposition, cell proliferation, and apoptosis as well as immunotherapy. In this chapter, the hitherto available immunogenetic-related reports on melanoma predisposition and progression are summed up.

Keywords

Melanoma · Immunogenetics · Genetic susceptibility · Pathogenesis

1 Introduction

There are three major types of skin cancer including basal cell carcinoma, squamous cell carcinoma, and melanoma. These types share some features; however, they are so different from etiology to progression. Non-melanoma skin cancers (basal cell and squamous cell carcinoma) are relatively considered to be non-lethal and curable malignancies. However, melanoma is the most dangerous and deadliest skin cancer because it often spreads to the lung, liver, brain, bone, and lymph nodes (Schadendorf et al. 2018).

In 2018, 287,723 new cases of melanoma (1.6% of all cancers) and 60,712 melanoma-related deaths (0.6% of all cancer-related death) have been reported in 185 countries (Bray et al. 2018). Melanoma is rare in people with darker skin and is more frequent in males than females.

Cutaneous malignant melanoma results from the interplay of genetic susceptibility and environmental factors (Anne 2018). Genetic factors that contribute to inherited susceptibility for melanoma are being progressively detected and introduced. Familial melanoma includes

F. Darbeheshti (✉)
Departments of Medical Genetics, School of Medicine, Tehran University of Medical Sciences, Tehran, Iran

Cancer Immunology Project (CIP), Universal Scientific and Research Network (USERN), Tehran, Iran

N. Rezaei and F. Rajabi (eds.), *The Immunogenetics of Dermatologic Diseases*, Advances in Experimental Medicine and Biology 1367,
https://doi.org/10.1007/978-3-030-92616-8_15

approximately 10% of cases (Halk et al. 2019). Several high and low penetrance mutations have been identified as underlying factors of heritable melanoma, such as CDKN2A, CDK4, BAP1, POT1, ACD, TERF2IP, and TERT (Hill et al. 2013). Nevertheless, in approximately 50% of familial melanoma cases, the underlying mutations are unexplained.

The majority of melanoma cases are sporadic and somatic genetic alterations are remarkably frequent in melanoma lesions. Activating somatic mutations in BRAF are approximately present in 60% of malignant melanomas (Brose et al. 2002). NRAS, KIT, PTEN, MITF, and AKT are other involved genes in sporadic melanoma (Singh et al. 2008). Melanoma is considered one of the most immunogenic tumors due to its higher mutation load compared with other cancers. Hence, it is one of the best-investigated cancers in terms of tumor/immune cell relationship (Passarelli et al. 2017).

Genetic variations in immune system components are involved in several aspects of melanoma including predisposition, cell proliferation, and apoptosis as well as immunotherapy. The first evidence regarding the importance of the immune system in determining the risk of skin cancer was recognized more than 40 years ago when it was observed that the incidence of skin cancer is greatly increased in patients receiving immunosuppressive drugs. Various studies in different countries have discovered that the prevalence of melanoma is 7 times higher, basal cell carcinoma 10 times higher, and squamous cell carcinoma 65–250 times higher in immunosuppressed patients compared with the general populations (Hart and Norval 2018). These observations indicate a pivotal role for the immune system in controlling skin cancers.

The most well-known environmental risk factor in melanoma is ultraviolet (UV) radiation present in sunlight. Interestingly, polymorphic genetic factors contribute to the damaging immune effects of UVB radiation and thereby alter an individual's risk of developing sunlight-induced skin cancers.

In this chapter, the hitherto available immunogenetic-related reports on melanoma predisposition and progression are summed up.

2 Human Leukocyte Antigen Polymorphisms; Is It a Definite Susceptibility Locus for Melanoma?

Human leukocyte antigen (HLA) is a cell surface glycoprotein specialized to present antigenic peptides to T-cell receptors. The most critical function of the HLA molecule is inducing and regulating immune responses. HLA genes region on chromosome 6 demonstrates high polymorphism. HLA genes are divided into three groups: class I, II, and III. Class I includes two subgroups named classical (HLA-A, -B, and -C) and non-classical (HLA-G, -E, and -F). Class I antigens are vital for the cytotoxic T lymphocytes to function in tumor cell recognition.

Currently, a large number of population studies are available concerning the association between particular HLA alleles and diseases; among the long list of human diseases, autoimmune diseases and malignancies are predominant.

Structural variants in HLA genes and dysregulation of their expression are some of the possible mechanisms that cause tumor cells to escape immune surveillance as well as various responses to immunotherapy drugs. Several studies have demonstrated HLA association with the risk of developing melanoma; however, the results are inconsistent and inconclusive.

2.1 HLA Genotype and Expression

Until now, several studies have been conducted to look for an association between specific HLA alleles and melanoma susceptibility in various countries. Although there is no consensus evidence in the related articles, some results indicate a potential effect of specific HLA genotype on

Table 1 Studies that have investigated the relationship between HLA genotype and melanoma

Article	Population	Technique	Results
Bateman et al. (1998)	UK British Caucasian 99 cases and 293 control	SSOP	HLA DQB1*0303 and DQB1*0301 alleles influence susceptibility to melanoma and act as prognostic factors
Kageshita et al. (1997)	Japan 96 cases and 136 controls	PCR–RFLP	HLA class II alleles may not contribute to susceptibility to melanoma
Lombardi et al. (1998)	Italy 132 cases and 102 controls	PCR-SSO	HLA class II alleles may not contribute to susceptibility to melanoma
Lulli et al. (1998)	Italy 53 cases and 53 controls	PCR-SSO	Protective role of DQBl*0301, DQB1'0302, and DQB1*0303 alleles
Marincola et al. (1995)	USA 74 cases and 105 controls	PCR-SSP	No association between HLA DQB1 * 0301 and patients with melanoma
Planelles et al. (2006)	Spain 117 cases and 301 controls	PCR-SSP	An increased homozygosity rate for DQA1*0505 and DQA1*0301 in patients
Kandilarova et al. (2016)	Poland 283 cases and 174 controls	PCR-SSP	Positive association of HLA-C*14 and negative association of HLA-C*02 with the disease

susceptibility or resistance to melanoma. Table 1 shows the studies that investigated the relationship between HLA alleles and melanoma.

As noted in Table 2, there are inconsistencies among the studies already published due to ethnic diversity and other variables that are involved in inter-population research. Although a definite susceptibility HLA allele has not been discovered for melanoma until now, it could be suggested that specific HLA haplotypes would function as an immune modulator in melanoma initiation and progression. For instance, the HLA DQB1*0303 allele.

According to previous studies, HLA expression in melanoma lesions affects melanoma prognosis and immunotherapy (Sottile et al. 2016). A strong negative association between HLA class I expression and progression of the metastatic lesions was reported by real-time PCR and immunohistological techniques (Carretero et al. 2008). Consistently, quantitative expression analysis of HLA-A, B, and C genes in melanoma tumors indicated higher HLA expression in regressing than in progressing metastases (Carretero et al. 2012). The loss of tumor HLA-A2 expression leads to the lack of T-cell functionality (Tjin et al. 2011). An integrated analysis of omics data on melanoma has indicated significant hypermethylation of HLA-C locus and its low gene expression. Samples that have hypermethylated HLA-C showed a poorer survival (Jiang et al. 2016).

According to previous researches, the downregulation of HLA class I is an important parameter in melanoma and can be linked to cancer immune escape mechanisms. It seems that alteration of HLA class I expression is the major factor determining the success or failure of immunotherapy, so it needs to be monitored.

An interesting subject concerning HLA is a link between non-classical HLA class I expression and cancer immunosuppression. This subgroup is characterized by low genetic diversity and specific expression patterns. Non-classical

HLA class I has a principal tolerance-inducing function and can develop tumors by inducing immune escape through binding to inhibitory receptors. A high frequency of non-classical HLA class I expression has been commonly detected in both hematological and solid tumors with a poorer prognosis (Kochan et al. 2013).

Several researches indicate the roles of non-classical HLA class I in melanoma progression. A study about HLA-G indicated high levels of HLA-G in melanoma samples compared with healthy controls (Paul et al. 1999). Another investigation revealed HLA-G expression to be significantly higher in melanoma than in nevi (benign), suggesting the role of HLA-G in malignant transformation in this cell type (Ibrahim et al. 2004). The high expression of HLA-G in melanoma tumors was associated with a bad prognosis (Melsted et al. 2017). It is suggested expression of HLA-G would protect the melanoma from NK cell-mediated lysis (Paul et al. 1998; Rebmann et al. 2007).

Also, HLA-E among 1477 immune response-related genes were ranked 19th overexpressed genes in melanoma by measuring the level of cDNAs. HLA-E has been detected in 57% and 67% primary and metastatic lesions, respectively, by immunohistochemistry, though it was mostly undetectable in normal skin and nevi biopsies (Tremante et al. 2014). A significantly high level of both soluble HLA-E and -G in serum samples of melanoma patients compared with healthy controls has been reported (Allard et al. 2011; Ugurel et al. 2001).

Taken together, it is possible to conclude the over-expression of non-classical HLA class I molecules in melanoma cells can be a mechanism to evade immune surveillance. Emerging evidence supports an important role of HLA-G and HLA-E in tumor progression. However, a basic question has remained unanswered: What is the molecular mechanism of HLA dysregulation in tumor cells? Is it regulated at the transcriptional or post-transcriptional levels?

3 The Inflammasome: A Link Between Innate Immunity and Susceptibility to Sporadic Melanoma

The inflammasome is a multiprotein cytoplasmic complex that contributes to the inflammatory process and plays a pivotal role in detecting pathogens as well as sterile stressors, such as cancers and autoimmune diseases (Davis et al. 2011; Lukens and Kanneganti 2014). Inflammasome activates the caspase-1-dependant secretion of highly pro-inflammatory interleukin (IL)-1β and IL-18 cytokines. It also induces a form of cell death named pyroptosis (Gross et al. 2011).

It is suggested inflammation is a double-edged sword in malignancies. It helps remove transformed cells while it makes cytokines and survival factors available for tumor growth. Recently, Inflammasomes have been given special attention in melanoma progression as being directly linked to IL-1β-mediated tumorigenesis.

There is an association between single nucleotide polymorphisms (SNP) in inflammasome genes and cancer development and/or its progression (Liu et al. 2010; Machado et al. 2001).

The NLRP1 and NLRP3 are components of the inflammasome. It is revealed that melanoma samples have a high expression of NLRP1 in the cytoplasm. After knocking down NLRP1, downregulation of caspase-1 activity, IL-1β production, and nuclear factor-κβ activity were observed. This evidence points out the role of the NLRP1 inflammasome in the metastasis process. Therefore, it is suggested that NLRP1 promotes melanoma tumorigenesis by activating inflammasomes and by suppressing apoptotic pathways (Zhai et al. 2017).

The association between NLRP3/NLRP1 polymorphisms and susceptibility of melanoma is seen in a Swedish case–control study. NLRP3 variant (rs35829419) was significantly more common in male patients compared with controls and the NLRP1 variant (rs12150220) was significantly more common in fair-skinned female patients (Verma et al. 2012). Although the immunogenetic association of NLRP polymorphisms with melanoma has not been strong, previous studies have provided valuable clues about the association between immunogenetic signatures in inflammasome and susceptibility for melanoma that needs to be further investigated.

Another study on inflammasome SNPs in Brazilian melanoma patients and healthy controls indicated that CARD8 rs6509365 was significantly more common in controls than in patients (Silva et al. 2016). Also, investigation of CARD8 expression revealed that its expression was increased in melanoma biopsies compared to healthy skin. It has been assumed the CARD8 rs6509365 A > G intronic variant could reduce CARD8 gene expression (Ko et al. 2009). CARD8 has been postulated to serve as an inhibitor of NLRP3-inflammasome activation. Moreover, CARD8 plays an anti-apoptotic role (Yamamoto et al. 2005). Taken together, a protective effect of the CARD8 rs6509365 variant against melanoma has been suggested.

4 The Crosstalk Between Immune System and UV Radiation

It is well-known that ultraviolet radiation (UVR) is one of the major risk factors involved in the development of melanoma as well as basal and squamous cell carcinoma (Hart and Norval 2018). It is postulated that genotoxic, inflammatory, and immunosuppressive properties of UVR contribute to melanoma pathophysiology (Arisi et al. 2018). The major solar UVR reaching the earth's surface is UVA and UVB. Both UV types cause DNA damage as well as immune suppression which play pivotal roles in skin carcinogenesis. UVA wavelengths have a greater ability to generate reactive oxygen and nitrogen species in skin cells which then causes oxidative DNA damages (Liu-Smith et al. 2017). On the other hand, UVB can be directly absorbed by DNA molecules and thus causes UV-signature DNA damages.

Xeroderma pigmentosa (XP) patients provide further evidence about the crosstalk among UVR, immune system, and skin cancers. These individuals have extreme photosensitivity caused by an inability to repair DNA following UVR exposure as well as immune abnormalities such as decreased circulating T lymphocytes and natural killer (NK) cell activity and reduction of IFN-γ production which are presumably involved in an increased risk for skin cancer.

UVR-related immune changes may be cumulative or redundant depending on the genetic background of an individual, the wavelengths and intensity of UVR, the time span of radiation exposure, and skin type. Acute, low-dose ultraviolet B radiation protocols in UVB-susceptible mice and humans impair induction of contact hypersensitivity to highly reactive haptens but not others (UVB-resistant). These observations suggest genetic features of an individual effect on sensitivity to UVR (Fig. 1).

4.1 Mast Cells

Innate immune background plays a role in determining skin cancer risk among individuals (Grimbaldeston et al. 2003). The density of mast cells is positively correlated with susceptibility to melanoma. Consistently, a case–control study reported prevalence of dermal mast cells was higher in the buttock skin from melanoma patients than in healthy controls (Grimbaldeston et al. 2004). It is suggested the immunomodulatory effects of mast cell products in UV-irradiated skin may contribute significantly to the initiation and development of melanoma. Some researches have demonstrated the important role of dermal mast cells in UV-induced immunosuppression (Biggs et al. 2010; Byrne et al. 2015; Damiani et al. 2015; Sarchio et al. 2014).

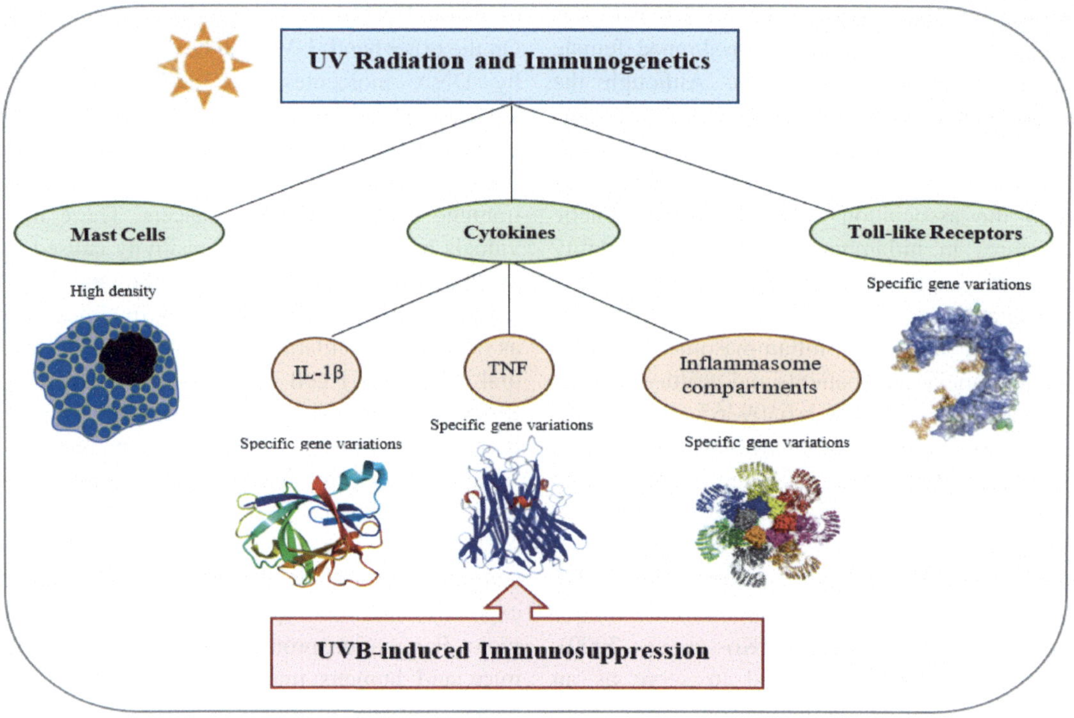

Fig. 1 The crosstalk between immunogenetics and UV radiation results in susceptibility for melanoma

4.2 Cytokines

Another immunogenetic factor concerning UVR susceptibility that was reported in previous studies is variants in tumor necrosis factor (TNF) genes. Both TNFα and TNFβ genes, located within the HLA class III region, produce cytokine proteins which play important roles in the regulation of inflammation and immunity. The region encoding these genes contains several SNP as well as microsatellites (dinucleotide repeat polymorphisms) (Jongeneel et al. 1991). TNFα secretion is associated with polymorphisms in the TNF region (Niizeki et al. 2001). On the other hand, TNF is a UVB-induced immune modulator (Vermeer and Streilein 1990; Yoshikawa and Streilein 1990) responsible for UVB-induced suppression of systemic immunity (Köck et al. 1990). UV radiation induces the up-expression of TNF-α in keratinocytes (Corsini et al. 1995) as well as TNF-α release from dermal mast cells (Alard et al. 1999).

In murine, the 5′ regulatory region of the TNFα gene has a $(CA)_n$ mini-repeat. An investigation revealed the TNFα allele of UVB-resistant (UVB-R) mice contains exactly 14 CA repeats, whereas the TNFα alleles of UVB-susceptible (UVB-S) mice display repeats that are either greater or less than 14 (Vincek et al. 1993). In humans, a study assessed the association between variants of TNF genes and UVB-S or UVB-R phenotype in healthy Caucasian volunteers. The microsatellite analysis demonstrated a significant increase in the frequencies of TNFα2 in UVB-S individuals and of TNFd3 in UVB-R individuals (Niizeki et al. 2001). According to the results, it is proposed that the TNF region is a strong candidate for containing genes that impose immune-damaging effects of UVB radiation in humans. Since examination of UVB-S or UVB-R phenotype by the same experimental protocol in ten melanoma cases showed all patients to be UVB-S (Streilein et al. 1994), the author has concluded UVB-S is a risk factor for sunlight-induced melanoma. Consistently, there is a significant increase in the frequencies of TNFa2 variant in UVB-S individuals and TNFd3 in UVB-R individuals (Niizeki et al. 2002).

Interestingly, the exposure to UVB significantly suppresses Ab responses to hepatitis B vaccine in individuals homozygous for the minor variant (TT) of the IL-1β (+3953 C/T) polymorphism (Sleijffers et al. 2003). The author has suggested that SNPs of the IL-1β gene which influence expression need to be considered as far as UV-susceptibility is concerned.

Interestingly, reactive oxygen species and damaged DNA are activators of inflammasomes. In HaCaT cells, an immortal keratinocyte cell line, UVB exposure induces activation of NLRP3 inflammasome and increases IL-1β secretion (Nasti and Timares 2012). As noted above, genetic variants of inflammasome components are potentially involved in susceptibility for melanoma. Accordingly, it can be proposed that there is an inflammasome-UVR axis to influence predisposition to melanoma which needs to be further investigated.

4.3 Toll-Like Receptors

Toll-like receptors (TLRs) are a component of innate immunity that links innate and acquired immunity. These receptors are important in detecting pathogens and cancer cells. After induction by pathogens, TLRs activate signaling pathways that result in TLR-induced inflammatory response such as the release of inflammatory cytokines and type I interferons (Kumar et al. 2009). Several studies in the past decade have dealt with the role of TLR polymorphisms in various cancers (El-Omar et al. 2008).

Taking into account the TLRs roles and UVB-induced immunosuppression, a study in mice revealed that TLR4-/- mice are resistant to UVB-induced immunosuppression compared with TLR4 + / + mice (Lewis et al. 2011). This observation indicates the role of TLR4 expression in immunosuppression by exposure to UVB.

A large case–control study has investigated 47 single nucleotide polymorphisms in 8 TLR genes and their potential impact on melanoma susceptibility and patient survival. Results of this study indicated a tendency (not statistically significant) to disease susceptibility in TLR2-rs3804099 and decreased risk in TLR4-rs2149356 polymorphism (Gast et al. 2011). Moreover, a significant association between improved overall survival and survival following metastasis was reported in carriers of the variant allele (D299G) of TLR4-rs4986790. This SNP can have functional consequences as located in the ectodomain of TLR4.

Melanoma biopsies show TLR3 upregulation; moreover, its activation results in melanoma cell migration both in vivo and in vitro (Goto et al. 2008). In Caucasian melanoma patients, rs3775292 in the intron region of TLR3 was significantly associated with sentinel lymph node metastasis as well as rs7668666 with melanoma-specific death (Park et al. 2013).

Another case–control study concerning TLR7 has not suggested an association between TLR7 Gln11Leu polymorphism and increased susceptibility to cutaneous melanoma (Elefanti et al. 2016).

Thus far, although it is known that different immunogenetic backgrounds affect the response to UV light, we cannot precisely determine its influence on the response to UV exposure yet. It seems that more investigation of polymorphisms of the TNF and cytokine genes may help develop eventually a simple genetic test to identify the UVB-S and UVB-R traits in humans.

5 Immunogenetics and Melanoma Prognosis

Melanoma is known as immunogenic cancer. This means that it manifests the ability to induce an immune response to prevent tumor growth (Gogas et al. 2006). Accordingly, several studies have proposed that germline variations in immune-modulating genes may be involved in melanoma prognosis (Blankenstein et al. 2012). Among them, inherited genetic alterations in interleukin-10 (IL10) are the most widely studied issue.

5.1 Interleukin-10 Expression; Influential Germline Variants

Some studies have reported an association between high levels of IL10 and anti-tumor response in melanoma (Fortis et al. 1996). It is proved that the promoter polymorphisms of the IL10 gene affect its expression which is defined as 'high-', 'medium-', and 'low'-expression genotypes (Perrey et al. 1998). The three linked polymorphisms located in the IL10 promoter were genotyped in melanoma patients. The high-expression genotype IL10−1082GG (rs1800896) is associated with noninvasive tumor growth and the low-expression genotype IL10−1082AA is associated with poor prognosis (Howell et al. 2001). The authors supposed that low expression of IL10 is a poor prognostic biomarker. This hypothesis was further confirmed by various independent studies (Alonso et al. 2005; Martinez-Escribano et al. 2002; Euw et al. 2008). Moreover, carriers of the minor allele (G) at IL10 rs1518111 have increased melanoma-related death (Park et al. 2013). It should be noted that a couple of studies have reported inconsistent results and melanoma tumors with higher expression of IL10 exhibited more aggressive progression (Itakura et al. 2011; Moore et al. 2001).

A large cohort study genotyped 72 SNPs within 44 immunomodulatory genes in melanoma patients. IL10 rs3024493 heterozygotes (GT) which is mid-secretors were significantly associated with better OS while low-secretors (TT) showed significantly worse disease outcome. The authors suggested IL10 may exert both anti- and pro-tumoral activities and the optimal balance of IL10 secretion determines immune response against melanoma (Rendleman et al. 2015). Interestingly, the low-expression genotype of rs3024493 was associated with the downregulation of interleukin-10 (IL10) secretion in CD4+ T cells (Rendleman et al. 2015).

5.2 The PD-1 Receptor and Its Ligands

Programmed cell death 1 (PD-1), also called CD279, is an inhibitory receptor that is expressed on the surface of antigen-stimulated T cells. PD-1 interacts with two ligands: PD-1 ligand 1 (PD-L1) and PD-L2. Both PD-L1 and PD-L2 can be expressed by tumor cells; however, PD-L1 is the dominant inhibitory ligand of PD-1 on T cells in the human tumor microenvironment, so PD-L1 regulates tolerance and autoimmunity. The expression of programmed death-ligand 1 (PD-L1) is frequently observed in human cancers. The binding of PD-L1 to its receptor PD-1 on activated T cells inhibits anti-tumor immunity by counteracting T cell-activating signals. The PD-L1-PD-1 pathway in malignancies is a remarkable issue because of its proven value as a therapeutic target in various types of cancer. At present, antibodies targeting the PD-L1-PD-1 axis have been approved for melanoma because inhibiting the PD-1-PD-L1 axis increases immune responses toward tumor cells (Postow et al. 2015; Weber et al. 2015). Immunotherapy with monoclonal antibodies (mAbs) that block PD-1/PD-L1 interactions on immune cells has remarkable success in the treatment of melanoma (Ugurel et al. 2016). However, about 25% of patients with melanoma who received PD-1 blockade therapy were initially responsive but developed resistance after about 21 months (Ribas et al. 2016). In 2019, the somatic loss of function mutation of JAK1 was identified as a mechanism of PD-1 blockade therapy by genome-wide CRISPR screening (Han et al. 2019).

5.2.1 PD-1/PD-L1 Expression and Melanoma Prognosis

A recent study based on Cancer Genome Atlas data interestingly showed DNA hypomethylation influences PD-L1 expression in melanoma and hence melanoma's ability to evade anti-tumor immune responses (Chatterjee et al. 2018). These results have implications for combining epigenetic therapy with immunotherapy.

PD-L1 expression in melanoma specimens, as well as PD-1 expression on T cells, was investigated in peripheral blood. In this study, PD-L1 expression had a positive association with tumor thickness. The overall survival rate of the high-expression group was significantly lower than that of the low-expression group. Patients with stage IV disease had high PD-1 expression on both CD8-positive and CD4-positive T cells in the peripheral blood (Hino et al. 2010). Consistently, cell-intrinsic PD-1 promotes melanoma tumorigenesis, even in mice lacking adaptive immunity. PD-1 inhibition on melanoma cells suppresses tumor growth in immunocompetent, immunocompromised, and PD-1-deficient tumor graft recipient mice (Kleffel et al. 2015).

The elevated PD-1 expression is associated with better survival according to the Cancer Genome Atlas data (Danilova et al. 2016). The overall survival of patients with PD-L1 positive metastatic melanoma was significantly prolonged compared with that of patients with PD-L1 negative metastatic melanoma (Taube et al. 2012).

5.2.2 Germline Immunogenetic Variants Affect on Response to PD-1 Blockade Therapy

The recent study regarding the association between autoimmune-related germline variants and response melanoma patients to anti-PD-1 has provided evidence that rs17388568, a risk variant for allergy, colitis, and type 1 diabetes, is associated with increased anti-PD-1 response. This variant maps to a locus of established immune-related genes: IL2 and IL21 (Chat et al. 2019).

5.3 Less-Investigated Germline Variants

Exploration of 94 SNP within 55 immuno-related loci in germline DNA of melanoma patients revealed SNP rs2796817 in TGFB2 has strong associations with both recurrence-free and overall survival (RFS and OS, respectively). Moreover, SNPs in IRF8 (rs4843861), CCL5 (rs4796120), and CD8A (rs3810831) are significantly associated with OS. The strongest SNP association with melanoma prognosis was located in TGFB2 which suppresses IL-2 dependent T-cell growth (Rendleman et al. 2013).

A study on 44 germline polymorphisms located in the type I interferon gene cluster on chromosome 9p22 revealed associations between two IFNW1 gene polymorphisms and survival. The carriers of the allele G and A of the rs10964859 and rs10964862 polymorphisms, respectively, were associated with reduced disease-free survival in both German and Spanish patients. Patients homozygous (G/G) for rs10964859 and rs10964862 (A/A) were associated with an increased risk of death following metastasis (Lenci et al. 2012).

CTLA-4 (cytotoxic T lymphocyte-associated antigen-4) receptor is known as a negative regulator of activation and effector functions of T cells. Anti-CTLA-4 therapies are currently used as a therapeutic approach in metastatic melanoma (Savoia et al. 2016). The analysis of six CTLA-4 single nucleotide polymorphisms in the Italian population revealed a significant association between rs11571316 (−1577G>A) and rs3087243 (CT60G>A, in the 3'UTR) genotypes and improved OS. Heterozygous patients for rs11571316 and rs3087243 were significantly correlated with a higher OS (Queirolo et al. 2013). The author had speculated that the heterozygous G/A genotypes at rs11571316 and rs3087243 loci might result in reduced levels of both CTLA-4 on T cells and circulating CTLA-4 in melanoma patients.

The investigation of SNPs in the CD28, CTLA4, and ICOS genes disclosed an association between CD28 rs3181098 (AA/AG) and reduced metastases-free survival as well as an association between AA genotype in the ICOS rs11571323 and reduced overall survival in German Melanoma patients (Bouwhuis et al. 2010). Although germline immune-related variants are not well-defined prognostic biomarkers in melanoma yet, they may eventually be used in personalized prognosis-based treatments at early stages.

6 Conclusion

In conclusion, these studies provide evidence for the underlying immunomodulatory genes in melanoma susceptibility and prognosis which can help to improve disease management. It should be noted that further investigations of SNPs at immune-related genes in additional independent case–control studies are necessary to unravel definite immune-related susceptibility loci in melanoma. It seems reasonable to expect that personalized medicine based on genetic variants and/or dysregulation of immune-modulatory genes will be developed in different aspects of melanoma management such as determining susceptibility, immunotherapy, and prognosis.

References

Alard P, Niizeki H, Hanninen L, Streilein JW (1999) Local ultraviolet B irradiation impairs contact hypersensitivity induction by triggering release of tumor necrosis factor-α from mast cells. Involvement of mast cells and Langerhans cells in susceptibility to ultraviolet B. J Investig Dermatol 113:983–990

Allard M, Oger R, Vignard V, Percier J-M, Fregni G, Périer A, Caignard A, Charreau B, Bernardeau K, Khammari A (2011) Serum soluble HLA-E in melanoma: a new potential immune-related marker in cancer. PLoS One 6:e21118

Alonso R, Suarez A, Castro P, Lacave AJ, Gutierrez C (2005) Influence of interleukin-10 genetic polymorphism on survival rates in melanoma patients with advanced disease. Melanoma Res 15:53–60

Anne E (2018) Melanoma–role of the environment and genetics. Photochem Photobiol Sci 17:1853–1860

Arisi M, Zane C, Caravello S, Rovati C, Zanca A, Venturini M, Calzavara-Pinton P (2018) Sun exposure and melanoma, certainties and weaknesses of the present knowledge. Front Med 5

Bateman A, Turner S, Theaker J, Howell W (1998) HLA-DQB1* 0303 and* 0301 alleles influence susceptibility to and prognosis in cutaneous malignant melanoma in the British Caucasian population. Tissue Antigens 52:67–73

Biggs L, Yu C, Fedoric B, Lopez AF, Galli SJ, Grimbaldeston MA (2010) Evidence that vitamin D3 promotes mast cell–dependent reduction of chronic UVB-induced skin pathology in mice. J Exp Med 207:455–463

Blankenstein T, Coulie PG, Gilboa E, Jaffee EM (2012) The determinants of tumour immunogenicity. Nat Rev Cancer 12:307

Bouwhuis MG, Gast A, Figl A, Eggermont AM, Hemminki K, Schadendorf D, Kumar R (2010) Polymorphisms in the CD28/CTLA4/ICOS genes: role in malignant melanoma susceptibility and prognosis? Cancer Immunol Immunother 59:303

Bray F, Ferlay J, Soerjomataram I, Siegel RL, Torre LA, Jemal A (2018) Global cancer statistics 2018: GLOBOCAN estimates of incidence and mortality worldwide for 36 cancers in 185 countries. CA: Cancer J Clin 68:394–424.

Brose MS, Volpe P, Feldman M, Kumar M, Rishi I, Gerrero R, Einhorn E, Herlyn M, Minna J, Nicholson A (2002) BRAF and RAS mutations in human lung cancer and melanoma. Can Res 62:6997–7000

Byrne SN, Hammond KJ, Chan CY-Y, Rogers LJ, Beaugie C, Rana S, Marsh-Wakefield F, Thurman JM, Halliday GM (2015) The alternative complement component factor B regulates UV-induced oedema, systemic suppression of contact and delayed hypersensitivity, and mast cell infiltration into the skin. Photochem Photobiol Sci 14:801–806

Carretero R, Romero JM, Ruiz-Cabello F, Maleno I, Rodriguez F, Camacho FM, Real LM, Garrido F, Cabrera T (2008) Analysis of HLA class I expression in progressing and regressing metastatic melanoma lesions after immunotherapy. Immunogenetics 60:439

Carretero R, Wang E, Rodriguez AI, Reinboth J, Ascierto ML, Engle AM, Liu H, Camacho FM, Marincola FM, Garrido F (2012) Regression of melanoma metastases after immunotherapy is associated with activation of antigen presentation and interferon-mediated rejection genes. Int J Cancer 131:387–395

Chat V, Ferguson R, Simpson D, Kazlow E, Lax R, Moran U, Pavlick A, Frederick D, Boland G, Sullivan R (2019) Autoimmune genetic risk variants as germline biomarkers of response to melanoma immune-checkpoint inhibition. Cancer Immunol Immunoth1-9

Chatterjee A, Rodger EJ, Ahn A, Stockwell PA, Parry M, Motwani J, Gallagher SJ, Shklovskaya E, Tiffen J, Eccles MR (2018) Marked global DNA hypomethylation is associated with constitutive PD-L1 expression in melanoma. iScience 4:312–325

Corsini E, Bruccoleri A, Marinovich M, Galli C (1995) In vitro mechanism (s) of ultraviolet-induced tumor necrosis factor-α release in a human keratinocyte cell line. Photodermatol Photoimmunol Photomed 11:112–118

da Silva WC, Oshiro TM, de Sá DC, Franco DD, Neto CF, Pontillo A (2016) Genotyping and differential expression analysis of inflammasome genes in sporadic malignant melanoma reveal novel contribution of CARD8, IL1B and IL18 in melanoma susceptibility and progression. Cancer genetics 209:474–480

Damiani E, Puebla-Osorio N, Gorbea E, Ullrich SE (2015) Platelet-activating factor induces epigenetic modifications in human mast cells. J Investig Dermatol 135:3034–3040

Danilova L, Wang H, Sunshine J, Kaunitz GJ, Cottrell TR, Xu H, Esandrio J, Anders RA, Cope L, Pardoll DM (2016) Association of PD-1/PD-L axis expression with cytolytic activity, mutational load, and prognosis in melanoma and other solid tumors. Proc Natl Acad Sci 113:E7769–E7777

Davis BK, Wen H, Ting JP-Y (2011) The inflammasome NLRs in immunity, inflammation, and associated diseases. Annu Rev Immunol 29:707–735

El-Omar E, Ng M, Hold G (2008) Polymorphisms in Toll-like receptor genes and risk of cancer. Oncogene 27:244

Elefanti L, Sacco G, Stagni C, Rastrelli M, Menin C, Russo I, Alaibac M (2016) TLR7 Gln11Leu single nucleotide polymorphism and susceptibility to cutaneous melanoma. Oncol Lett 12:275–280

Fortis C, Foppoli M, Gianotti L, Galli L, Citterio G, Consogno G, Gentilini O, Braga M (1996) Increased interleukin-10 serum levels in patients with solid tumours. Cancer Lett 104:1–5

Gast A, Bermejo JL, Claus R, Brandt A, Weires M, Weber A, Plass C, Sucker A, Hemminki K, Schadendorf D (2011) Association of inherited variation in Toll-like receptor genes with malignant melanoma susceptibility and survival. PLoS One 6:e24370.

Gogas H, Ioannovich J, Dafni U, Stavropoulou-Giokas C, Frangia K, Tsoutsos D, Panagiotou P, Polyzos A, Papadopoulos O, Stratigos A (2006) Prognostic significance of autoimmunity during treatment of melanoma with interferon. N Engl J Med 354:709–718

Goto Y, Arigami T, Kitago M, Nguyen SL, Narita N, Ferrone S, Morton DL, Irie RF, Hoon DS (2008) Activation of Toll-like receptors 2, 3, and 4 on human melanoma cells induces inflammatory factors. Mol Cancer Ther 7:3642–3653

Grimbaldeston M, Pearce A, Robertson B, Coventry B, Marshman G, Finlay-Jones J, Hart P (2004) Association between melanoma and dermal mast cell prevalence in sun-unexposed skin. Br J Dermatol 150:895–903

Grimbaldeston MA, Green A, Darlington S, Robertson BO, Marshman G, Finlay-Jones JJ, Hart PH (2003) Susceptibility to basal cell carcinoma is associated with high dermal mast cell prevalence in non–sun-exposed skin for an Australian population. Photochem Photobiol 78:633–639

Gross O, Thomas CJ, Guarda G, Tschopp J (2011) The inflammasome: an integrated view. Immunol Rev 243:136–151

Halk A, Potjer T, Kukutsch N, Vasen H, Hes F, van Doorn R (2019) Surveillance for familial melanoma: recommendations from a national centre of expertise. Br J Dermatol

Han P, Dai Q, Fan L, Zhang X, Li F, Yang X (2019) Genome-wide CRISPR screening identifies JAK1 deficiency as a mechanism of T-cell resistance. Front Immunol 10:251

Hart PH, Norval M (2018) Ultraviolet radiation-induced immunosuppression and its relevance for skin carcinogenesis. Photochem Photobiol Sci 17:1872–1884

Hill VK, Gartner JJ, Samuels Y, Goldstein AM (2013) The genetics of melanoma: recent advances. Annu Rev Genomics Hum Genet 14:257–279

Hino R, Kabashima K, Kato Y, Yagi H, Nakamura M, Honjo T, Okazaki T, Tokura Y (2010) Tumor cell expression of programmed cell death-1 ligand 1 is a prognostic factor for malignant melanoma. Cancer: Interdiscip Int J Am Cancer Soc 116:1757–1766

Howell W, Turner S, Bateman A, Theaker J (2001) IL-10 promoter polymorphisms influence tumour development in cutaneous malignant melanoma. Genes Immun 2:25

Ibrahim EC, Aractingi S, Allory Y, Borrini F, Dupuy A, Duvillard P, Carosella ED, Avril MF, Paul P (2004) Analysis of HLA antigen expression in benign and malignant melanocytic lesions reveals that upregulation of HLA-G expression correlates with malignant transformation, high inflammatory infiltration and HLA-A1 genotype. Int J Cancer 108:243–250

Itakura E, Huang R-R, Wen D-R, Paul E, Wünsch PH, Cochran AJ (2011) IL-10 expression by primary tumor cells correlates with melanoma progression from radial to vertical growth phase and development of metastatic competence. Mod Pathol 24:801

Jiang Y, Shi X, Zhao Q, Krauthammer M, Rothberg BEG, Ma S (2016) Integrated analysis of multidimensional omics data on cutaneous melanoma prognosis. Genomics 107:223–230

Jongeneel CV, Briant L, Udalova IA, Sevin A, Nedospasov SA, Cambon-Thomsen A (1991) Extensive genetic polymorphism in the human tumor necrosis factor region and relation to extended HLA haplotypes. Proc Natl Acad Sci 88:9717–9721

Kageshila T, Naruse T, Hiral S, Ono T, Horikoshi T, Nakagawa H, Tamaki K, Hayashibe K, Ichihashi M, Nakayama J (1997) Molecular genetic analysis of HLA class II alleles in Japanese patients with melanoma. Tissue Antigens 49:466–470

Kandilarova SM, Paschen A, Mihaylova A, Ivanova M, Schadendorf D, Naumova E (2016) The influence of HLA and KIR genes on malignant melanoma development and progression. Arch Immunol Ther Exp 64:73–81

Kleffel S, Posch C, Barthel SR, Mueller H, Schlapbach C, Guenova E, Elco CP, Lee N, Juneja VR, Zhan Q (2015) Melanoma cell-intrinsic PD-1 receptor functions promote tumor growth. Cell 162:1242–1256

Ko DC, Shukla KP, Fong C, Wasnick M, Brittnacher MJ, Wurfel MM, Holden TD, O'Keefe GE, Van Yserloo B, Akey JM (2009) A genome-wide in vitro bacterial-infection screen reveals human variation in the host response associated with inflammatory disease. Am J Human Genet 85:214–227

Kochan G, Escors D, Breckpot K, Guerrero-Setas D (2013) Role of non-classical MHC class I molecules in cancer immunosuppression. Oncoimmunology 2: e26491

Köck A, Schwarz T, Kirnbauer R, Urbanski A, Perry P, Ansel J, Luger T (1990) Human keratinocytes are a source for tumor necrosis factor alpha: evidence for synthesis and release upon stimulation with endotoxin or ultraviolet light. J Exp Med 172:1609–1614

Kumar H, Kawai T, Akira S (2009) Toll-like receptors and innate immunity. Biochem Biophys Res Commun 388:621–625

Lenci RE, Bevier M, Brandt A, Bermejo JL, Sucker A, Moll I, Planelles D, Requena C, Nagore E, Hemminki K (2012) Influence of genetic variants in type I interferon genes on melanoma survival and therapy. PLoS One 7:e50692

Lewis W, Simanyi E, Li H, Thompson CA, Nasti TH, Jaleel T, Xu H, Yusuf N (2011) Regulation of ultraviolet radiation induced cutaneous photoimmunosuppression by toll-like receptor-4. Arch Biochem Biophys 508:171–177

Liu-Smith F, Jia J, Zheng Y (2017) UV-induced molecular signaling differences in melanoma and non-melanoma skin cancer. In: Ultraviolet light in human health, diseases and environment. Springer, pp 27–40

Liu X, Wang Z, Yu J, Lei G, Wang S (2010) Three polymorphisms in interleukin-1β gene and risk for breast cancer: a meta-analysis. Breast Cancer Res Treat 124:821–825

Lombardi ML, Mercuro O, Pirozzi G, Ionna F, Lombari V, Mozzillo N, Manzo C (1998) Molecular analysis of HLA DRB1 and DQB1 polymorphism in Italian melanoma patients. J Immunother (Hagerstown, Md.: 1997) 21:435–439

Lukens JR, Kanneganti T-D (2014) Beyond canonical inflammasomes: emerging pathways in IL-1-mediated autoinflammatory disease. In: Seminars in immunopathology. Springer, pp 595–609

Lulli P, Grammatico P, Brioli G, Catricala C, Morellini M, Roccella M, Mariani B, Pennesi G, Roccella F, Cappellacci S (1998) HLA-DR and-DQ alleles in Italian patients with melanoma. Tissue Antigens 51:276–280

Machado JC, Pharoah P, Sousa S, Carvalho R, Oliveira C, Figueiredo C, Amorim A, Seruca R, Caldas C, Carneiro F (2001) Interleukin 1B and interleukin 1RN polymorphisms are associated with increased risk of gastric carcinoma. Gastroenterology 121:823–829

Marincola FM, Shamamian P, Rivoltini L, Salgaller M, Cormier J, Restifo NP, Simonis TB, Venzon D, White DE, Parkinson DR (1995) HLA associations in the antitumor response against malignant melanoma. J Immunother Emphas Tumor Immunol: Off J Soc Biol Ther 18:242

Martinez-Escribano J, Moya-Quiles M, Muro M, Montes-Ares O, Hernandez-Caselles T, Frias J, Alvarez-Lopez M (2002) Interleukin-10, interleukin-6 and interferon-γ gene polymorphisms in melanoma patients. Melanoma Res 12:465–469

Melsted WN, Johansen LL, Lock-Andersen J, Behrendt N, Eriksen JO, Bzorek M, Scheike T, Hviid TVF (2017) HLA class Ia and Ib molecules and FOXP3+ TILs in relation to the prognosis of malignant melanoma patients. Clin Immunol 183:191–197

Moore KW, de Waal MR, Coffman RL, O'Garra A (2001) Interleukin-10 and the interleukin-10 receptor. Annu Rev Immunol 19:683–765

Nasti TH, Timares L (2012) Inflammasome activation of IL-1 family mediators in response to cutaneous photodamage. Photochem Photobiol 88:1111–1125

Niizeki H, Inoko H, Streilein JW (2002) Polymorphisms in the TNF region confer susceptibility to UVB-induced impairment of contact hypersensitivity induction in mice and humans. Methods 28:46–54

Niizeki H, Naruse T, Hecker K, Taylor J, Kurimoto I, Shimizu T, Yamasaki Y, Inoko H, Streilein J (2001) Polymorphisms in the tumor necrosis factor (TNF) genes are associated with susceptibility to effects of ultraviolet-B radiation on induction of contact hypersensitivity. Tissue Antigens 58:369–378

Park JY, Amankwah EK, Anic GM, Lin H-Y, Walls B, Park H, Krebs K, Madden M, Maddox K, Marzban S (2013) Gene variants in angiogenesis and lymphangiogenesis and cutaneous melanoma progression. Cancer Epidemiol Prev Biomark 22:827–834

Passarelli A, Mannavola F, Stucci LS, Tucci M, Silvestris F (2017) Immune system and melanoma biology: a balance between immunosurveillance and immune escape. Oncotarget 8:106132.

Paul P, Cabestré FA, Le Gal F-A, Khalil-Daher I, Le Danff C, Schmid M, Mercier S, Avril M-F, Dausset J, Guillet J-G (1999) Heterogeneity of HLA-G gene transcription and protein expression in malignant melanoma biopsies. Can Res 59:1954–1960

Paul P, Rouas-Freiss N, Khalil-Daher I, Moreau P, Riteau B, Le Gal FA, Avril MF, Dausset J, Guillet JG, Carosella ED (1998) HLA-G expression in melanoma: a way for tumor cells to escape from immunosurveillance. Proc Natl Acad Sci 95:4510–4515

Perrey C, Pravica V, Sinnott PJ, Hutchinson IV (1998) Genotyping for polymorphisms in interferon-γ, interleukin-10, transforming growth factor-β1 and tumour necrosis factor-α genes: a technical report. Transpl Immunol 6:193–197

Planelles D, Nagore E, Moret A, Botella-Estrada R, Vila E, Guillén C, Montoro J (2006) HLA class II polymorphisms in Spanish melanoma patients: homozygosity for HLA-DQA1 locus can be a potential melanoma risk factor. Br J Dermatol 154:261–266

Postow MA, Callahan MK, Wolchok JD (2015) Immune checkpoint blockade in cancer therapy. J Clin Oncol 33:1974

Queirolo P, Morabito A, Laurent S, Lastraioli S, Piccioli P, Ascierto P, Gentilcore G, Serra M, Marasco A, Tornari E (2013) Association of CTLA-4 polymorphisms with improved overall survival in melanoma patients treated with CTLA-4 blockade: a pilot study. Cancer Invest 31:336–345

Rebmann V, Wagner S, Grosse-Wilde H (2007) HLA-G expression in malignant melanoma. In: Seminars in cancer biology. Elsevier, pp 422–429

Rendleman J, Shang S, Shields J, Adaniel C, Fleming NH, Shapiro R, Berman RS, Pavlick AC, Shao Y, Osman I (2013) Genetic variation in immunomodulatory genes as markers of melanoma recurrence-free and overall survival. American Society of Clinical Oncology, City

Rendleman J, Vogelsang M, Bapodra A, Adaniel C, Silva I, Moogk D, Martinez CN, Fleming N, Shields J, Shapiro R (2015) Genetic associations of the interleukin locus at 1q32. 1 with clinical outcomes of cutaneous melanoma. J Med Genet 52:231–239

Ribas A, Hamid O, Daud A, Hodi FS, Wolchok JD, Kefford R, Joshua AM, Patnaik A, Hwu W-J, Weber JS (2016) Association of pembrolizumab with tumor response and survival among patients with advanced melanoma. JAMA 315:1600–1609

Sarchio SN, Scolyer RA, Beaugie C, McDonald D, Marsh-Wakefield F, Halliday GM, Byrne SN (2014) Pharmacologically antagonizing the CXCR4-CXCL12 chemokine pathway with AMD3100 inhibits sunlight-induced skin cancer. J Investig Dermatol 134:1091–1100

Savoia P, Astrua C, Fava P (2016) Ipilimumab (Anti-Ctla-4 Mab) in the treatment of metastatic melanoma: effectiveness and toxicity management. Hum Vaccin Immunother 12:1092–1101

Schadendorf D, van Akkooi AC, Berking C, Griewank KG, Gutzmer R, Hauschild A, Stang A, Roesch A, Ugurel S (2018) Melanoma. The Lancet 392:971–984

Singh M, Lin J, Hocker T, Tsao H (2008) Genetics of melanoma tumorigenesis. Br J Dermatol 158:15–21

Sleijffers A, Yucesoy B, Kashon M, Garssen J, De Gruijl FR, Boland GJ, Van Hattum J, Luster MI, Van Loveren H (2003) Cytokine polymorphisms play a role in susceptibility to ultraviolet B-induced modulation of immune responses after hepatitis B vaccination. J Immunol 170:3423–3428

Sottile R, Pangigadde PN, Tan T, Anichini A, Sabbatino F, Trecroci F, Favoino E, Orgiano L, Roberts J, Ferrone S (2016) HLA class I downregulation is associated with enhanced NK-cell killing of melanoma cells with acquired drug resistance to BRAF inhibitors. Eur J Immunol 46:409–419

Streilein JW, Taylor JR, Vincek V, Kurimoto I, Richardson J, Tie C, Medema J-P, Golomb C (1994) Relationship between ultraviolet radiation-induced immunosuppression and carcinogenesis. J Investig Dermatol 103:107–111

Taube JM, Anders RA, Young GD, Xu H, Sharma R, McMiller TL, Chen S, Klein AP, Pardoll DM, Topalian SL (2012) Colocalization of inflammatory response with B7-h1 expression in human melanocytic lesions supports an adaptive resistance mechanism of immune escape. Sci Transl Med 4:127ra137–127ra137

Tjin EP, Konijnenberg D, Krebbers G, Mallo H, Drijfhout JW, Franken KL, van der Horst CM, Bos JD, Nieweg OE, Kroon BB (2011) T-cell immune function in tumor, skin, and peripheral blood of advanced stage melanoma patients: implications for immunotherapy. Clin Cancer Res 17:5736–5747

Tremante E, Ginebri A, Lo Monaco E, Benassi B, Frascione P, Grammatico P, Cappellacci S, Catricalà C, Arcelli D, Natali PG (2014) A melanoma immune response signature including Human Leukocyte Antigen-E. Pigment Cell Melanoma Res 27:103–112

Ugurel S, Rebmann V, Ferrone S, Tilgen W, Grosse-Wilde H, Reinhold U (2001) Soluble human leukocyte antigen–G serum level is elevated in melanoma patients and is further increased by interferon-α immunotherapy. Cancer: Interdiscipl Int J Am Cancer Soc 92:369–376.

Ugurel S, Röhmel J, Ascierto PA, Flaherty KT, Grob JJ, Hauschild A, Larkin J, Long GV, Lorigan P, McArthur GA (2016) Survival of patients with advanced metastatic melanoma: the impact of novel therapies. Eur J Cancer 53:125–134

Verma D, Bivik C, Farahani E, Synnerstad I, Fredrikson M, Enerbäck C, Rosdahl I, Söderkvist P (2012) Inflammasome polymorphisms confer susceptibility to sporadic malignant melanoma. Pigment Cell Melanoma Res 25:506–513

Vermeer M, Streilein J (1990) Ultraviolet B light-induced alterations in epidermal Langerhans cells are mediated in part by tumor necrosis factor-alpha. Photodermatol Photoimmunol Photomed 7:258–265

Vincek V, Kurimoto I, Medema JP, Prieto E, Streilein JW (1993) Tumor necrosis factor α polymorphism correlates with deleterious effects of ultraviolet B light on cutaneous immunity. Can Res 53:728–732

von Euw EM, Barrio MM, Furman D, Levy EM, Bianchini M, Peguillet I, Lantz O, Vellice A, Kohan A, Chacón M (2008) A phase I clinical study of vaccination of melanoma patients with dendritic cells loaded with allogeneic apoptotic/necrotic melanoma cells. Analysis of toxicity and immune response to the vaccine and of IL-10-1082 promoter genotype as predictor of disease progression. J Trans Med 6:6

Weber JS, D'Angelo SP, Minor D, Hodi FS, Gutzmer R, Neyns B, Hoeller C, Khushalani NI, Miller WH Jr, Lao CD (2015) Nivolumab versus chemotherapy in patients with advanced melanoma who progressed after anti-CTLA-4 treatment (CheckMate 037): a randomised, controlled, open-label, phase 3 trial. Lancet Oncol 16:375–384

Yamamoto M, Torigoe T, Kamiguchi K, Hirohashi Y, Nakanishi K, Nabeta C, Asanuma H, Tsuruma T, Sato T, Hata F (2005) A novel isoform of TUCAN is overexpressed in human cancer tissues and suppresses both caspase-8–and caspase-9–mediated apoptosis. Can Res 65:8706–8714

Yoshikawa T, Streilein JW (1990) Genetic basis of the effects of ultraviolet light B on cutaneous immunity. Evidence that polymorphism at the Tnfa and Lps loci governs susceptibility. Immunogenetics 32:398–405

Zhai Z, Liu W, Kaur M, Luo Y, Domenico J, Samson JM, Shellman YG, Norris DA, Dinarello CA, Spritz RA (2017) NLRP1 promotes tumor growth by enhancing inflammasome activation and suppressing apoptosis in metastatic melanoma. Oncogene 36:3820

The Immunogenetics of Non-melanoma Skin Cancer

Sabha Mushtaq

Abstract

Non-melanoma skin cancer (NMSC) is the most common malignancy seen in Caucasians and includes basal cell carcinoma (BCC) and squamous cell carcinoma (SCC). The incidence of NMSC is showing an increasing trend which is attributed to the increased use of sunbeds, recreational sun exposure, aging population, and partly to improved screening and reporting. Ultraviolet (UV) radiation plays the most crucial role in the pathogenesis of both BCC and SCC by inducing DNA damage and mutagenic photoproducts. Other risk factors are fair skin, old age, genetic predisposition, immunosuppression, ionizing radiation, organic chemicals, and HPV infection. The role of genomic instability, genetic mutations/aberrations, and host immunity has been fairly illustrated in several studies. This chapter aims to discuss these aspects of NMSC in detail.

Keywords

Non-melanoma skin cancer · SCC · BCC · HLA · Genetics · Immunogenetics · PTCH · p53 · RAS · Pathogenesis

1 Introduction

Non-melanoma skin cancer (NMSC) is a broad group of skin cancers that largely includes basal cell carcinoma (BCC) and squamous cell carcinoma (SCC). In Caucasians, NMSC is the most common malignancy with BCCs constituting 75% and SCCs 25% of NMSCs (Leiter et al. 2014). Due to population aging, use of sunbeds, and recreational exposure to UV radiation, the incidence of NMSCs has shown an increasing trend worldwide (Griffin et al. 2016). The rising trend can also be attributed to improved screening measures. The etiopathogenesis of NMSCs involves a complex interplay between the host of factors and environmental triggers of which ultraviolet (UV) radiation is the most important. Exposure to ionizing radiation, organic chemicals, immunosuppression, human papillomavirus infection, and genetic predisposition are some other risk factors (Didona et al. 2018). The role of genetics in the pathogenesis of NMSCs has been put forth by several studies in the recent past (Bonamigo et al. 2012; Asgari et al. 2016; Yesantharao et al. 2017; Glover et al. 1993; Vineretsky et al. 2016).

S. Mushtaq (✉)
Department of Dermatology, Venereology, and Leprology, Government Medical College & Associated Hospitals, University of Jammu, Jammu, J&K 180001, India

N. Rezaei and F. Rajabi (eds.), *The Immunogenetics of Dermatologic Diseases*, Advances in Experimental Medicine and Biology 1367,
https://doi.org/10.1007/978-3-030-92616-8_16

2 Epidemiology

NMSC occurs throughout the world in different races. The incidence rates of NMSC may be under-reported as these neoplasms are not routinely included in cancer registries. A wide geographical variation is observed in the incidence of NMSC worldwide. In a systematic review, the highest rates were found in Australia (>1000/100,000 person-years for BCC) and the lowest in Africa (<1/100,000 person-years for BCC) (Lomas et al. 2012). In the US, the total number of NMSCs is estimated to be 5.4 million cases in 2012 as compared to 3.5 million cases in 2006 (Rogers et al. 2015, 2010). The incidence rate of BCC in the Netherlands quadrupled from 1973 to 2009 with a 6.8% annual increase for men and 7.9% for women between 2002 and 2009 (Flohil et al. 2013). The wide variation in the distribution of NMSCs can be attributed to the amount of ambient sun irradiance and skin type. The solar irradiance is in turn determined by the geographical latitude and proximity to the equator (Soyer et al. 2012).

The intrinsic factors predisposing to the development of NMSCs are age and skin phenotype. The incidence of both BCC and SCC increases with age with 80% of cases of BCC occurring in individuals aged 60 and above (Garcovich et al. 2017). Whites have a higher incidence of NMSC than Hispanics (Harris et al. 2001). Patients with a history of BCC have high chances of a subsequent one with a 5-year cumulative risk of 29.2% (Flohil et al. 2013).

3 Clinical Features

BCC, also known as rodent ulcer or basal epithelioma, is a slowly progressive neoplasm arising within the photodamaged skin. It is a locally invasive tumor with limited potential for metastasis. The five common clinical types described are superficial, nodular, morpheaform, pigmented, and fibroepithelial polyp of Pinkus. Nodular BCC is the most common type accounting for more than 50% of all BCCs. It begins as a smooth translucent pearly white papule or nodule with surface telangiectasias and may progress to develop central ulceration (Fig. 1) (Griffin et al. 2016).

SCC arises predominantly in an area of photodamaged skin exposed maximally to solar irradiation such as bald scalp, dorsal hand and forearm, pinna, and lower lip. It can present in a variety of morphologies—papulonodular, plaque-like, verrucous, exophytic, tumid, or ulcerated, with all types of lesions demonstrating induration when palpated (Fig. 2). Secondary changes like erosions and crusting may also be seen. SCCs usually arise from pre-malignant skin lesions like Bowen's disease and actinic keratosis and show a more rapid progression and distant metastases when compared to BCC (Griffin et al. 2016; Soyer et al. 2012).

4 Pathogenesis of BCC

The pathophysiology of BCC involves a complex interplay between genetic and environmental factors. The risk factors can be intrinsic like genetic predisposition, old age, and Fitzpatrick skin type or extrinsic like sun exposure, ionizing radiation, phototherapy, and iatrogenic immunosuppression (Griffin et al. 2016; Didona et al. 2018). Of these, sun exposure appears to be of etiologic importance in the development of BCC. Solar UV radiation, both UV-A and UV-B, are mutagenic and can cause DNA damage by different mechanisms. UV-A causes DNA damage indirectly by forming reactive oxygen species which interact with proteins, lipids, and DNA and form intermediate molecules which in turn interact with DNA. UV-B radiation induces covalent bond formation between adjoining pyrimidines leading to the generation of mutagenic photoproducts like cyclopyrimidine dimers (TT) and pyrimidine-pyrimidine (6–4) adducts. UV-B radiation, therefore, results in direct DNA and RNA damage. The majority of the mutations seen in BCC are UV-signature mutations (Narayanan et al. 2010).

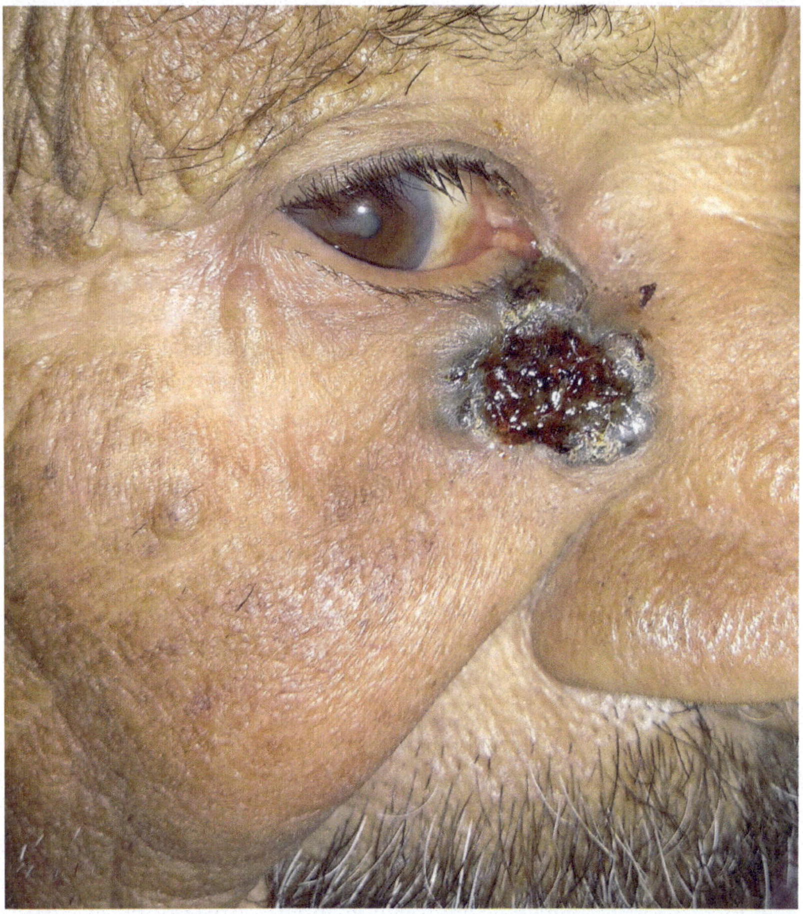

Fig. 1 Well-defined ulcerated plaque with rolled out pigmented borders in a patient with basal cell carcinoma (BCC) over the face

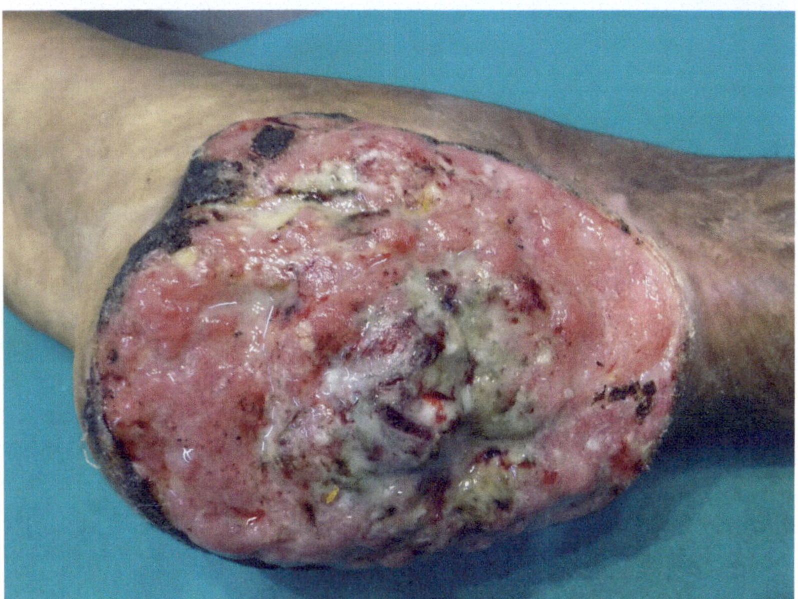

Fig. 2 Ulcerated fungating growth over the heel in a patient with squamous cell carcinoma (SCC)

5 Role of Genetics in the Pathogenesis of BCC

Oncogenes and tumor suppressor genes are two broad groups of genes whose mutation contributes to the development of cancer. Several such genes have been implicated in the pathogenesis of BCC (Tsao 2001). The evidence for genetics playing a role in BCC pathogenesis initially came from a study of patients with Basal cell nevus syndrome or Gorlin syndrome, who were found to carry mutations in the *PTCH1* gene, an important component of the Hedgehog (HH) signaling pathway (Acocella et al. 2009). The HH signaling pathway is important during embryonic development with a minimal role in normal adult tissues. However, activation of the HH signaling pathway is known to occur in a variety of neoplasms including BCC. The role of other genetic components of the HH signaling pathway like smoothened (*SMO*) and glioma-associated oncogene (*GLI*) in BCC has also been investigated (Acocella et al. 2009; Caro and Low 2010). Genomic studies in the recent past have also pointed out the role of additional genetic mutations affecting other signaling pathways (*NOTCH, WNT, and mTOR)* to be associated with BCC. Genetic alterations are found in about 90% of BCC cases in various reports (Shi et al. 2017; Tampa et al. 2020).

PTCH

The patched genes were initially identified in *Drosophila melanogaster.* The human homolog of the patched gene, *PTCH1,* is a "gatekeeper" tumor suppressor gene located on chromosome 9q. The *PTCH1* gene is an important component of the HH signaling pathway which plays a vital role in the regulation of cellular proliferation. In the skin, the HH pathway is essential for maintaining the stem cell niche and regulating the development of the pilosebaceous unit. The *PTCH1* gene is 35 kb in length and consists of 35 exons. The protein product of the PTCH1 gene is patched-1 which acts as a receptor for the Sonic Hedgehog (ligand) (Pellegrini et al. 2017; Zhang et al. 2001). When Sonic Hedgehog (SHH) is not bound to patched-1, the latter prevents cellular proliferation by inhibiting a G-protein receptor called Smoothened (SMO). Upon binding with SHH, SMO is released from repression, thus, allowing downstream signal transduction via transcription factor Gli coded by glioma-associated oncogene (*GLI).* Due to inactivating mutations in the *PTCH1* gene, the mutated patched protein fails to suppress SMO and thereby cellular proliferation (Daya-Grosjean and Couve-Privat 2005; Otsuka et al. 2015).

PTCH1 mutations leading to sustained/aberrant activation of the SHH pathway are reported both in hereditary and sporadic BCC. Most BCCs with *PTCH1* mutations show loss of heterozygosity with a deletion in one allele and a truncated mutation in the other (Tsao 2001; Pellegrini et al. 2017).

SMO

Activating mutations in the *SMO* gene can be present in 10–20% of sporadic BCCs and up to 50% of patients with BCC resistant to Hedgehog pathway inhibitors (HPI) (Pellegrini et al. 2017; Atwood et al. 2015). In sporadic BCC, the mutations are mainly missense affecting the codon 535. In treatment-resistant BCCs, *D473A SMO* mutation decreases the affinity of both Vismodegib and Sonidegib for their molecular target whereas *E518A* mutation decreases the affinity of Vismodegib only (Wang et al. 2014).

SUFU

SUFU gene located on chromosome 10q24.32 consists of 12 exons. It encodes a component of the Sonic Hedgehog/Patched signaling pathway called the suppressor of fused (Sufu) which negatively regulates the HHP by inhibiting the transcriptional activity of Gli1. Inactivating mutations of the *SUFU* gene resulting in increased Gli transcription have been detected in sporadic BCC and up to 5% cases of Nevoid

BCC/Gorlin syndrome (GS). *SUFU* mutation-positive GS patients have about 20 times higher risk of medulloblastoma when compared to *PTCH1* mutation-positive patients. Monitoring by brain MRI in childhood is, therefore, suggested in *SUFU*-related cases of GS (Smith et al. 2014).

Tp53

Tumor suppressor gene *Tp53*, also known as "guardian of the genome""is located on chromosome 17 (17p13.1). It codes for a 53-kDa tumor protein *p53* which plays a key role in cell cycle regulation, DNA repair, and apoptosis. Genetic alteration in *the Tp53* gene is seen in about 30–70% of cases of BCC with the majority of the mutations being UV-signature missense mutations at dipyrimidine sites (CC → TT or C → T). *Tp53* mutations can be present in BCC independent of mutations in the components of the HH signaling pathway (Jayaraman et al. 2014; Reifenberger et al. 2005).

RAS

Mutations in the *RAS* oncogene family (H-ras, K-ras, N-ras) play an important role in human cancers. Although located on different chromosomes, the three *RAS* genes code for the same 21-kDa protein called p21-ras protein. When bound to GTP, the p21-ras protein is active and interacts with protein kinase raf1 to initiate a kinase cascade, resulting in various cellular events. Activating point mutations in *RAS* oncogenes lead to a constitutively active ras protein that promotes cellular proliferation and survival. The frequency of *RAS* mutations in BCC varies from 0–30% in different studies (Tsao 2001; Schroeff et al. 1990).

FOXP1

FOXP1 gene codes for forkhead box protein 1 which has a role in normal organ development and immune responses including regulation of B-cell development and monocyte differentiation. Its overexpression and role in tumorigenesis have been reported in esophageal cancers and cutaneous B-cell lymphomas, wherein it acts as an oncogene. In some cancers like the prostate, it acts as a tumor suppressor (Levine et al. 2013; Koon et al. 2007; Takayama et al. 2014). The results of a two-stage GWAS of BCC involving 17,187 cases and 287,054 controls revealed significant overexpression of *FOXP1* in BCC compared with normal controls (Chahal et al. 2016).

TNS3

*TNS3 (*Tensin 3*)* located on chromosome 7p12.3 is a protein-coding gene belonging to the tensin family of adhesion proteins (Tensin 1–4) which acts as a bridge between the actin cytoskeleton and extracellular matrix. Tensins are expressed widely in normal tissues and play a role in mediating cytoskeletal integrity and cellular motility. The role in cellular motility and migration has been proposed to be implicated in their metastasis suppressor role in renal cell carcinoma, wherein all four tensins are reported to be under-expressed (Martuszewska et al. 2009). However, in BCC, *TNS3* expression is significantly upregulated (Chahal et al. 2016).

CASC15

The *CASC15* (Cancer susceptibility candidate 15) long non-coding RNA locus on chromosome 6p22.3 has been shown to be involved in cellular proliferation, migration, invasion, and apoptosis. Upregulation of *CASC15* in melanoma is associated with metastasis and disease progression (Sand et al. 2016). The role of *CASC15* in the development of BCC is supported by its significant overexpression in the latter which has been confirmed by GWAS (Chahal et al. 2016).

Single nucleotide polymorphisms (SNPs)

GWASs have identified many immune-regulatory loci involved in the increased susceptibility to BCC. Single nucleotide polymorphism (SNP), rs191177147, located within an intron of the *lipoma preferred partner* (*LPP*) gene which is also associated with hair color has been identified in BCC and may contribute to BCC development by altering pigmentation phenotypes (Chahal et al. 2016). The *LPP* gene located on chromosome 3q27-q28 encodes LIM domain proteins which are expressed in the cell periphery and play a role in cellular adhesion and motility. The encoded proteins also shuttle from the focal adhesion sites to the nucleus and are believed to regulate transcription (Petit et al. 2000). Other immune-related SNPs which have been identified include rs10425559 at 19p13.3 which is intergenic and flanked by *TICAM1* and *PLIN3*, rs9267650 at 6p21.3 0.5 kb downstream of *NEU1,* and rs11993814 at 8q21.13 which lies 9 *kb* upstream of *ZBTB10* (Chahal et al. 2016).

HLA genes

The human leukocyte antigen (HLA) system is a group of proteins, encoded by the HLA gene complex located on the short arm of chromosome 6. HLA genes are grouped into three classes.

Class I HLA genes (HLA-A, HLA-B, and HLA-C) are expressed on the surface of all nucleated cells, class II (HLA-DR, DQ, and DP) are expressed on immune cells only, and class III encode molecules that are not involved in antigen presentation but are related to the immune system. These include complement components, cytokines, and other signaling molecules.

The activation of the immune system can induce spontaneous regression in BCC (Leiter et al. 2014; Asgari et al. 2016; Rogers et al. 2010; Zhang et al. 2001). BCC lesions mainly are often infiltrated by CD8 + T-cells that express T-cell receptor (TCR) αβ, perforin, Interleukin-2 receptor, and HLA-DR that are able to lyse the malignant cells (Bonamigo et al. 2012; Asgari et al. 2016; Lomas et al. 2012; Rogers et al. 2010; Soyer et al. 2012; Atwood et al. 2015).

Reduced HLA expression along with loss of expression of tumor antigens allows the neoplastic cells to escape the T-cell-mediated immune surveillance. Lowering the expression of adhesion molecules and Interferon-γ receptors and releasing tolerogenic cytokines such as interleukin-10 and TGF-β are other mechanisms by which these cells escape the immune system (Harris et al. 2001; Narayanan et al. 2010; Tsao 2001; Acocella et al. 2009; Pellegrini et al. 2017).

The role of HLA in the pathophysiology of NMSC is also reflected in the higher incidence in immunocompromised transplant patients when compared to immunocompetent patients (Bonamigo et al. 2012). BCC is positively associated with HLA-DR1 and HLA-DR7 and negatively associated with HLA-DR4 (Bonamigo et al. 2012; Bavinck et al. 2000).

Two immune-related single nucleotide polymorphisms (SNPs) in the HLA region, one lying within an exon of HLA-B at 6p21.33 (rs1050529) and the other at 6p21.32 located 24 kb upstream of *HLA-DQA2* (rs9275642), have also been identified in GWAS (Chahal et al. 2016). HLA-B which encodes the heavy chain component of the MHC class I molecules plays a crucial role in the T-cell-mediated immune responses. MHC class I downregulation is found to be associated with immune evasion by the tumor cells from destruction by the T-cells (Mendez et al. 2009).

PDCD1

The *PDCD1* gene is located at 2q37.3 and encodes a member of the CD28 family of inhibitory immune checkpoint receptors known as PD1. This receptor is involved in the maintenance of both central and peripheral tolerance. PD1 is expressed on T-cells following TCR-MHC interaction and by binding to its receptors inhibits T-cells activation and relays apoptotic signals. The expression of PD1 ligands on cancer cells allows them to escape the immune surveillance by inducing apoptosis in invading T-cells (Fathi et al. 2021). Polymorphisms in the PDCD1 gene have been linked to BCC development. The PD1.3G allele within the transcription factor binding site and the AC haplotype of PD1.3/PD1.5 have been shown to confer susceptibility to BCC (Fathi et al. 2019).

6 Pathogenesis of SCC

SCC, the second most common skin cancer after BCC, originates from the suprabasal epidermal keratinocytes. Unlike BCC which is believed to occur de novo, the development of cutaneous SCCs is a multistage process. Actinic keratosis (AK) is the most common pre-malignant lesion but the risk of transformation of a single AK to an SCC over 10 years is only 10% (Griffin et al. 2016; Didona et al. 2018). Genetic injury caused by solar ultraviolet radiation is considered a major etiological factor in the development of cutaneous SCC. The total cumulative dose of UV radiation exposure from sunlight and artificial sources like tanning lamps and PUVA therapy carries the highest risk in the causation of SCC (Wang et al. 2014). Aside from its mutagenic properties, ultraviolet exposure promotes immune suppression by reducing antigen presentation and up-regulating the number and function of suppressor T-cells in the skin (Tampa et al. 2020; Otsuka et al. 2015). The fact that individuals with an exaggerated immune response to UV light such as those with polymorphic light eruption develop fewer keratinocyte-derived cancers points to the importance of local immune suppression in the pathogenesis of NMSC, especially SCC, that may even compensate for mutagenic properties of UV exposure (Shi et al. 2017). SCC development is associated with an increase in the number of regulatory T-cells, suppression of type I interferon production, and downregulation of E-selectin on nearby endothelial cells (Griffin et al. 2016; Garcovich et al. 2017).

Other predisposing factors for SCC include Fitzpatrick skin type 1 and 2, exposure to ionizing radiation and chemical carcinogens, human papillomavirus infection, immunosuppression, and genetic syndromes like xeroderma pigmentosum and epidermodysplasia verruciformis (Didona et al. 2018; Rogers et al. 2015; Caro and Low 2010).

7 Role of Genetics in the Pathogenesis of SCC

Genetic studies have revealed the role of various genes and HLA associations in the pathogenesis of SCC. The burden of genetic mutations and genomic instability in SCC is cumulative and very high, resulting in aberrations in various cell signaling pathways responsible for regulating the cell cycle, cell survival, apoptosis, and genomic stability (Dotto and Rustgi 2016). The role of genes associated with SCC is discussed in detail below:

Tp53

Mutations in the tumor suppressor gene *Tp53* which codes for tumor suppressor protein *p*53 are seen in up to 90% of SCCs. The majority of these mutations are UV-signature mutations, CC → TT or C → T. The result of these mutations is the defect in repair of UV radiation-induced DNA damage and cellular apoptosis when the damage exceeds the capacity of the repairing mechanisms (Dotto and Rustgi 2016; Brash et al. 1991). Downregulation of *Tp53* mRNA by the aberrant activation of *Fyn*, an epidermal growth factor receptor belonging to the Src family of tyrosine kinase, is another mechanism by which the tumor suppressor function of the *Tp53* gene is impaired in SCC (Ratushny et al. 2012). HPV proteins E6 and E7 are also suggested to play a synergistic role in UV-induced DNA damage by inhibiting *p53*-mediated transcription of genes (Fischer et al. 2017; Aldabagh et al. 2013). Alteration in the *p53* pathway is proposed to be an early event in the pathogenesis of SCC (Tsao 2001; Dotto and Rustgi 2016).

Under non-stressed conditions, the wild-type *Tp53* proteins are present at low levels in normal tissues. This is due to the labile nature of the wild-type *Tp53* proteins and their rapid proteasomal degradation mediated predominantly by ubiquitin ligase MDM2 which is a key negative regulator of *p53* (Dotto and Rustgi 2016; Maki et al. 1996). It has been observed that in cutaneous SCCs, the mutant-type *Tp53* proteins gain stability with prolonged half-life and accumulate in the cell cytoplasm, unlike normal tissues where it is rapidly degraded. This overexpression of the mutant-type *Tp53* correlates with sun exposure and may be responsible for alteration in MHC presentation of wild-type epitopes. Also, the role of *p53* acting as a tumor-associated antigen (TAA) and its role in the immunobiology of cutaneous SCCs are an area of research. Breakthrough in this area can lead us to a vaccine against *p53* which could be useful in a variety of tumors with *p53* overexpression (Black and Ogg 2003).

CDKN2A gene

The *CDKN2A* gene on chromosome 9p21 which codes for cyclin-dependent kinase inhibitor protein p16 normally functions to cause cell cycle arrest in the G1 phase. Inactivation of p16 results in uncontrolled cell cycle progression and, therefore, carcinogenesis. *CDKN2A/p16* inactivation most commonly occurs by promoter methylation and is considered a late event in the pathogenesis of SCC. Mutations in *CDKN2A* have been reported in approximately 24% of SCCs (Tsao 2001; Pacifico and Leone 2007). Saridaki et al. conducted mutational and allelic imbalance analysis of CDKN2A genes in cutaneous SCC patients and observed mutations and loss of heterozygosity of 9p in 52% of the samples, implying inactivation of CDKN2A genes via either allelic loss or UV-induced mutation (Saridaki et al. 2003).

RAS

Activating mutations in the *RAS* oncogenes have been reported in 10–50% of SCCs (Tsao 2001). The variable frequency is attributed to the differences in the experimental technique used and the part of the tumor tested. Catalog of Somatic mutations in Cancer (COSMIC) data shows that mutations in at least one of the three genes (Hras, Nras, and Kras) are present in 21% of the SCCs with Hras mutations (9%) more common than Nras (7%) and Kras (5%) (Bamford et al. 2004; Lazar et al. 2020). *HRAS* mutations have been more commonly documented in well-differentiated, rapidly developing cutaneous SCCs in patients on BRAF inhibitors than sporadic SCCs. The mitogen-activated protein kinase (MAPK)/extracellular signal-related kinase (ERK) pathway activation, which is regulated by negative feedback in normal cells, leads to cellular growth and differentiation. The pathway involves RAS protein and three protein kinases, RAF, MEK, ERK, and is initiated by binding of the ligand to a receptor tyrosine kinase and subsequent activation of RAS. The activation of this signaling pathway culminates in the translocation of ERK/MAPK to the nucleus where activation of transcription factors results in gene expression. In melanoma cells with *BRAF V600E* mutation, there is dysregulation and persistent activation of MAPK signaling, independent of upstream signals from RAS resulting in enhanced cellular proliferation, survival, and invasion. BRAF inhibitors act by inhibition of the MAPK signaling pathway but in cells harboring *RAS* mutations, paradoxical activation of the MAPK signaling pathway results in increased prevalence of cutaneous SCCs. (Su et al. 2012).

c-Myc* and *c-Fos

Zheng et al. analyzed 73 cases of cutaneous SCCs for *c-Myc and c-Fos* genes and observed significantly higher expression (72.60% and 83.56%, respectively) compared with the control group. They also demonstrated that the expression of *c-Myc* was negatively associated with the differentiation of cutaneous SCC while *c-Fos* expression was positively associated with the differentiation of cutaneous SCC (Zheng et al. 2014). Similar findings were reported in another study that documented *Myc* genomic aberrations in 63% of SCCs with higher frequency in poorly differentiated SCCs (Toll et al. 2009).

NOTCH

NOTCH signaling pathway plays a role in normal epidermal development by regulating cellular proliferation, differentiation, stem cell maintenance, apoptosis, and cell survival. Out of the four mammalian *NOTCH* proteins, *NOTCH1* and *NOTCH2* are expressed in the human epidermis (Ratushny et al. 2012). In a study by Wang et al., whole-exome sequencing of cutaneous SCCs identified *NOTCH 1* and *NOTCH 2* mutations in up to 75% of the cases (Wang et al. 2011).

Pigmentary genes

The genetic variability in the melanocortin-1 receptor potentiates the UV sensitivity of the skin and the risk of SCC. Single nucleotide polymorphisms in genes responsible for pigmentation and related to the pigmentation pathway, such as tyrosinase *(TYR)* on chromosome 11q14, *SLC45A2* on chromosome 5p13, and *IRF4* on chromosome 6p25, are associated with SCC risk (Asgari et al. 2016). Oculocutaneus albinism patients with pigmentary gene mutations show an increased risk of developing cutaneous SCC (Didona et al. 2018).

GWAS meta-analysis of 19,149 SCC cases and 680,049 controls identified eight new susceptibility loci which corresponded to genes involved in immune regulation (*BACH2*), keratinocyte differentiation (*TRPS*, *KRT5*), cancer progression (*SETDB1*, *CASP8/ALS2CR12*, *WEE1*), and pigmentation (*TYRP1*). The immunoregulatory gene *BACH2* which plays a role in tumor immunosuppression is underexpressed in SCC as compared to normal skin and could be responsible for evasion of the cancer cells from immune surveillance (Sarin et al. 2020). In addition, a transcriptome-wide association study (TWAS) validated five susceptibility loci including eight genes in SCC: *CASP8* at 2q33; *ORMDL3* at 17q21; *AHI1* at 6q23; *CTSS*, *HORMAD1*, *GOLPH3L*, and *ANXA9* at 1q21; and *HAL* at 12q23. Lower imputed expression levels of *CASP8* (caspase 8) which is involved in cellular apoptosis are negatively associated with cutaneous SCC. *ORMDL3 (*ORMDL sphingolipid biosynthesis regulator 3) is involved in calcium homeostasis and its increased expression in SCC interferes with activation of T-lymphocytes, thereby promoting tumor evasion. *AHI1* is an oncogene and its imputed expression levels are positively associated with cutaneous SCC. *HAL* (histidine ammonia-lyase) is involved in the synthesis of urocanic acid which protects against UV-mediated DNA damage. Individuals with a high imputed expression of *HAL* are associated with decreased risk of cutaneous SCC. *CTSS*, *HORMAD1*, *GOLPH3L*, and *ANXA9* are all negatively associated with cutaneous SCC (Ioannidis NM, Wang W, Furlotte NA, Hinds DA, andMe Research T, Bustamante CD, Jorgenson E, Asgari MM, Whittemore AS 2018).

HLA genes

Multiple HLA genes and alleles are associated with a higher risk of cutaneous SCC. HLA genes and MHC proteins are involved in the tumor antigen presentation to immune cells which plays a role in host defense against tumorigenesis (Yesantharao et al. 2017; Glover et al. 1993; Vineretsky et al. 2016).

Many studies have shown that HLA-SCC associations are heterogeneous depending upon the immune status of the patients (Yesantharao et al. 2017; Glover et al. 1993; Bouwes Bavinck et al. 1991). A systematic review conducted by Yesentharao et al. concluded that immunity plays a crucial role in the development of SCC and that distinct HLA-SCC associations are present in immunocompetent and immunocompromised hosts. This review documented that class I HLA alleles *HLA B*58* and *Bw4* were found to be negatively associated with cutaneous SCC in immunocompetent patients whereas *HLA A*03*, *HLA A*11,* and *HLA B*27* showed a variable association in immunocompromised patients. The positively associated HLA class II alleles with cutaneous SCC in immunocompetent patients included *HLA DRB1*01*, *HLA DRB1*07*, *HLA DQB1*, and *HLA DQA1*. The *HLA DRB1*07* and *HLA DQA1*01* confer risk to SCC in immunosuppressed patients (Yesantharao et al. 2017). The HLA-SCC associations showed a geographical variability which reflected the differences in patient population, methodology, immunosuppression protocol, and other unidentified factors. The same review observed that there was more evidence for class I HLA-SCC associations in immunosuppressed patients than in immunocompetent patients. The methods of HLA typing which was employed in most studies were based on serological typing which fails to adequately distinguish between different HLA alleles. The review suggested the use of more precise methods for typing HLA alleles associated with SCC as alleles within the same allele group can differ in their efficacy in antigen presentation. The underlying mechanism by which HLA allelic variants play a role in the pathogenesis of SCC is proposed to be related to the impairment in the presentation of cutaneous SCC tumor antigens to T-lymphocytes (Yesantharao et al. 2017). The role of HPV infection in influencing the HLA-SCC associations in immunosuppressed patients has also been studied. The allele group HLA DRB1*07 is believed to be associated with the impaired presentation of HPV 8 antigen L1 to CD4 + T-lymphocytes, which results in an ineffective immune response (Yesantharao et al. 2017; Bavinck et al. 1993).

Besides the association between germline HLA variants and cutaneous SCC, abnormal cell surface expression of HLA proteins on tumor cells is also seen. Unlike melanoma and BCC, which have complete loss of class I HLA proteins, cutaneous SCCs show an aberrant, heterogeneous, and reduced expression of these proteins. The HLA presentation of SCC does not have a prognostic value and it is not associated with the degree of tumor invasion. Class II HLA alleles on the other hand are overexpressed on the cell surface in cutaneous SCCs and correlate with the histopathological type and cellular differentiation (Yesantharao et al. 2017; Garcia-Plata et al. 1993; Hua et al. 1985; Markey et al. 1990).

The risk of skin cancers including NMSC can be predicted by polygenic risk scores (PRS) for skin cancer. PRS are developed using GWAS data and are useful in risk stratification with improved prediction ability. A review conducted by Roberts et al. included GWAS and PRS studies on skin cancer. The study observed that the PRS for cutaneous squamous cell carcinoma and BCC showed a two- and three-fold increase in risk, respectively, and a 2% increase in prediction ability. The clinical utility and implementation of PRS for cutaneous SCC and BCC, however, need to be further substantiated by larger, more comprehensive studies (Roberts et al. 2019).

8 Conclusion

Non-melanoma skin cancers are on the rise owing to a range of factors including an aging population, increased recreational sun exposure, and efficient skin cancer screening methods. Ultraviolet radiation (UV)-mediated DNAdamage and genetic mutations in both tumor suppressors and proto-oncogenes are central to the pathogenesis of NMSCs. Genome-wide association studies have also identified numerous immune-regulatory genes and single nucleotide polymorphisms which confer increased susceptibility to the development of NMSCs. Polygenic risk scores have emerged as better predictors of skin cancer susceptibility by combining multiple susceptibility variants and can be used in addition to the existing prediction models for skin cancers.

References

Leiter U, Eigentler T, Garbe C (2014) Epidemiology of skin cancer. Adv Exp Med Biol 810:120–140

Griffin LL, Ali FR, Lear JT (2016) Non-Melanoma Skin Cancer. Clin Med (lond) 16:62–65

Didona D, Paolino G, Bottoni U, Cantisani C (2018) Non Melanoma Skin Cancer Pathogenesis Overview. Biomedicines 6.

Bonamigo RR, Carvalho AV, Sebastiani VR, Silva CM, Pinto AC (2012) HLA and skin cancer. An Bras Dermatol 87:9–16; quiz 17–18.

Asgari MM, Wang W, Ioannidis NM, Itnyre J, Hoffmann T, Jorgenson E, Whittemore AS (2016) Identification of Susceptibility Loci for Cutaneous Squamous Cell Carcinoma. J Invest Dermatol 136:930–937

Yesantharao P, Wang W, Ioannidis NM, Demehri S, Whittemore AS, Asgari MM (2017) Cutaneous squamous cell cancer (cSCC) risk and the human leukocyte antigen (HLA) system. Hum Immunol 78:327–335

Glover MT, Bodmer J, Bodmer W, Kennedy LJ, Brown J, Navarrete C, Kwan JT, Leigh IM (1993) HLA antigen frequencies in renal transplant recipients and non-immunosuppressed patients with non-melanoma skin cancer. Eur J Cancer 29A:520–524

Vineretsky KA, Karagas MR, Christensen BC, Kuriger-Laber JK, Perry AE, Storm CA, Nelson HH (2016) Skin Cancer Risk Is Modified by KIR/HLA Interactions That Influence the Activation of Natural Killer Immune Cells. Cancer Res 76:370–376

Lomas A, Leonardi-Bee J, Bath-Hextall F (2012) A systematic review of worldwide incidence of non-melanoma skin cancer. Br J Dermatol 166:1069–1080

Rogers HW, Weinstock MA, Feldman SR, Coldiron BM (2015) Incidence Estimate of Nonmelanoma Skin Cancer (Keratinocyte Carcinomas) in the U.S. Population, 2012. JAMA Dermatol 151:1081–1086

Rogers HW, Weinstock MA, Harris AR, Hinckley MR, Feldman SR, Fleischer AB, Coldiron BM (2010) Incidence estimate of nonmelanoma skin cancer in the United States, 2006. Arch Dermatol 146:283–287

Flohil SC, Seubring I, van Rossum MM, Coebergh JW, de Vries E, Nijsten T (2013) Trends in Basal cell carcinoma incidence rates: a 37-year Dutch observational study. J Invest Dermatol 133:913–918

Soyer HP, Rigel D, Wurm EM (2012) Actinic keratosis, basal cell carcinoma and squamous cell carcinoma. In: JL B, JL J, J S (eds) Dermatology, 3rd ed edn. Elsevier-Saunders, Philadelphia, pp 1773–1795.

Garcovich S, Colloca G, Sollena P, Andrea B, Balducci L, Cho WC, Bernabei R, Peris K (2017) Skin Cancer Epidemics in the Elderly as An Emerging Issue in Geriatric Oncology. Aging Dis 8:643–661

Harris RB, Griffith K, Moon TE (2001) Trends in the incidence of nonmelanoma skin cancers in southeastern Arizona, 1985–1996. J Am Acad Dermatol 45:528–536

Narayanan DL, Saladi RN, Fox JL (2010) Ultraviolet radiation and skin cancer. Int J Dermatol 49:978–986

Tsao H (2001) Genetics of nonmelanoma skin cancer. Arch Dermatol 137:1486–1492

Acocella A, Sacco R, Bertolai R, Sacco N (2009) Genetic and clinicopathologic aspects of Gorlin-Goltz syndrome (NBCCS): presentation of two case reports and literature review. Minerva Stomatol 58:43–53

Caro I, Low JA (2010) The role of the hedgehog signaling pathway in the development of basal cell carcinoma and opportunities for treatment. Clin Cancer Res 16:3335–3339

Shi FT, Yu M, Zloty D, Bell RH, Wang E, Akhoundsadegh N, Leung G, Haegert A, Carr N, Shapiro J, McElwee KJ (2017) Notch signaling is significantly suppressed in basal cell carcinomas and activation induces basal cell carcinoma cell apoptosis. Mol Med Rep 15:1441–1454

Tampa M, Georgescu SR, Mitran CI, Mitran MI, Matei C, Scheau C, Constantin C, Neagu M (2020) Recent Advances in Signaling Pathways Comprehension as Carcinogenesis Triggers in Basal Cell Carcinoma. J Clin Med 9.

Pellegrini C, Maturo MG, Di Nardo L, Ciciarelli V, Gutierrez Garcia-Rodrigo C, Fargnoli MC (2017) Understanding the Molecular Genetics of Basal Cell Carcinoma. Int J Mol Sci 18.

Zhang H, Ping XL, Lee PK, Wu XL, Yao YJ, Zhang MJ, Silvers DN, Ratner D, Malhotra R, Peacocke M, Tsou HC (2001) Role of PTCH and p53 genes in early-onset basal cell carcinoma. Am J Pathol 158:381–385

Daya-Grosjean L, Couve-Privat S (2005) Sonic hedgehog signaling in basal cell carcinomas. Cancer Lett 225:181–192

Otsuka A, Levesque MP, Dummer R, Kabashima K (2015) Hedgehog signaling in basal cell carcinoma. J Dermatol Sci 78:95–100

Atwood SX, Sarin KY, Whitson RJ, Li JR, Kim G, Rezaee M, Ally MS, Kim J, Yao C, Chang AL, Oro AE, Tang JY (2015) Smoothened variants explain the majority of drug resistance in basal cell carcinoma. Cancer Cell 27:342–353

Wang C, Wu H, Evron T, Vardy E, Han GW, Huang XP, Hufeisen SJ, Mangano TJ, Urban DJ, Katritch V, Cherezov V, Caron MG, Roth BL, Stevens RC (2014) Structural basis for Smoothened receptor modulation and chemoresistance to anticancer drugs. Nat Commun 5:4355

Smith MJ, Beetz C, Williams SG, Bhaskar SS, O'Sullivan J, Anderson B, Daly SB, Urquhart JE, Bholah Z, Oudit D, Cheesman E, Kelsey A, McCabe MG, Newman WG, Evans DG (2014) Germline mutations in SUFU cause Gorlin syndrome-associated childhood medulloblastoma and redefine the risk associated with PTCH1 mutations. J Clin Oncol 32:4155–4161

Jayaraman SS, Rayhan DJ, Hazany S, Kolodney MS (2014) Mutational landscape of basal cell carcinomas by whole-exome sequencing. J Invest Dermatol 134:213–220

Reifenberger J, Wolter M, Knobbe CB, Kohler B, Schonicke A, Scharwachter C, Kumar K, Blaschke B, Ruzicka T, Reifenberger G (2005) Somatic mutations in the PTCH, SMOH, SUFUH and TP53 genes in sporadic basal cell carcinomas. Br J Dermatol 152:43–51

van der Schroeff JG, Evers LM, Boot AJ, Bos JL (1990) Ras oncogene mutations in basal cell carcinomas and squamous cell carcinomas of human skin. J Invest Dermatol 94:423–425

Levine DM, Ek WE, Zhang R, Liu X, Onstad L, Sather C, Lao-Sirieix P, Gammon MD, Corley DA, Shaheen NJ, Bird NC, Hardie LJ, Murray LJ, Reid BJ, Chow WH, Risch HA, Nyren O, Ye W, Liu G, Romero Y, Bernstein L, Wu AH, Casson AG, Chanock SJ, Harrington P, Caldas I, Debiram-Beecham I, Caldas C, Hayward NK, Pharoah PD, Fitzgerald RC, Macgregor S, Whiteman DC, Vaughan TL (2013) A genome-wide association study identifies new susceptibility loci for esophageal adenocarcinoma and Barrett's esophagus. Nat Genet 45:1487–1493

Koon HB, Ippolito GC, Banham AH, Tucker PW (2007) FOXP1: a potential therapeutic target in cancer. Expert Opin Ther Targets 11:955–965

Takayama K, Suzuki T, Tsutsumi S, Fujimura T, Takahashi S, Homma Y, Urano T, Aburatani H, Inoue S (2014) Integrative analysis of FOXP1 function reveals a tumor-suppressive effect in prostate cancer. Mol Endocrinol 28:2012–2024

Chahal HS, Wu W, Ransohoff KJ, Yang L, Hedlin H, Desai M, Lin Y, Dai HJ, Qureshi AA, Li WQ, Kraft P, Hinds DA, Tang JY, Han J, Sarin KY (2016) Genome-wide association study identifies 14 novel risk alleles associated with basal cell carcinoma. Nat Commun 7:12510

Martuszewska D, Ljungberg B, Johansson M, Landberg G, Oslakovic C, Dahlback B, Hafizi S (2009) Tensin3 is a negative regulator of cell migration and all four Tensin family members are downregulated in human kidney cancer. PLoS One 4:e4350.

Sand M, Bechara FG, Sand D, Gambichler T, Hahn SA, Bromba M, Stockfleth E, Hessam S (2016) Long-noncoding RNAs in basal cell carcinoma. Tumour Biol 37:10595–10608

Petit MM, Fradelizi J, Golsteyn RM, Ayoubi TA, Menichi B, Louvard D, Van de Ven WJ, Friederich E (2000) LPP, an actin cytoskeleton protein related to zyxin, harbors a nuclear export signal and transcriptional activation capacity. Mol Biol Cell 11:117–129

Bavinck JN, Bastiaens MT, Marugg ME, Beckers RC, Westendorp RG, Vermeer BJ, Claas FH (2000) Further evidence for an association of HLA-DR7 with basal cell carcinoma on the tropical island of Saba. Arch Dermatol 136:1019–1022

Mendez R, Aptsiauri N, Del Campo A, Maleno I, Cabrera T, Ruiz-Cabello F, Garrido F, Garcia-Lora A (2009) HLA and melanoma: multiple alterations in HLA class I and II expression in human melanoma cell lines from ESTDAB cell bank. Cancer Immunol Immunother 58:1507–1515

Fathi F, Zamani B, Piroozmand A, Mozafarpoor S, Seyedhashemi E, ArefNezhad R, Motedayyen H (2021) Programmed cell death 1 (PDCD1) gene haplotypes and susceptibility of patients to basal cell carcinoma. Mol Biol Rep 48:2047–2052

Fathi F, Ebrahimi M, Eslami A, Hafezi H, Eskandari N, Motedayyen H (2019) Association of programmed death-1 gene polymorphisms with the risk of basal cell carcinoma. Int J Immunogenet 46:444–450

Dotto GP, Rustgi AK (2016) Squamous Cell Cancers: A Unified Perspective on Biology and Genetics. Cancer Cell 29:622–637

Brash DE, Rudolph JA, Simon JA, Lin A, McKenna GJ, Baden HP, Halperin AJ, Ponten J (1991) A role for sunlight in skin cancer: UV-induced p53 mutations in squamous cell carcinoma. Proc Natl Acad Sci U S A 88:10124–10128

Ratushny V, Gober MD, Hick R, Ridky TW, Seykora JT (2012) From keratinocyte to cancer: the pathogenesis and modeling of cutaneous squamous cell carcinoma. J Clin Invest 122:464–472

Fischer M, Uxa S, Stanko C, Magin TM, Engeland K (2017) Human papilloma virus E7 oncoprotein abrogates the p53–p21-DREAM pathway. Sci Rep 7:2603

Aldabagh B, Angeles JG, Cardones AR, Arron ST (2013) Cutaneous squamous cell carcinoma and human papillomavirus: is there an association? Dermatol Surg 39:1–23

Maki CG, Huibregtse JM, Howley PM (1996) In vivo ubiquitination and proteasome-mediated degradation of p53(1). Cancer Res 56:2649–2654

Black AP, Ogg GS (2003) The role of p53 in the immunobiology of cutaneous squamous cell carcinoma. Clin Exp Immunol 132:379–384

Pacifico A, Leone G (2007) Role of p53 and CDKN2A inactivation in human squamous cell carcinomas. J Biomed Biotechnol 2007:43418

Saridaki Z, Liloglou T, Zafiropoulos A, Koumantaki E, Zoras O, Spandidos DA (2003) Mutational analysis of CDKN2A genes in patients with squamous cell carcinoma of the skin. Br J Dermatol 148:638–648

Bamford S, Dawson E, Forbes S, Clements J, Pettett R, Dogan A, Flanagan A, Teague J, Futreal PA, Stratton MR, Wooster R (2004) The COSMIC (Catalogue of Somatic Mutations in Cancer) database and website. Br J Cancer 91:355–358

Lazar AD, Dinescu S, Costache M (2020) Deciphering the Molecular Landscape of Cutaneous Squamous Cell Carcinoma for Better Diagnosis and Treatment. J Clin Med 9.

Su F, Viros A, Milagre C, Trunzer K, Bollag G, Spleiss O, Reis-Filho JS, Kong X, Koya RC, Flaherty KT, Chapman PB, Kim MJ, Hayward R, Martin M, Yang H, Wang Q, Hilton H, Hang JS, Noe J, Lambros M, Geyer F, Dhomen N, Niculescu-Duvaz I, Zambon A, Niculescu-Duvaz D, Preece N, Robert L, Otte NJ, Mok S, Kee D, Ma Y, Zhang C, Habets G, Burton EA, Wong B, Nguyen H, Kockx M,

Andries L, Lestini B, Nolop KB, Lee RJ, Joe AK, Troy JL, Gonzalez R, Hutson TE, Puzanov I, Chmielowski B, Springer CJ, McArthur GA, Sosman JA, Lo RS, Ribas A, Marais R (2012) RAS mutations in cutaneous squamous-cell carcinomas in patients treated with BRAF inhibitors. N Engl J Med 366:207–215

Zheng Y, Wang GR, Jia JJ, Luo SJ, Wang H, Xiao SX (2014) Expressions of oncogenes c-fos and c-myc in skin lesion of cutaneous squamous cell carcinoma. Asian Pac J Trop Med 7:761–764

Toll A, Salgado R, Yebenes M, Martin-Ezquerra G, Gilaberte M, Baro T, Sole F, Alameda F, Espinet B, Pujol RM (2009) MYC gene numerical aberrations in actinic keratosis and cutaneous squamous cell carcinoma. Br J Dermatol 161:1112–1118

Wang NJ, Sanborn Z, Arnett KL, Bayston LJ, Liao W, Proby CM, Leigh IM, Collisson EA, Gordon PB, Jakkula L, Pennypacker S, Zou Y, Sharma M, North JP, Vemula SS, Mauro TM, Neuhaus IM, Leboit PE, Hur JS, Park K, Huh N, Kwok PY, Arron ST, Massion PP, Bale AE, Haussler D, Cleaver JE, Gray JW, Spellman PT, South AP, Aster JC, Blacklow SC, Cho RJ (2011) Loss-of-function mutations in Notch receptors in cutaneous and lung squamous cell carcinoma. Proc Natl Acad Sci U S A 108:17761–17766

Sarin KY, Lin Y, Daneshjou R, Ziyatdinov A, Thorleifsson G, Rubin A, Pardo LM, Wu W, Khavari PA, Uitterlinden A, Nijsten T, Toland AE, Olafsson JH, Sigurgeirsson B, Thorisdottir K, Jorgensen E, Whittemore AS, Kraft P, Stacey SN, Stefansson K, Asgari MM, Han J (2020) Genome-wide meta-analysis identifies eight new susceptibility loci for cutaneous squamous cell carcinoma. Nat Commun 11:820

Ioannidis NM, Wang W, Furlotte NA, Hinds DA, andMe Research T, Bustamante CD, Jorgenson E, Asgari MM, Whittemore AS (2018) Gene expression imputation identifies candidate genes and susceptibility loci associated with cutaneous squamous cell carcinoma. Nat Commun 9:4264

Bouwes Bavinck JN, Vermeer BJ, van der Woude FJ, Vandenbroucke JP, Schreuder GM, Thorogood J, Persijn GG, Claas FH (1991) Relation between skin cancer and HLA antigens in renal-transplant recipients. N Engl J Med 325:843–848

Bavinck JN, Gissmann L, Claas FH, Van der Woude FJ, Persijn GG, Ter Schegget J, Vermeer BJ, Jochmus I, Muller M, Steger G et al (1993) Relation between skin cancer, humoral responses to human papillomaviruses, and HLA class II molecules in renal transplant recipients. J Immunol 151:1579–1586

Garcia-Plata D, Mozos E, Carrasco L, Solana R (1993) HLA molecule expression in cutaneous squamous cell carcinomas: an immunopathological study and clinical-immunohistopathological correlations. Histol Histopathol 8:219–226

Hua LA, Kagen CN, Carpenter RJ, Goltz RW (1985) HLA and beta 2-microglobulin expression in basal and squamous cell carcinomas of the skin. Int J Dermatol 24:660–663

Markey AC, Churchill LJ, MacDonald DM (1990) Altered expression of major histocompatibility complex (MHC) antigens by epidermal tumours. J Cutan Pathol 17:65–71

Roberts MR, Asgari MM, Toland AE (2019) Genome-wide association studies and polygenic risk scores for skin cancer: clinically useful yet? Br J Dermatol 181:1146–1155

The Immunogenetics of Cutaneous Drug Reactions

Neda Khalili

Abstract

Adverse drug reactions (ADRs) are the cause of nearly three to six percent of inpatient admissions and are associated with high morbidity and mortality rates. Cutaneous adverse drug reactions (cADRs) represent the most frequent ADRs observed among patients during hospital stay. Recent investigations have found that various HLA genotypes have a significant association with ADRs, especially immune-mediated ADRs. This chapter is devoted to the description of the immunopathogenic mechanism of these reactions and the specific HLA-drug associations. Also, we discuss the association of other non-HLA genes with the development of cADRs and provide a summary of the currently approved recommendations on pre-treatment HLA genotyping tests.

Keywords

Adverse drug reactions · HLA antigens · Cutaneous adverse drug reaction · Genotyping

1 Introduction

The World Health Organization (WHO) defines an adverse drug reaction (ADR) as "a response to a medicinal product which is *noxious and unintended* and which occurs *at doses normally used in man* for the prophylaxis, diagnosis or therapy of disease or the restoration, correction or modification of physiological function" (Edwards and Biriell 1994). However, considerable heterogeneity exists regarding the definition of ADR across published literature. ADRs represent a major cause of morbidity and mortality and entail a remarkable burden on health-care systems. These reactions are the cause of nearly three to six percent of inpatient admissions, which account for five to ten percent of inpatient costs. It has been approximated that ADRs are the fifth most frequent cause of mortality in the hospital setting while about 50% of these reactions are preventable (Beijer and Blaey 2002; Carr and Pirmohamed 2018; Giardina et al. 2018; Hakkarainen et al. 2012; Kongkaew et al. 2008; Lazarou et al. 1998; Pirmohamed et al. 2004; Saedder et al. 2015). Antiplatelet drugs, diuretics, nonsteroidal anti-inflammatory drugs (NSAIDs), and anticoagulants are the main drugs associated with preventable ADRs (Mjorndal et al. 2002; Pirmohamed 2012; Ruiter et al. 2012; Hooft et al. 2008). ADRs can have various clinical manifestations, which mostly affect the skin and mucosa, the liver, and the circulatory system. Cutaneous

N. Khalili (✉)
Cancer Immunology Project (CIP), Universal Scientific Education and Research Network (USERN), Tehran, Iran
e-mail: nkhalili@alumnus.tums.ac.ir

N. Rezaei and F. Rajabi (eds.), *The Immunogenetics of Dermatologic Diseases*, Advances in Experimental Medicine and Biology 1367,
https://doi.org/10.1007/978-3-030-92616-8_17

adverse drug reactions (cADRs) are mainly present in hospital ADRs rather than ADRs leading to hospitalization. These reactions represent the most common ADRs observed in patients during hospital stays (Giardina et al. 2018). ADRs are commonly classified into two types: type A reactions that are dose-dependent and predictable based on the pharmacological properties of the drug, and type B reactions that are unpredictable, idiosyncratic, and immune-mediated (IM) (comprising both B-cell and T cell-mediated reactions). Reviews investigating the risk factors for serious ADRs are currently very limited. In a study by Saedder et al., the number of medications used by an individual was a risk factor for ADRs among adult and elderly inpatients (Saedder et al. 2015). Other studies have also confirmed that polypharmacy contributes to an increased risk for ADR (Davies et al. 2009; Nguyen et al. 2006). Besides, several additional risk factors including female gender, increased age, specific drug classes, and comorbidities have been generally accepted as predictors of ADR occurrence (Giardina et al. 2018; Wolfe et al. 2018). Genetic factors can play a pivotal role in the pharmacokinetics and pharmacodynamics of drugs in addition to susceptibility to immunologic reactions such as hypersensitivity responses. Recently, various HLA genotypes have been found to be highly associated with adverse drug reactions, precisely IM-ADRs, such as carbamazepine-induced Stevens-Johnson syndrome (SJS) in patients carrying *HLA-B*15:02* and abacavir-induced hypersensitivity syndrome (HSS) in patients carrying *HLA-B*57:01* (Locharernkul et al. 2008b; Mallal et al. 2008a). This has led to an increasing number of FDA-approved drug labels recommending HLA genetic testing before prescribing certain types of medications. However, HLA alleles are not the only genetic factors associated with cADRs. The association of non-HLA genes with cADRs has been studied to a lesser extent, for instance, genes involved in cytokine signaling, those involved in production and release of pre-formed or newly formed mediators, and other immune-related genes such as *Transporter Antigen Processing (TAP1/2)*, *MHC class I related chain A/B (MICA/MICB)*, *hemochromatosis gene (High Fe, HFE)*, *T-cell receptors genes (TCRs)*, *B-cell receptors genes (BCRs)*, and *killer cell immunoglobulin-like receptors (KIRs)* (Böhm and Cascorbi 2016; Daly 2013; Karnes et al. 2019).

The *HLA genes* are located on chromosome 6p21.3 and are highly polymorphic. They play a key role in normal immunological functions and are also linked to various diseases related to the immune system. Initiation of antigen-specific immune responses requires the presentation of endogenous and exogenous peptide antigens to T-cells by HLA molecules. HLA molecules that are expressed on the surface of various cell lines could display bound peptides, leading to their recognition by T-cells via surface TCRs. Class I MHC molecules (HLA-A, HLA-B, and HLA-C) are expressed on all nucleated cells and are involved in the activation of CD8 + cytotoxic T-cells, whereas class II MHC molecules (HLA-DP, HLA-DQ, and HLA-DR) are expressed only by professional antigen-presenting cells (dendritic cells, B-cells, and macrophages) and can trigger the activation of CD4 + helper T-cells. Herein, we mainly focus on the best-studied IM-ADRs that are associated with specific HLA-risk alleles. These T cell-mediated IM-ADRs include delayed exanthema without systemic symptoms as in maculopapular eruption (MPE), contact dermatitis, drug-induced hypersensitivity syndrome (DIHS)/HHS/drug reaction with eosinophilia and systemic symptoms (DRESS), SJS/toxic epidermal necrolysis (TEN), fixed drug eruption (FDE), acute generalized exanthematous pustulosis (AGEP), single organ involvement pathologies such as drug-induced liver disease (DILI), and the abacavir hypersensitivity syndrome (AHS) (Pirmohamed et al. 2011a, b).

2 The Immunopathogenic Mechanism

Currently, five immunologic models exist that explain how small drug molecules elicit T cell-mediated immune responses: (a) the hapten and pro-hapten model, (b) the pharmacological interaction with immune receptors (p-i) model, (c) the altered peptide repertoire model, (d) the altered TCR repertoire model, and (e) the danger hypothesis (Illing et al. 2016; Yun et al. 2016) (Fig. 1). These models are only able to describe the initial steps of ADR and there is no prediction for whether the T cell-mediated immune reaction will result in humoral or cellular immune responses. Furthermore, there is little correlation between these models and the actual clinical phenotype of the ADR (Yun et al. 2016).

According to model (a), small molecule drugs that are incapable of inducing a direct immunologic response could covalently bind to larger peptides (albumin or other intra/extracellular proteins) and generate complexes that act as neoantigens and trigger T-cell responses. These interactions could either happen inside the cellular environment that requires subsequent processing by antigen-presenting cells or at the cell surface level. In the pro-hapten model, a reactive metabolite of the drug may act as the hapten.

Model (b) proposes that drugs bind noncovalently to either the MHC or TCR molecules, directly activating T-cells. This interaction happens at the cell surface level and does not require antigen processing. Since TCRs/MHCs are activated directly, subsequent B-cell responses are not expected. The activation could occur via strengthening the TCR interaction with the HLA/peptide complex. The drug can also bind to TCR or MHC directly activating it independent of the peptide that is being presented. Alternatively, the drug can change the TCR configuration in a manner that makes it more susceptible to recognize self-antigens (allosterism) (Yun et al. 2016).

Model (c) postulates that drugs change the structure of the MHC-I binding cleft by noncovalently binding to the peptide repertoire. The neo-epitopes are then able to present specific self-peptides that are otherwise never identified by the immune system as non-self molecules and thus stimulate a T cell-mediated immune response (Ostrov et al. 2012).

Model (d) implies that the binding of drugs to specific TCRs leads to conformational changes that enable them to recognize self-peptide-HLA complexes as non-self (foreign) antigens (Watkins and Pichler 2013).

Finally, based on model (e), drugs provoke cellular damage via chemical reactions. The distressed and injured cells would then release

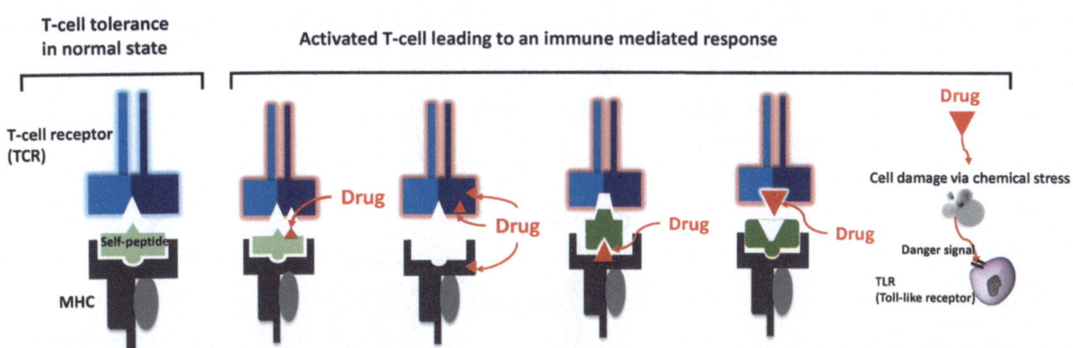

Mechanism	(a) Hapten/ pro-hapten	(b) p-i concept	(c) Altered peptide repertoire	(d) Altered TCR repertoire	(e) danger hypothesis
Site of drug complex formation	Intracellular/ Cell surface	Cell surface	Intracellular	Cell surface	NA
Mechanism	Drug attaches to an inert peptide turning it neo-antigen	Drug directly interacts with TCR or MHC independent of the immune repertoire	Drug changes the peptide repertoire enabling it to present self-peptides	Interaction with the drug changes the TCR allowing it react to self antigens	Drug causes cell damage by provoking a chemical stress. Stress related molecules activate the TLRs.

Fig. 1 An overview of the five models explaining drug-mediated immune responses

alarm signals, such as TNF-α, CD40L, IFN-α, and IL-1β, which are able to produce an immune response by activating Toll-like receptors (TLRs) (Pradeu and Cooper 2012). After epidemiologic studies found an association between viral infections and ADRs, investigations on the immunopathogenic role of these pathogens in the development of ADRs began. First proposed by White et al., the heterologous immunity model proposed a cross-reaction between drug-altered self-peptides and memory T-cells that had been formed earlier in life by exposure to prevalent viral pathogens (particularly HHV) as the initiator of an inappropriate immune response (White et al. 2015b). Based on this model, the location of pre-existing memory T-cells defines the tissues involved after drug exposure. Memory T-cells have been divided into three categories: (1) Central memory T-cells (TCM): These cells, which move freely through lymph nodes, express the following molecules: CD45RO, L-selectin, and CCR7; (2) Effector memory T-cells (TEM): These cells that are present in tissues and the peripheral circulation only express CD45R0; (3) Tissue-resident memory T-cells (TRM): These cells express CD69, CD103, and CD45RO and are restricted to the tissues. Herpes simplex virus (HSV) could repeatedly trigger the TRM T-cells residing within the mucocutaneous tissue, thus potentially explaining the limited skin and mucosal involvement of drug reactions (e.g., SJS/TEN) in individuals with HLA-B*15:02 using carbamazepine. In contrast, systemic viruses such as cytomegalovirus (CMV) and Ebstein-Barr virus (EBV) trigger the TEM T-cells and could thus explain the multiorgan features of abacavir hypersensitivity syndrome (Pavlos et al. 2014; White et al. 2015a).

The integration of the heterologous immunity model with the aforementioned immunologic concepts may be able to provide a more detailed explanation of the ADR pathogenesis (Fig. 2) (Duong et al. 2017). However, this model should not be confused with virus reactivation in the setting of ADR that commonly occurs with human herpes virus-6 (HHV-6) in the setting of DRESS syndrome (Adler et al. 2017).

Polymorphisms in genes encoding drug-metabolizing enzymes, MHC genes, and other immune-related genes could have a determining effect on ADRs' mechanisms.

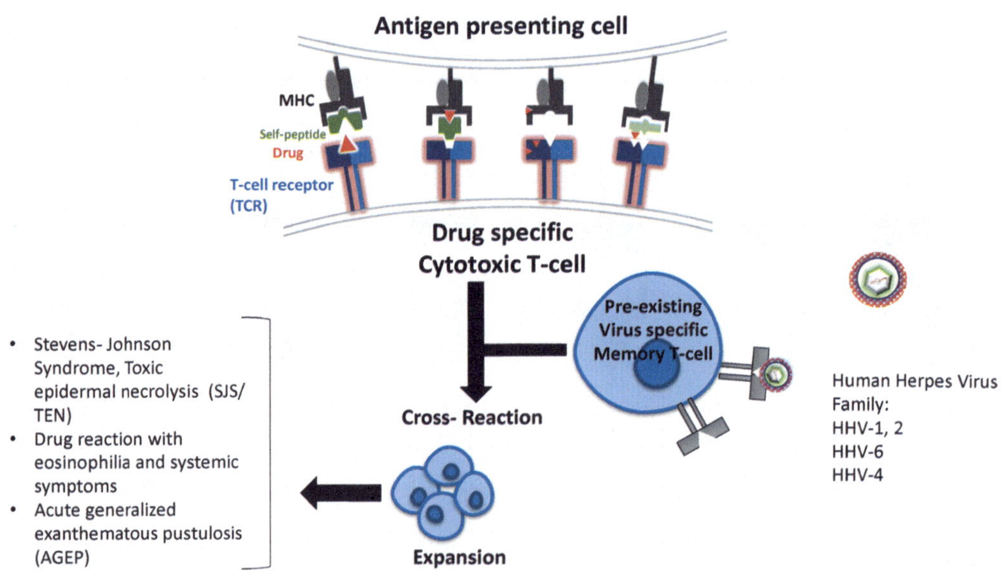

Fig. 2 A schematic diagram of the heterologous immunity model. This model explains the association between viral infections and cutaneous adverse drug reactions

3 HLA Alleles and Cutaneous Adverse Drug Reactions

In 1987, HLA alleles were reported to be associated with cADRs for the first time (Roujeau et al. 1987). To date, abacavir, carbamazepine, and allopurinol have been found to have the strongest HLA associations for developing ADR. Table 1 provides further details on the HLA alleles associated with cutaneous ADRs.

4 Non-HLA Alleles and Cutaneous Adverse Drug Reactions

In addition to HLA alleles, other genes can impact drug-induced adverse events. Such findings make it evident that several other factors are involved in the etiology of ADRs that can be used to form a panel of markers for the prediction of what was previously thought of as "unpredictable" reactions. These genes may be involved in cytokine signaling (*TGFB1*, *IFNGR1*, *IL18*, *IL4R*, *IL4*, *TNF IL13*, *NOD2*, and *IL10*), production and release of newly created mediators (*LTC4S*, *TBXA2R*, *PTGER4*, *ALOX5*, *ALOX5AP*, *TBXAS1*, *PTGDR*, and *CYSLTR1*), or production and release of pre-formed mediators (*HNMT*, *LGALS3*, *FCER1A*, *FCER1G*, and *MS4A2*). Table 2 presents the most recent associations found between non-HLA immune-related genes and cutaneous ADRs.

5 Databases with HLA Alleles and Adverse Drug Reactions

Currently, two databases have been designed to facilitate the data gathering of studies on HLA-ADR associations (Du et al. 2015; Ghattaoraya et al. 2016). The HLA and Adverse Drug Reaction Database, which is available at http://www.allelefrequencies.net/hla-adr/, is a part of the Allele Frequencies Net Database (AFND). This open database lists known adverse drug reactions with HLA alleles and covers the information of approximately 48 drugs and 318 HLA alleles in various populations. Also, this centralized resource presents information on ethnicity, the disease of interest, and the proportion of cases and controls with the HLA allele involved in developing ADRs. The second database is named the Human Leukocyte Antigen-Adverse Drug Reaction (HLADR) database and is available at http://pgx.fudan.edu.cn/hladr/. It is an open and freely accessible database that currently consists of more than 50 FDA-approved drugs and 450 HLA alleles. Each study report provides useful information including ADRs, drugs, HLA alleles, the ethnic and geographic origins of the study population, a 2×2 contingency table showing the performance metrics (odds ratio, p-value, positive predictive value (PPV), negative predictive value (NPV), sensitivity, and specificity), and FDA drug label changes that are the result of the respective HLA-drug associations.

6 Specific Drugs and cADRs

6.1 Abacavir

Abacavir is a nucleoside (guanosine analog) reverse transcriptase inhibitor (NRTI) that is used as an antiretroviral medication for HIV treatment in combination with other drugs. Based on the literature, five percent of patients receiving this drug develop hypersensitivity reactions (Hetherington et al. 2001; Martin and Kroetz 2013). The clinical features of AHS differ from that of DRESS; its onset is more rapid and it lacks an association with eosinophilia and organ involvement. This syndrome features at least two of these symptoms: fever, lethargy, malaise, rash, headache, myalgia, arthralgia, respiratory symptoms (dyspnea and cough), and gastrointestinal symptoms (abdominal pain, nausea, and vomiting). These symptoms are most likely observed within six weeks after administration of the drug; nevertheless, immunologically confirmed or patch test positive AHS usually appears 1.5 days to three weeks after the introduction of the culprit drug (Hetherington et al. 2001; Redwood et al. 2018). Once these clinical symptoms are present,

Table 1 Key HLA-associated cutaneous adverse drug reactions

Drug	*HLA*	ADR	Ethnicity	Reference
Abacavir	*B*57:01*	AHS	Caucasian/Afro-American/Thai/Hispanic/European	(Hetherington et al. 2002; Mallal et al. 2002, 2008b; Saag et al. 2008)
Allopurinol	*B*58:01*	SJS/TEN/DIHS/MPE/DISI	Korean/Han Chinese/Thai/Caucasian/Japanese/European	(Gonçalo et al. 2013; Hung et al. 2005; Kang et al. 2011; Kaniwa et al. 2008; Lonjou et al. 2008; Tassaneeyakul et al. 2009)
	*C*03:02*	SJS/TEN/DIHS	Korean/Han Chinese/Caucasian	(Cristallo et al. 2011; Hung et al. 2005; Kang et al. 2011)
	*A*33:03*	SJS/TEN/DIHS/DISI	Korean/Han Chinese/Caucasian	(Cristallo et al. 2011; Hung et al. 2005; Kang et al. 2011)
	*DRB1*03:01*	SJS/TEN/DIHS	Han Chinese	(Negrini and Becquemont 2017)
Antituberculosis drugs (Isoniazid, Rifampin, Ethambutol, and Pyrazinamide)	*C*04:01*	HHS	Korean	(Kim et al. 2013)
	*A*11:01*	HHS	Korean	(Kim et al. 2013)
	*B*15:01*	HHS	Korean	(Kim et al. 2013)
Aspirin	*DPB1*03:01*	AIU	Korean	(Kim et al. 2006)
	*DQB1*06:09*	AIU	Korean	(Kim et al. 2005)
	*DRB1*13:02*	AIU	Korean	(Kim et al. 2005)
Carbamazepine	*A*31:01*	SJS/TEN/DIHS/MPE	Japanese/Han Chinese/European/Caucasian/Korean/Norwegian	(Hung et al. 2006; McCormack et al. 2011; Ozeki et al. 2011)
	*B*15:02*	SJS/TEN/MPE	Indian/Thai/Han Chinese/Malay	(Chung et al. 2004; Locharernkul et al. 2008a; Mehta et al. 2009; Tassaneeyakul et al. 2010; Then et al. 2011)
	*B*15:11*	SJS/TEN	Japanese/Han Chinese/Korean	(Kaniwa et al. 2010; Kim et al. 2011)
	*B*51:01*	SJS/TEN/DIHS/MPE	Japanese/Han Chinese	(Hsiao et al. 2014; Niihara et al. 2012)
	*A*02:01*	MPE/DIHS	Han Chinese	(Li et al. 2013)

(continued)

Table 1 (continued)

Drug	*HLA*	ADR	Ethnicity	Reference
Oxcarbazepine	*B*38:02*	MPE	Han Chinese	(Lv et al. 2013)
	*B*15:02*	MPE/SJS	Han Chinese/Thai	(Chen et al. 2017; Chu et al. 2011; Hung et al. 2010)
	*B*27:04*	MPE	Han Chinese	(He et al. 2012)
	*B*13:02*	MPE	Han Chinese	(He et al. 2012)
Dapsone	*B*13:01*	HHS	Han Chinese	(Wang et al. 2013; Zhang et al. 2013)
	*C*03:04*	HHS	Han Chinese	(Zhang et al. 2013)
Lamotrigine	*A*30:01*	MPE	Han Chinese	(Li et al. 2013)
	*A*24:01*	MPE/non-bullous cADRs	Korean/Norwegian	(Moon et al. 2015; Shirzadi et al. 2015)
	*B*15:19*	MPE	Han Chinese	(Shi et al. 2011)
	*B*15:02*	SJS/TEN	Han Chinese	(Negrini and Becquemont 2017)
	*B*38:01*	SJS/TEN	Europeans	(Lonjou et al. 2008)
Nevirapine	*B *35:01*	DIHS	Asian	(Keane et al. 2014)
	*DRB1*01:01*	Skin rash	Caucasian	(Martin et al. 2005; Vitezica et al. 2008)
	*B*35:05*	MPE/DRESS	Thai	(Chantarangsu et al. 2009)
	*Cw*08*	DIHS/Skin rash	Japanese/Italian	(Gatanaga et al. 2007; Littera et al. 2006)
	*C*04:01*	SJS/TEN	Black/Malawian	(Carr et al. 2013)
	*DRB1*01:02*	DIHS	Caucasian	(Littera et al. 2006)
NSAIDs	*A*02:06*	SJS/TEN	Korean/Japanese	(Ueta et al. 2014a, 2014b)
	*DRB1*11*	Anaphylactoid reaction	European	(Quiralte et al. 1999)
	*B*44:03*	SJS/TEN	Japanese/Indian/Brazilian	(Oussalah et al. 2016; Ueta et al. 2014a, 2014b)

(continued)

Table 1 (continued)

Drug	*HLA*	ADR	Ethnicity	Reference
Phenytoin	*B*13:01*	SJS/TEN	Han Chinese	(Yampayon et al. 2017)
	*B*15:02*	SJS/TEN	Han Chinese/Thai/Malay	(Chang et al. 2016; Cheung et al. 2013; Chung W–H, Chang W–C, Lee Y-S, Wu Y-Y, Yang C-H, Ho H-C, Chen M-J, Lin J-Y, Hui RC-Y, Ho J-C, Wu W-M, Chen T-J, Wu T, Wu Y-R, Hsih M-S, Tu P–H, Chang C-N, Hsu C-N, Wu T-L, Choon S-E, Hsu C-K, Chen D-Y, Liu C-S, Lin C-Y, Kaniwa N, Saito Y, Takahashi Y, Nakamura R, Azukizawa H, Shi Y, Wang T-H, Chuang S–S, Tsai S-F, Chang C-J, Chang Y-S, Hung S-I, Consortium ftTSCAR, Consortium tJPDS 2014; Hung et al. 2010; Locharernkul et al. 2008a; Man et al. 2007)
	*C*08:01*	SJS/TEN/MPE	Han Chinese/Mexican mestizos	(Fricke-Galindo et al. 2014; Hung et al. 2010)
	*B*15:13*	SJS/TEN/DIHS	Malay	(Chang et al. 2016)
Phenobarbital	*B*13:01*	SJS/TEN/DRESS/rash	Thai	(Manuyakorn et al. 2016)
	*B*51:01*	SJS/TEN	Japanese	(Kaniwa et al. 2013)
	*A*01:01*	SJS/TEN/DRESS/rash	Thai	(Manuyakorn et al. 2016)
Sulfamethoxazole	*C*08:01*	SJS/TEN	Thai	(Kongpan et al. 2015)
	*C*06:02*	SJS/TEN	Thai	(Kongpan et al. 2015)
	*B*15:02*	SJS/TEN	Thai	(Kongpan et al. 2015)
	*B*38*	SJS/TEN	European	(Lonjou et al. 2008)
	*A*30*	FDE	Turkish	(Ozkaya-Bayazit and Akar 2001)
Sulfonamides	*A*29*	SJS/TEN	N/A	(Roujeau et al. 1987)
	*B*12*	SJS/TEN	N/A	(Roujeau et al. 1987)
	*DR*7*	SJS/TEN	N/A	(Roujeau et al. 1987)

(continued)

Table 1 (continued)

Drug	*HLA*	ADR	Ethnicity	Reference
Sulfasalazine	*B*13:01*	DIHS	Han Chinese	(Yang et al. 2014)
	*B*15:05*	DIHS	Han Chinese	(Yang et al. 2014)
	*B*58:01*	DIHS	Han Chinese	(Yang et al. 2014)
	*B*07:02*	DIHS	Han Chinese	(Yang et al. 2014)
	*B*39:01*	DIHS	Han Chinese	(Yang et al. 2014)
Feprazone	*B*22*	FDE	Scandinavian	(Pellicano et al. 1997)
Methazolamide	*B*59:01*	SJS/TEN	Korean/Chinese	(Kim et al. 2010; Yang et al. 2016)
	*C*01:02*	SJS/TEN	Korean/Chinese	(Kim et al. 2010; Yang et al. 2016)
Oxicam	*B*73:01*	SJS/TEN	European	(Lonjou et al. 2008)
Vancomycin	*A*32:01*	DRESS	European	(Konvinse et al. 2019)
Acetaminophen	*DQB1*02:02*	SJS/TEN	Caucasian	(Negrini and Becquemont 2017)
Acetazolamide	*B*59:01*	SJS/TEN	Korean	(Her et al. 2011; Park et al. 2015)
Clindamycin	*B*51:01*	Not Specified	Han Chinese	(Yang et al. 2017)
	*B*15:27*	Not Specified	Han Chinese	(Yang et al. 2017)
Trichloroethylene	*B*13:01*	Dermatitis	Chinese	(Negrini and Becquemont 2017)
Zonisamide	*A*02:07*	SJS/TEN	Japanese	(Kaniwa et al. 2013)
β-lactam penicillins	*A*2 and DRw52*	MPE	Not Specified	(Romano et al. 1998)
	DRB9	Urticaria	Han Chinese	(Yang et al. 2006)

HLA, human leukocyte antigen; ADR, adverse drug reaction; AHS, abacavir hypersensitivity syndrome; SJS, Stevens-Johnson syndrome; TEN, toxic epidermal necrolysis; DIHS, drug-induced hypersensitivity syndrome; MPE, maculopapular exanthema; DISI, drug-induced skin reaction; AIU, aspirin-induced urticaria; AGEP, acute generalized exanthematous pustulosis; FDE, fixed-drug eruption; HSS, hypersensitivity syndrome; NSAIDs, nonsteroidal anti-inflammatory drugs; N/A, not available

Table 2 Key Non-HLA-associations of cutaneous adverse drug reactions

Drug	Gene	ADR	Ethnicity	Reference
Penicillin	*IL-4Ralpha Q576R, IL-4Ralpha I75V, STAT6 in 2SNP3, IL-10 promoter, E237G variant of the FcεRIβ gene, LGALS3, IL4, IL13, TNF, IFNGR1, IL18, NOD2*	Urticaria/Anaphylactic shock/Immediate allergic reactions	Chinese/Not Specified	(Guglielmi et al. 2006; Huang et al. 2009, 2012; Oussalah et al. 2016; Qiao et al. 2004, 2005)
NSAIDs	*ALOX5, ALOX5AP, ALOX15, TBXAS1, PTGDR, CYSLTR1, LTC4S, FCERIA, TGFB1, TNFA, HNMT, IL18, CEP68, PTGER4*	Urticaria	Korean/Not Specified	(Choi et al. 2009; Kim et al. 2006; Oussalah et al. 2016; Park et al. 2008)
Aspirin	*LTC4S, TBXA2R, PTGER4, FCER1A, MS4A2, FCER1G, HNMT, TGFB1, TNF, IL18*	Non-specific reactions	Not Specified	(Bae et al. 2007; Oussalah et al. 2016)
Carbamazepine	*TNF2*	Hypersensitivity reactions	White	(Pirmohamed et al. 2001)
Allopurinol	*rs2734583 in BAT1, rs3094011 in HCP5 and GA005234 in MICC*	SJS/TEN	Japanese	(Tohkin et al. 2013)
Abacavir	*rs2395029 in HCP5*	AHS	European	(Colombo et al. 2008)
N/A	*IL1-beta-511C > T, IL1-RN (intron2-VNTR) and IL10-592C > A*	DRESS	Not Specified	(Barbaud et al. 2014)
NMBAs	*MRGPRX2*	Anaphylactoid reactions	Not Specified	(McNeil et al. 2014; Navines-Ferrer et al. 2018)
N/A	*TLR3, IL4R*	SJS/TEN (with ocular manifestations)	Japanese	(Ueta et al. 2007a, 2007b)

ADR, adverse drug reaction; NSAIDs, nonsteroidal anti-inflammatory drugs; NMBAs, neuromuscular blocking agents; AHS,abacavir hypersensitivity syndrome; SJS, Stevens-Johnson syndrome; TEN, toxic epidermal necrolysis; DRESS, drug reactionwith eosinophilia and systemic symptoms

it is mandatory to discontinue the drug immediately. It is important to note that rechallenge can be fatal because symptoms can reappear within hours. The first evidence of a robust association between the occurrence of AHS and carrying an HLA class I allele, specifically *HLA-B*57:01*, was initially described in 2002 (Hetherington et al. 2002; Mallal et al. 2002). Other studies also demonstrated similar results leading to the final confirmation of this association in 2008 by the PREDICT-1 trial (Hughes et al. 2008). This study revealed that screening for the presence of the *HLA-B*57:01* genotype could help in preventing the occurrence of abacavir-related hypersensitivity reactions in patients (Mallal et al. 2008b). In the same year, a case–control study, namely the SHAPE study, also demonstrated a 100% NPV of *HLA-B*57:01* testing for abacavir hypersensitivity among different ethnicities, further generalizing the findings of the PREDICT-1 study (Saag et al. 2008). The PPV of *HLA-B*57:01* genetic screening is nearly 50%, indicating that although this allele should be present to trigger AHS, it is not sufficient because this reaction does not occur in all those who carry *HLA-B*57:01*.

6.2 Carbamazepine

Carbamazepine is an aromatic antiepileptic drug (AED) mainly used to treat epilepsy, trigeminal neuralgia, bipolar disorder, and carpal tunnel syndrome (CTS) (Barbarino et al. 2015). It has an association with various cADRs including DIHS, MPE, rarely SJS/TEN, and APEG. Except for AGEP, which occurs relatively early, other cADRs usually occur within two to eight weeks after drug initiation (Amstutz et al. 2014). It is estimated that approximately ten percent of patients develop such reactions after exposure to carbamazepine (Simper et al. 2018). In 2004, an investigation among the Han-Chinese population showed that a strong relationship exists between *HLA-B*15:02* and carbamazepine-induced SJS (Chung et al. 2004). Several other studies noted this association among Thai, Malay, Korean, Indian, and Vietnamese populations. These results eventually led to the recommendation of genetic screening for *HLA-B*15:02* before treatment initiation as it is not as expensive as treating patients with carbamazepine-induced SJS (Chen et al. 2011; Chung et al. 2004; Locharernkul et al. 2008a, 2011; Mehta et al. 2009; Tassaneeyakul et al. 2010; Then et al. 2011). Other HLA genotypes have also demonstrated a robust association with carbamazepine-induced cADRs, including *HLA-A*31:01* and *HLA-B75* family members (*HLA-B*15:11, HLA-B*15:21*, and *HLA-B*15:08*), especially among Han-Chinese, Japanese and European populations (Ikeda et al. 2010; Jaruthamsophon et al. 2017; Kaniwa et al. 2010). Conversely, some alleles (*HLA-A*24:02* and *HLA-B*40:01*) are assumed to offer protection against carbamazepine-induced cADRs (Grover and Kukreti 2014; Hsiao et al. 2014). Furthermore, a number of studies have proposed that the development of carbamazepine-related ADR is dependent on both specific HLA alleles and TCR clonotypes (Ko and Chen 2012; Ko et al. 2011; Wei et al. 2012).

6.3 Allopurinol

Allopurinol is a xanthine oxidase inhibitor commonly prescribed for gout, uric acid kidney stones, and tumor lysis syndrome-related hyperuricemia. Many studies have stated that a relationship exists between *HLA-B*58:01* and allopurinol-related cADRs (e.g., SJS/TEN, DIHS, and MPE) in different ethnicities (Cao et al. 2012; Hung et al. 2005; Kaniwa et al. 2008; Lonjou et al. 2008; Tassaneeyakul et al. 2009; Tohkin et al. 2013). These reactions are speculated to occur in 0.1–0.4% of exposed patients (Hershfield et al. 2013; Ramasamy et al. 2013). Studies have shown that both allopurinol and oxypurinol, its main metabolite, could reactivate CD8 + T-cells (Yun et al. 2014). Since the PPV of possessing *HLA-B*58:01* is relatively low, one can assume that other factors, including renal insufficiency, higher plasma levels of oxypurinol, and other risk alleles (*HLA-DRB1*03:01, HLA-A*33:03*, and *HLA-C*03:02*), also may contribute to the pathogenesis of allopurinol-related cADRs (Kang et al. 2011). However, the NPV is 100% among Asians (Phillips and Mallal 2010; Tassaneeyakul et al. 2009). Unlike other drug-associated IM-ADRs, allopurinol reacts in a dose-dependent manner, with higher initial doses resulting in a higher risk of cADRs (Sousa-Pinto et al. 2016). Chung et al. have suggested that as well as *HLA-B*58:01*, clonotype-specific T-cells play a role in the development of cADRs induced by allopurinol as demonstrated by the higher expression of granulysin after oxypurinol induction (Chung et al. 2015).

6.4 Nevirapine

Nevirapine is an oral non-nucleoside reverse transcriptase inhibitor (NNRTI) that is part of the antiretroviral therapy for HIV. It is thought that about five to ten percent of patients who use nevirapine develop a cADR a few weeks after initiating treatment (Carr et al. 2017; Cornejo Castro et al. 2015; Keane et al. 2014; Shubber et al. 2013; Wit et al. 2008). The first study to show a relationship between *HLA-DRB1*01:01* carriage and DRESS was performed among Western Australian (Caucasian) patients in 2005. In this study, multisystem hypersensitivity reactions were seen in patients with a CD4 percentage of more than 25%, implying that lower CD4 counts abolished nevirapine-related ADRs involving multiple organs. In contrast, patients with lower CD4 + T-cell percentages developed isolated rash (Martin et al. 2005). The results of this study suggested that nevirapine-specific immune reactions might be dependent on the proportion of available CD4 + T-cells; however, later studies have shown the association of nevirapine-related ADRs with MHC class I alleles, namely *HLA-C*08*, *HLA-B*35*, and *HLA-C*04* (Chantarangsu et al. 2009; Cornejo Castro et al. 2015; Dickinson et al. 2014; Gatanaga et al. 2007; Phillips et al. 2010).

6.5 Monoclonal Antibodies

Although no associations between ADRs induced by checkpoint inhibitors and certain HLA alleles have been reported so far, the increasing evidence of immune-related adverse reactions with these drugs supports the need for further research in this field (Camacho 2015; Sibaud et al. 2016).

7 HLA Genotyping Before Drug Prescription

The high impact of ADRs on mortality, morbidity, and disease burden provides a strong rationale for the establishment of pharmacogenetic and immunologic tests that have the potential to distinguish individuals at high risk of developing IM-ADRs before treatment initiation. It has been approximated that pharmacogenetic testing could prevent 20–30% of ADRs (Ingelman-Sundberg 2001); thus, this field proves to be a translational research priority aimed at preventing the onset of drug-related reactions. However, the implementation of these interventions should be strongly supported by scientific evidence. The main attributes in the decision to use these screening tests in routine clinical practice are as follows: the negative predictive value (preferably 100%), the respective frequency of the IM-ADR, and the risk allele in the intended population, the number needed to test (preferably low), the scarcity of safe and effective alternative therapies, the cost-effectiveness of the test, and the economic burden of the disease.

After the results of the PREDICT-1 trial and the SHAPE study were published in 2008, the US Food and Drug Administration (FDA), the European Medicines Agency (EMA), the US Department of Health and Human Services (HHS), the Clinical Pharmacogenetics Implementation Consortium (CPIC), and several international HIV organizations recommended the mandatory *HLA-B*57:01* genetic testing prior to abacavir treatment in patients of all ethnicities. Initial studies aimed at reducing AHS via a *HLA-B*57:01* genetic screening test before abacavir initiation have shown promising results (Aberg et al. 2014; Churchill et al. 2016; Phillips and Mallal 2009; Rauch et al. 2006; Yip et al. 2015; Zucman et al. 2007). As for carbamazepine, Taiwan FDA as well as the US FDA have stated that *HLA-B*15:02* screening genetic tests should be carried out before starting therapy in patients with origins from populations that *HLA-B*15:02* might be present. The US FDA has also recommended avoiding carbamazepine therapy in all patients of any ethnic group who carry *HLA-B*15:02*, except only when the therapeutics benefits of using carbamazepine are greater than the risk of developing ADR (Ferrell and McLeod 2008). Other organizations such as the EMA, Hong Kong Department of Health, and the Singapore Ministry of Health also have restricted pre-treatment *HLA-B*15:02* genotyping for carbamazepine only to patients with a specific Asian ancestry. Based on CPIC's recommendation, for those of any age or ancestry who have at least one copy of the *HLA-B*15:02* allele, an alternative medication should be used based on the underlying disease. However, if the benefits of employing treatment far outweigh the risks, this recommendation can be disregarded (Leckband et al. 2013). The US FDA and EMA currently do not recommend pre-treatment genotyping for the *HLA-A*31:01* allele in patients planning to initiate carbamazepine (Phillips et al. 2018). Additionally, with regards to alternative antiepileptic therapy, the FDA and CPIC recommend avoiding phenytoin, and, in certain circumstances, lamotrigine, eslicarbazepine acetate, and oxcarbazepine in patients carrying *HLA-B*15:02* (Caudle et al. 2014). Since allopurinol's main use is for rheumatologic diseases, the American College of Rheumatology has recommended *HLA-B*58:01* genotyping prior to using allopurinol for the first time in patients with advanced renal failure and those with specific Asian ancestry (Ke et al. 2017).

8 Future Directions

The discovery of HLA-drug associations resulted in the consideration that certain allergy reactions are actually preventable, some of which were previously thought to be unpredictable.

Despite recent breakthroughs in developing clinically useful preemptive genotyping tests, the process of drug hypersensitivity remains elusive. Although HLA alleles are shown to play an imperative part in ADRs' development, the contribution of other factors such as epigenetic changes and microRNAs in predisposing individuals to hypersensitivity reactions to drugs remains unknown. The majority of the HLA-risk alleles that have an association with specific ADRs are reported to have a low PPV (<10%). The low PPV indicates that other factors in addition to or other than the MHC result in the occurrence of an IM-ADR. Some of these factors that have been partly studied are the effects of abnormal hepatic and/or renal function and polymorphisms in genes responsible for cytokine production or the regulation of drug transport and metabolism. Elucidation of additional patient-specific variables can introduce new horizons in the immunopathogenic mechanisms of IM-ADRs.

As discussed earlier, a number of investigations have concluded that HLA testing before drug prescription is cost-effective; nevertheless, others have suggested HLA genotyping to be performed after the initiation of certain vital drugs, such as vancomycin. Vancomycin is prescribed for patients with life-threatening infections along with other antibiotics, such as β-lactams or fluoroquinolone, as an empirical regimen. Konvinse et al. have suggested the use of HLA typing, *HLA-A* 32:01* in this particular instance, after vancomycin has been started and the results of bacterial cultures are at hand. Delayed testing could also benefit patients who are candidates for longer or multiple treatment courses since most cADRs occur two weeks after the initiation of the drug (Konvinse et al. 2019). In fact, pre-treatment genotyping may lead to restrictions in current and future antibiotic choices. This can eventually result in the employment of excessively broad-spectrum or inferior antibiotics, which can jeopardize safety at the patient and public level.

Moreover, since a significant percentage of the respective studies were conducted in Asian countries, additional HLA alleles may be in association with ADRs among other ethnic populations that have not been investigated so far. Also, immunogenetic associations with ADRs are still undiscovered for many commonly used drugs. Therefore, further pharmacogenomic research on this topic should be pursued.

References

Aberg JA, Gallant JE, Ghanem KG, Emmanuel P, Zingman BS, Horberg MA (2014) Primary care guidelines for the management of persons infected with HIV: 2013 update by the HIV medicine association of the infectious diseases society of America. Clin Infect Dis 58:e1-34

Adler N, Aung A, Ergen E, Trubiano J, Goh M, Phillips E (2017) Recent advances in the understanding of severe cutaneous adverse reactions. Br J Dermatol 177:1234–1247

Amstutz U, Shear NH, Rieder MJ, Hwang S, Fung V, Nakamura H, Connolly MB, Ito S, Carleton BC (2014) Recommendations for HLA-B*15:02 and HLA-A*31:01 genetic testing to reduce the risk of carbamazepine-induced hypersensitivity reactions. Epilepsia 55:496–506

Bae JS, Kim SH, Ye YM, Yoon HJ, Suh CH, Nahm DH, Park HS (2007) Significant association of FcepsilonRIalpha promoter polymorphisms with aspirin-intolerant chronic urticaria. J Allergy Clin Immunol 119:449–456

Barbarino JM, Kroetz DL, Klein TE, Altman RB (2015) PharmGKB summary: very important pharmacogene information for human leukocyte antigen B. Pharmacogenet Genom 25:205–221

Barbaud A, Waton J, Herbeth B, Bursztejn AC, Bollaert M, Schmutz JL, Gueant-Rodriguez RM, Namour F, Gueant JL, Aimone-Gastin I (2014) Comparison of cytokine gene polymorphism in drug-induced maculopapular eruption, urticaria and drug reaction with eosinophilia and systemic symptoms (DRESS). J Eur Acad Dermatol Venereol 28:491–499

Beijer HJ, de Blaey CJ (2002) Hospitalisations caused by adverse drug reactions (ADR): a meta-analysis of observational studies. Pharm World Sci 24:46–54

Böhm R, Cascorbi I (2016) Pharmacogenetics and predictive testing of drug hypersensitivity reactions. Front Pharmacol 7:396–396

Camacho LH (2015) CTLA-4 blockade with ipilimumab: biology, safety, efficacy, and future considerations. Cancer Med 4:661–672

Cao ZH, Wei ZY, Zhu QY, Zhang JY, Yang L, Qin SY, Shao LY, Zhang YT, Xuan JK, Li QL, Xu JH, Xu F, Ma L, Huang HY, Xing QH, Luo XQ (2012) HLA-B*58:01 allele is associated with augmented risk for both mild and severe cutaneous adverse reactions induced by allopurinol in Han Chinese. Pharmacogenomics 13:1193–1201

Carr DF, Bourgeois S, Chaponda M, Takeshita LY, Morris AP, Castro EM, Alfirevic A, Jones AR, Rigden DJ, Haldenby S, Khoo S, Lalloo DG, Heyderman RS, Dandara C, Kampira E, van Oosterhout JJ, Ssali F, Munderi P, Novelli G, Borgiani P, Nelson MR, Holden A, Deloukas P, Pirmohamed M (2017) Genome-wide association study of nevirapine hypersensitivity in a sub-Saharan African HIV-infected population. J Antimicrob Chemother 72:1152–1162

Carr DF, Chaponda M, Jorgensen AL, Castro EC, van Oosterhout JJ, Khoo SH, Lalloo DG, Heyderman RS, Alfirevic A, Pirmohamed M (2013) Association of human leukocyte antigen alleles and nevirapine hypersensitivity in a Malawian HIV-infected population. Clin Infect Dis 56:1330–1339

Carr DF, Pirmohamed M (2018) Biomarkers of adverse drug reactions. Exp Biol Med (Maywood) 243:291–299

Caudle KE, Rettie AE, Whirl-Carrillo M, Smith LH, Mintzer S, Lee MT, Klein TE, Callaghan JT (2014) Clinical pharmacogenetics implementation consortium guidelines for CYP2C9 and HLA-B genotypes and phenytoin dosing. Clin Pharmacol Ther 96:542–548

Chang CC, Ng CC, Too CL, Choon SE, Lee CK, Chung WH, Hussein SH, Lim KS, Murad S (2016) Association of HLA-B*15:13 and HLA-B*15:02 with phenytoin-induced severe cutaneous adverse reactions in a Malay population. Pharmacogen J 17:170

Chantarangsu S, Mushiroda T, Mahasirimongkol S, Kiertiburanakul S, Sungkanuparph S, Manosuthi W, Tantisiriwat W, Charoenyingwattana A, Sura T, Chantratita W, Nakamura Y (2009) HLA-B*3505 allele is a strong predictor for nevirapine-induced skin adverse drug reactions in HIV-infected Thai patients. Pharmacogenet Genom 19:139–146

Chen CB, Hsiao YH, Wu T, Hsih MS, Tassaneeyakul W, Jorns TP, Sukasem C, Hsu CN, Su SC, Chang WC, Hui RC, Chu CY, Chen YJ, Wu CY, Hsu CK, Chiu TM, Sun PL, Lee HE, Yang CY, Kao PH, Yang CH, Ho HC, Lin JY, Chang YC, Chen MJ, Lu CW, Ng CY, Kuo KL, Lin CY, Yang CS, Chen DP, Chang PY, Wu TL, Lin YJ, Weng YC, Kuo TT, Hung SI, Chung WH (2017) Risk and association of HLA with oxcarbazepine-induced cutaneous adverse reactions in Asians. Neurology 88:78–86

Chen P, Lin JJ, Lu CS, Ong CT, Hsieh PF, Yang CC, Tai CT, Wu SL, Lu CH, Hsu YC, Yu HY, Ro LS, Lu CT, Chu CC, Tsai JJ, Su YH, Lan SH, Sung SF, Lin SY, Chuang HP, Huang LC, Chen YJ, Tsai PJ, Liao HT, Lin YH, Chen CH, Chung WH, Hung SI, Wu JY, Chang CF, Chen L, Chen YT, Shen CY (2011) Carbamazepine-induced toxic effects and HLA-B*1502 screening in Taiwan. N Engl J Med 364:1126–1133

Cheung YK, Cheng SH, Chan EJ, Lo SV, Ng MH, Kwan P (2013) HLA-B alleles associated with severe cutaneous reactions to antiepileptic drugs in Han Chinese. Epilepsia 54:1307–1314

Choi JH, Kim SH, Cho BY, Lee SK, Kim SH, Suh CH, Park HS (2009) Association of TNF-alpha promoter polymorphisms with aspirin-induced urticaria. J Clin Pharm Ther 34:231–238

Chu M, Yang P, Hou S, Li F, Chen Y, Kijlstra A (2011) Behçet's disease exhibits an increased osteopontin serum level in active stage but no association with osteopontin and its receptor gene polymorphisms. Hum Immunol 72:525–529

Chung W-H, Chang W-C, Lee Y-S, Wu Y-Y, Yang C-H, Ho H-C, Chen M-J, Lin J-Y, Hui RC-Y, Ho J-C, Wu W-M, Chen T-J, Wu T, Wu Y-R, Hsih M-S, Tu P-H, Chang C-N, Hsu C-N, Wu T-L, Choon S-E, Hsu C-K, Chen D-Y, Liu C-S, Lin C-Y, Kaniwa N, Saito Y, Takahashi Y, Nakamura R, Azukizawa H, Shi Y, Wang T-H, Chuang S-S, Tsai S-F, Chang C-J, Chang Y-S, Hung S-I, Consortium ftTSCAR, Consortium tJPDS (2014) Genetic variants associated with phenytoin-related severe cutaneous adverse reactionsphenytoin-related severe cutaneous adverse reactionsphenytoin-related severe cutaneous adverse reactions. JAMA 312:525–534

Chung WH, Hung SI, Hong HS, Hsih MS, Yang LC, Ho HC, Wu JY, Chen YT (2004) Medical genetics: a marker for Stevens-Johnson syndrome. Nature 428:486

Chung WH, Pan RY, Chu MT, Chin SW, Huang YL, Wang WC, Chang JY, Hung SI (2015) Oxypurinol-specific T cells possess preferential TCR clonotypes and express granulysin in allopurinol-induced severe cutaneous adverse reactions. J Invest Dermatol 135:2237–2248

Churchill D, Waters L, Ahmed N, Angus B, Boffito M, Bower M, Dunn D, Edwards S, Emerson C, Fidler S, Fisher M, Horne R, Khoo S, Leen C, Mackie N, Marshall N, Monteiro F, Nelson M, Orkin C, Palfreeman A, Pett S, Phillips A, Post F, Pozniak A, Reeves I, Sabin C, Trevelion R, Walsh J, Wilkins E, Williams I, Winston A (2016) British HIV Association guidelines for the treatment of HIV-1-positive adults with antiretroviral therapy 2015. HIV Med 17:s2–s104

Colombo S, Rauch A, Rotger M, Fellay J, Martinez R, Fux C, Thurnheer C, Gunthard HF, Goldstein DB, Furrer H, Telenti A (2008) The HCP5 single-nucleotide polymorphism: a simple screening tool for prediction of hypersensitivity reaction to abacavir. J Infect Dis 198:864–867

Cornejo Castro EM, Carr DF, Jorgensen AL, Alfirevic A, Pirmohamed M (2015) HLA-allelotype associations with nevirapine-induced hypersensitivity reactions and hepatotoxicity: a systematic review of the literature and meta-analysis. Pharmacogenet Genom 25:186–198

Cristallo AF, Schroeder J, Citterio A, Santori G, Ferrioli GM, Rossi U, Bertani G, Cassano S, Gottardi P, Ceschini N, Barocci F, Ribizzi G, Cutrupi V, Cairoli R, Rapisarda V, Pastorello EA, Barocci S (2011) A study of HLA class I and class II 4-digit allele level in Stevens-Johnson syndrome and toxic epidermal necrolysis. Int J Immunogenet 38:303–309

Daly AK (2013) Pharmacogenomics of adverse drug reactions. Genome Med 5:5–5

Davies EC, Green CF, Taylor S, Williamson PR, Mottram DR, Pirmohamed M (2009) Adverse drug reactions in hospital in-patients: a prospective analysis of 3695 patient-episodes. PLoS One 4:e4439

Dickinson L, Chaponda M, Carr DF, van Oosterhout JJ, Kumwenda J, Lalloo DG, Pirmohamed M, Heyderman RS, Khoo SH (2014) Population pharmacokinetic and pharmacogenetic analysis of nevirapine in hypersensitive and tolerant HIV-infected patients from Malawi. Antimicrob Agents Chemother 58:706–712

Du T, Yang L, Luo H, Zhou P, Mei H, Xuan J, Xing Q, Ning B, Mendrick DL, Shi L (2015) HLADR: a database system for enhancing the discovery of biomarkers for predicting human leukocyte antigen-mediated idiosyncratic adverse drug reactions. Biomark Med 9:1079–1093

Duong TA, Valeyrie-Allanore L, Wolkenstein P, Chosidow O (2017) Severe cutaneous adverse reactions to drugs. The Lancet 390:1996–2011

Edwards IR, Biriell C (1994) Harmonisation in pharmacovigilance. Drug Saf 10:93–102

Ferrell PB Jr, McLeod HL (2008) Carbamazepine, HLA-B*1502 and risk of Stevens-Johnson syndrome and toxic epidermal necrolysis: US FDA recommendations. Pharmacogenomics 9:1543–1546

Fricke-Galindo I, Martinez-Juarez IE, Monroy-Jaramillo N, Jung-Cook H, Falfan-Valencia R, Ortega-Vazquez A, Alonso-Vilatela ME, Lopez-Lopez M (2014) HLA-A*02:01:01/-B*35:01:01/-C*04:01:01 haplotype associated with lamotrigine-induced maculopapular exanthema in Mexican Mestizo patients. Pharmacogenomics 15:1881–1891

Gatanaga H, Yazaki H, Tanuma J, Honda M, Genka I, Teruya K, Tachikawa N, Kikuchi Y, Oka S (2007) HLA-Cw8 primarily associated with hypersensitivity to nevirapine. AIDS 21:264–265

Ghattaoraya GS, Dundar Y, González-Galarza FF, Maia MHT, Santos EJM, da Silva ALS, McCabe A, Middleton D, Alfirevic A, Dickson R, Jones AR (2016) A web resource for mining HLA associations with adverse drug reactions: HLA-ADR. Database 2016

Giardina C, Cutroneo PM, Mocciaro E, Russo GT, Mandraffino G, Basile G, Rapisarda F, Ferrara R, Spina E, Arcoraci V (2018) Adverse drug reactions in hospitalized patients: results of the FORWARD (Facilitation of Reporting in Hospital Ward) study. Front Pharmacol 9:350

Gonçalo M, Coutinho I, Teixeira V, Gameiro AR, Brites MM, Nunes R, Martinho A (2013) HLA-B*58:01 is a risk factor for allopurinol-induced DRESS and Stevens-Johnson syndrome/toxic epidermal necrolysis in a Portuguese population. Br J Dermatol 169:660–665

Grover S, Kukreti R (2014) HLA alleles and hypersensitivity to carbamazepine: an updated systematic review with meta-analysis. Pharmacogenet Genom 24:94–112

Guglielmi L, Fontaine C, Gougat C, Avinens O, Eliaou JF, Guglielmi P, Demoly P (2006) IL-10 promoter and IL4-Ralpha gene SNPs are associated with immediate beta-lactam allergy in atopic women. Allergy 61:921–927

Hakkarainen KM, Hedna K, Petzold M, Hagg S (2012) Percentage of patients with preventable adverse drug reactions and preventability of adverse drug reactions–a meta-analysis. PLoS One 7:e33236

He N, Min FL, Shi YW, Guo J, Liu XR, Li BM, Zhou JH, Ou YM, Liao JX, Liao WP (2012) Cutaneous reactions induced by oxcarbazepine in Southern Han Chinese: incidence, features, risk factors and relation to HLA-B alleles. Seizure 21:614–618

Her Y, Kil MS, Park JH, Kim CW, Kim SS (2011) Stevens-Johnson syndrome induced by acetazolamide. J Dermatol 38:272–275

Hershfield MS, Callaghan JT, Tassaneeyakul W, Mushiroda T, Thorn CF, Klein TE, Lee MT (2013) Clinical pharmacogenetics implementation consortium guidelines for human leukocyte antigen-B genotype and allopurinol dosing. Clin Pharmacol Ther 93:153–158

Hetherington S, Hughes AR, Mosteller M, Shortino D, Baker KL, Spreen W, Lai E, Davies K, Handley A, Dow DJ, Fling ME, Stocum M, Bowman C, Thurmond LM, Roses AD (2002) Genetic variations in

HLA-B region and hypersensitivity reactions to abacavir. Lancet 359:1121–1122

Hetherington S, McGuirk S, Powell G, Cutrell A, Naderer O, Spreen B, Lafon S, Pearce G, Steel H (2001) Hypersensitivity reactions during therapy with the nucleoside reverse transcriptase inhibitor abacavir. Clin Ther 23:1603–1614

Hsiao YH, Hui RC, Wu T, Chang WC, Hsih MS, Yang CH, Ho HC, Chang YG, Chen MJ, Lin JY, Chen DP, Chang PY, Wu TL, Hung SI, Chung WH (2014) Genotype-phenotype association between HLA and carbamazepine-induced hypersensitivity reactions: strength and clinical correlations. J Dermatol Sci 73:101–109

Huang CZ, Yang J, Qiao HL, Jia LJ (2009) Polymorphisms and haplotype analysis of IL-4Ralpha Q576R and I75V in patients with penicillin allergy. Eur J Clin Pharmacol 65:895–902

Huang CZ, Zou D, Yang J, Qiao HL (2012) Polymorphisms of STAT6 and specific serum IgE levels in patients with penicillin allergy. Int J Clin Pharmacol Ther 50:461–467

Hughes S, Hughes A, Brothers C, Spreen W, Thorborn D (2008) PREDICT-1 (CNA106030): the first powered, prospective trial of pharmacogenetic screening to reduce drug adverse events. Pharm Stat J Appl Stat Pharm Ind 7:121–129

Hung S-I, Chung W-H, Liou L-B, Chu C-C, Lin M, Huang H-P, Lin Y-L, Lan J-L, Yang L-C, Hong H-S, Chen M-J, Lai P-C, Wu M-S, Chu C-Y, Wang K-H, Chen C-H, Fann CSJ, Wu J-Y, Chen Y-T (2005) HLA-B*5801 allele as a genetic marker for severe cutaneous adverse reactions caused by allopurinol. Proc Natl Acad Sci USA 102:4134–4139

Hung SI, Chung WH, Jee SH, Chen WC, Chang YT, Lee WR, Hu SL, Wu MT, Chen GS, Wong TW, Hsiao PF, Chen WH, Shih HY, Fang WH, Wei CY, Lou YH, Huang YL, Lin JJ, Chen YT (2006) Genetic susceptibility to carbamazepine-induced cutaneous adverse drug reactions. Pharmacogenet Genom 16:297–306

Hung SI, Chung WH, Liu ZS, Chen CH, Hsih MS, Hui RC, Chu CY, Chen YT (2010) Common risk allele in aromatic antiepileptic-drug induced Stevens-Johnson syndrome and toxic epidermal necrolysis in Han Chinese. Pharmacogenomics 11:349–356

Ikeda H, Takahashi Y, Yamazaki E, Fujiwara T, Kaniwa N, Saito Y, Aihara M, Kashiwagi M, Muramatsu M (2010) HLA class I markers in Japanese patients with carbamazepine-induced cutaneous adverse reactions. Epilepsia 51:297–300

Illing PT, Mifsud NA, Purcell AW (2016) Allotype specific interactions of drugs and HLA molecules in hypersensitivity reactions. Curr Opin Immunol 42:31–40

Ingelman-Sundberg M (2001) Pharmacogenetics: an opportunity for a safer and more efficient pharmacotherapy. J Intern Med 250:186–200

Jaruthamsophon K, Tipmanee V, Sangiemchoey A, Sukasem C, Limprasert P (2017) HLA-B*15:21 and carbamazepine-induced Stevens-Johnson syndrome: pooled-data and in silico analysis. Sci Rep 7:45553

Kang HR, Jee YK, Kim YS, Lee CH, Jung JW, Kim SH, Park HW, Chang YS, Jang IJ, Cho SH, Min KU, Kim SH, Lee KW (2011) Positive and negative associations of HLA class I alleles with allopurinol-induced SCARs in Koreans. Pharmacogenet Genom 21:303–307

Kaniwa N, Saito Y, Aihara M, Matsunaga K, Tohkin M, Kurose K, Furuya H, Takahashi Y, Muramatsu M, Kinoshita S, Abe M, Ikeda H, Kashiwagi M, Song Y, Ueta M, Sotozono C, Ikezawa Z, Hasegawa R (2010) HLA-B*1511 is a risk factor for carbamazepine-induced Stevens-Johnson syndrome and toxic epidermal necrolysis in Japanese patients. Epilepsia 51:2461–2465

Kaniwa N, Saito Y, Aihara M, Matsunaga K, Tohkin M, Kurose K, Sawada J, Furuya H, Takahashi Y, Muramatsu M, Kinoshita S, Abe M, Ikeda H, Kashiwagi M, Song Y, Ueta M, Sotozono C, Ikezawa Z, Hasegawa R (2008) HLA-B locus in Japanese patients with anti-epileptics and allopurinol-related Stevens-Johnson syndrome and toxic epidermal necrolysis. Pharmacogenomics 9:1617–1622

Kaniwa N, Sugiyama E, Saito Y, Kurose K, Maekawa K, Hasegawa R, Furuya H, Ikeda H, Takahashi Y, Muramatsu M, Tohkin M, Ozeki T, Mushiroda T, Kubo M, Kamatani N, Abe M, Yagami A, Ueta M, Sotozono C, Kinoshita S, Ikezawa Z, Matsunaga K, Aihara M (2013) Specific HLA types are associated with antiepileptic drug-induced Stevens-Johnson syndrome and toxic epidermal necrolysis in Japanese subjects. Pharmacogenomics 14:1821–1831

Karnes JH, Miller MA, White KD, Konvinse KC, Pavlos RK, Redwood AJ, Peter JG, Lehloenya R, Mallal SA, Phillips EJ (2019) Applications of immunopharmacogenomics: predicting, preventing, and understanding immune-mediated adverse drug reactions. Annu Rev Pharmacol Toxicol 59:463–486

Ke CH, Chung WH, Wen YH, Huang YB, Chuang HY, Tain YL, Wang YL, Wu CC, Hsu CN (2017) Cost-effectiveness analysis for genotyping before allopurinol treatment to prevent severe cutaneous adverse drug reactions. J Rheumatol 44:835–843

Keane NM, Pavlos RK, McKinnon E, Lucas A, Rive C, Blyth CC, Dunn D, Lucas M, Mallal S, Phillips E (2014) HLA Class I restricted CD8+ and Class II restricted CD4+ T cells are implicated in the pathogenesis of nevirapine hypersensitivity. AIDS 28:1891–1901

Kim SH, Choi JH, Lee KW, Kim SH, Shin ES, Oh HB, Suh CH, Nahm DH, Park HS (2005) The human leucocyte antigen-DRB1*1302-DQB1*0609-DPB1*0201 haplotype may be a strong genetic marker for aspirin-induced urticaria. Clin Exp Allergy 35:339–344

Kim SH, Kim M, Lee KW, Kim SH, Kang HR, Park HW, Jee YK (2010) HLA-B*5901 is strongly associated with methazolamide-induced Stevens-Johnson syndrome/toxic epidermal necrolysis. Pharmacogenomics 11:879–884

Kim SH, Lee KW, Song WJ, Kim SH, Jee YK, Lee SM, Kang HR, Park HW, Cho SH, Park SH, Min KU, Chang YS (2011) Carbamazepine-induced severe cutaneous adverse reactions and HLA genotypes in Koreans. Epilepsy Res 97:190–197

Kim SH, Lee SK, Kim SH, Park HW, Chang YS, Lee KW, Jee YK (2013) Antituberculosis drug-induced hypersensitivity syndrome and its association with human leukocyte antigen. Tuberculosis (Edinb) 93:270–274

Kim SH, Ye YM, Lee SK, Choi JH, Holloway JW, Park CS, Park HS (2006) Association of TNF-alpha genetic polymorphism with HLA DPB1*0301. Clin Exp Allergy 36:1247–1253

Ko TM, Chen YT (2012) T-cell receptor and carbamazepine-induced Stevens-Johnson syndrome and toxic epidermal necrolysis: understanding a hypersensitivity reaction. Expert Rev Clin Immunol 8:467–477

Ko TM, Chung WH, Wei CY, Shih HY, Chen JK, Lin CH, Chen YT, Hung SI (2011) Shared and restricted T-cell receptor use is crucial for carbamazepine-induced Stevens-Johnson syndrome. J Allergy Clin Immunol 128:1266-1276.e1211

Kongkaew C, Noyce PR, Ashcroft DM (2008) Hospital admissions associated with adverse drug reactions: a systematic review of prospective observational studies. Ann Pharmacother 42:1017–1025

Kongpan T, Mahasirimongkol S, Konyoung P, Kanjanawart S, Chumworathayi P, Wichukchinda N, Kidkeukarun R, Preechakul S, Khunarkornsiri U, Bamrungram W, Supharatwattanakun B, Mootsikapun P, Kwangsukstid S, Denjanta S, Vannaprasaht S, Rungapiromnan W, Suwankesawong W, Tassaneeyakul W, Tassaneeyakul W (2015) Candidate HLA genes for prediction of co-trimoxazole-induced severe cutaneous reactions. Pharmacogenet Genom 25:402–411

Konvinse KC, Trubiano JA, Pavlos R, James I, Shaffer CM, Bejan CA, Schutte RJ, Ostrov DA, Pilkinton MA, Rosenbach M, Zwerner JP, Williams KB, Bourke J, Martinez P, Rwandamuriye F, Chopra A, Watson M, Redwood AJ, White KD, Mallal SA, Phillips EJ (2019) HLA-A*32:01 is strongly associated with vancomycin-induced drug reaction with eosinophilia and systemic symptoms. J Allergy Clin Immunol

Lazarou J, Pomeranz BH, Corey PN (1998) Incidence of adverse drug reactions in hospitalized patients: a meta-analysis of prospective studies. JAMA 279:1200–1205

Leckband SG, Kelsoe JR, Dunnenberger HM, George AL Jr, Tran E, Berger R, Muller DJ, Whirl-Carrillo M, Caudle KE, Pirmohamed M (2013) Clinical pharmacogenetics implementation consortium guidelines for HLA-B genotype and carbamazepine dosing. Clin Pharmacol Ther 94:324–328

Li LJ, Hu FY, Wu XT, An DM, Yan B, Zhou D (2013) Predictive markers for carbamazepine and lamotrigine-induced maculopapular exanthema in Han Chinese. Epilepsy Res 106:296–300

Littera R, Carcassi C, Masala A, Piano P, Serra P, Ortu F, Corso N, Casula B, La Nasa G, Contu L, Manconi PE (2006) HLA-dependent hypersensitivity to nevirapine in Sardinian HIV patients. AIDS 20:1621–1626

Locharernkul C, Loplumlert J, Limotai C, Korkij W, Desudchit T, Tongkobpetch S, Kangwanshiratada O, Hirankarn N, Suphapeetiporn K, Shotelersuk V (2008a) Carbamazepine and phenytoin induced Stevens-Johnson syndrome is associated with HLA-B*1502 allele in Thai population. Epilepsia 49:2087–2091

Locharernkul C, Loplumlert J, Limotai C, Korkij W, Desudchit T, Tongkobpetch S, Kangwanshiratada O, Hirankarn N, Suphapeetiporn K, Shotelersuk V (2008b) Carbamazepine and phenytoin induced Stevens-Johnson syndrome is associated with HLA-B* 1502 allele in Thai population. Epilepsia 49:2087–2091

Locharernkul C, Shotelersuk V, Hirankarn N (2011) Pharmacogenetic screening of carbamazepine-induced severe cutaneous allergic reactions. J Clin Neurosci 18:1289–1294

Lonjou C, Borot N, Sekula P, Ledger N, Thomas L, Halevy S, Naldi L, Bouwes-Bavinck JN, Sidoroff A, de Toma C, Schumacher M, Roujeau JC, Hovnanian A, Mockenhaupt M (2008) A European study of HLA-B in Stevens-Johnson syndrome and toxic epidermal necrolysis related to five high-risk drugs. Pharmacogenet Genom 18:99–107

Lv YD, Min FL, Liao WP, He N, Zeng T, Ma DH, Shi YW (2013) The association between oxcarbazepine-induced maculopapular eruption and HLA-B alleles in a northern Han Chinese population. BMC Neurol 13:75

Mallal S, Nolan D, Witt C, Masel G, Martin AM, Moore C, Sayer D, Castley A, Mamotte C, Maxwell D, James I, Christiansen FT (2002) Association between presence of HLA-B*5701, HLA-DR7, and HLA-DQ3 and hypersensitivity to HIV-1 reverse-transcriptase inhibitor abacavir. Lancet 359:727–732

Mallal S, Phillips E, Carosi G, Molina J-M, Workman C, Tomažič J, Jägel-Guedes E, Rugina S, Kozyrev O, Cid JF (2008a) HLA-B* 5701 screening for hypersensitivity to abacavir. N Engl J Med 358:568–579

Mallal S, Phillips E, Carosi G, Molina JM, Workman C, Tomazic J, Jagel-Guedes E, Rugina S, Kozyrev O, Cid JF, Hay P, Nolan D, Hughes S, Hughes A, Ryan S, Fitch N, Thorborn D, Benbow A (2008b) HLA-B*5701 screening for hypersensitivity to abacavir. N Engl J Med 358:568–579

Man CB, Kwan P, Baum L, Yu E, Lau KM, Cheng AS, Ng MH (2007) Association between HLA-B*1502 allele and antiepileptic drug-induced cutaneous reactions in Han Chinese. Epilepsia 48:1015–1018

Manuyakorn W, Mahasirimongkol S, Likkasittipan P, Kamchaisatian W, Wattanapokayakit S, Inunchot W, Visudtibhan A, Wichukchinda N, Benjaponpitak S (2016) Association of HLA genotypes with phenobarbital hypersensitivity in children. Epilepsia 57:1610–1616

Martin AM, Nolan D, James I, Cameron P, Keller J, Moore C, Phillips E, Christiansen FT, Mallal S (2005) Predisposition to nevirapine hypersensitivity associated with HLA-DRB1*0101 and abrogated by low CD4 T-cell counts. AIDS 19:97–99

Martin MA, Kroetz DL (2013) Abacavir pharmacogenetics–from initial reports to standard of care. Pharmacotherapy 33:765–775

McCormack M, Alfirevic A, Bourgeois S, Farrell JJ, Kasperaviciute D, Carrington M, Sills GJ, Marson T, Jia X, de Bakker PI, Chinthapalli K, Molokhia M, Johnson MR, O'Connor GD, Chaila E, Alhusaini S, Shianna KV, Radtke RA, Heinzen EL, Walley N, Pandolfo M, Pichler W, Park BK, Depondt C, Sisodiya SM, Goldstein DB, Deloukas P, Delanty N, Cavalleri GL, Pirmohamed M (2011) HLA-A*3101 and carbamazepine-induced hypersensitivity reactions in Europeans. N Engl J Med 364:1134–1143

McNeil BD, Pundir P, Meeker S, Han L, Undem BJ, Kulka M, Dong X (2014) Identification of a mast-cell-specific receptor crucial for pseudo-allergic drug reactions. Nature 519:237

Mehta TY, Prajapati LM, Mittal B, Joshi CG, Sheth JJ, Patel DB, Dave DM, Goyal RK (2009) Association of HLA-B*1502 allele and carbamazepine-induced Stevens-Johnson syndrome among Indians. Indian J Dermatol Venereol Leprol 75:579–582

Mjorndal T, Boman MD, Hagg S, Backstrom M, Wiholm BE, Wahlin A, Dahlqvist R (2002) Adverse drug reactions as a cause for admissions to a department of internal medicine. Pharmacoepidemiol Drug Saf 11:65–72

Moon J, Park HK, Chu K, Sunwoo JS, Byun JI, Lim JA, Kim TJ, Shin JW, Lee ST, Jung KH, Jung KY, Jeon D, Kim DW, Yu KS, Jang IJ, Kang HR, Park HW, Lee SK (2015) The HLA-A*2402/Cw*0102 haplotype is associated with lamotrigine-induced maculopapular eruption in the Korean population. Epilepsia 56:e161-167

Navines-Ferrer A, Serrano-Candelas E, Lafuente A, Munoz-Cano R, Martin M (2018) MRGPRX2-mediated mast cell response to drugs used in perioperative procedures and anaesthesia. 8:11628

Negrini S, Becquemont L (2017) HLA-associated drug hypersensitivity and the prediction of adverse drug reactions. Pharmacogenomics 18:1441–1457

Nguyen JK, Fouts MM, Kotabe SE, Lo E (2006) Polypharmacy as a risk factor for adverse drug reactions in geriatric nursing home residents. Am J Geriatr Pharmacother 4:36–41

Niihara H, Kakamu T, Fujita Y, Kaneko S, Morita E (2012) HLA-A31 strongly associates with carbamazepine-induced adverse drug reactions but not with carbamazepine-induced lymphocyte proliferation in a Japanese population. J Dermatol 39:594–601

Ostrov DA, Grant BJ, Pompeu YA, Sidney J, Harndahl M, Southwood S, Oseroff C, Lu S, Jakoncic J, de Oliveira CAF (2012) Drug hypersensitivity caused by alteration of the MHC-presented self-peptide repertoire. Proc Natl Acad Sci 109:9959–9964

Oussalah A, Mayorga C, Blanca M, Barbaud A, Nakonechna A, Cernadas J, Gotua M, Brockow K, Caubet JC, Bircher A, Atanaskovic M, Demoly P, LK Tanno, Terreehorst I, Laguna JJ, Romano A, Gueant JL (2016) Genetic variants associated with drugs-induced immediate hypersensitivity reactions: a PRISMA-compliant systematic review. Allergy 71:443–462

Ozeki T, Mushiroda T, Yowang A, Takahashi A, Kubo M, Shirakata Y, Ikezawa Z, Iijima M, Shiohara T, Hashimoto K, Kamatani N, Nakamura Y (2011) Genome-wide association study identifies HLA-A*3101 allele as a genetic risk factor for carbamazepine-induced cutaneous adverse drug reactions in Japanese population. Hum Mol Genet 20:1034–1041

Ozkaya-Bayazit E, Akar U (2001) Fixed drug eruption induced by trimethoprim-sulfamethoxazole: evidence for a link to HLA-A30 B13 Cw6 haplotype. J Am Acad Dermatol 45:712–717

Park HJ, Kim SR, Leem DW, Moon IJ, Koh BS, Park KH, Park JW, Lee JH (2015) Clinical features of and genetic predisposition to drug-induced Stevens-Johnson syndrome and toxic epidermal necrolysis in a single Korean tertiary institution patients-investigating the relation between the HLA -B*4403 allele and lamotrigine. Eur J Clin Pharmacol 71:35–41

Park HJ, Ye YM, Hur GY, Kim SH, Park HS (2008) Association between a TGFbeta1 promoter polymorphism and the phenotype of aspirin-intolerant chronic urticaria in a Korean population. J Clin Pharm Ther 33:691–697

Pavlos R, Mallal S, Ostrov D, Pompeu Y, Phillips E (2014) Fever, rash, and systemic symptoms: understanding the role of virus and HLA in severe cutaneous drug allergy. J Allergy Clin Immunol Pract 2:21–33

Pellicano R, Lomuto M, Ciavarella G, Di Giorgio G, Gasparini P (1997) Fixed drug eruptions with feprazone are linked to HLA-B22. J Am Acad Dermatol 36:782–784

Phillips E, Lucas M, Keane N, Lucas A, McKinnon E, Mallal S (2010) HLA-B*35 is associated with nevirapine hypersensitivity in the contemporary Western Australian HIV cohort study. In: 4th international drug hypersensitivity meeting. Rome, Italy

Phillips E, Mallal S (2009) Successful translation of pharmacogenetics into the clinic: the abacavir example. Mol Diagn Ther 13:1–9

Phillips EJ, Mallal SA (2010) Pharmacogenetics of drug hypersensitivity. Pharmacogenomics 11:973–987

Phillips EJ, Sukasem C, Whirl-Carrillo M, Müller DJ, Dunnenberger HM, Chantratita W, Goldspiel B, Chen

Y-T, Carleton BC, George AL Jr, Mushiroda T, Klein T, Gammal RS, Pirmohamed M (2018) Clinical pharmacogenetics implementation consortium guideline for HLA genotype and use of carbamazepine and oxcarbazepine: 2017 update. Clin Pharmacol Ther 103:574–581

Pirmohamed M (2012) Genetics and the potential for predictive tests in adverse drug reactions. Chem Immunol Allergy 97:18–31

Pirmohamed M, Aithal GP, Behr E, Daly A, Roden D (2011a) The phenotype standardization project: improving pharmacogenetic studies of serious adverse drug reactions. Clin Pharmacol Ther 89:784–785

Pirmohamed M, Friedmann PS, Molokhia M, Loke YK, Smith C, Phillips E, La Grenade L, Carleton B, Papaluca-Amati M, Demoly P, Shear NH (2011b) Phenotype standardization for immune-mediated drug-induced skin injury. Clin Pharmacol Ther 89:896–901

Pirmohamed M, James S, Meakin S, Green C, Scott AK, Walley TJ, Farrar K, Park BK, Breckenridge AM (2004) Adverse drug reactions as cause of admission to hospital: prospective analysis of 18 820 patients. BMJ 329:15–19

Pirmohamed M, Lin K, Chadwick D, Park BK (2001) TNFalpha promoter region gene polymorphisms in carbamazepine-hypersensitive patients. Neurology 56:890–896

Pradeu T, Cooper EL (2012) The danger theory: 20 years later. Front Immunol 3:287

Qiao H-L, Yang J, Zhang Y-W (2004) Specific serum IgE levels and FcεRIβ genetic polymorphism in patients with penicillins allergy. Allergy 59:1326–1332

Qiao HL, Yang J, Zhang YW (2005) Relationships between specific serum IgE, cytokines and polymorphisms in the IL-4, IL-4Ralpha in patients with penicillins allergy. Allergy 60:1053–1059

Quiralte J, Sanchez-Garcia F, Torres MJ, Blanco C, Castillo R, Ortega N, de Castro FR, Perez-Aciego P, Carrillo T (1999) Association of HLA-DR11 with the anaphylactoid reaction caused by nonsteroidal anti-inflammatory drugs. J Allergy Clin Immunol 103:685–689

Ramasamy SN, Korb-Wells CS, Kannangara DR, Smith MW, Wang N, Roberts DM, Graham GG, Williams KM, Day RO (2013) Allopurinol hypersensitivity: a systematic review of all published cases, 1950–2012. Drug Saf 36:953–980

Rauch A, Nolan D, Martin A, McKinnon E, Almeida C, Mallal S (2006) Prospective genetic screening decreases the incidence of abacavir hypersensitivity reactions in the Western Australian HIV cohort study. Clin Infect Dis 43:99–102

Redwood AJ, Pavlos RK, White KD, Phillips EJ (2018) HLAs: key regulators of T-cell-mediated drug hypersensitivity. Hla 91:3–16

Romano A, De Santis A, Romito A, Di Fonso M, Venuti A, Gasbarrini GB, Manna R (1998) Delayed hypersensitivity to aminopenicillins is related to major histocompatibility complex genes. Ann Allergy Asthma Immunol 80:433–437

Roujeau JC, Huynh TN, Bracq C, Guillaume JC, Revuz J, Touraine R (1987) Genetic susceptibility to toxic epidermal necrolysis. Arch Dermatol 123:1171–1173

Ruiter R, Visser LE, Rodenburg EM, Trifiro G, Ziere G, Stricker BH (2012) Adverse drug reaction-related hospitalizations in persons aged 55 years and over: a population-based study in the Netherlands. Drugs Aging 29:225–232

Saag M, Balu R, Phillips E, Brachman P, Martorell C, Burman W, Stancil B, Mosteller M, Brothers C, Wannamaker P, Hughes A, Sutherland-Phillips D, Mallal S, Shaefer M (2008) High sensitivity of human leukocyte antigen-b*5701 as a marker for immunologically confirmed abacavir hypersensitivity in white and black patients. Clin Infect Dis 46:1111–1118

Saedder EA, Lisby M, Nielsen LP, Bonnerup DK, Brock B (2015) Number of drugs most frequently found to be independent risk factors for serious adverse reactions: a systematic literature review. Br J Clin Pharmacol 80:808–817

Shi YW, Min FL, Liu XR, Zan LX, Gao MM, Yu MJ, Liao WP (2011) Hla-B alleles and lamotrigine-induced cutaneous adverse drug reactions in the Han Chinese population. Basic Clin Pharmacol Toxicol 109:42–46

Shirzadi M, Thorstensen K, Helde G, Moen T, Brodtkorb E (2015) Do HLA-A markers predict skin-reactions from aromatic antiepileptic drugs in a Norwegian population? A case control study. Epilepsy Res 118:5–9

Shubber Z, Calmy A, Andrieux-Meyer I, Vitoria M, Renaud-Thery F, Shaffer N, Hargreaves S, Mills EJ, Ford N (2013) Adverse events associated with nevirapine and efavirenz-based first-line antiretroviral therapy: a systematic review and meta-analysis. AIDS 27:1403–1412

Sibaud V, Meyer N, Lamant L, Vigarios E, Mazieres J, Delord JP (2016) Dermatologic complications of anti-PD-1/PD-L1 immune checkpoint antibodies. Curr Opin Oncol 28:254–263

Simper GS, Ho GT, Celik AA, Huyton T, Kuhn J (2018) Carbamazepine-Mediated Adverse Drug Reactions: CBZ-10,11-epoxide but Not Carbamazepine Induces the Alteration of Peptides Presented by HLA-B *15:02. 2018:5086503

Sousa-Pinto B, Correia C, Gomes L, Gil-Mata S, Araujo L, Correia O, Delgado L (2016) HLA and delayed drug-induced hypersensitivity. Int Arch Allergy Immunol 170:163–179

Tassaneeyakul W, Jantararoungtong T, Chen P, Lin PY, Tiamkao S, Khunarkornsiri U, Chucherd P, Konyoung P, Vannaprasaht S, Choonhakarn C, Pisuttimarn P, Sangviroon A, Tassaneeyakul W (2009) Strong association between HLA-B*5801 and allopurinol-induced Stevens-Johnson syndrome and toxic epidermal necrolysis in a Thai population. Pharmacogenet Genomics 19:704–709

Tassaneeyakul W, Tiamkao S, Jantararoungtong T, Chen P, Lin S-Y, Chen W-H, Konyoung P, Khunarkornsiri U, Auvichayapat N, Pavakul K,

Kulkantrakorn K, Choonhakarn C, Phonhiamhan S, Piyatrakul N, Aungaree T, Pongpakdee S, Yodnopaglaw P (2010) Association between HLA-B*1502 and carbamazepine-induced severe cutaneous adverse drug reactions in a Thai population. Epilepsia 51:926–930

Then SM, Rani ZZ, Raymond AA, Ratnaningrum S, Jamal R (2011) Frequency of the HLA-B*1502 allele contributing to carbamazepine-induced hypersensitivity reactions in a cohort of Malaysian epilepsy patients. Asian Pac J Allergy Immunol 29:290–293

Tohkin M, Kaniwa N, Saito Y, Sugiyama E, Kurose K, Nishikawa J, Hasegawa R, Aihara M, Matsunaga K, Abe M, Furuya H, Takahashi Y, Ikeda H, Muramatsu M, Ueta M, Sotozono C, Kinoshita S, Ikezawa Z (2013) A whole-genome association study of major determinants for allopurinol-related Stevens-Johnson syndrome and toxic epidermal necrolysis in Japanese patients. Pharmacogenomics J 13:60–69

Ueta M, Kaniwa N, Sotozono C, Tokunaga K, Saito Y, Sawai H, Miyadera H, Sugiyama E, Maekawa K, Nakamura R, Nagato M, Aihara M, Matsunaga K, Takahashi Y, Furuya H, Muramatsu M, Ikezawa Z, Kinoshita S (2014a) Independent strong association of HLA-A*02:06 and HLA-B*44:03 with cold medicine-related Stevens-Johnson syndrome with severe mucosal involvement. Sci Rep 4:4862

Ueta M, Kannabiran C, Wakamatsu TH, Kim MK, Yoon KC, Seo KY, Joo CK, Sangwan V, Rathi V, Basu S, Shamaila A, Lee HS, Yoon S, Sotozono C, Gomes JA, Tokunaga K, Kinoshita S (2014b) Trans-ethnic study confirmed independent associations of HLA-A*02:06 and HLA-B*44:03 with cold medicine-related Stevens-Johnson syndrome with severe ocular surface complications. Sci Rep 4:5981

Ueta M, Sotozono C, Inatomi T, Kojima K, Hamuro J, Kinoshita S (2007a) Association of IL4R polymorphisms with Stevens-Johnson syndrome. Journal of Allergy and Clinical Immunology 120:1457–1459

Ueta M, Sotozono C, Inatomi T, Kojima K, Tashiro K, Hamuro J, Kinoshita S (2007b) Toll-like receptor 3 gene polymorphisms in Japanese patients with Stevens-Johnson syndrome. Br J Ophthalmol 91:962–965

van der Hooft CS, Dieleman JP, Siemes C, Aarnoudse AJ, Verhamme KM, Stricker BH, Sturkenboom MC (2008) Adverse drug reaction-related hospitalisations: a population-based cohort study. Pharmacoepidemiol Drug Saf 17:365–371

Vitezica ZG, Milpied B, Lonjou C, Borot N, Ledger TN, Lefebvre A, Hovnanian A (2008) HLA-DRB1*01 associated with cutaneous hypersensitivity induced by nevirapine and efavirenz. AIDS 22:540–541

Wang H, Yan L, Zhang G, Chen X, Yang J, Li M, Shen J, Yu M, Huo R, Wang B (2013) Association between HLA-B*1301 and dapsone-induced hypersensitivity reactions among leprosy patients in China. J Invest Dermatol 133:2642–2644

Watkins S, Pichler WJ (2013) Sulfamethoxazole induces a switch mechanism in T cell receptors containing TCRVβ20–1, altering pHLA recognition. PLoS One 8

Wei CY, Chung WH, Huang HW, Chen YT, Hung SI (2012) Direct interaction between HLA-B and carbamazepine activates T cells in patients with Stevens-Johnson syndrome. J Allergy Clin Immunol 129:1562-1569.e1565

White KD, Chung W-H, Hung S-I, Mallal S, Phillips EJ (2015a) Evolving models of the immunopathogenesis of T cell–mediated drug allergy: the role of host, pathogens, and drug response. Journal of Allergy and Clinical Immunology 136:219–234

White KD, Chung WH, Hung SI, Mallal S, Phillips EJ (2015) Evolving models of the immunopathogenesis of T cell-mediated drug allergy: the role of host, pathogens, and drug response. J Allergy Clin Immunol 136:219–234; quiz 235.

Wit FW, Kesselring AM, Gras L, Richter C, van der Ende ME, Brinkman K, Lange JM, de Wolf F, Reiss P (2008) Discontinuation of nevirapine because of hypersensitivity reactions in patients with prior treatment experience, compared with treatment-naive patients: the ATHENA cohort study. Clin Infect Dis 46:933–940

Wolfe D, Yazdi F, Kanji S, Burry L, Beck A (2018) Incidence, causes, and consequences of preventable adverse drug reactions occurring in inpatients: a systematic review of systematic reviews. 13:e0205426

Yampayon K, Sukasem C, Limwongse C, Chinvarun Y, Tempark T, Rerkpattanapipat T, Kijsanayotin P (2017) Influence of genetic and non-genetic factors on phenytoin-induced severe cutaneous adverse drug reactions. Eur J Clin Pharmacol 73:855–865

Yang F, Gu B, Zhang L, Xuan J, Luo H, Zhou P, Zhu Q, Yan S, Chen S-a, Cao Z, Xu J, Xing Q, Luo X (2014) HLA-B*13:01 is associated with salazosulfapyridine-induced drug rash with eosinophilia and systemic symptoms in Chinese Han population. Pharmacogenomics 15:1461–1469

Yang F, Xuan J, Chen J, Zhong H, Luo H, Zhou P, Sun X, He L, Chen S, Cao Z, Luo X, Xing Q (2016) HLA-B*59:01: a marker for Stevens-Johnson syndrome/toxic epidermal necrolysis caused by methazolamide in Han Chinese. Pharmacogenomics J 16:83–87

Yang J, Qiao HL, Zhang YW, Jia LJ, Tian X, Gao N (2006) HLA-DRB genotype and specific IgE responses in patients with allergies to penicillins. Chin Med J (engl) 119:458–466

Yang Y, Chen S, Yang F, Zhang L, Alterovitz G, Zhu H, Xuan J, Yang X, Luo H, Mu J, He L, Luo X, Xing Q (2017) HLA-B*51:01 is strongly associated with clindamycin-related cutaneous adverse drug reactions. Pharmacogenomics J 17:501–505

Yip VL, Hawcutt DB, Pirmohamed M (2015) Pharmacogenetic markers of drug efficacy and toxicity. Clin Pharmacol Ther 98:61–70

Yun J, Cai F, Lee FJ, Pichler WJ (2016) T-cell-mediated drug hypersensitivity: immune mechanisms and their clinical relevance. Asia Pac Allergy 6:77–89

Yun J, Marcaida MJ, Eriksson KK, Jamin H, Fontana S, Pichler WJ, Yerly D (2014) Oxypurinol directly and immediately activates the drug-specific T cells via the preferential use of HLA-B*58:01. J Immunol 192:2984–2993

Zhang F-R, Liu H, Irwanto A, Fu X-A, Li Y, Yu G-Q, Yu Y-X, Chen M-F, Low H-Q, Li J-H, Bao F-F, Foo J-N, Bei J-X, Jia X-M, Liu J, Liany H, Wang N, Niu G-Y, Wang Z-Z, Shi B-Q, Tian H-Q, Liu H-X, Ma S-S, Zhou Y, You J-B, Yang Q, Wang C, Chu T-S, Liu D-C, Yu X-L, Sun Y-H, Ning Y, Wei Z-H, Chen S-L, Chen X-C, Zhang Z-X, Liu Y-X, Pulit SL, Wu W-B, Zheng Z-Y, Yang R-D, Long H, Liu Z-S, Wang J-Q, Li M, Zhang L-H, Wang H, Wang L-M, Xiao P, Li J-L, Huang Z-M, Huang J-X, Li Z, Liu J, Xiong L, Yang J, Wang X-D, Yu D-B, Lu X-M, Zhou G-Z, Yan L-B, Shen J-P, Zhang G-C, Zeng Y-X, de Bakker PIW, Chen S-M, Liu J-J (2013) HLA-B*13:01 and the dapsone hypersensitivity syndrome. N Engl J Med 369:1620–1628

Zucman D, Truchis P, Majerholc C, Stegman S, Caillat-Zucman S (2007) Prospective screening for human leukocyte antigen-B*5701 avoids abacavir hypersensitivity reaction in the ethnically mixed French HIV population. J Acquir Immune Defic Syndr 45:1–3

The Immunogenetic Aspects of Photodynamic Therapy

Chaw-Ning Lee and Tak-Wah Wong

Abstract

Photodynamic therapy (PDT) has become the first-line treatment of actinic keratosis, superficial basal cell carcinoma, and squamous cell carcinoma in situ (Bowen's disease) in dermatology. The off-label use of PDT has also escalated in recent years owing to its applications in the treatment of various non-neoplastic skin diseases such as acne vulgaris, vascular lesions, rejuvenation, and chronic wounds. Daylight PDT that uses natural sunlight to activate a photosensitizer with advantages such as low cost and reduced pain is widely used in Europe. This chapter reviews the applications and immunogenetic aspects of PDT. However, the studies of immunity and genetic changes in human tissue after PDT are limited.

C.-N. Lee · T.-W. Wong (✉)
Departments of Dermatology, College of Medicine, National Cheng Kung University Hospital, Tainan, Taiwan
e-mail: twwong@mail.ncku.edu.tw

T.-W. Wong
Department of Biochemistry & Molecular Biology, College of Medicine, Tainan, Taiwan

Center of Applied Nanomedicine, National Cheng Kung University, Tainan, Taiwan

1 History of Photodynamic Therapy

In 1978, Dougherty et al. reported the first large case series of 25 patients with 113 primary or secondary skin tumors successfully treated with photodynamic therapy (PDT). They applied a hematoporphyrin derivative (HpD) on the tumors and irradiated them with red light from a xenon arc lamp for 24–168 h (Ackroyd et al. 2001). The first US Food and Drug Administration (FDA) approval for PDT was issued in 1995 for esophageal cancer using porfimer sodium (Photofrin) as the photosensitizer (Huang 2005). Thereafter, PDT was widely used in different benign diseases and malignant tumors such as age-related macular degeneration (AMD), acne, verruca, bladder cancer, and skin cancer. The most commonly used topical photosensitizers in dermatology include 5-aminolevulinic acid (ALA) and methyl aminolevulinate (MAL). ALA-mediated PDT was approved by the FDA in treating actinic keratosis in 1999. MAL-PDT was approved in Europe for treating superficial skin cancers long before it was commercially available in the USA.

2 Mechanisms

Photosensitizers (PS), visible light, and oxygen are the three key components of PDT. PS can be administrated via intravenous, topical, or intralesional routes. Specific wavelengths of light

N. Rezaei and F. Rajabi (eds.), *The Immunogenetics of Dermatologic Diseases*, Advances in Experimental Medicine and Biology 1367,
https://doi.org/10.1007/978-3-030-92616-8_18

trigger the excitement of the PS to a triplet state that leads to either type-I or type-II reactions depending on the type of PS used and the concentrations of substrate and oxygen (Castano et al. 2004). These two types of reactions both involve oxygen and should be differentiated from the main photochemical reaction in psoralen-ultraviolet A (PUVA) that involves DNA-psoralen covalent adducts. In type-I reaction, when the excited triplet PS returns to its ground state, it transfers an electron to oxygen in the tissues to form reactive oxygen species including radical anion and radical cation (e.g., $O_2^{\bullet -}$, H2O2, and HO$^{\bullet}$) (Fig. 1). In type-II reaction, excited PS directly transfers its energy to molecular oxygen to form singlet oxygen (Castano et al. 2004). These ROS and/or singlet oxygen induce necrosis and apoptosis in tumor cells (Noodt et al. 1996).

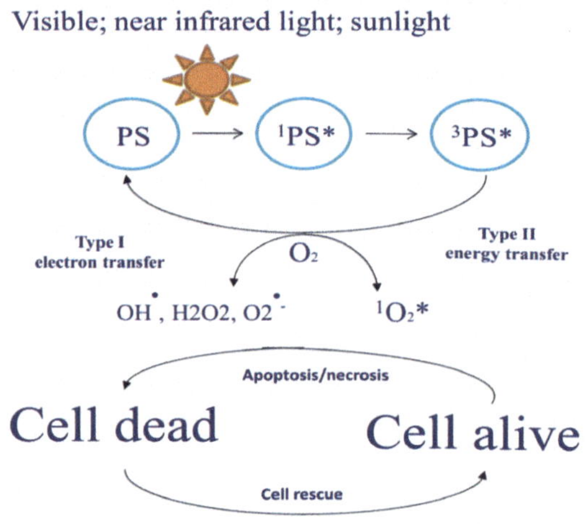

Fig. 1 Schematic diagram showing type-I and type-II reactions of photodynamic therapy. PS: photosensitizer

The most commonly used PSs in dermatology are aminolevulinic acid (ALA), methyl-ALA (MAL), and a new nanoemulsion 10% ALA hydrogel (BF-200 ALA) (Reinhold et al. 2016). ALA is a prodrug that is converted into protoporphyrin IX (PpIX) in cell mitochondria via the intrinsic cellular heme biosynthetic pathway. Exogenous administration of ALA leads to higher levels of PpIX in tumor cells compared to normal cells. Although several explanations have been provided for this phenomenon, the mechanism remains unclear (Yang et al. 2015). It has been suggested that increased PpIX in cancerous cells might result from alterations in enzymes and transporters that allow the exogenous ALA to bypass natural inhibitory pathways of heme synthesis and lead to the accumulation of PpIX. For instance, cancer cells have higher porphobilinogen deaminase activity that leads to PpIX formation and a lower ferrochelatase activity that turns PpIX into heme. This results in higher and longer retention of PpIX in these tumoral cells (Collaud et al. 2004; Hinnen et al. 1998; Ohgari et al. 2005).

Another explanation is the increased expression of low-density lipoprotein (LDL) receptors on cancer cells. This leads to increased abortion of hydrophobic photosensitizing drugs and is carried by lipoproteins such as LDL (Maziere et al. 1991). Intracellularly, hydrophilic photosensitizers have a preference for accumulation in lysosomes and cytoplasm, while hydrophobic ones tend to concentrate in organelles membranes, such as the mitochondrial membrane, endoplasmic reticulum membrane, and the cell membrane (Kongshaug et al. 1989). The diffusion area for ROS and singlet oxygen is around a micrometer and it disappears within milliseconds. Therefore, the damage it causes is within the organelle level (Fig. 2).

PpIX has absorption peaks at 410, 510, 545, 580, 630, 670, and 700 nm wavelengths (Fig. 3). The light-emitting diode (LED) has been widely used as the light source to excite PSs in dermatology. Though the Soret band (extreme intense band) of PpIX is 410 nm (blue light), the 635 nm wavelength (bright red light) is used in the clinic for deeper tissue penetration. Approximately 3 h after ALA application on the cancerous or precancerous skin lesions, a bright red fluorescence of PpIX can be observed under Wood's lamp (365 nm). Subclinical atypical cells can also be visualized in this manner which is termed "photodynamic diagnosis" (Fig. 4). Irradiation should be continued until the disappearance of fluorescence (photobleaching). The light dose applied for topical ALA-PDT depends on whether the target disease is benign or malignant, ranging from 37 to 200 J/cm^2 (higher light doses are used

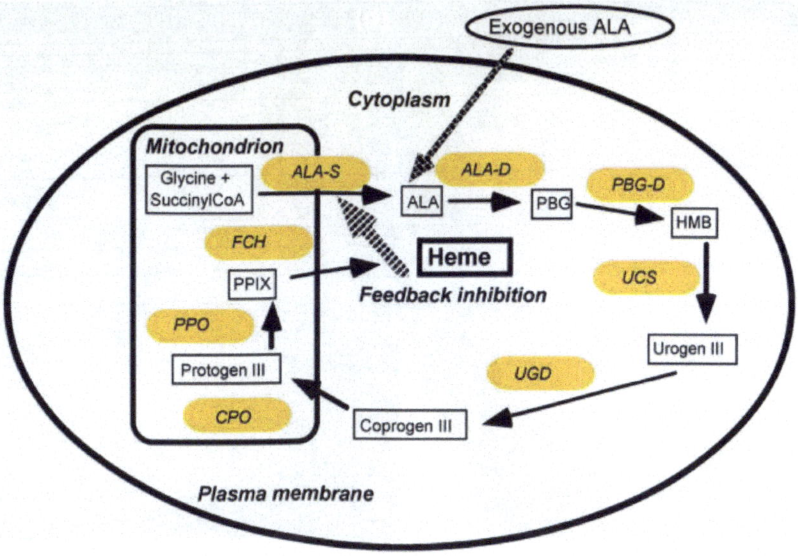

Fig. 2 The heme synthesis pathway in a cell. Administration of exogenous aminolevulinic acid (ALA) bypasses the regular feedback inhibition pathway and results in protoporphyrin IX (PpIX) accumulation in a mitochondrion. Abbreviations are ALA-D: ALA dehydratase; ALA-S: ALA synthetase; Coprogen III: coproporphyrinogen III; CPO: coproporphyrinogen oxidase; FCH: ferrochelatase; HMB: hydroxymethylbilane, PBG-D: porphobilinogen deaminase; protogen III: protoporphyrinogen; PPO: protoporphyrinogen oxidase; Urogen III: uroporphyrinogen III; UCS: uroporphyrinogen synthase, UGD: uroporphyrinogen decarboxylase. From Castano et al. Photodiagnosis Photodyn Ther 2004. 1: 279–293 with permission

to treat malignant diseases). In general, the light dose in systemic PDT should be controlled more precisely since the cytotoxicity, inflammation, and pain are more profound. The choice of wavelength to excite PS depends on tumor thickness. Blue light can penetrate about 1 mm into the skin and is used to treat actinic keratosis, while red light can penetrate up to 3 mm (Ash et al. 2017). Curettage or laser abrasion before ALA-PDT can facilitate PS absorption into deeper tissue and improve the efficacy of PDT.

In recent years intravenous administration of photosensitizers is finding its place in dermatology for the treatment of vascular lesions such as port-wine stain (PWS). The principles and methods used in these procedures have been adopted from ophthalmologic studies on the management of age-related macular degeneration (AMD) (Huang 2005). One of the main photosensitizers utilized for this matter is hematoporphyrin monomethyl ether (HMME). Within 30 min after HMME administration, while the photosensitizer is still circulating in the vessels, the lesions are irradiated. The hydrophobic photosensitizer is absorbed by endothelial cells via LDL receptors. This leads to damage to the endothelial lining of the vessels which then promotes intravascular thrombosis and obstruction (Schmidt-Erfurth and Hasan 2000; Yuan et al. 2008).

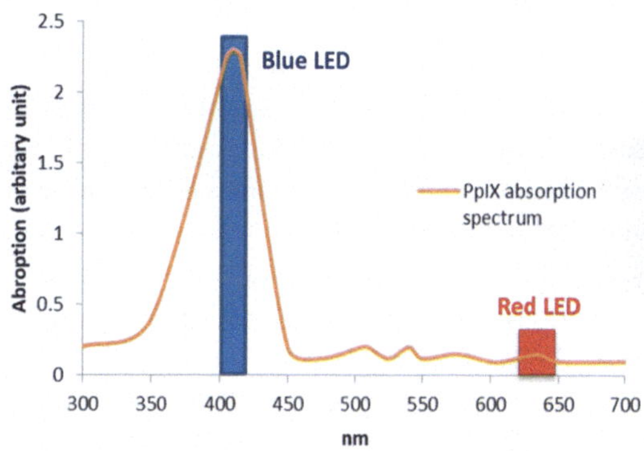

Fig. 3 The spectrums of commercial blue and red light-emitting diode (LED), and the protoporphyrin IX (PpIX) absorption spectrum (orange line). The absorption of PpIX peaks at 410 (Soret band), 505, 540, 580, and 635 nm

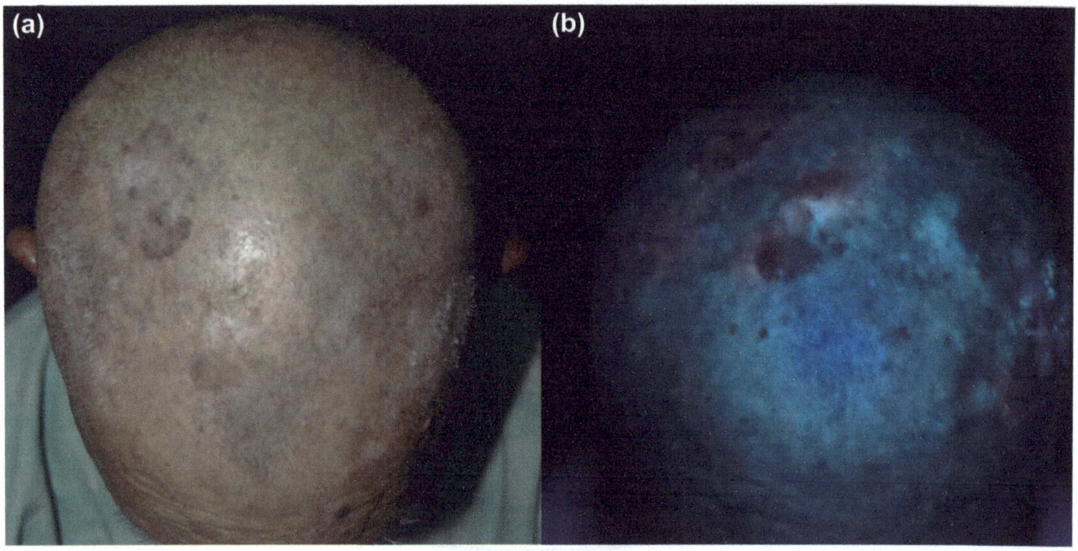

Fig. 4 **a** Actinic keratosis on the scalp of a 73-year-old male scalp is visualized under white light. **b** Red fluorescence on clinical and subclinical lesions of actinic keratosis is visualized under Wood's lamp illumination after three-hour incubation with methyl-aminolevulinic acid indicates the selective acumination of protoporphyrin IX (PpIX) in atypical cells

3 Different Light Sources Used in PDT

Usually, an incoherent light source is used to excite PS in the field of dermatology. Albeit in recent years lasers have also gained popularity especially for treating cutaneous vascular lesions with PDT (Qin et al. 2007).

In 1904, Kromayer used a mercury lamp in a projector as the light source for PDT (McDonagh 2001). Later, a high output xenon arc lamp (300–1200 nm) was used in nonmelanoma skin cancer and other benign skin disorders (Brancaleon and Moseley 2002). In 2001, Wong et al. used a homemade light-emitting diode (LED) to treat digital Bowen disease successfully. They were probably the first to use this light source in a clinical setting (Wong et al. 2001).

Lasers including Argon laser, dye laser, metal vapor laser, Nd: YAG lasers, and diode lasers are also used as PDT light sources. However, the treatment area of a laser beam is small and a beam expander which may reduce the fluence rate has to be used to expand the irradiation area (Brancaleon and Moseley 2002). A diode laser with a continuous mode or intense pulsed mode (picosecond to the millisecond) is more widely used in treating skin cancer. The red blood cells in the vascular component of basal cell carcinoma (BCC) absorb dye laser selectively which makes this laser an ideal weapon to target tumors with high vascularity (Soleymani et al. 2017). Shah et al. used a 595-nm pulse dye laser to treat 20 superficial and nodular BCCs with a high success rate in tumors smaller than 1.5 cm in diameter (Shah et al. 2009).

Intense pulse light (IPL) is a polychromatic non-coherent light covering a wide spectrum ranging from 500 to 1,200 nm depending on the cut-off filter and this includes the absorption spectrum of PpIX. A 95% complete response rate was reported in 31 patients with actinic keratosis (AK) treated with IPL-PDT (accompanied by a 640-nm filter) (Michelini 2018). IPL-PDT was also studied in patients with Bowen's disease (BD), superficial BCC, and photorejuvenation (Hall et al. 2004; Piccolo and Kostaki 2018). It was reported that IPL-PDT is less time-consuming and less painful than conventional PDT.

Interstitial lasers such as PDL are the newer modalities that have been employed for more precise targeting of vascular anomalies (Jerjes et al. 2011).

4 Gene Expressions Modified by PDT

Field cancerization is a term used in cancers with high risk to develop in multiple sites. This term was first coined by Slaughter in 1953 for describing multicentric squamous cell carcinoma of the oral cavity (Slaughter et al. 1953). The same phrase could also be applied to multicentric clinical and subclinical neoplastic skin lesions (AK, BD, and SCC) in UV-exposed skin. Since only a small percentage (0.1% to 20%) of photodamaged skin will eventually become malignant, the term "actinic field damage" was proposed instead (Marks et al. 1988; Neugebauer et al. 2019; Philipp-Dormston et al. 2016).

Studies have shown that MAL-PDT reverses actinic skin damage and photoaging by decreasing the severity and extent of keratinocyte atypia as well as decreasing the expression of *Ki-67* and mutated *p53* (Bagazgoitia et al. 2011; Wiegell et al. 2012). However, multiple sessions of PDT may be needed to clear the dysplastic skin completely (Bagazgoitia et al. 2011). Joly *et al.* reported the correction of abnormal cancer-associated gene expression and the induction of remodeling in photodamaged skin in seven organ transplant recipients whose AKs were treated with MAL-PDT (Joly et al. 2018). They used whole-genome gene expression profiling and found that MAL-PDT corrected aberrantly expressed cancer-associated genes (such as *APOBEC3A* and *TYMP*). MAL-PDT also induced the expression of dermal extracellular matrix genes in sun-exposed skin. They also highlighted the 15 most dysregulated genes which were normalized after MAL-PDT. These cancer-associated genes may be useful in the future as biomarkers to predict and monitor the efficacy of PDT.

In a recent article, Rybarski et al. have proposed eight genes (*MMP1, SPRR 1B, KLK6, CDH3, PI3, SPP1, FN1,* and *INHBA*) to be associated with the neoplastic process involved in the SCC formation. They have suggested that further studies on the effects of daylight PDT on these genes would be of great value in predicting the outcome of treatment (Rybarski et al. 2018).

5 Host Immunity in PDT

The PDT acts in multiple manners. It can cause cellular necrosis in the target tissue via radical oxygens and it could cause vascular thrombosis that eventually leads to reduced oxygen and nutrition supply. Moreover, the host immune response toward PDT is one of the key factors in treatment success that is also believed to attribute to the long-term suppression of tumor growth following PDT (Gollnick et al. 2003). Tumor-cell necrosis or apoptosis following PDT therapy leads to the release of different sets of damage-associated molecular patterns (DAMPs) depending on the type of tumor and photosensitizer (Hsieh et al. 2003; Korbelik et al. 2005). These DAMPs trigger the innate immune response by activating neutrophils, macrophages, and dendritic cells that engulf the cellular remnants (Krosl et al. 1995). After PDT, leucocytes, predominantly neutrophils, are the main immune cells that infiltrate the tumor and its surrounding tissue. With the help of DAMPs, the tumor-derived antigens are expressed on the surface of dendritic cells via major histocompatibility complexes leading to the activation of the adaptive immune system (Jalili et al. 2004; Mroz et al. 2011; Reginato et al. 2014). Cytotoxic T-cells (CD8+), helper T-cells (CD4+), and immunoglobulin-producing B-cells are all involved in the systemic antitumor response that controls distant tumors following local PDT (Kabingu et al. 2007; Preise et al. 2009). As for the cytokines involved in the PDT-related immune response, intravenous ALA-PDT has been reported to increase TNF-α, interleukin (IL)-6, and IL-10 in the irradiated area. IL-6 is a proinflammatory cytokine that acts in antitumoral immune responses, whereas TNF-α is the main cytokine found in healthy skin treated with topical ALA-PDT (Gollnick et al. 1997). Wong et al. revealed that

PDT reduces the cellular response to IL-6 and epidermal growth factor (EGF) in both normal and tumor cells which could eventually affect the outcome of PDT (Wong et al. 2003). A follow-up study showed that soluble IL-6 receptor-α (sIL-6Rα) and IL-6 were released by leucocytes in the presence of PDT-treated tumor cells (Wei et al. 2007). The same team compared local and systemic inflammation elicited by a second-generation photosensitizer, 2-[1-hexyloxyethyl]-2-devinyl pyropheophorbide-a (HPPH), to Photofrin in mice. They found that HPPH-PDT-induced neutrophil recruitment is dependent on the presence of macrophage inflammatory protein (MIP)-2 and E-selectin, but not on IL-6 or keratinocyte chemoattractants. This suggested that different PSs may induce a similar inflammatory response but the severity of the reactions is distinct (Gollnick et al. 2003).

6 Impacts of Genetic Polymorphisms on PDT Efficacy

Most studies in this regard have been conducted in ophthalmologic conditions where PDT is frequently used for targeting vessels. Genetic polymorphisms that can influence the PDT responsiveness are either related to the pathogenesis of the diseases being targeted or have pharmacologic impacts that are related to the functions of the photosensitizers. Since the principles that govern the mechanism of action in PDT are constant regardless of the site that is being treated, we could assume that the same set of genetic polymorphisms could affect the success rate of PDT in dermatologic conditions where vessels are being targeted.

As mentioned earlier, in the systemic administration of photosensitizers, the main mechanism is endothelial cell injury that leads to vascular coagulation. Hence, single nucleotide polymorphisms of genes encoding the coagulation/fibrinolytic pathways could greatly impact the outcome of PDT (Parmeggiani et al. 2007). In a study of patients with exudative age-related macular degeneration (AMD), three genetic polymorphisms were found to positively influence PDT outcome: the *methylenetetrahydrofolate reductase (MTHFR) 677 T* variant that results in hyperhomocysteinema and the 1691A allele of *FV* gene and the 20210A allele of *FII* gene both of which cause a prothrombotic state. The only polymorphism that negatively correlated with PDT responsiveness was the *FXIII* 185 T allele. This variant is associated with the increased fibrinolytic activity of factor XIII that presumably reduces fibrin-clot stability (Parmeggiani et al. 2007).

Genetic polymorphisms of *vascular endothelial growth factor (VEGF)* are another group that has been found to influence PDT outcomes in AMD. VEGF is expressed as a result of PDT-induced ischemia and promotes neovascularization, an undesired consequence, especially in the treatment of vascular lesions (Tammela et al. 2005). The CC genotypes of the rs699947 in the promoter region and the rs2146323 in the intron 2 region of *VEGF* are associated with PDT failure (Immonen et al. 2010). The rs699947-CC genotype has been shown to correlate with higher VEGF production (Shahbazi et al. 2002).

7 Applications of PDT in Dermatology

PDT with topical application of a PS has become one of the first-line treatments in precancerous diseases and superficial nonmelanocytic skin cancers (Cohen and Lee 2016). It has also been utilized as an off-label treatment in various neoplastic and non-neoplastic skin diseases (Table 1) (Wen et al. 2017). The most common topical PSs are ALA and MAL. Certain PSs were approved by the US FDA in the dermatologic field. A less official but clinically approved photosensitizer is indocyanine green (ICG) that has been utilized in the treatment of acne (Tuchin et al. 2003). ICG-PDT has also shown promising results in treating chorioretinopathy and hepatocellular carcinoma. In the treatment of acne, ICG-PDT has shown

Table 1 Application of photodynamic therapy in dermatology

Precancerous lesions and cancer	Benign lesions	Infectious diseases
Actinic Keratosis (AK)	Rosacea	Cutaneous leishmaniasis
Bowen's disease (BD)	Oily skin	Condyloma acuminatum
Basal cell carcinoma (BCC)	Skin rejuvenation	Acne vulgaris
Cutaneous T-Cell lymphoma	Psoriasis vulgaris (PV)	Verruca vulgaris
Melanoma	Vulvar lichen sclerosis et atrophicus (VLSA)	
Superficial squamous cell carcinoma	Vascular lesions	
Extramammary Paget's disease		

better bactericidal and clinical efficacy than ALA-PDT (Choi et al. 2018). ICG has several advantages, it is relatively inexpensive compared to other PSs and it absorbs near-infrared (NIR) light which allows a deeper tissue penetration (Wong et al. 2018). Moreover, ICG-PDT drives methicillin-resistant *Staphylococcus aureus* toward a drug-sensitive phenotype (Wong et al. 2019). ICG-PDT was also able to enhance wound healing in a mouse model (Chiu et al. 2019). These results suggest that ICG-PDT may have potential clinical use in the treatment of infectious diseases and chronic wounds.

In the USA, two drug/light combinations are approved for the treatment of non-hyperkeratotic AK. ALA 20% solution (Levulan Kerastick®) that is activated with blue light and 16.8% methyl-ALA cream (Metvix®) that is activated with red light. However, Metvix® is no longer available in the US market. A 10% ALA nanoemulsion gel (Ameluz®) used with red light irradiation is approved for superficial non-melanoma skin cancers in Europe, Canada, Australia, and several other countries, and has recently been expanded to the treatment of BCC and SCC in situ in the USA (Nestor et al. 2019).

Several systemic PSs are available mainly for targeting vascular lesions. Porfimer sodium (Photofrin), HpD, and the second-generation fast-clearing benzoporphyrin derivatives (such as Verteporfin) and chlorins are among the most used intravenous PSs (Zane et al. 2001).

7.1 Precancerous Lesions and Superficial Skin Cancer

7.1.1 Actinic Keratosis (AK) and Bowen's Disease (BD)

A systemic review and meta-analysis of 2174 AKs treated with cryotherapy and 2170 AKs treated with PDT found superiority of PDT over cryotherapy for treatment of thin AKs on the face and scalp with a 14% better chance of complete clearance after a three-month interval (Patel et al. 2014; Wen et al. 2017).

For more aggressive lesions such as BD, repeated sessions and monitoring are recommended because a single session of ALA-PDT allows only 53% of patients to achieve relapse-free survival at five years (Souza et al. 2009). In Brazil, a retrospective study reported a 53.8% recurrence rate in 31 BD patients who received MAL-PDT (Cabete et al. 2015), similar to what had been reported for ALA-PDT (Tarstedt et al. 2016). Nevertheless, PDT is still recommended as an alternative treatment for BD due to advantages such as being non-invasive, clinical feasibility with multiple lesions treated in one session, and superior esthetical results (Cohen and Lee 2016; Wong et al. 2001).

7.1.2 Basal Cell Carcinoma (BCC)

MAL-PDT is considered as an effective and safe therapy for patients with multiple BCCs such as Gorlin syndrome (Basset-Seguin et al. 2014).

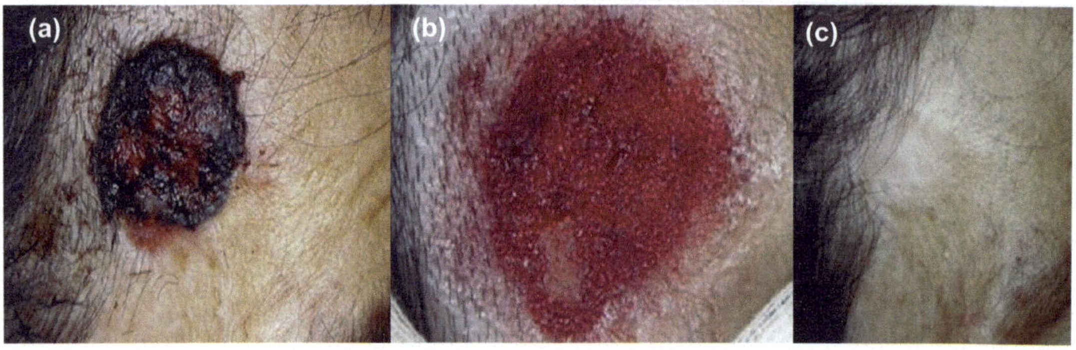

Fig. 5 **a**, **b** A 74-year-old woman with a large pigmented basal cell carcinoma on the forehead treated with ALA-PDT after debulking the main tumor. **c** Note that minimal scar after wound healing. The patient was clinically free of tumor at a three-year follow-up

This is especially true for superficial or small BCCs since thicker nodular BCCs may require a combination therapy such as debulking plus PDT to achieve complete clearance (Thissen et al. 2000) (Fig. 5 shows a case of nodular BCC treated with combination therapy by the authors). Another option for treating nodular BCC is intralesional PDT (I-PDT). In I-PDT the irradiation is delivered via insertion of a 630-nm laser beam in the tumor after letting the local injection of one percent ALA (0.2 mL/cm^2) incubate for two hours (Rodriguez-Prieto et al. 2012). In a study by Rodriguez-Prieto et al. 19 out of 20 patients treated with this strategy were free of tumor after a median follow-up of six years. The team treated another 18 BCCs successfully with this approach and analyzed the inflammatory response and cytokine levels in the tumor after I-PDT (Suarez-Valladares et al. 2018). They observed an increase in IL-1β, IL-6, and IL-8 levels after treatment (Gollnick et al. 1997; Suarez-Valladares et al. 2018).

7.1.3 Cutaneous T-Cell Lymphoma

Rodrigues *et al*. reported the first successful case of PDT treatment in lymphomatoid papulosis (LyP) lesions resistant to traditional treatments (Rodrigues et al. 2009). A study group in Japan successfully treated mycosis fungoides (MF) with PDT (Kabata et al. 2017). This team was also able to successfully treat LyP and prevent its recurrences with PDT (Arimatsu et al. 2019). They found increased expression of high mobility group box 1 (HMGB1) protein, one of the immunogenic cell death (ICD) proteins responsible for self-defense against malignant neoplasm, on the immunostaining of the PDT-treated LyP lesions (Showalter et al. 2017). These findings suggested that ICD might play an important role in PDT-induced cell death.

7.1.4 In Situ Photo-Immunotherapy (ISPI) in Melanoma

PDT alone is not recommended for treating melanoma because melanin absorbs most of the irradiated photons. However, another method known as in situ photo-immunotherapy (ISPI) is effective. ISPI comprises of topical application of an immune modifier such as imiquimod before, during, and after PDT to boost the host's immune response. ICG-photothermal therapy and/or PDT with an 805-nm laser showed great effects in local and distant tumor control in late-stage melanoma (Li et al. 2010; Naylor et al. 2006). Li et al. (2010) reported complete local response in eight out of 11 late-stage melanoma patients with one or multiple six-week cycles of ISPI.

7.1.5 Extramammary Paget's Disease (EMPD)

PDT is a non-invasive treatment for EMPD with a similar outcome compared to conventional therapy (Shieh et al. 2002). PDT combined with imiquimod can enhance the efficacy of PDT by

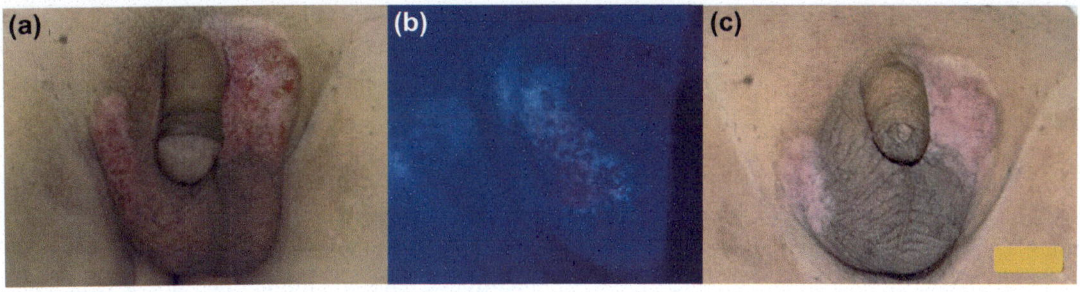

Fig. 6 **a** 65-year-old man with extramammary Paget's disease on the scrotum successfully treated with ALA-PDT. A Large lesions on the scrotum before treatment. **b** Vivid fluorescence was observed under Wood's lamp illumination which highlighted the tumor after one-hour incubation with BF-200 ALA. **c** Clinically free of tumor at two months after eight PDT sessions in two weeks (white light 100 J/cm^2 each, totally 800 J/cm^2) followed by ten days of topical application of imiquimod

boosting the immune response against EMPD (Bauman et al. 2018; Jing et al. 2014). A multicentric retrospective study on vulvar Paget's disease involving six hospitals in France reported 15% complete response and 38% partial response with PDT that is similar to other therapies (Rioli et al. 2018). ALA-PDT is also applied in secondary EMPD as a palliative treatment (Shen et al. 2018). The authors have also successfully treated EMPD with ALA-PDT using the same approach (Fig. 6, unpublished data).

7.2 Benign Lesions

7.2.1 Vascular Malformation

Most reports on the use of PDT in the treatment of PWS are from China. Qin et al. reported the use of PDT in 1,385 patients with PWS using different photosensitizers such as HMME, HpD, and photocarcinorin (PsD-007) with argon laser as the light source. They were able to demonstrate fair to excellent results in 92.3% after one session of PDT (Qiu et al. 2011). These findings were in line with their previous study on 238 patients treated with PsD-007 and a copper-vapor laser that had a 98% response rate after two to four sessions of PDT (excellent response in 29%, good in 32%, and fair in 37%) (Qin et al. 2007).

In a study including 581 individuals with PWS, the efficacy of PDT coupled with copper-vapor laser (510.6 and 578.2 nm), as the light source, was higher than conventional pulsed dye laser (PDL) with lower rates of complications reported for PDT (Yuan et al. 2008). PDT has also been used in combination with PDL to minimize the adverse effects and achieve a higher efficacy. Benzoporphyrin derivative monoacid ring (BPD-MA) was used as the photosensitizer in this treatment strategy (Kelly et al. 2004; Tournas et al. 2009).

Very few studies have also reported the use of PDT on vascular anomalies other than PWS. In a study by Jerjes et al., 43 individuals with different types of arteriovenous malformation were treated with meta-tetra hydroxyphenyl chlorine (mTHPC and temoporfin)-mediated PDT which resulted in >50% reduction in the size of the lesions in 15 patients, <50% reduction in 11 patients, <25% reduction in 12 patients, and five non-responders (Jerjes et al. 2011).

Likewise, cutaneous vascular tumors have also been targeted with PDT. In a mouse model, BPD-MA-mediated PDT with a 690-nm laser as the light source was able to eradicate tumors (Middelkamp-Hup et al. 2003). Moreover, successful treatment of Kaposi sarcoma and angiosarcoma have been achieved with PDT in a few case reports and a small case series (Chin et al. 2008; Tardivo et al. 2006; Thong et al. 2007).

7.2.2 Rosacea

Twenty patients with the diagnosis of rosacea that underwent four sessions of ALA-PDT showed significant improvements in flushing, erythema, and papule/pustules with transient adverse events including erythema and swelling being in the acceptable range (Fan et al. 2018). The possible mechanism of PDT in the treatment of rosacea might be related to its effects on increasing the toll-like receptor (TLR) expression, downregulating cytokine secretion, and killing Demodex species (Gilaberte et al. 2009; Ma et al. 2016).

7.2.3 Acne Vulgaris

ALA is selectively absorbed by the pilosebaceous unit and metabolized to PpIX in sebocytes. When excited with light, the formation of ROS/singlet oxygen causes apoptosis of sebocytes (Endly and Miller 2017). ALA-PDT had shown anti-inflammatory, immune-regulatory, and antibacterial effects in the treatment of acne. Recent randomized trials showed that ALA-PDT is more effective in reducing inflammation and total lesion count in acne patients compared to traditional oral doxycycline plus topical adapalene (Nicklas et al. 2019). A proof-of-concept study of a new formulation of five percent ALA thermosetting gel also showed significant improvements in inflammatory acne (Serini et al. 2019). However, high-quality evidence-based studies of PDT treatment for acne are lacking (Barbaric et al. 2016).

7.2.4 Skin Rejuvenation

A new application of PDT is in skin rejuvenation. PDT reduces fine wrinkles, skin roughness, actinic elastosis, and mottled hyperpigmentation (Karrer et al. 2013; Philipp-Dormston 2018). Kim et al. showed that conditioned media from PDT-treated keratinocytes or dermal fibroblasts had reduced melanin content and tyrosinase activity without any effect on the survival in melanocytes (Kim et al. 2018).

7.2.5 Cutaneous Leishmaniasis (CL)

Recently, a meta-analysis of six studies utilizing ALA or MAL-PDT in the treatment of CL showed promising results. Nevertheless, most cases needed several sessions to achieve complete resolution (Snoek et al. 2008). A randomized controlled trial showed a superior effect of ALA-PDT in treating CL compared to paromomycin and placebo (Asilian and Davami 2006). All patients in the ALA-PDT group were amastigote-free.

7.2.6 Condyloma Acuminatum (CA) and Verruca

ALA-PDT could significantly reduce both CA recurrence rates and human papilloma viral loads (Hu et al. 2018; Ying et al. 2013). Applying ALA-PDT immediately after CO_2 laser evaporation can improve the absorption of ALA and increase the effectiveness of PDT (Zhang et al. 2019).

Li *et al.* reported an overall clearance of more than 60% in 6,146 verruca lesions treated with ALA-PDT (Li et al. 2014). Qian *et al.* (Qian et al. 2014) and Yang *et al.* (Yang et al. 2016) also reported excellent results after several sessions of ALA-PDT in recalcitrant facial verruca. A preliminary study of ALA-PDT on recalcitrant facial verruca pretreated with pulsed CO_2 laser showed complete clearance of the lesions (Gao et al. 2016). Recalcitrant verruca vulgaris on the hands and feet are also responsive to PDT (Stender et al. 1999).

7.2.7 Miscellaneous Conditions

Hypericin, a natural chromophore found in *Hypericum perforatum* L. (St. John's wort) has attracted attention as a photosensitizer for PDT in recent years due to its selective accumulation in neoplastic tissue. A phase II placebo-controlled clinical study of PDT with topical hypericin was conducted in patients with patch/plaque stage MF and plaque-type psoriasis and found a positive response in 50% and 60-80% of cases, respectively (Rook et al. 2010).

In a study consisting of ten patients with vulvar lichen sclerosis et atrophicus (VLSA), all patients reported some degree of satisfaction after ALA-PDT (Lan et al. 2018). Olejek *et al.* reported a decrease in inflammation and an increase in the number of microvessels in VLSA lesions after PDT (Olejek et al. 2009). A systematic review showed that VLSA lesions improved after PDT in most studies but the histologic outcomes were inconsistent and thus further research on the mechanism of PDT in this disease is needed (Prodromidou et al. 2018).

Two new off-label indications of PDT are localized scleroderma and keloid (Wen et al. 2017).

8 Adverse Events

The major drawback of PDT is intolerable burning or stinging pain that occurs during treatment especially in areas with abundant sensory neurons like the nipple, genitalia, fingers, and toes (Kennedy and Pottier 1992). The treated area becomes inflamed and edematous. Fortunately, the discomfort usually lasts for only one to two days after treatment.

9 The New Era of PDT

9.1 Daylight PDT

In order to overcome the disadvantages (pain) and limitations (size of irradiation) of conventional PDT (cPDT), natural daylight PDT (dPDT) emerged in Europe around 2006 (Wiegell et al. 2008). The dPDT is more convenient and less painful and has fewer cutaneous adverse effects while being comparable in efficacy to cPDT (Rubel et al. 2014; Wiegell et al. 2008). Many studies revealed dPDT to be significantly less painful than cPDT referring to it as a "gain without pain" treatment (Mei et al. 2018; Zhao et al. 2018). A prospective study revealed an inferior efficacy for dPDT in treating grade II AK on the face/scalp compared to cPDT. Their complete remission rates (CR) were 36% and 61%, respectively (Fargnoli et al. 2015). In a meta-analysis of randomized controlled trials comparing cPDT (using MAL and red light) with dPDT (2-2.5 h' daylight illumination after MAL application) (Mei et al. 2018), the CR of high-grade AK after three to 12 months was significantly lower in the dPDT group compared to the cPDT group. However, in low-grade AK (I-II), the two methods of PDT had comparable results. These reports suggest that the therapeutic efficacy of dPDT in high-grade AK should be further studied (Mei et al. 2018). On the other hand, a consensus published by international experts recommended dPDT for the therapy of "actinic field damage" under the concept of "field cancerization" (Philipp-Dormston et al. 2016).

9.2 Combination Therapy

Several reports have shown that combining chemotherapy with PDT enhances treatment efficacy. Topical five percent 5-fluorouracil (5-FU) cream combined with dPDT in 24 AK patients showed a significantly higher response rate than dPDT alone (Nissen et al. 2017). Pretreatment with 5-FU for three days could enhance ALA-PDT efficacy in mouse models of SCC (Anand et al. 2017). In vitro and in vivo experiments revealed temozolomide-loaded carboxylated poly amido-amine combined with PDT could be used in melanoma (Tang et al. 2018). The authors have reported a case of recalcitrant lip verrucous carcinoma treated successfully with a combination of cryo-immunotherapy, CO_2 laser, acitretin, and ALA-PDT (Lee et al. 2018). The efficacy of this combination may be related to the release of damage-associated molecular patterns (DAMPs) (Luo et al. 2018).

10 Conclusion

In conclusion, PDT has been used to treat various benign and malignant skin diseases with promising results. The adverse events can be reduced by different modifications of the irradiation protocols. Hypothetically, the effectiveness of PDT treatment, especially in vascular lesions, may be influenced by genetic polymorphisms but further studies are needed to confirm this theory.

References

Ackroyd R, Kelty C, Brown N, Reed M (2001) The history of photodetection and photodynamic therapy. Photochem Photobiol 74:656–669

Anand S, Rollakanti KR, Brankov N, Brash DE, Hasan T, Maytin EV (2017) Fluorouracil enhances photodynamic therapy of squamous cell carcinoma via a p53-independent mechanism that increases protoporphyrin IX levels and tumor cell death. Mol Cancer Ther 16:1092–1101

Arimatsu A, Tomii K, Fujiwara H, Hasegawa G, Shigehara Y, Tachibana T (2019) Photodynamic therapy prevented the recurrence of lymphomatoid papulosis. Photodiagn Photodyn Ther

Ash C, Dubec M, Donne K, Bashford T (2017) Effect of wavelength and beam width on penetration in light-tissue interaction using computational methods. Lasers Med Sci 32:1909–1918

Asilian A, Davami M (2006) Comparison between the efficacy of photodynamic therapy and topical paromomycin in the treatment of Old World cutaneous leishmaniasis: a placebo-controlled, randomized clinical trial. Clin Exp Dermatol 31:634–637

Bagazgoitia L, Cuevas Santos J, Juarranz A, Jaen P (2011) Photodynamic therapy reduces the histological features of actinic damage and the expression of early oncogenic markers. Br J Dermatol 165:144–151

Barbaric J, Abbott R, Posadzki P, Car M, Gunn LH, Layton AM, Majeed A, Car J (2016) Light therapies for acne. Cochrane Database Syst Rev 9:CD007917

Basset-Seguin N, Bissonnette R, Girard C, Haedersdal M, Lear JT, Paul C, Piaserico S (2014) Consensus recommendations for the treatment of basal cell carcinomas in Gorlin syndrome with topical methylaminolaevulinate-photodynamic therapy. J Eur Acad Dermatol Venereol 28:626–632

Bauman TM, Rosman IS, Sheinbein DM (2018) Extramammary Paget's disease of the scrotum with complete response to imiquimod and photodynamic therapy. BMJ Case Rep 2018

Brancaleon L, Moseley H (2002) Laser and non-laser light sources for photodynamic therapy. Lasers Med Sci 17:173–186

Cabete J, Rafael M, Cravo M, Moura C, Sachse F, Pecegueiro M (2015) Long-term recurrence of non-melanoma skin cancer after topical methylaminolevulinate photodynamic therapy in a dermato-oncology department. An Bras Dermatol 90:846–850

Castano AP, Demidova TN, Hamblin MR (2004) Mechanisms in photodynamic therapy: part one-photosensitizers, photochemistry and cellular localization. Photodiagn Photodyn Ther 1:279–293

Chin WWL, Heng PWS, Thong PSP, Bhuvaneswari R, Hirt W, Kuenzel S, Soo KC, Olivo M (2008) Improved formulation of photosensitizer chlorin e6 polyvinylpyrrolidone for fluorescence diagnostic imaging and photodynamic therapy of human cancer. Eur J Pharm Biopharm 69:1083–1093

Chiu W-T, Tran T-TV, Pan S-C, Huang H-K, Chen Y-C, Wong T-W (2019) Cystic fibrosis transmembrane conductance regulator: a possible new target for photodynamic therapy enhances wound healing. Adv Wound Care

Choi SH, Seo JW, Kim KH (2018) Comparative study of the bactericidal effects of indocyanine green- and methyl aminolevulinate-based photodynamic therapy on Propionibacterium acnes as a new treatment for acne. J Dermatol 45:824–829

Cohen DK, Lee PK (2016) Photodynamic therapy for non-melanoma skin cancers. Cancers 8:90

Collaud S, Juzeniene A, Moan J, Lange N (2004) On the selectivity of 5-aminolevulinic acid-induced protoporphyrin IX formation. Curr Med Chem Anticancer Agents 4:301–316

Endly DC, Miller RA (2017) Oily skin: a review of treatment options. J Clin Aesthet Dermatol 10:49–55

Fan L, Yin R, Lan T, Hamblin MR (2018) Photodynamic therapy for rosacea in Chinese patients. Photodiagn Photodyn Ther 24:82–87

Fargnoli MC, Piccioni A, Neri L, Tambone S, Pellegrini C, Peris K (2015) Conventional versus daylight methyl aminolevulinate photodynamic therapy for actinic keratosis of the face and scalp: an intra-patient, prospective, comparison study in Italy. J Eur Acad Dermatol Venereol 29:1926–1932

Gao J, Shen C, Ko R, Zheng X, Wang Z, Liu S, Li Y, Tang M, Yin W, Yang C, Zhang X (2016) Combination effect of super pulsed carbon dioxide laser and photodynamic therapy for recalcitrant facial flat warts: a preliminary study. J Cosmet Laser Ther 18:56–57

Gilaberte Y, Frias MP, Rezusta A, Vera-Alvarez J (2009) Photodynamic therapy with methyl aminolevulinate for resistant scalp folliculitis secondary to Demodex infestation. J Eur Acad Dermatol Venereol 23:718–719

Gollnick SO, Evans SS, Baumann H, Owczarczak B, Maier P, Vaughan L, Wang WC, Unger E, Henderson BW (2003) Role of cytokines in photodynamic therapy-induced local and systemic inflammation. Br J Cancer 88:1772–1779

Gollnick SO, Liu X, Owczarczak B, Musser DA, Henderson BW (1997) Altered expression of interleukin 6 and interleukin 10 as a result of photodynamic therapy in vivo. Cancer Res 57:3904–3909

Hall JA, Keller PJ, Keller GS (2004) Dose response of combination photorejuvenation using intense pulsed light-activated photodynamic therapy and radiofrequency energy. Arch Facial Plast Surg 6:374–378

Hinnen P, de Rooij FW, van Velthuysen ML, Edixhoven A, van Hillegersberg R, Tilanus HW, Wilson JH, Siersema PD (1998) Biochemical basis of 5-aminolaevulinic acid-induced protoporphyrin IX accumulation: a study in patients with (pre)malignant lesions of the oesophagus. Br J Cancer 78:679–682

Hsieh YJ, Wu CC, Chang CJ, Yu JS (2003) Subcellular localization of Photofrin® determines the death phenotype of human epidermoid carcinoma A431 cells triggered by photodynamic therapy: when plasma membranes are the main targets. J Cell Physiol 194:363–375

Hu Z, Liu L, Zhang W, Liu H, Li J, Jiang L, Zeng K (2018) Dynamics of HPV viral loads reflect the treatment effect of photodynamic therapy in genital warts. Photodiagn Photodyn Ther 21:86–90

Huang Z (2005) A review of progress in clinical photodynamic therapy. Technol Cancer Res Treat 4:283–293

Immonen I, Seitsonen S, Tommila P, Kangas-Kontio T, Kakko S, Savolainen E-R, Savolainen MJ, Liinamaa MJ (2010) Vascular endothelial growth factor gene variation and the response to photodynamic therapy in age-related macular degeneration. Ophthalmology 117:103–108

Jalili A, Makowski M, Świtaj T, Nowis D, Wilczyński GM, Wilczek E, Chorąży-Massalska M, Radzikowska A, Maśliński W, Biały Ł (2004) Effective photoimmunotherapy of murine colon carcinoma induced by the combination of photodynamic therapy and dendritic cells. Clin Cancer Res 10:4498–4508

Jerjes W, Upile T, Hamdoon Z, Mosse CA, Akram S, Morley S, Hopper C (2011) Interstitial PDT for vascular anomalies. Lasers Surg Med 43:357–365

Jing W, Juan X, Li X, Jiayuan C, Qin H, Qing L, Shengmei X (2014) Complete remission of two patients with recurrent and wide spread extramammary Paget disease obtained from 5-aminolevulinic acid-based photodynamic therapy and imiquimod combination treatment. Photodiagn Photodyn Ther 11:434–440

Joly F, Deret S, Gamboa B, Menigot C, Fogel P, Mounier C, Reiniche P, Sidou F, Aubert J, Lear J, Fryer AA, Zolezzi F, Voegel JJ (2018) Photodynamic therapy corrects abnormal cancer-associated gene expression observed in actinic keratosis lesions and induces a remodeling effect in photodamaged skin. J Dermatol Sci

Kabata Y, Shimomura Y, Matsuo Y, Fujiwara H, Abe R (2017) Photodynamic therapy with intradermal application of 5-aminolevulinic acid successfully improved tumor lesions of mycosis fungoides. Int J Dermatol 56:e81–e82

Kabingu E, Vaughan L, Owczarczak B, Ramsey K, Gollnick S (2007) CD8+ T cell-mediated control of distant tumours following local photodynamic therapy is independent of CD4+ T cells and dependent on natural killer cells. Br J Cancer 96:1839

Karrer S, Kohl E, Feise K, Hiepe-Wegener D, Lischner S, Philipp-Dormston W, Podda M, Prager W, Walker T, Szeimies RM (2013) Photodynamic therapy for skin rejuvenation: review and summary of the literature–results of a consensus conference of an expert group for aesthetic photodynamic therapy. J Dtsch Dermatol Ges 11:137–148

Kelly KM, Kimel S, Smith T, Stacy A, Hammer-Wilson MJ, Svaasand LO, Nelson JS (2004) Combined photodynamic and photothermal induced injury enhances damage to in vivo model blood vessels. Lasers Surg Med: Off J Am Soc Laser Med Surg 34:407–413

Kennedy JC, Pottier RH (1992) Endogenous protoporphyrin IX, a clinically useful photosensitizer for photodynamic therapy. J Photochem Photobiol B 14:275–292

Kim SK, Oh SJ, Park SY, Kim WJ, Kim YS, Kim YC (2018) Photodynamic therapy inhibits melanogenesis through paracrine effects by keratinocytes and fibroblasts. Pigment Cell Melanoma Res 31:277–286

Kongshaug M, Moan J, Brown SB (1989) The distribution of porphyrins with different tumour localising ability among human plasma proteins. Br J Cancer 59:184–188

Korbelik M, Sun J, Cecic I (2005) Photodynamic therapy–induced cell surface expression and release of heat shock proteins: relevance for tumor response. Cancer Res 65:1018–1026

Krosl G, Korbelik M, Dougherty G (1995) Induction of immune cell infiltration into murine SCCVII tumour by photofrin-based photodynamic therapy. Br J Cancer 71:549

Lan T, Zou Y, Hamblin MR, Yin R (2018) 5-Aminolevulinic acid photodynamic therapy in refractory vulvar lichen sclerosus et atrophicus: series of ten cases. Photodiagn Photodyn Ther 21:234–238

Lee CN, Huang CC, Lin IC, Lee JY, Ou CY, Wong TW (2018) Recalcitrant lip verrucous carcinoma successfully treated with acitretin after carbon dioxide laser ablation. JAAD Case Rep 4:576–578

Li Q, Jiao B, Zhou F, Tan Q, Ma Y, Luo L, Zhai J, Luan Q, Li C, Wang G, Gao T (2014) Comparative study of photodynamic therapy with 5%, 10% and 20% aminolevulinic acid in the treatment of generalized recalcitrant facial verruca plana: a randomized clinical trial. J Eur Acad Dermatol Venereol 28:1821–1826

Li X, Naylor MF, Le H, Nordquist RE, Teague TK, Howard CA, Murray C, Chen WR (2010) Clinical effects of in situ photoimmunotherapy on late-stage melanoma patients: a preliminary study. Cancer Biol Ther 10:1081–1087

Luo M, Shi L, Zhang F, Zhou F, Zhang L, Wang B, Wang P, Zhang Y, Zhang H, Yang D, Zhang G, Chen WR, Wang X (2018) Laser immunotherapy for cutaneous squamous cell carcinoma with optimal thermal effects to enhance tumour immunogenicity. Int J Hyperthermia 34:1337–1350

Ma Y, Chen Q, Liu Y, Wang Q, Huang Z, Xiang L (2016) Effects of 5-aminolevulinic acid photodynamic therapy on TLRs in acne lesions and keratinocytes co-cultured with P. acnes. Photodiagn Photodyn Ther 15:172–181

Marks R, Rennie G, Selwood TS (1988) Malignant transformation of solar keratoses to squamous cell carcinoma. Lancet 1:795–797

Maziere J, Morliere P, Santus R (1991) The role of the low density lipoprotein receptor pathway in the delivery of lipophilic photosensitizers in the photodynamic therapy of tumours. Journal of photochemistry and photobiology. B, Biology 8:351–360

McDonagh AF (2001) Phototherapy: from ancient Egypt to the new millennium. J Perinatol 21(Suppl 1):S7–S12
Mei X, Wang L, Zhang R, Zhong S (2018) Daylight versus conventional photodynamic therapy for the treatment of actinic keratosis: a meta-analysis of randomized controlled trials. Photodiagn Photodyn Ther
Michelini M (2018) Photodynamic therapy activated by intense pulsed light in the treatment of actinic keratosis. G Ital Dermatol Venereol
Middelkamp-Hup MA, Sánchez-Carpintero I, Kossodo S, Waterman P, González S, Mihm MC Jr, Anderson RR (2003) Photodynamic therapy for cutaneous proliferative vascular tumors in a mouse model. J Investig Dermatol 121:634–639
Mroz P, Hashmi JT, Huang Y-Y, Lange N, Hamblin MR (2011) Stimulation of anti-tumor immunity by photodynamic therapy. Expert Rev Clin Immunol 7:75–91
Naylor MF, Chen WR, Teague TK, Perry LA, Nordquist RE (2006) In situ photoimmunotherapy: a tumour-directed treatment for melanoma. Br J Dermatol 155:1287–1292
Nestor MS, Berman B, Patel J, Lawson A (2019) Safety and efficacy of aminolevulinic acid 10% topical gel versus aminolevulinic acid 20% topical solution followed by blue-light photodynamic therapy for the treatment of actinic keratosis on the face and scalp: a randomized, double-blind study. J Clin Aesthet Dermatol 12:32–38
Neugebauer R, Su KA, Zhu Z, Sokil M, Chren MM, Friedman GD, Asgari MM (2019) Comparative effectiveness of treatment of actinic keratosis with topical fluorouracil and imiquimod in the prevention of keratinocyte carcinoma: a cohort study. J Am Acad Dermatol 80:998–1005
Nicklas C, Rubio R, Cardenas C, Hasson A (2019) Comparison of efficacy of aminolaevulinic acid photodynamic therapy vs. adapalene gel plus oral doxycycline for treatment of moderate acne vulgaris-A simple, blind, randomized, and controlled trial. Photodermatol Photoimmunol Photomed 35:3–10
Nissen CV, Heerfordt IM, Wiegell SR, Mikkelsen CS, Wulf HC (2017) Pretreatment with 5-fluorouracil cream enhances the efficacy of daylight-mediated photodynamic therapy for actinic keratosis. Acta Derm Venereol 97:617–621
Noodt BB, Berg K, Stokke T, Peng Q, Nesland JM (1996) Apoptosis and necrosis induced with light and 5-aminolaevulinic acid-derived protoporphyrin IX. Br J Cancer 74:22–29
Ohgari Y, Nakayasu Y, Kitajima S, Sawamoto M, Mori H, Shimokawa O, Matsui H, Taketani S (2005) Mechanisms involved in delta-aminolevulinic acid (ALA)-induced photosensitivity of tumor cells: relation of ferrochelatase and uptake of ALA to the accumulation of protoporphyrin. Biochem Pharmacol 71:42–49
Olejek A, Kozak-Darmas I, Kellas-Sleczka S, Steplewska K, Biniszkiewicz T, Birkner B, Jarek A, Nowak L, Stencel-Gabriel K, Sieron A (2009) Effectiveness of photodynamic therapy in the treatment of lichen sclerosus: cell changes in immunohistochemistry. Neuro Endocrinol Lett 30:547–551
Parmeggiani F, Costagliola C, Gemmati D, D'Angelo S, Perri P, Scapoli GL, Catozzi L, Federici F, Sebastiani A, Incorvaia C (2007) Predictive role of coagulation-balance gene polymorphisms in the efficacy of photodynamic therapy with verteporfin for classic choroidal neovascularization secondary to age-related macular degeneration. Pharmacogenet Genomics 17:1039–1046
Patel G, Armstrong AW, Eisen DB (2014) Efficacy of photodynamic therapy vs other interventions in randomized clinical trials for the treatment of actinic keratoses: a systematic review and meta-analysis. JAMA Dermatol 150:1281–1288
Philipp-Dormston WG (2018) Photodynamic therapy for aesthetic-cosmetic indications. G Ital Dermatol Venereol 153:817–826
Philipp-Dormston WG, Sanclemente G, Torezan L, Tretti Clementoni M, Le Pillouer-Prost A, Cartier H, Szeimies RM, Bjerring P (2016) Daylight photodynamic therapy with MAL cream for large-scale photodamaged skin based on the concept of "actinic field damage": recommendations of an international expert group. J Eur Acad Dermatol Venereol 30:8–15
Piccolo D, Kostaki D (2018) Photodynamic therapy activated by intense pulsed light in the treatment of nonmelanoma skin cancer. Biomedicines 6
Preise D, Oren R, Glinert I, Kalchenko V, Jung S, Scherz A, Salomon Y (2009) Systemic antitumor protection by vascular-targeted photodynamic therapy involves cellular and humoral immunity. Cancer Immunol Immunother 58:71–84
Prodromidou A, Chatziioannou E, Daskalakis G, Stergios K, Pergialiotis V (2018) Photodynamic therapy for vulvar lichen sclerosus-a systematic review. J Low Genit Tract Dis 22:58–65
Qian G, Wang S, Deng D, Yang G (2014) Is the step-up therapy of topical 5-aminolevulinic acid photodynamic therapy effective and safe for the patients with recalcitrant facial flat wart? Dermatol Ther 27:83–88
Qin Z-P, Li K-L, Ren L, Liu X-J (2007) Photodynamic therapy of port wine stains—a report of 238 cases. Photodiagn Photodyn Ther 4:53–59
Qiu H, Gu Y, Wang Y, Huang N (2011) Twenty years of clinical experience with a new modality of vascular-targeted photodynamic therapy for port wine stains. Dermatol Surg 37:1603–1610
Reginato E, Wolf P, Hamblin MR (2014) Immune response after photodynamic therapy increases anti-cancer and anti-bacterial effects. World J Immunol 4:1
Reinhold U, Dirschka T, Ostendorf R, Aschoff R, Berking C, Philipp-Dormston WG, Hahn S, Lau K, Jager A, Schmitz B, Lubbert H, Szeimies RM (2016) A randomized, double-blind, phase III, multicentre study to evaluate the safety and efficacy of BF-200 ALA (Ameluz((R))) versus placebo in the field-directed treatment of mild-to-moderate actinic keratosis with photodynamic therapy (PDT) when using the BF-RhodoLED((R)) lamp. Br J Dermatol 175:696–705

Rioli DI, Samimi M, Beneton N, Hainaut E, Martin L, Misery L, Quereux G (2018) Efficacy and tolerance of photodynamic therapy for vulvar Paget's disease: a multicentric retrospective study. Eur J Dermatol 28:351–355

Rodrigues M, McCormack C, Yap LM, Prince HM, Roberts H, Williams R, Foley P (2009) Successful treatment of lymphomatoid papulosis with photodynamic therapy. Australas J Dermatol 50:129–132

Rodriguez-Prieto MA, Gonzalez-Sixto B, Perez-Bustillo A, Alonso-Alonso T, Ortega-Valin L, Martinez-Valderrabano V, Gonzalez-Moran A, Garcia Doval I (2012) Photodynamic therapy with intralesional photosensitizer and laser beam application: an alternative treatment for nodular basal cell carcinoma. J Am Acad Dermatol 67:e134-136

Rook AH, Wood GS, Duvic M, Vonderheid EC, Tobia A, Cabana B (2010) A phase II placebo-controlled study of photodynamic therapy with topical hypericin and visible light irradiation in the treatment of cutaneous T-cell lymphoma and psoriasis. J Am Acad Dermatol 63:984–990

Rubel DM, Spelman L, Murrell DF, See JA, Hewitt D, Foley P, Bosc C, Kerob D, Kerrouche N, Wulf HC, Shumack S (2014) Daylight photodynamic therapy with methyl aminolevulinate cream as a convenient, similarly effective, nearly painless alternative to conventional photodynamic therapy in actinic keratosis treatment: a randomized controlled trial. Br J Dermatol 171:1164–1171

Rybarski M, Schmitz L, Novak B, Dirschka T (2018) Daylight photodynamic therapy for field cancerization: lessons from molecular biology. G Ital Dermatol Venereol 153:806–810

Schmidt-Erfurth U, Hasan T (2000) Mechanisms of action of photodynamic therapy with verteporfin for the treatment of age-related macular degeneration. Surv Ophthalmol 45:195–214

Serini SM, Cannizzaro MV, Dattola A, Garofalo V, Del Duca E, Ventura A, Milani M, Campione E, Bianchi L (2019) The efficacy and tolerability of 5-aminolevulinic acid 5% thermosetting gel photodynamic therapy (PDT) in the treatment of mild-to-moderate acne vulgaris. A two-center, prospective assessor-blinded, proof-of-concept study. J Cosmet Dermatol 18:156–162

Shah SM, Konnikov N, Duncan LM, Tannous ZS (2009) The effect of 595 nm pulsed dye laser on superficial and nodular basal cell carcinomas. Lasers Surg Med 41:417–422

Shahbazi M, Fryer AA, Pravica V, Brogan IJ, Ramsay HM, Hutchinson IV, Harden PN (2002) Vascular endothelial growth factor gene polymorphisms are associated with acute renal allograft rejection. J Am Soc Nephrol 13:260–264

Shen S, Zhang G, Wang P, Zhang Y, Keyal U, Ji J, Wang X (2018) ALA-PDT as palliative care in a patient with secondary perineum EMPD. Photodiagn Photodyn Ther 22:166–168

Shieh S, Dee AS, Cheney RT, Frawley NP, Zeitouni NC, Oseroff AR (2002) Photodynamic therapy for the treatment of extramammary Paget's disease. Br J Dermatol 146:1000–1005

Showalter A, Limaye A, Oyer JL, Igarashi R, Kittipatarin C, Copik AJ, Khaled AR (2017) Cytokines in immunogenic cell death: applications for cancer immunotherapy. Cytokine 97:123–132

Slaughter DP, Southwick HW, Smejkal W (1953) Field cancerization in oral stratified squamous epithelium; clinical implications of multicentric origin. Cancer 6:963–968

Soleymani T, Abrouk M, Kelly KM (2017) An Analysis of laser therapy for the treatment of nonmelanoma skin cancer. Dermatol Surg 43:615–624

Souza CS, Felicio LB, Ferreira J, Kurachi C, Bentley MV, Tedesco AC, Bagnato VS (2009) Long-term follow-up of topical 5-aminolaevulinic acid photodynamic therapy diode laser single session for non-melanoma skin cancer. Photodiagn Photodyn Ther 6:207–213

Stender IM, Lock-Andersen J, Wulf HC (1999) Recalcitrant hand and foot warts successfully treated with photodynamic therapy with topical 5-aminolaevulinic acid: a pilot study. Clin Exp Dermatol 24:154–159

Suarez-Valladares MJ, Calleja-Antolin SM, Ruiz G, de Morales JM, Rodriguez Prieto MA, Vega-Gutierrez J (2018) Inflammatory response and cytokine levels induced by intralesional photodynamic therapy and 630-nm laser in a case series of basal cell carcinoma. J Am Acad Dermatol 79:580–582

Tammela T, Enholm B, Alitalo K, Paavonen K (2005) The biology of vascular endothelial growth factors. Cardiovasc Res 65:550–563

Tang J, Zhou H, Hou X, Wang L, Li Y, Pang Y, Chen C, Jiang G, Liu Y (2018) Enhanced anti-tumor efficacy of temozolomide-loaded carboxylated poly(amido-amine) combined with photothermal/photodynamic therapy for melanoma treatment. Cancer Lett 423:16–26

Tardivo JP, Giglio AD, Paschoal LH, Baptista MS (2006) New photodynamic therapy protocol to treat AIDS-related Kaposi's sarcoma. Photomed Laser Ther 24:528–531

Tarstedt M, Gillstedt M, Wennberg Larko AM, Paoli J (2016) Aminolevulinic acid and methyl aminolevulinate equally effective in topical photodynamic therapy for non-melanoma skin cancers. J Eur Acad Dermatol Venereol 30:420–423

Thissen MR, Schroeter CA, Neumann HA (2000) Photodynamic therapy with delta-aminolaevulinic acid for nodular basal cell carcinomas using a prior debulking technique. Br J Dermatol 142:338–339

Thong PS-P, Ong K-W, Goh NS-G, Kho K-W, Manivasager V, Bhuvaneswari R, Olivo M, Soo K-C (2007) Photodynamic-therapy-activated immune response against distant untreated tumours in recurrent angiosarcoma. Lancet Oncol 8:950–952

Tournas JA, Lai J, Truitt A, Huang Y, Osann KE, Choi B, Kelly KM (2009) Combined benzoporphyrin derivative monoacid ring photodynamic therapy and pulsed dye laser for port wine stain birthmarks. Photodiagn Photodyn Ther 6:195–199

Tuchin VV, Genina EA, Bashkatov AN, Simonenko GV, Odoevskaya OD, Altshuler GB (2003) A pilot study of ICG laser therapy of acne vulgaris: photodynamic and photothermolysis treatment. Lasers Surg Med 33:296–310

van der Snoek EM, Robinson DJ, van Hellemond JJ, Neumann HA (2008) A review of photodynamic therapy in cutaneous leishmaniasis. J Eur Acad Dermatol Venereol 22:918–922

Wei LH, Baumann H, Tracy E, Wang Y, Hutson A, Rose-John S, Henderson BW (2007) Interleukin-6 trans signalling enhances photodynamic therapy by modulating cell cycling. Br J Cancer 97:1513–1522

Wen X, Li Y, Hamblin MR (2017) Photodynamic therapy in dermatology beyond non-melanoma cancer: an update. Photodiagn Photodyn Ther 19:140–152

Wiegell SR, Haedersdal M, Philipsen PA, Eriksen P, Enk CD, Wulf HC (2008) Continuous activation of PpIX by daylight is as effective as and less painful than conventional photodynamic therapy for actinic keratoses; a randomized, controlled, single-blinded study. Br J Dermatol 158:740–746

Wiegell SR, Wulf HC, Szeimies RM, Basset-Seguin N, Bissonnette R, Gerritsen MJ, Gilaberte Y, Calzavara-Pinton P, Morton CA, Sidoroff A, Braathen LR (2012) Daylight photodynamic therapy for actinic keratosis: an international consensus: international society for photodynamic therapy in dermatology. J Eur Acad Dermatol Venereol 26:673–679

Wong T-W, Wu E-C, Ko W-C, Lee C-C, Hor L-I, Huang IH (2018) Photodynamic inactivation of methicillin-resistant Staphylococcus aureus by indocyanine green and near infrared light. Dermatol Sin 36:8–15

Wong TW, Liao SZ, Ko WC, Wu CJ, Wu SB, Chuang YC, Huang IH (2019) Indocyanine green-mediated photodynamic therapy reduces methicillin-resistant staphylococcus aureus drug resistance. J Clin Med 8

Wong TW, Sheu HM, Lee JY, Fletcher RJ (2001) Photodynamic therapy for Bowen's disease (squamous cell carcinoma in situ) of the digit. Dermatol Surg 27:452–456

Wong TW, Tracy E, Oseroff AR, Baumann H (2003) Photodynamic therapy mediates immediate loss of cellular responsiveness to cytokines and growth factors. Cancer Res 63:3812–3818

Yang X, Palasuberniam P, Kraus D, Chen B (2015) Aminolevulinic acid-based tumor detection and therapy: molecular mechanisms and strategies for enhancement. Int J Mol Sci 16:25865–25880

Yang YL, Sang J, Liao NX, Wei F, Liao W, Chen JH (2016) Off-label photodynamic therapy for recalcitrant facial flat warts using topical 5-aminolevulinic acid. Lasers Med Sci 31:929–936

Ying Z, Li X, Dang H (2013) 5-aminolevulinic acid-based photodynamic therapy for the treatment of condylomata acuminata in Chinese patients: a meta-analysis. Photodermatol Photoimmunol Photomed 29:149–159

Yuan K-H, Li Q, Yu W-L, Zeng D, Zhang C, Huang Z (2008) Comparison of photodynamic therapy and pulsed dye laser in patients with port wine stain birthmarks: a retrospective analysis. Photodiagn Photodyn Ther 5:50–57

Zane C, De Panfilis G, Calzavara-Pinton P (2001) Photosensitizers—systemic sensitization. In: Comprehensive series in photosciences. Elsevier, pp 101–114

Zhang L, Li X, Liu X, Gao Y, Tang Q (2019) Treatment of multi-position condyloma acuminatum with topical CO2 laser combined photodynamic therapy—Report of 6 cases. Photodiagn Photodyn Ther

Zhao W, Guan M, Nong X, Li Q, Chen Z (2018) The safety and efficacy of daylight photodynamic therapy in the treatment of actinic keratoses: a systematic review and meta-analysis. Int J Dermatol

Subject Index

N. Rezaei and F. Rajabi (eds.), *The Immunogenetics of Dermatologic Diseases*,
Advances in Experimental Medicine and Biology 1367,
https://doi.org/10.1007/978-3-030-92616-8

The manufacturer's authorised representative in the EU is Springer Nature Customer Service Centre GmbH, Europaplatz 3, 69115 Heidelberg, Germany. If you have any concerns regarding our products, please contact ProductSafety@springernature.com

Printed and bound by CPI Group (UK) Ltd, Croydon, CR0 4YY
30/09/2026
02225496-0019